Anatomy: A Complete Help Guide For Identifying The Human Body For Anatomy Class

Black And White Edition

I0482152

By K.R. Lefkowitz

ISBN: 10:153352906X
ISBN-13: 978-1533529060

How To Use....

This book is mean't to be used for you to label and practice the components of the cardiovascular system. In going through your anatomy class and later in medical field you will need to know how to label the components, pictures of each system and know it inside and out. The best way is for you to label all the components that you know yourself and research the areas that you don't. Can you label all parts of the heart, ventricles, parties, veins, etc...? Can you recognize a picture and know immediately what it is? You can find the corresponding picture in the table of contents. Nothing is labeled on purpose. This is for you to label. For you to know. And what you don't know for you to research in your texts and find the answers. Through this way of learning and researching the parts you don't know, allows you to actually learn it and have it stored in long term memory. This active way of learning will in the long term be beneficial beyond belief in your future career or knowledge. Mark the pages, make notes, and use this practice book and pictures to help you understand the parts of the anatomy.

TABLE OF CONTENTS:

MUSCULAR SYSTEM - PAGE 3 -70

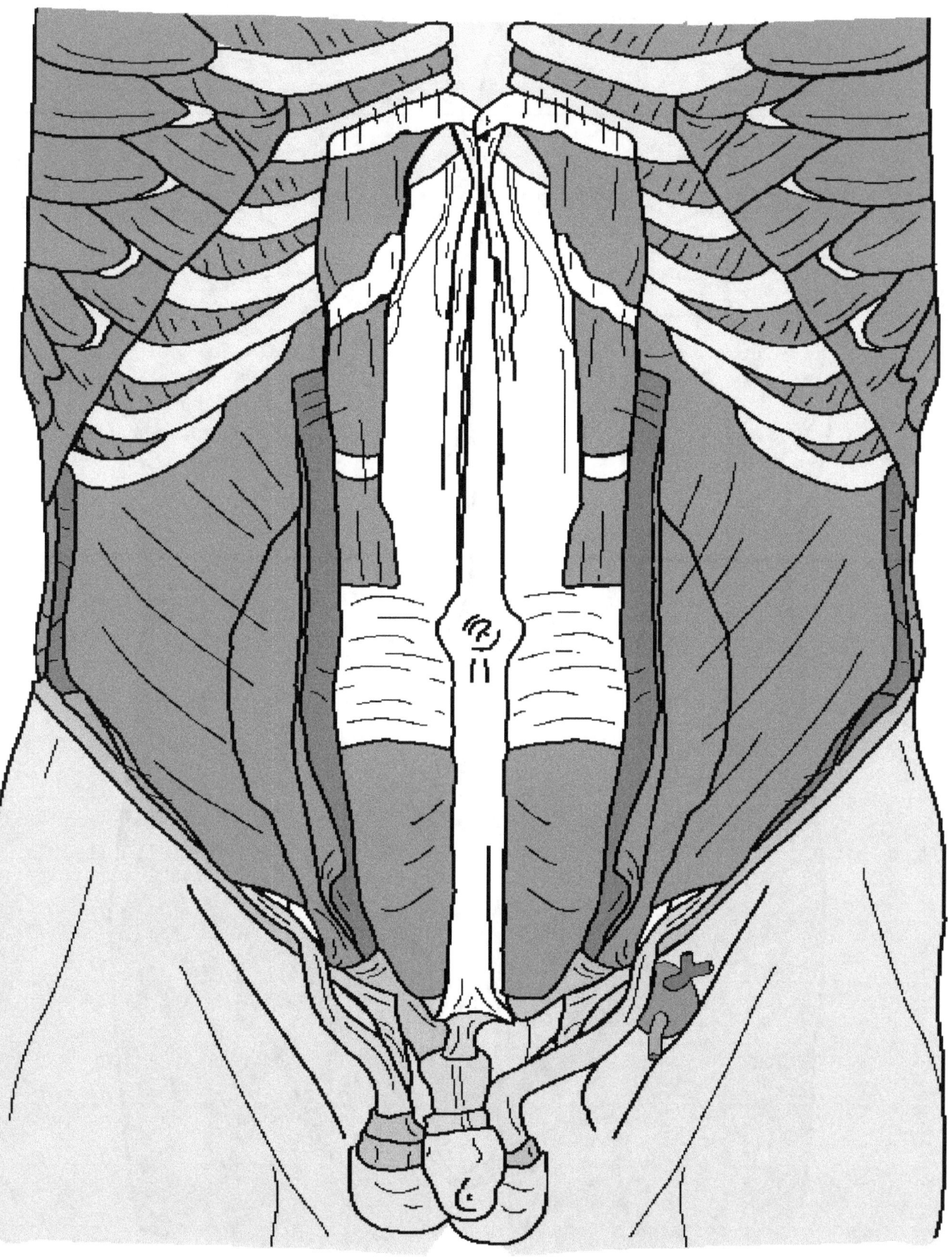

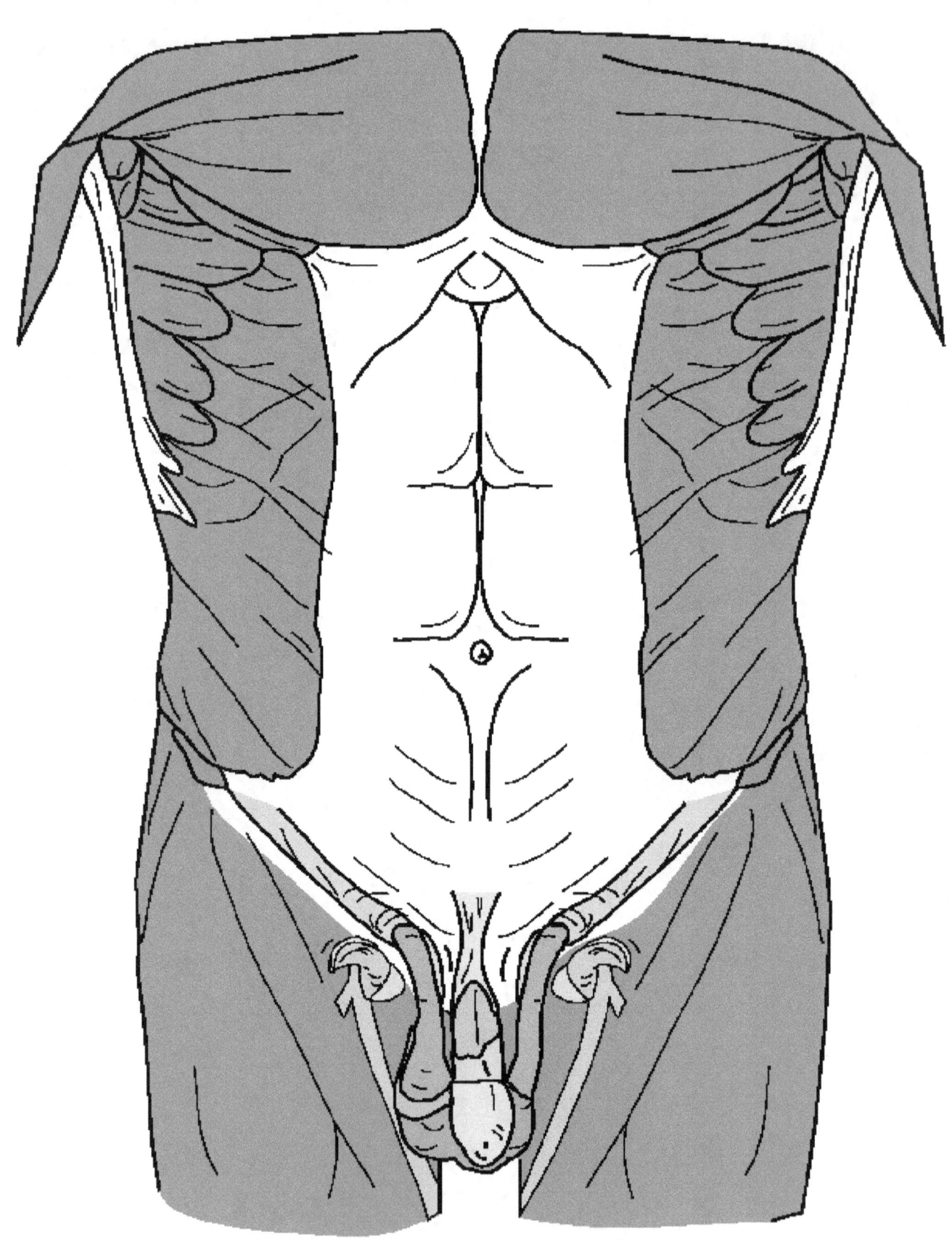

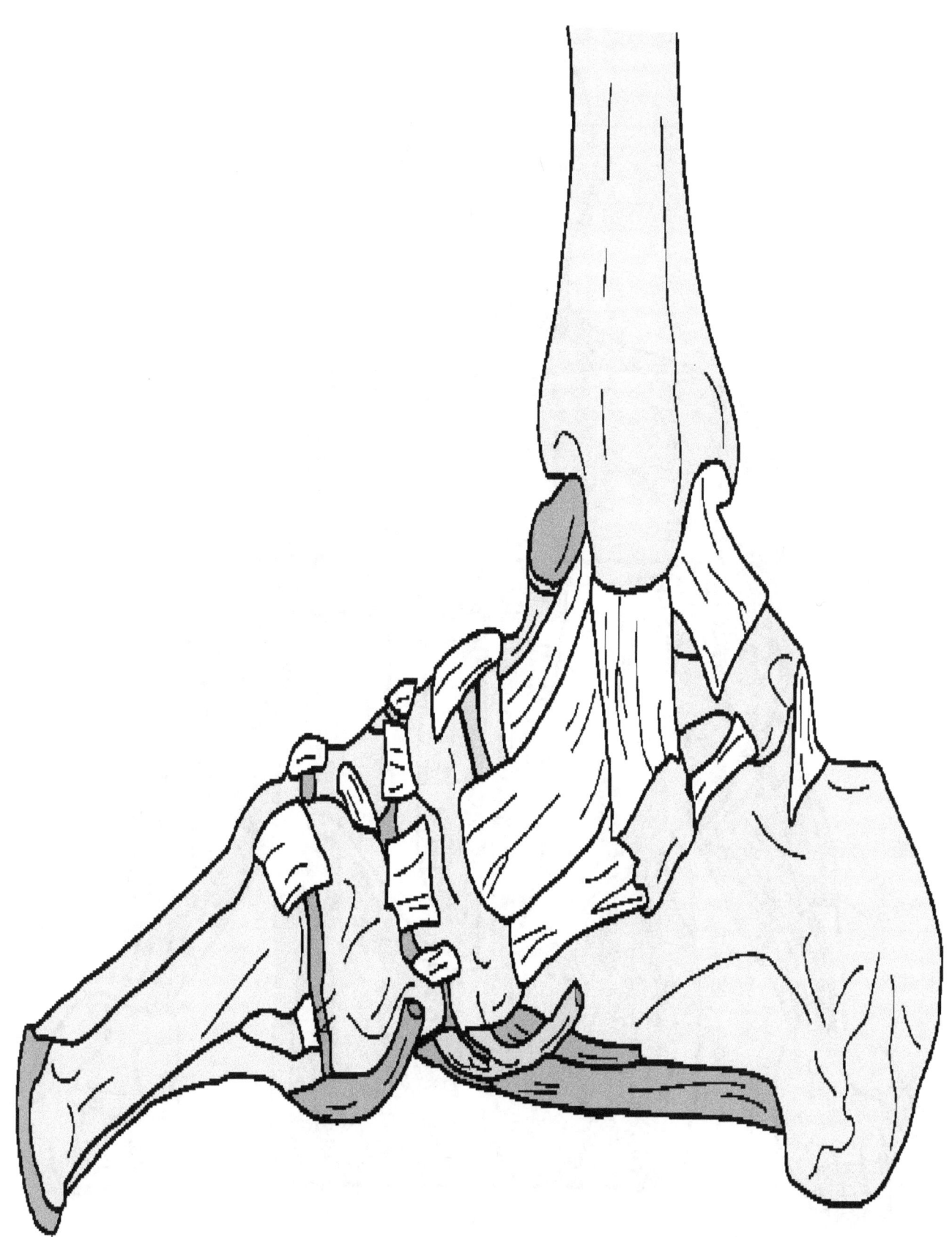

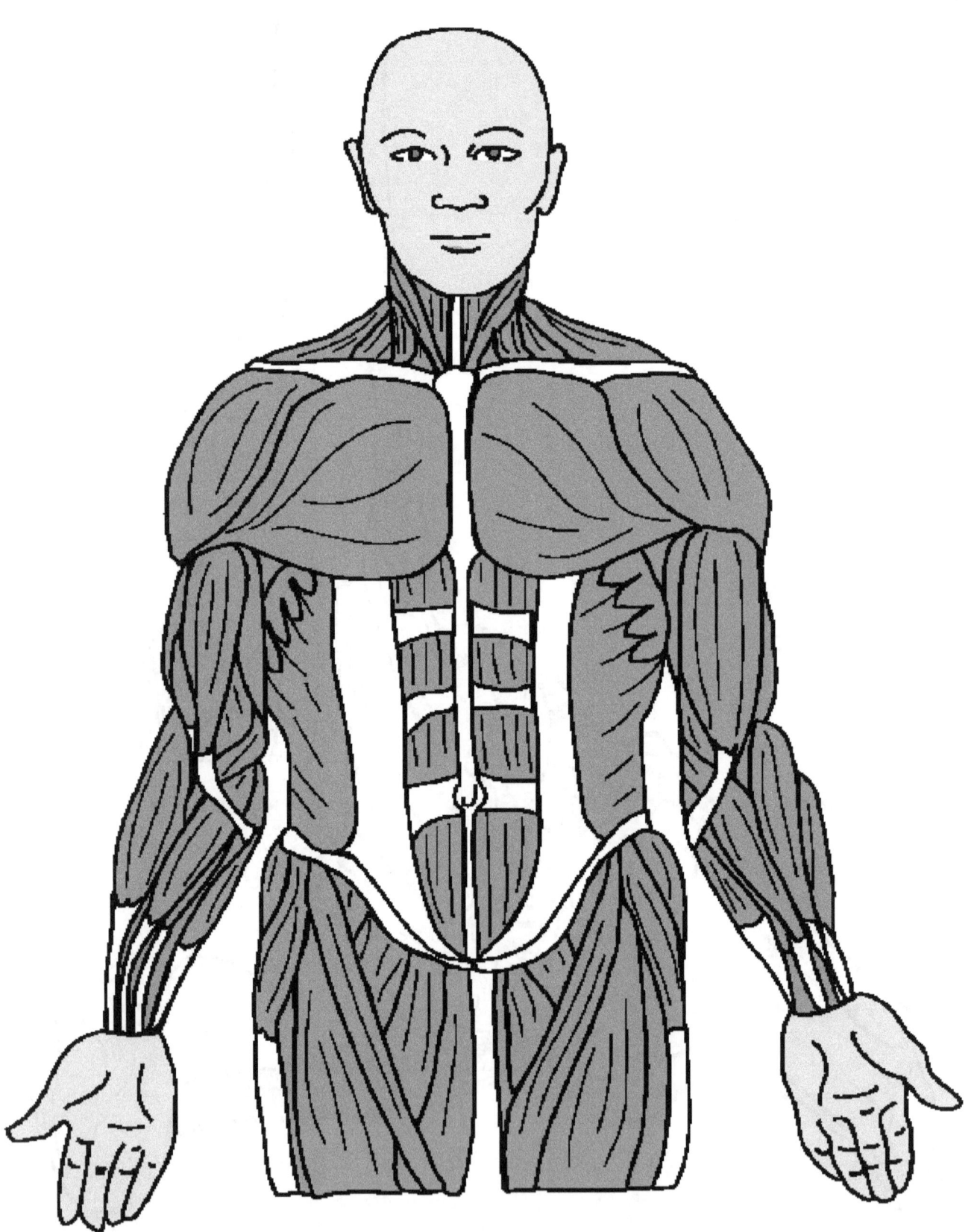

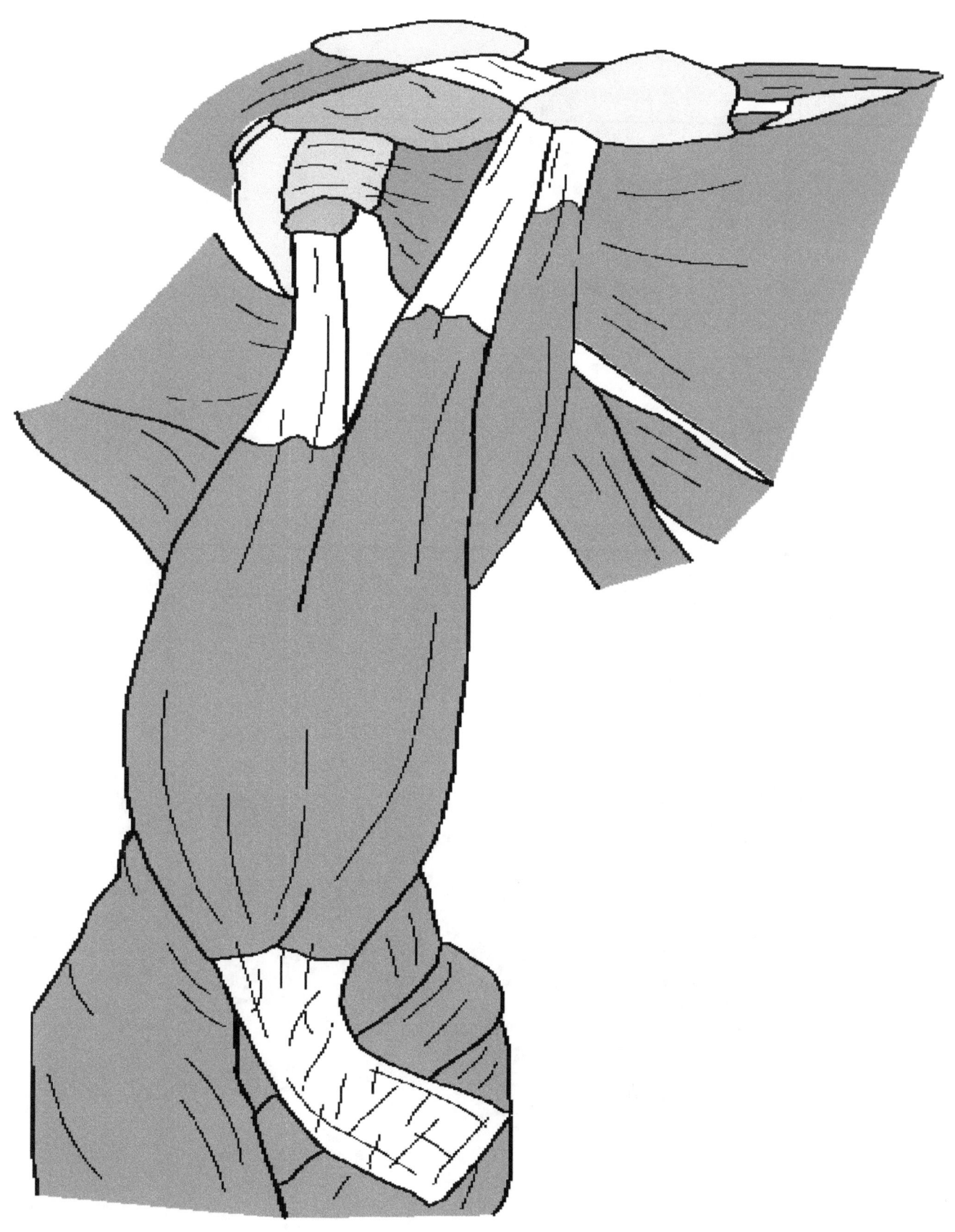

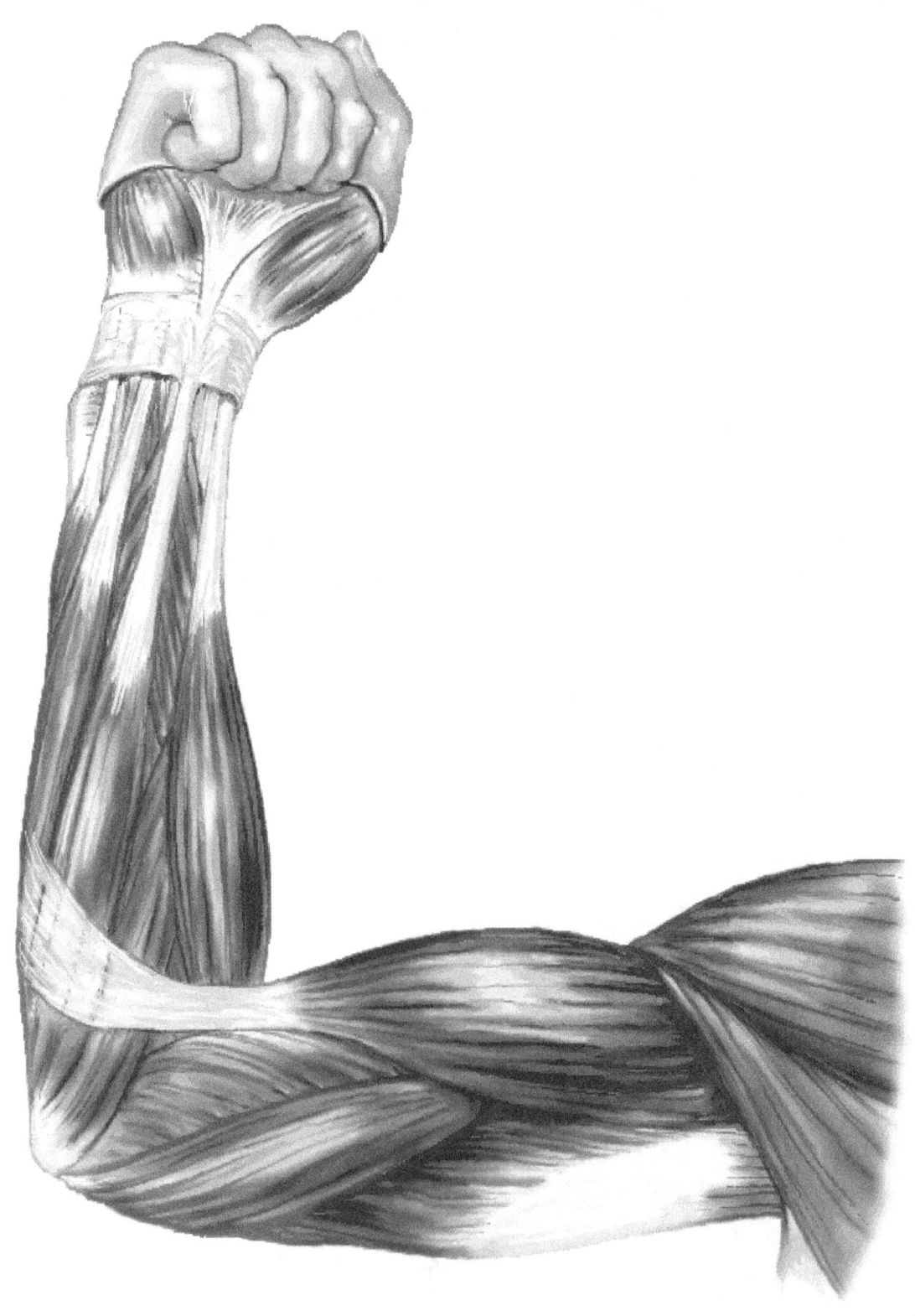

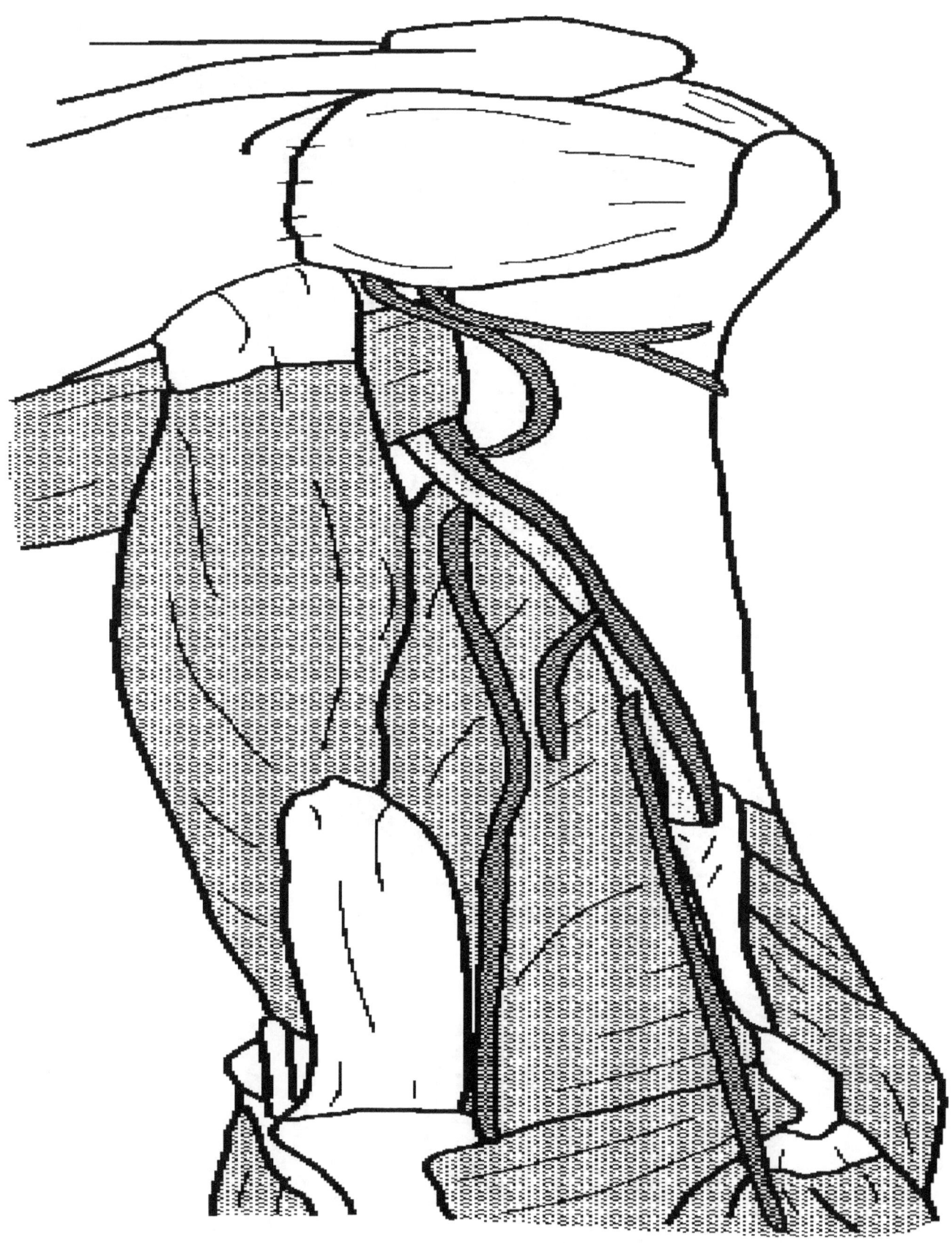

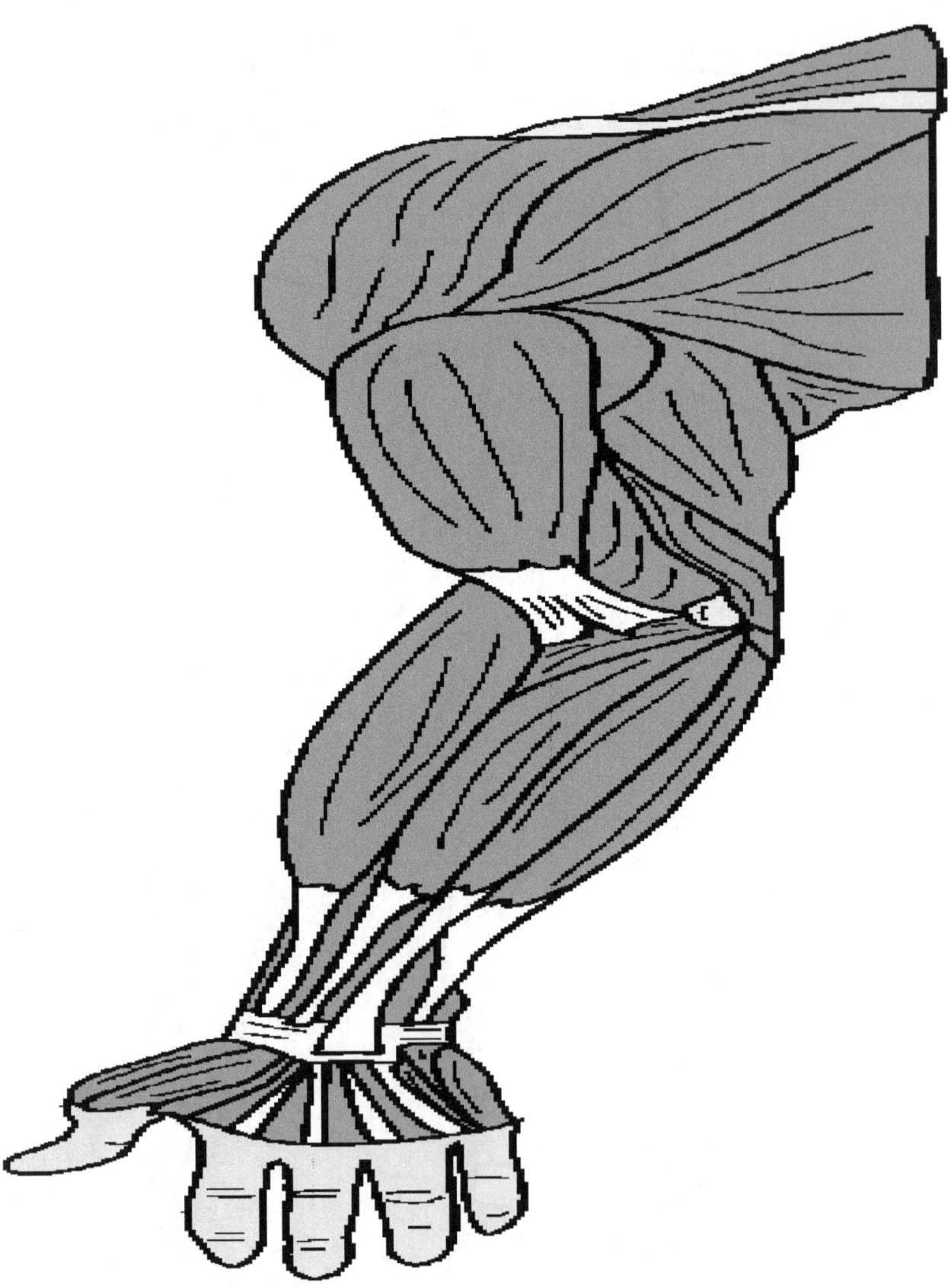

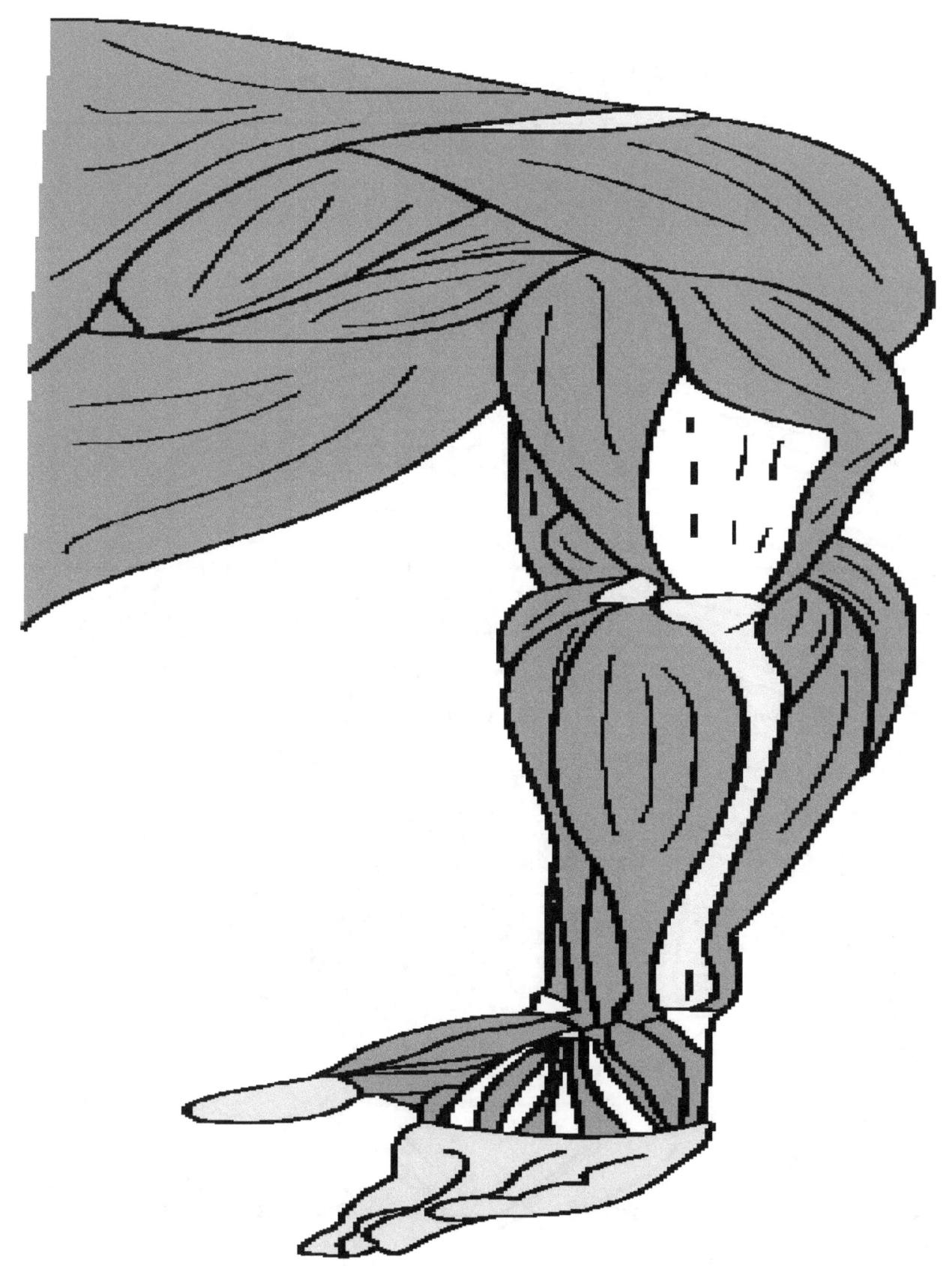

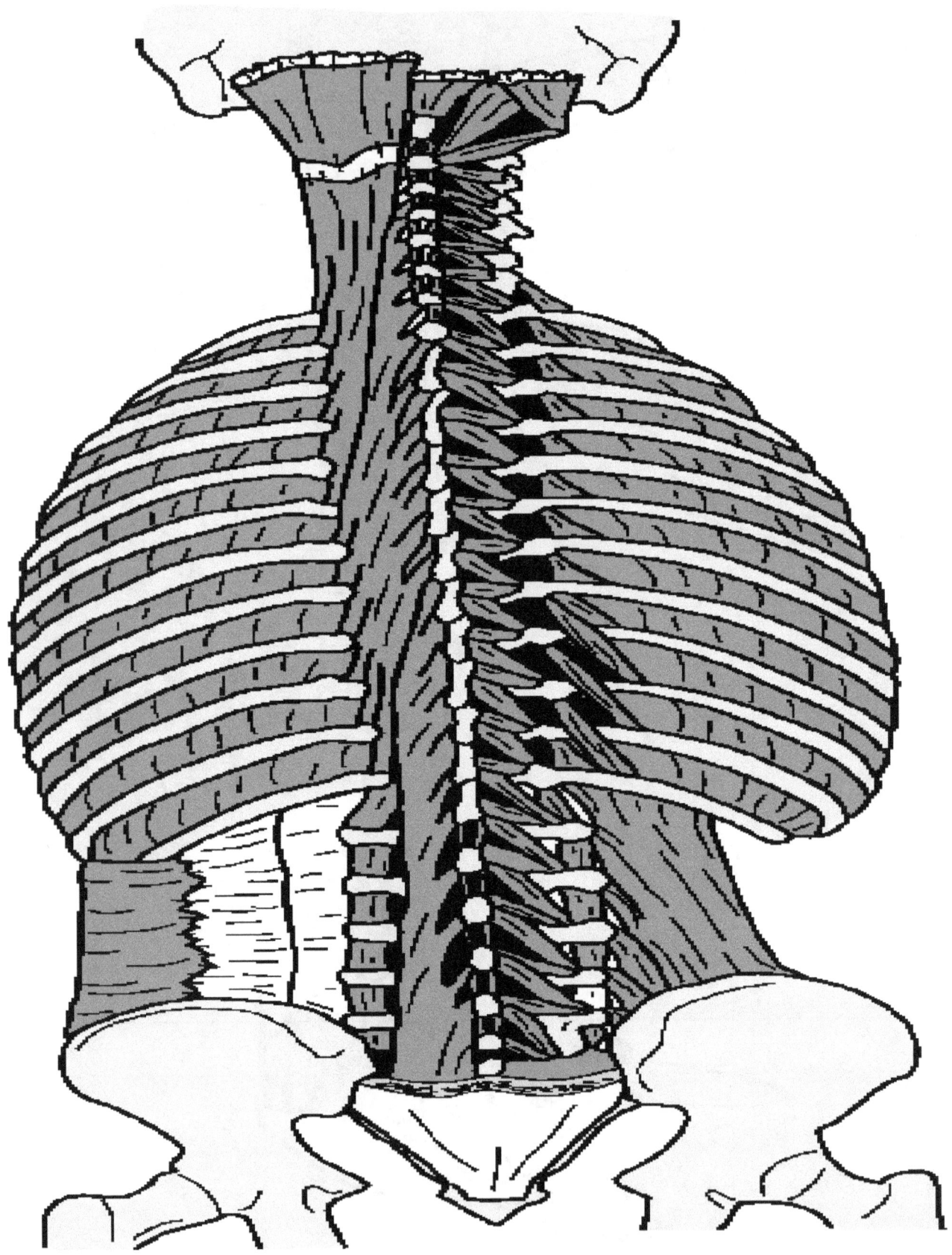

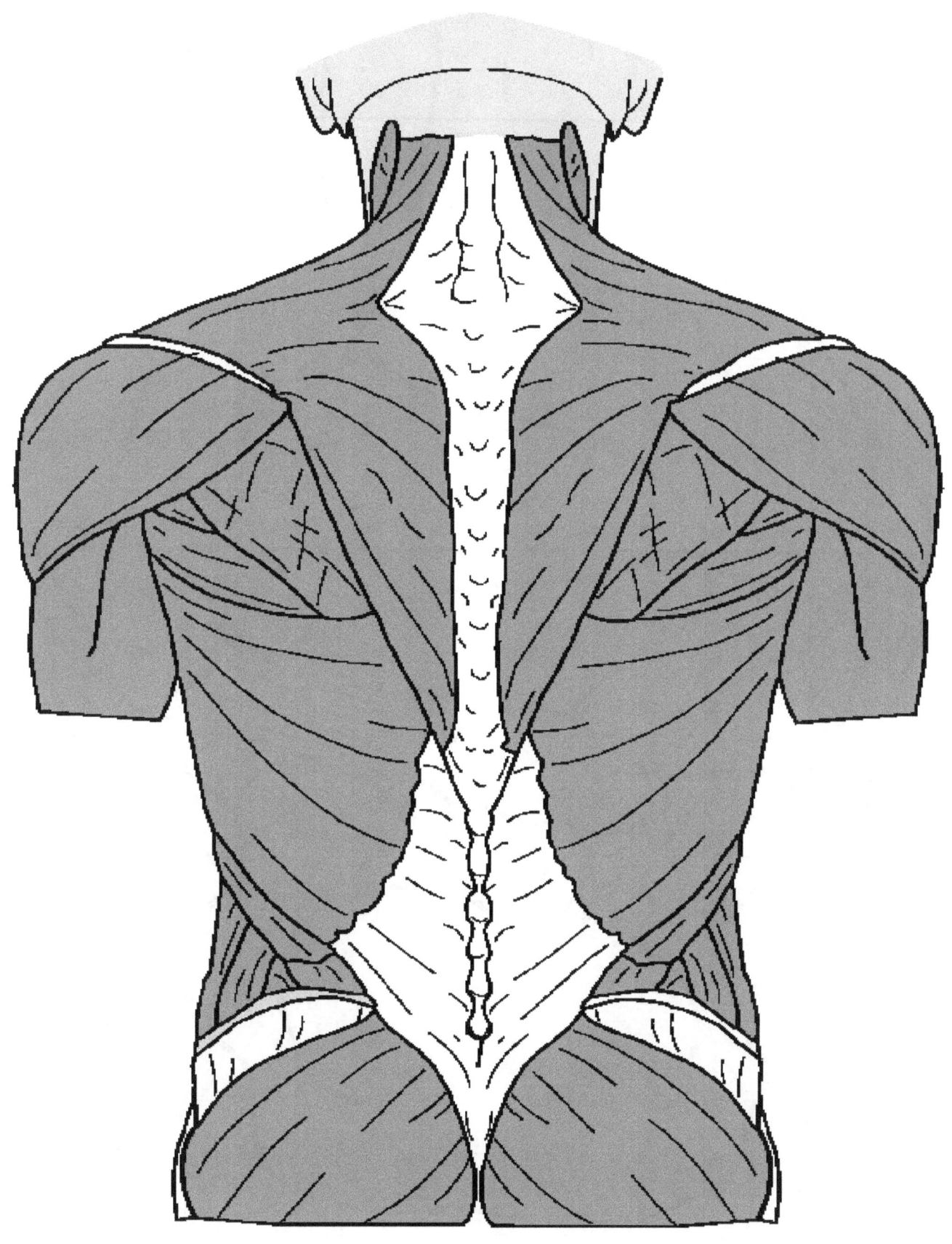

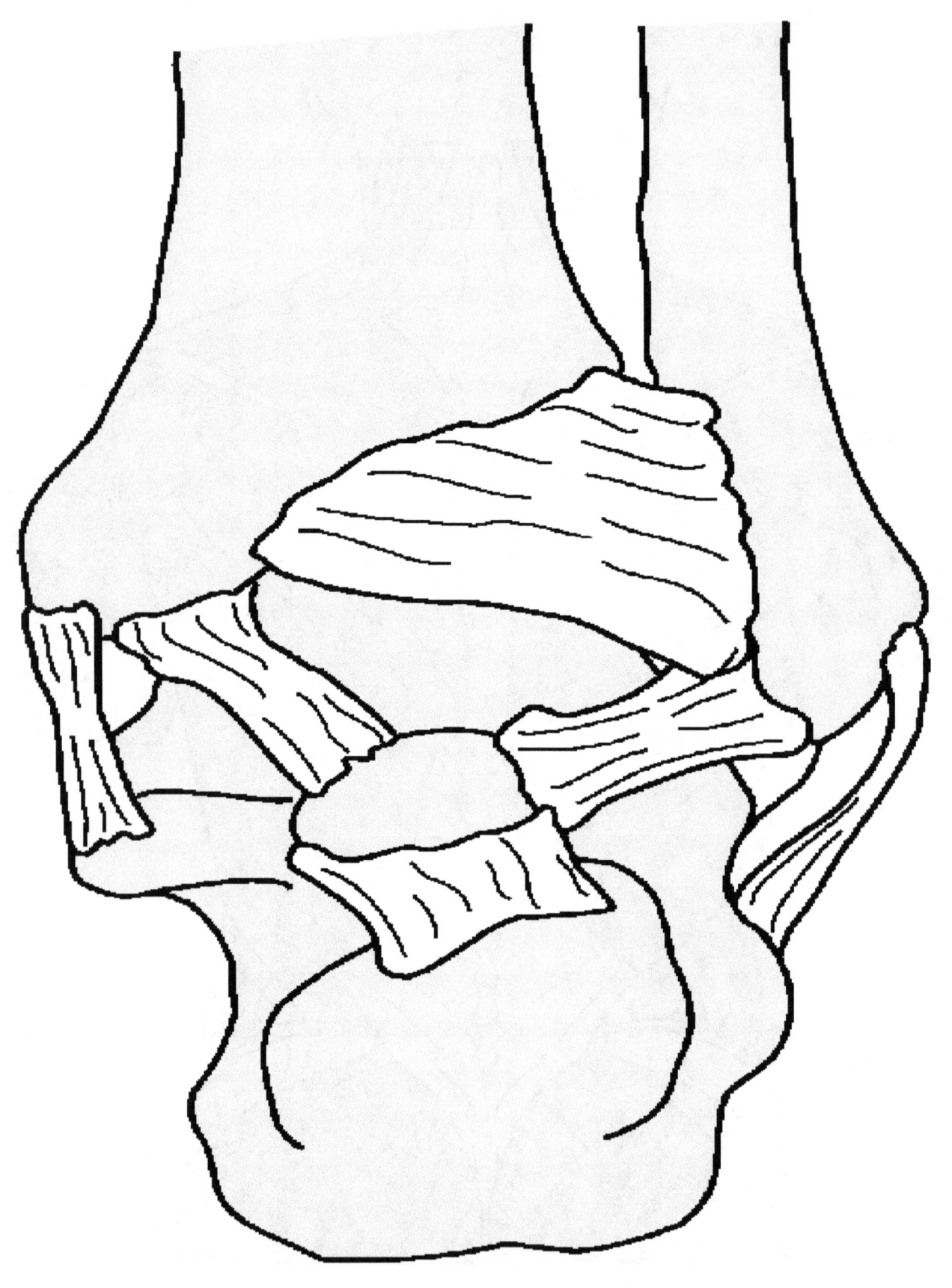

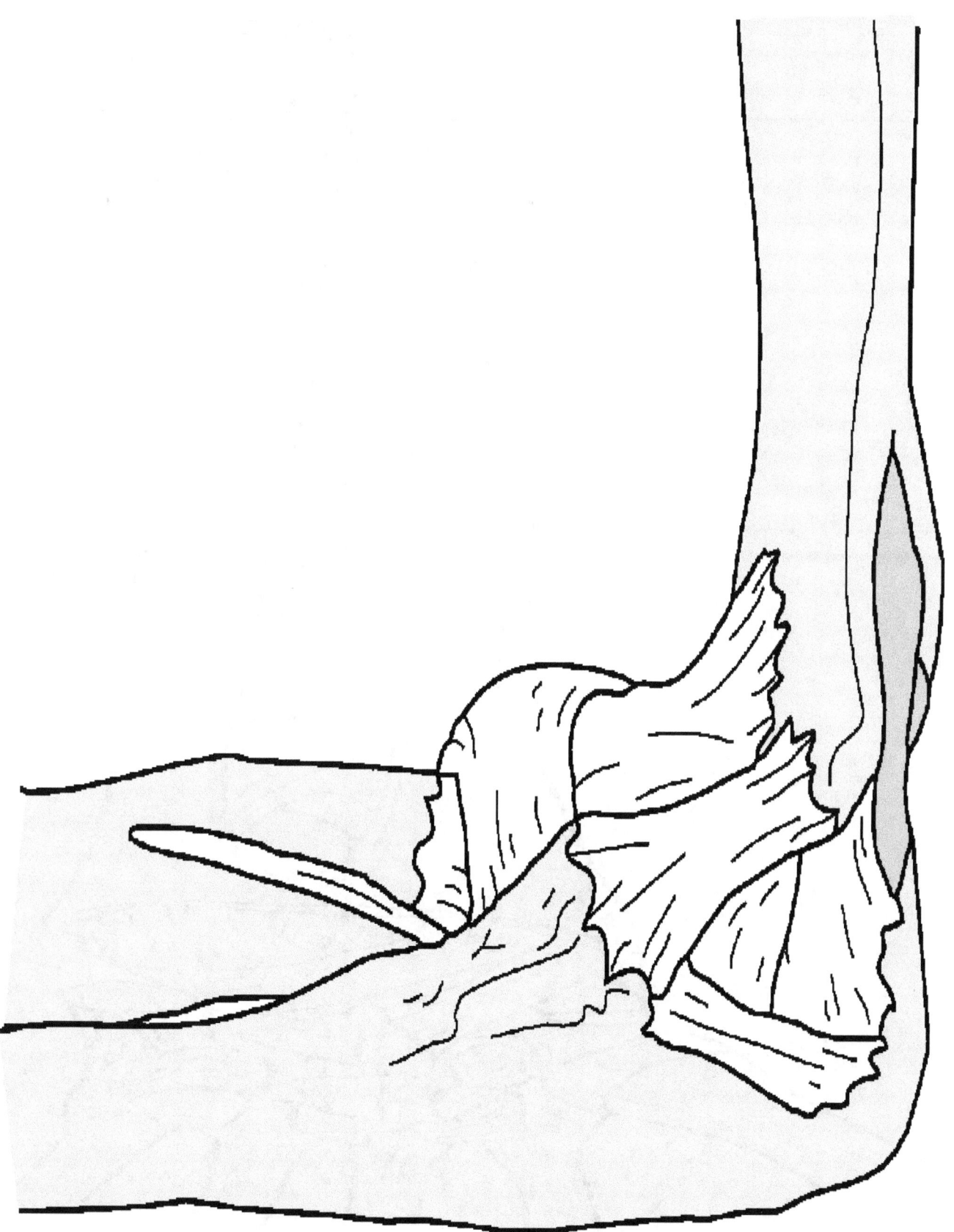

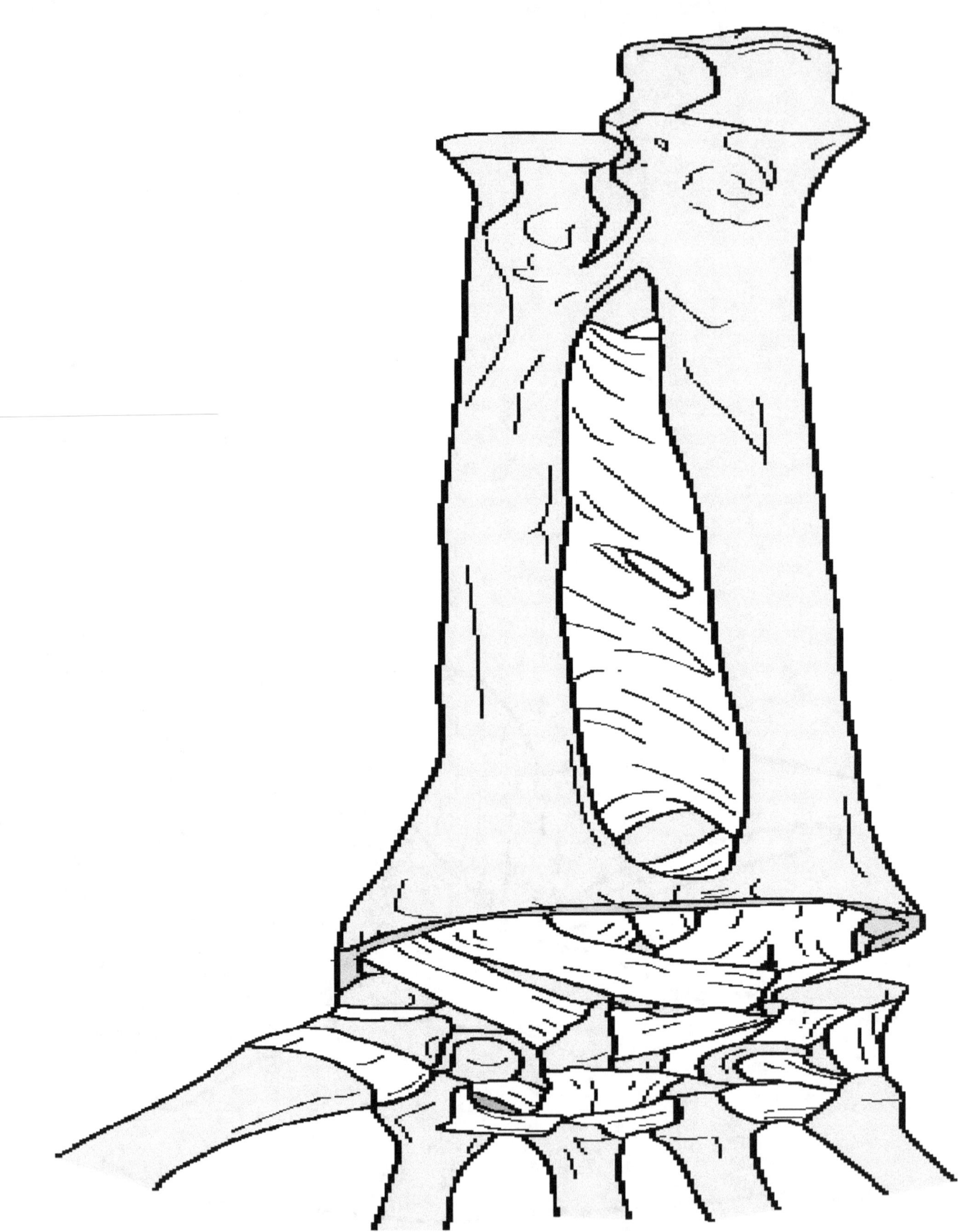

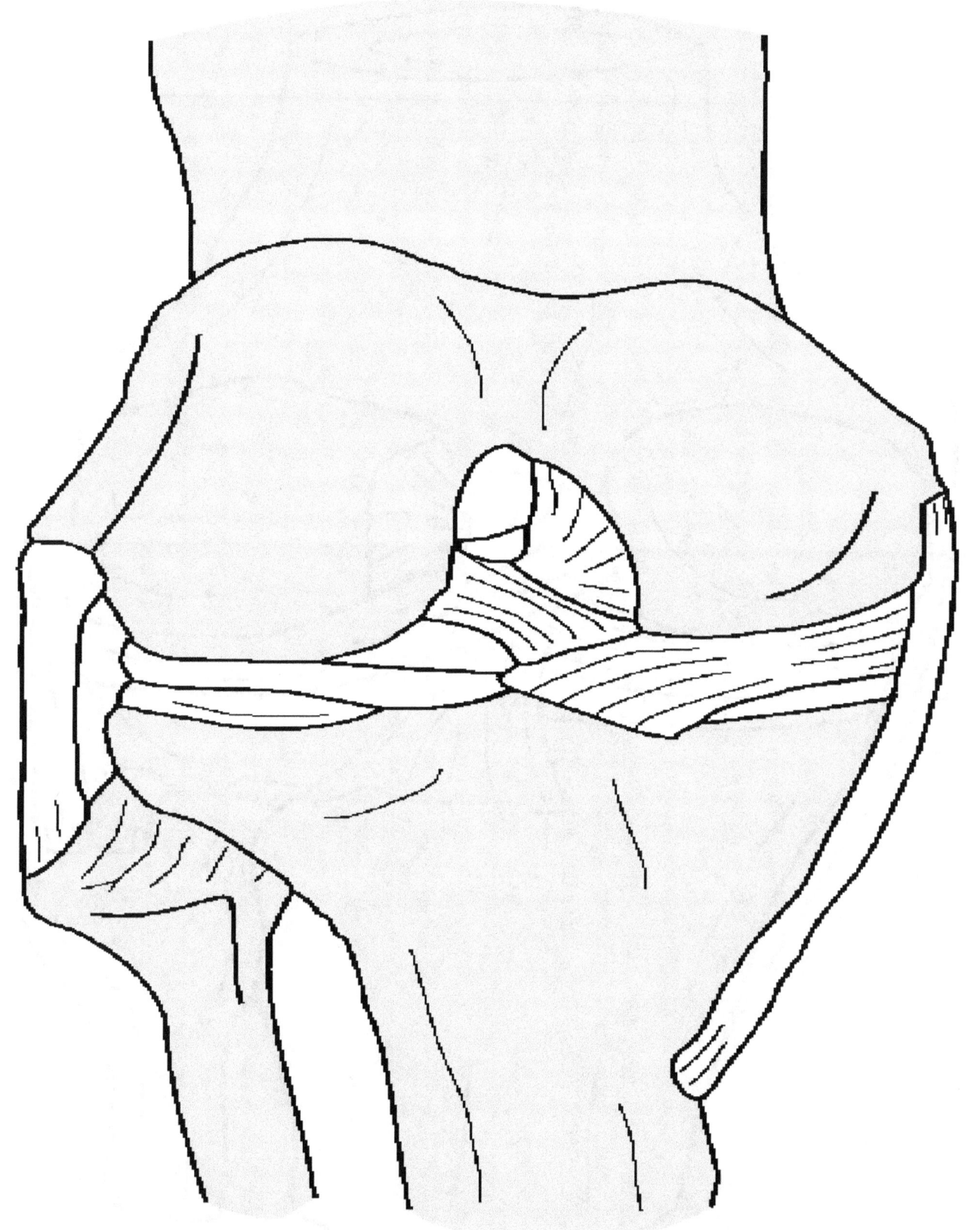

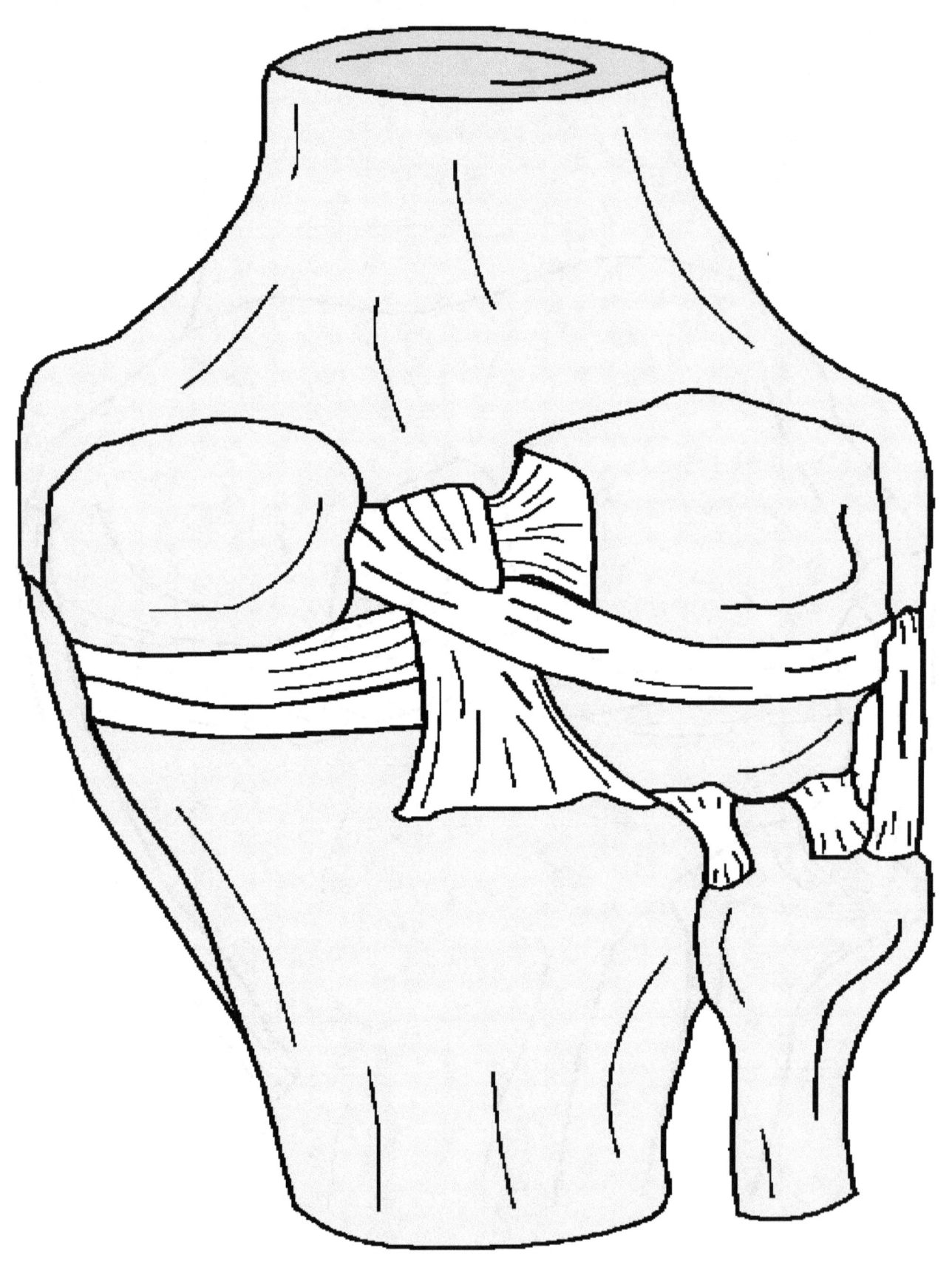

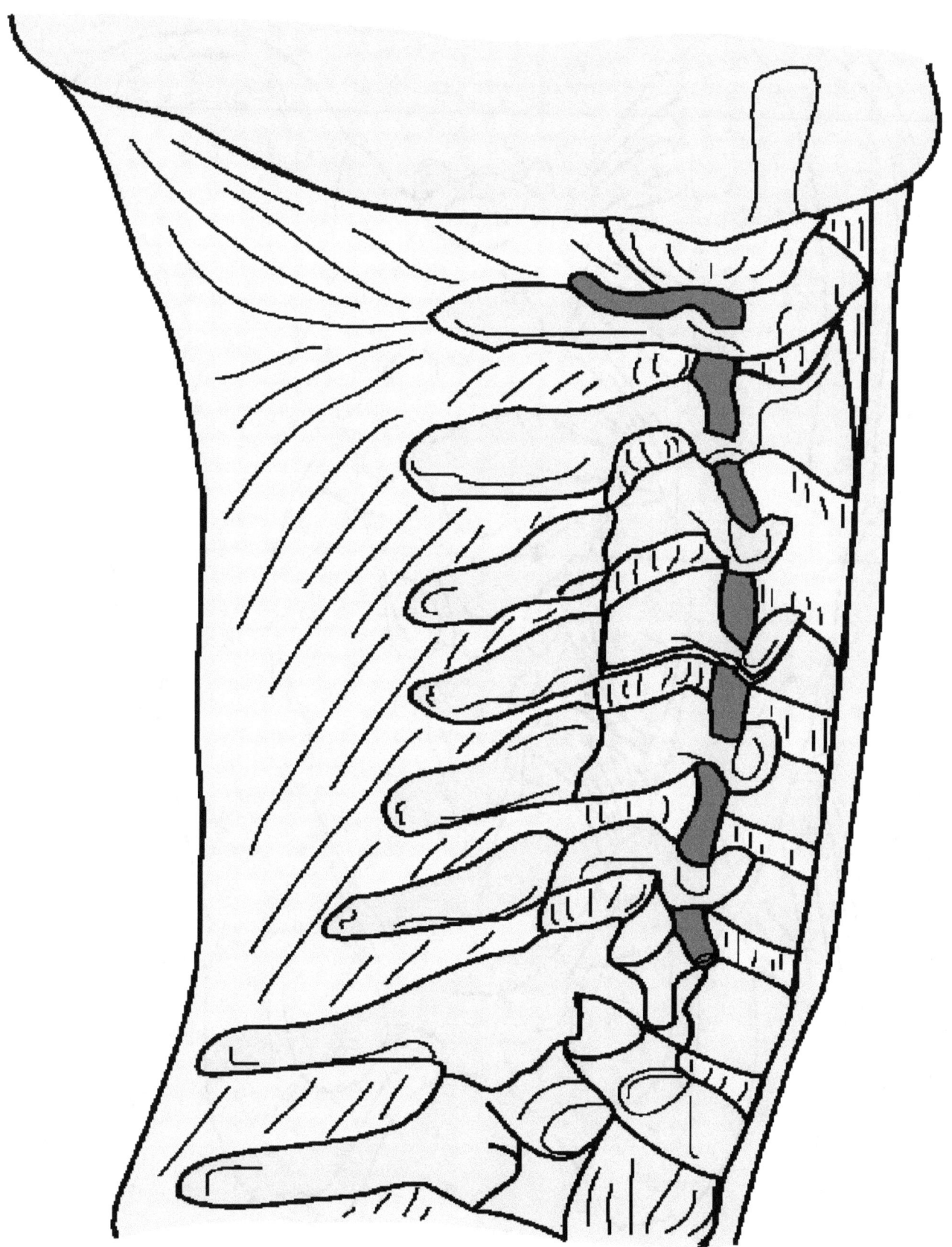

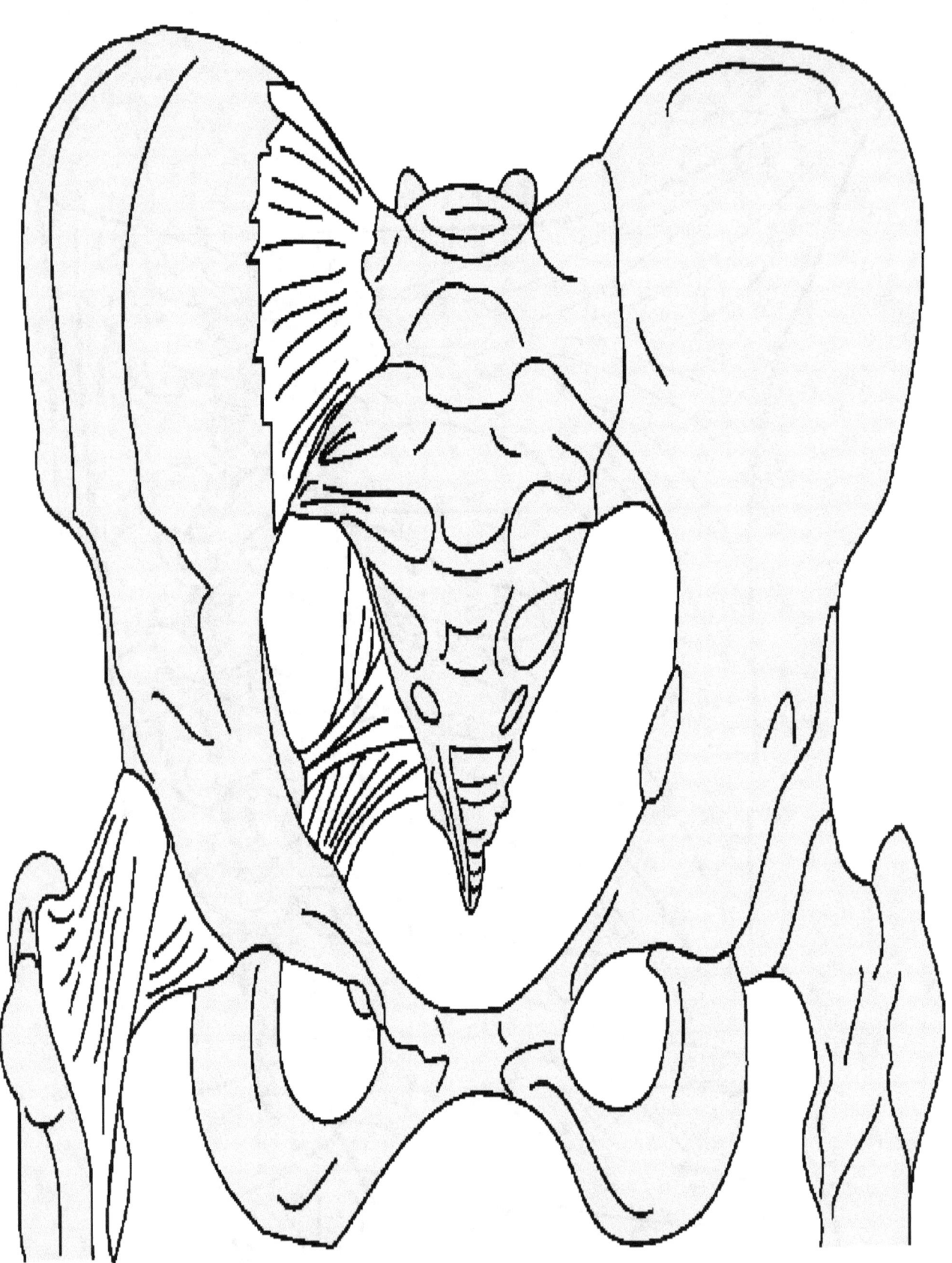

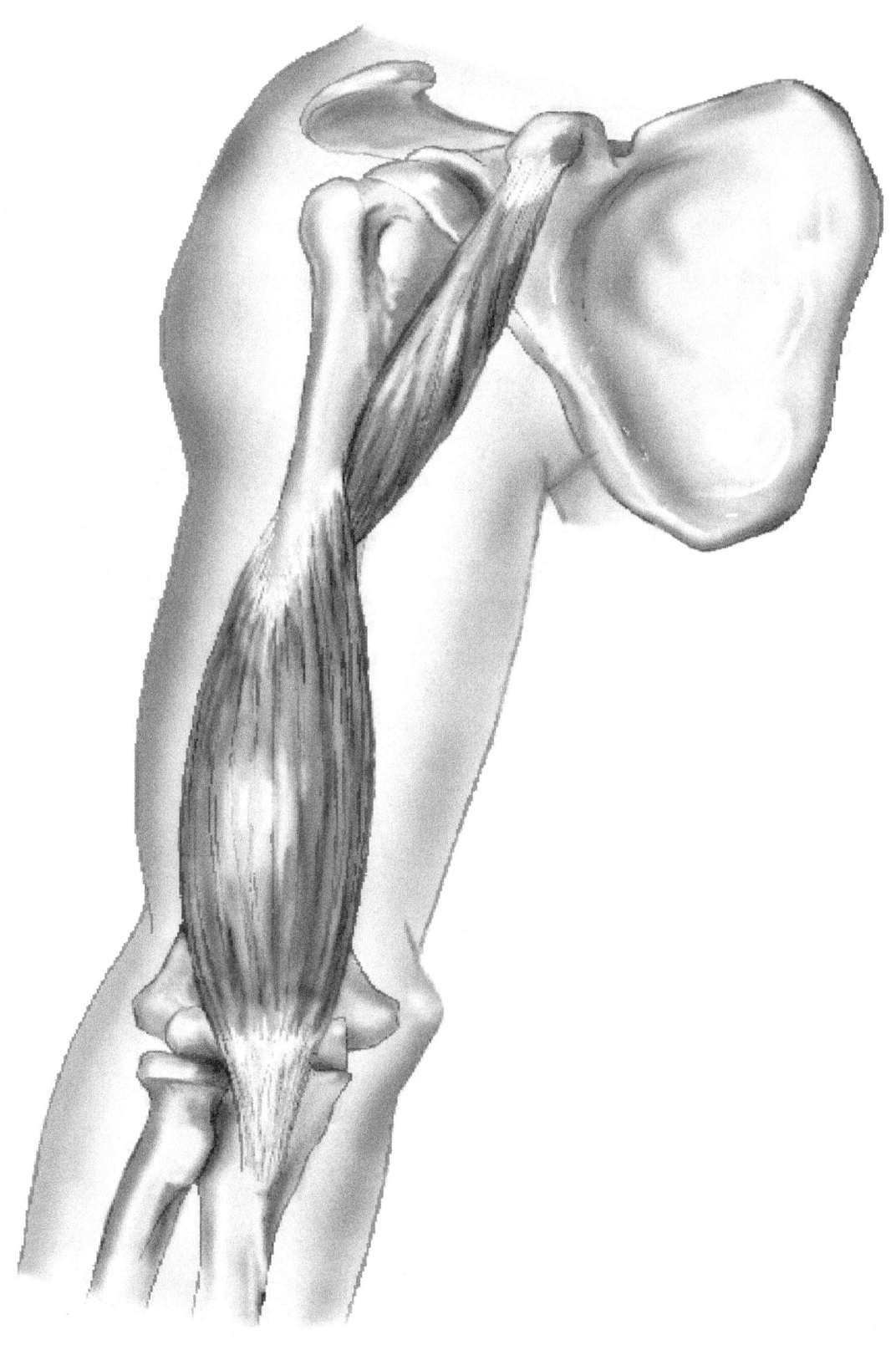

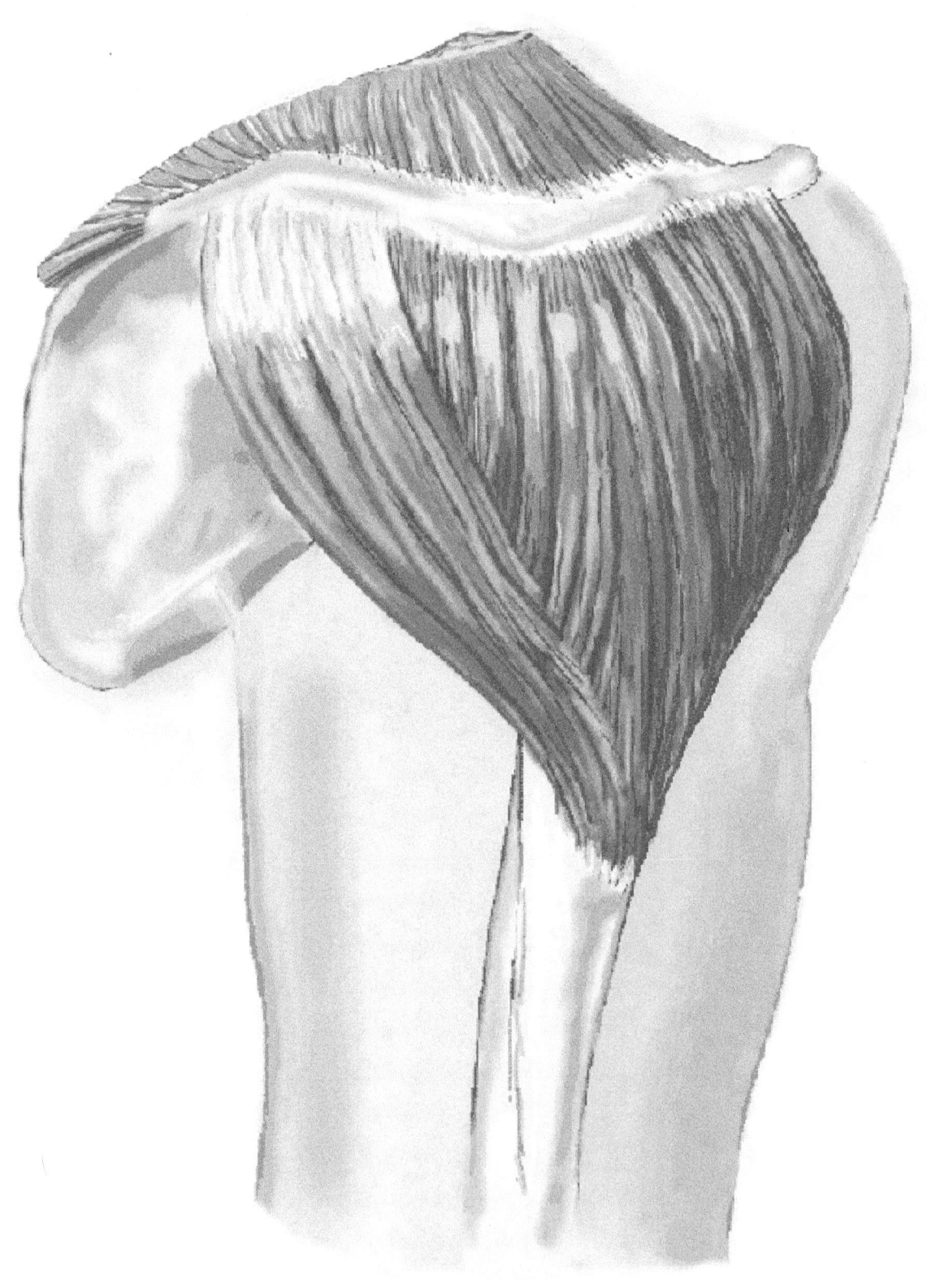

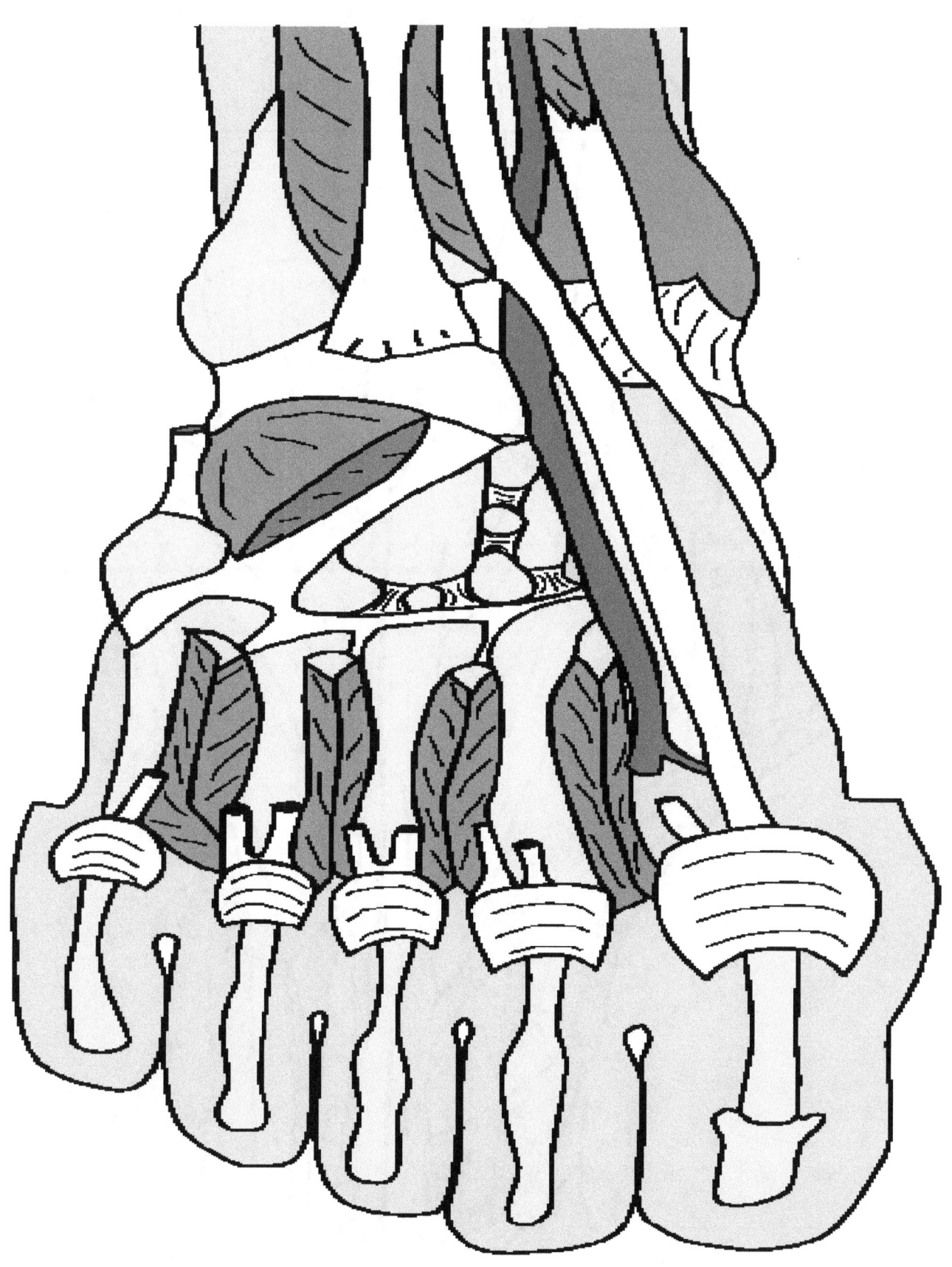

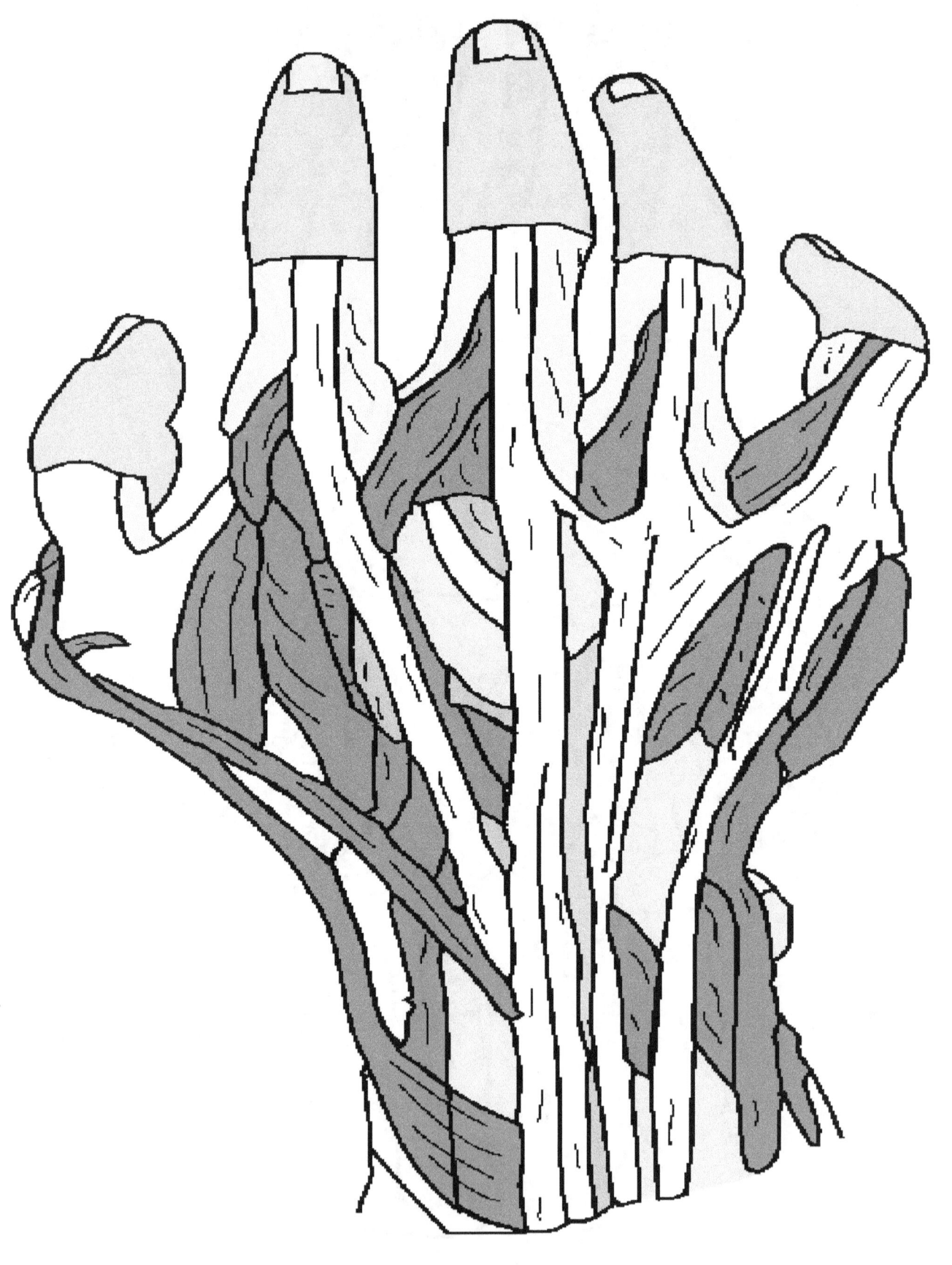

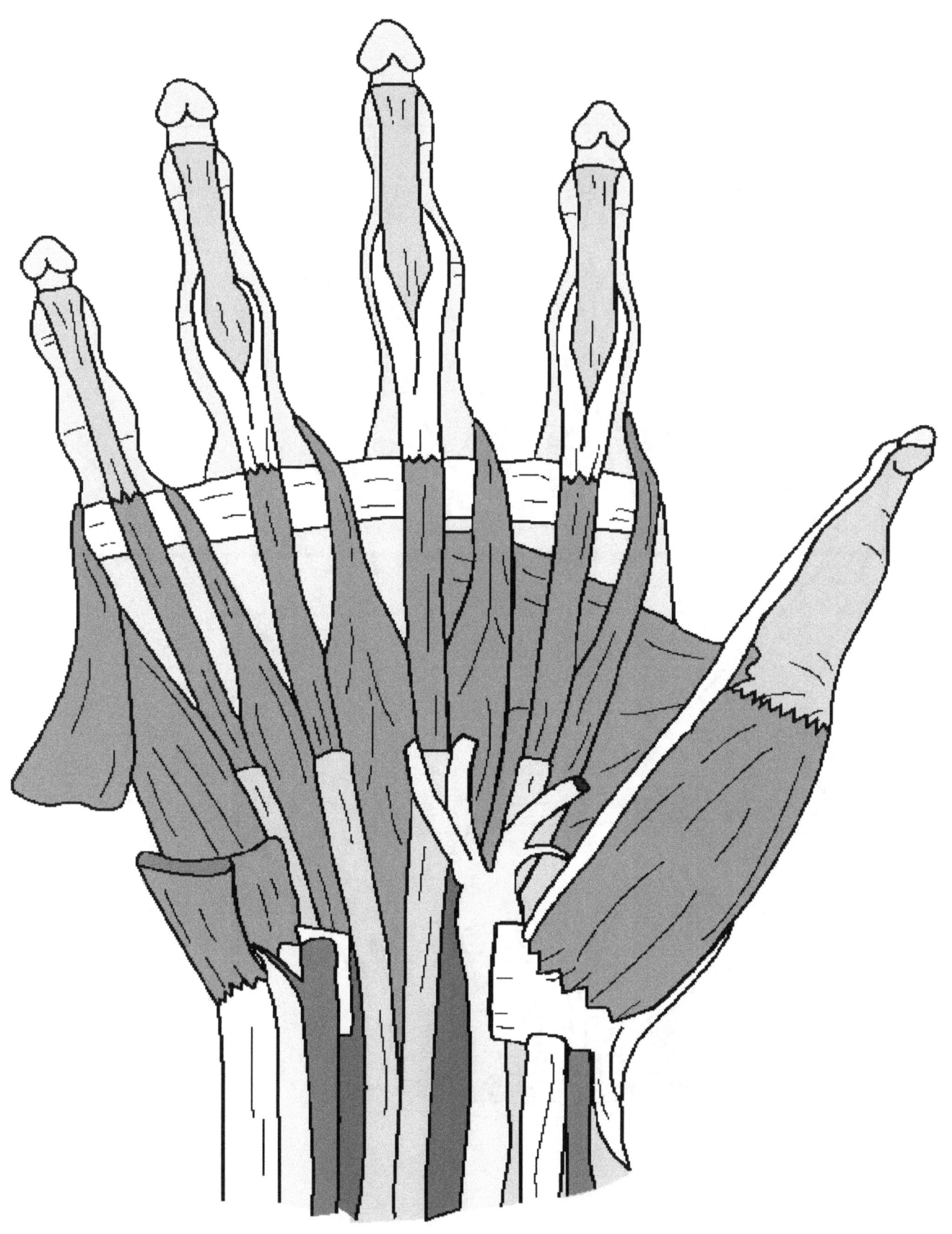

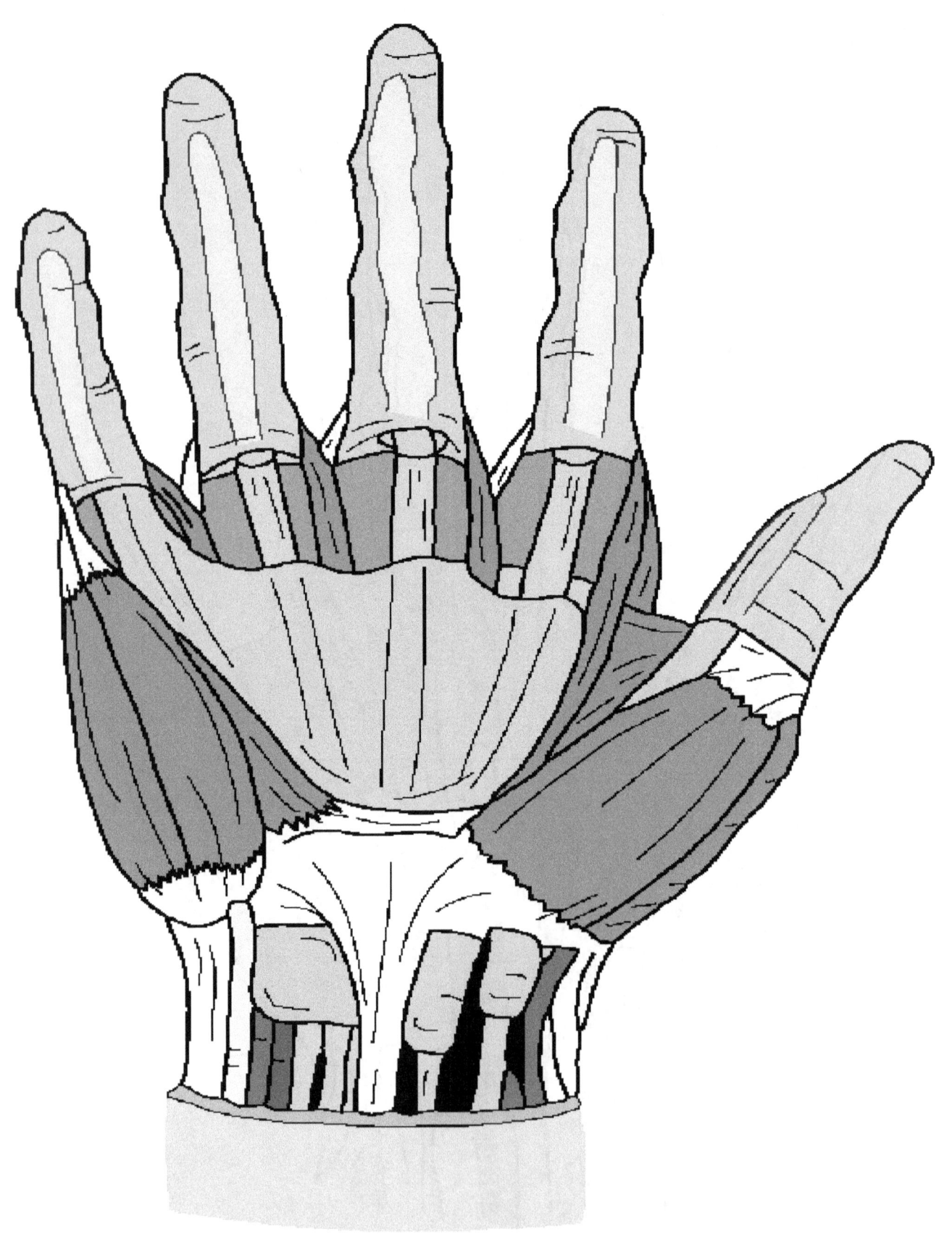

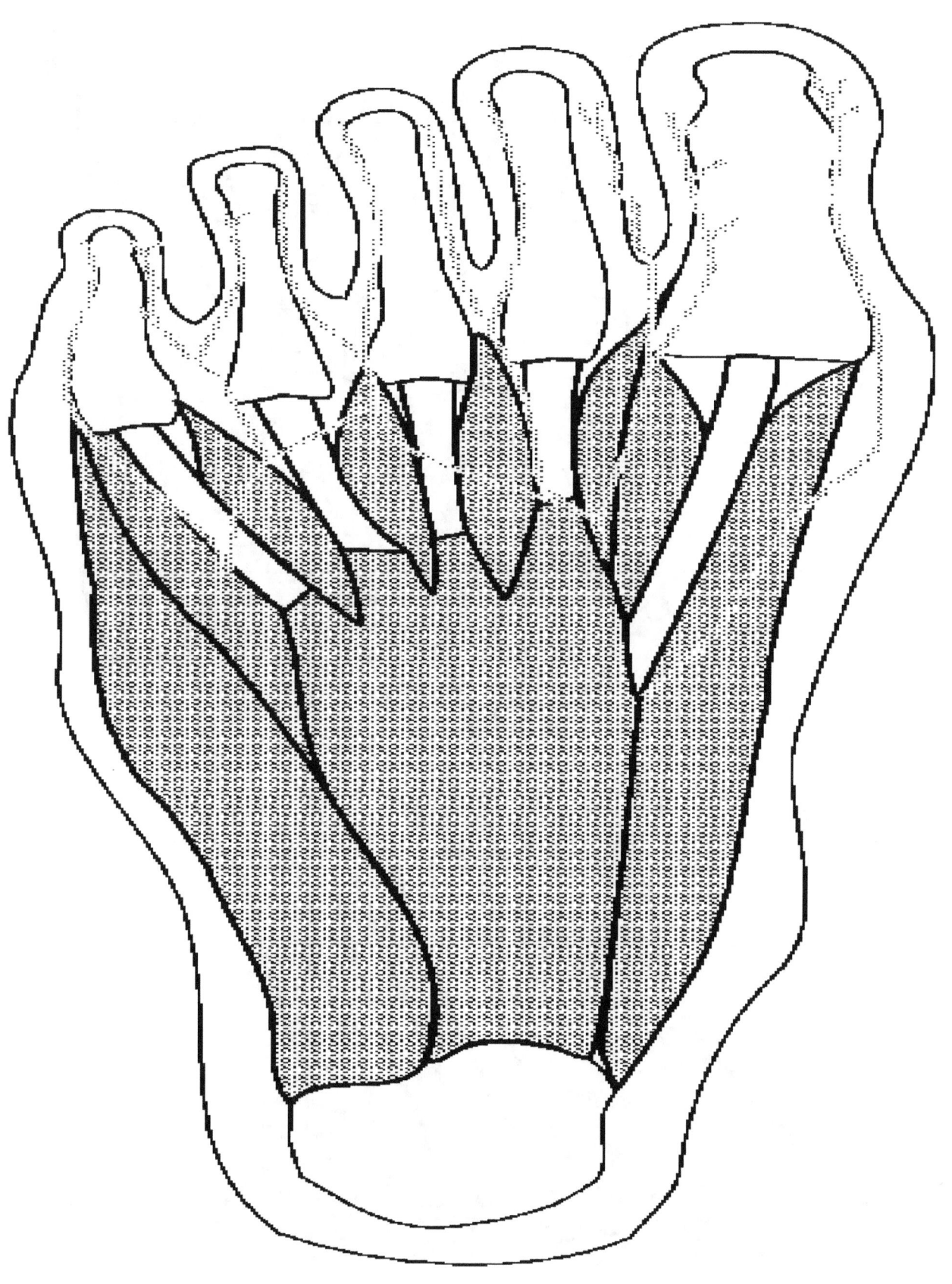

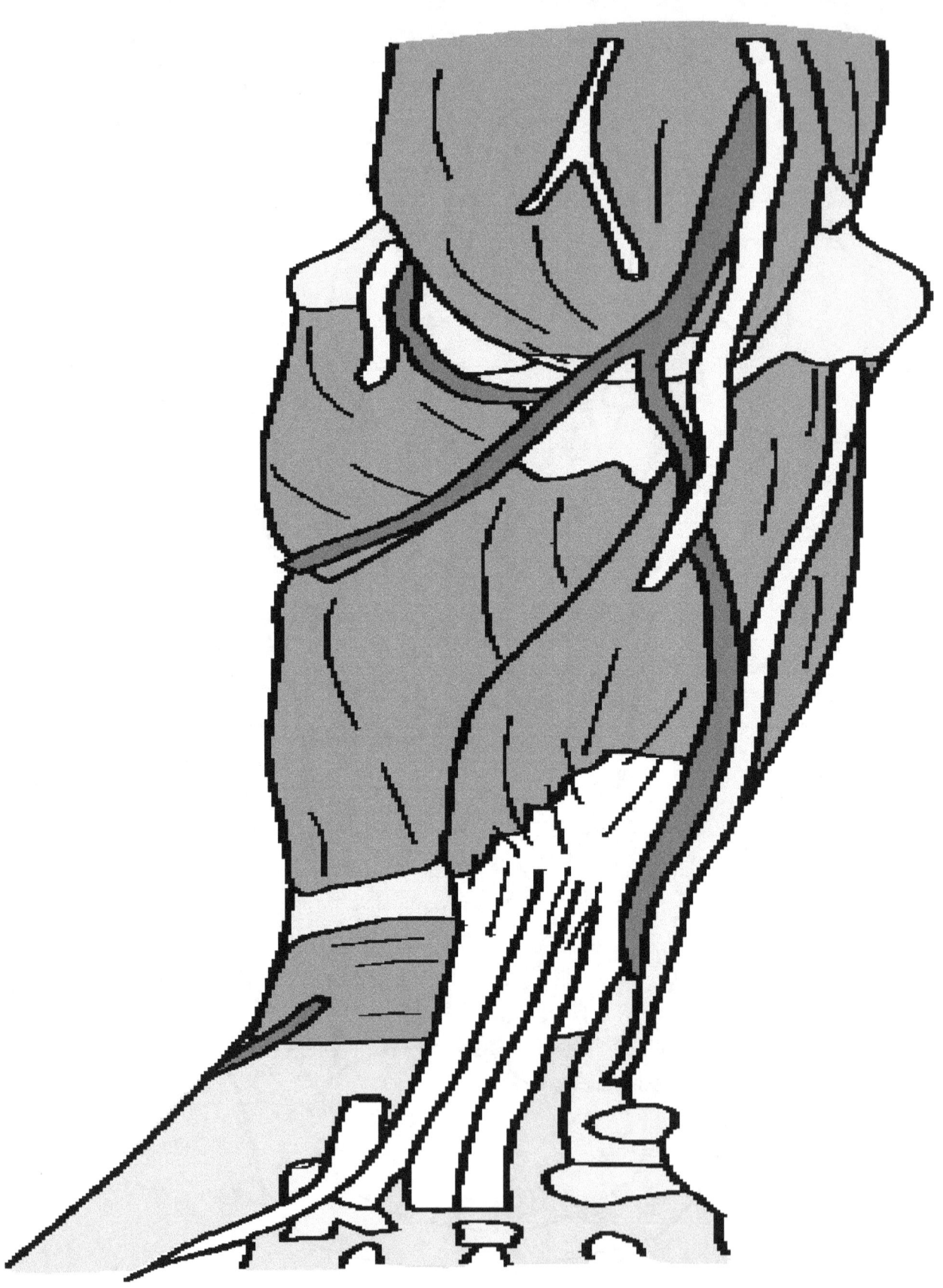

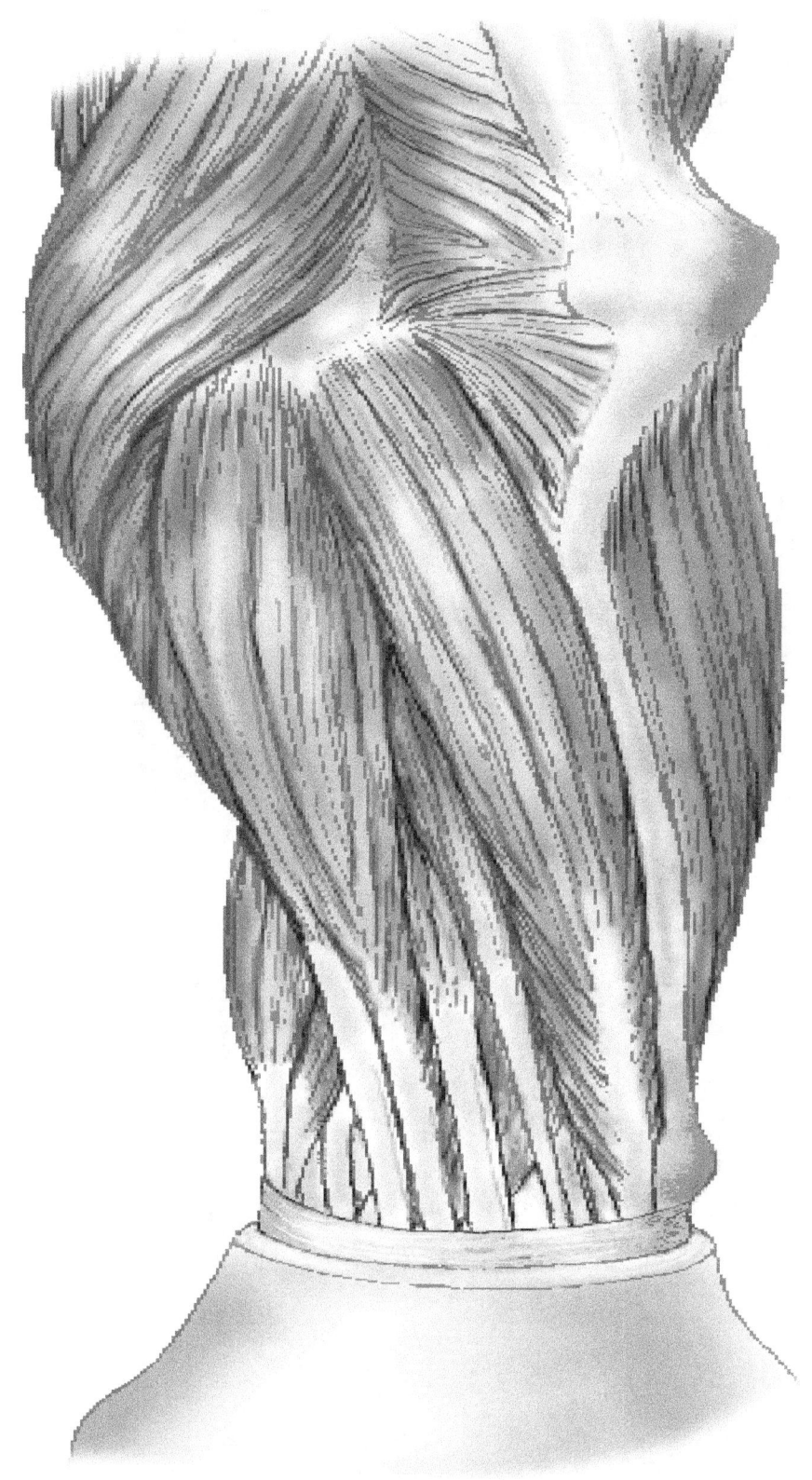

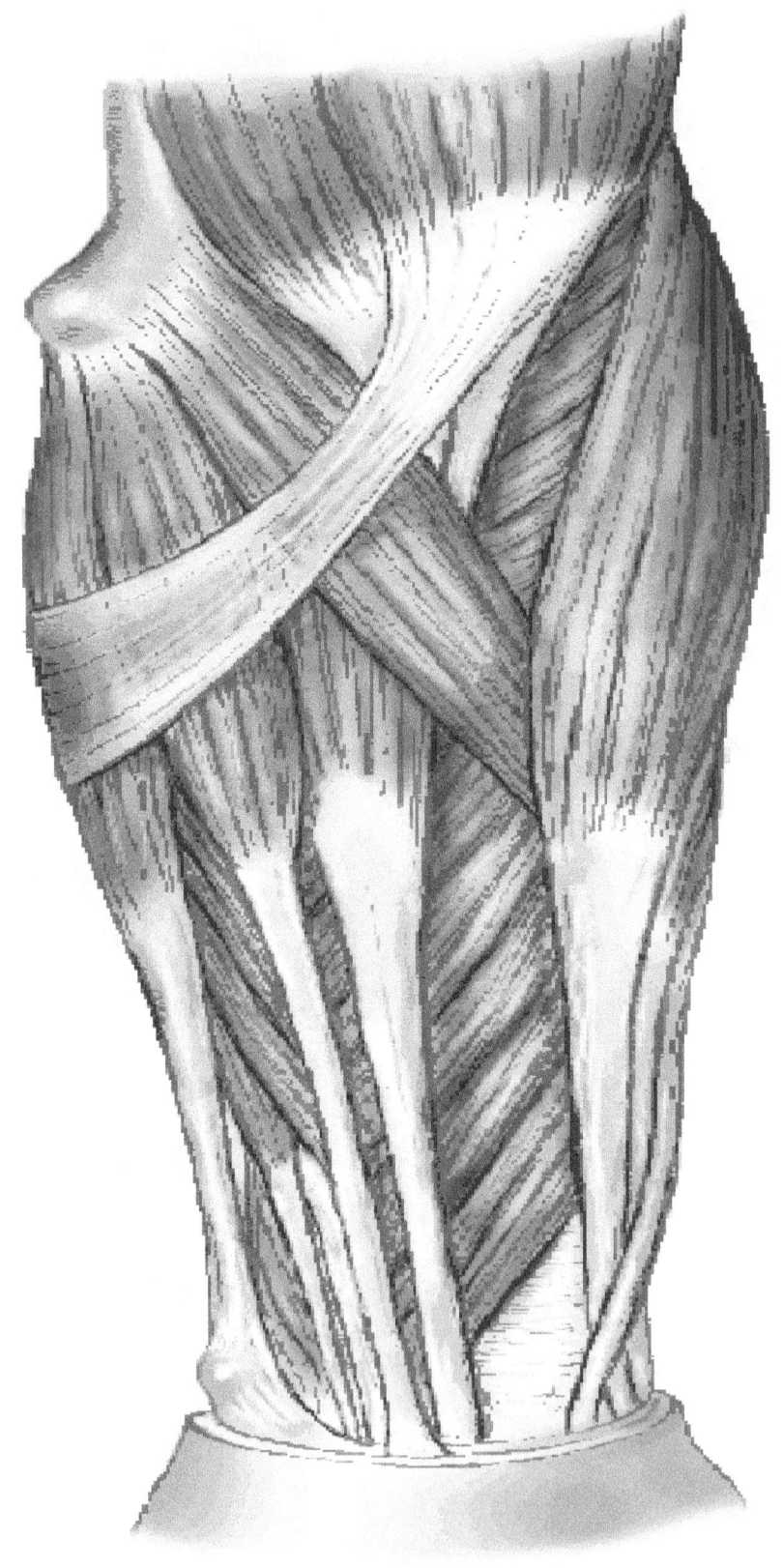

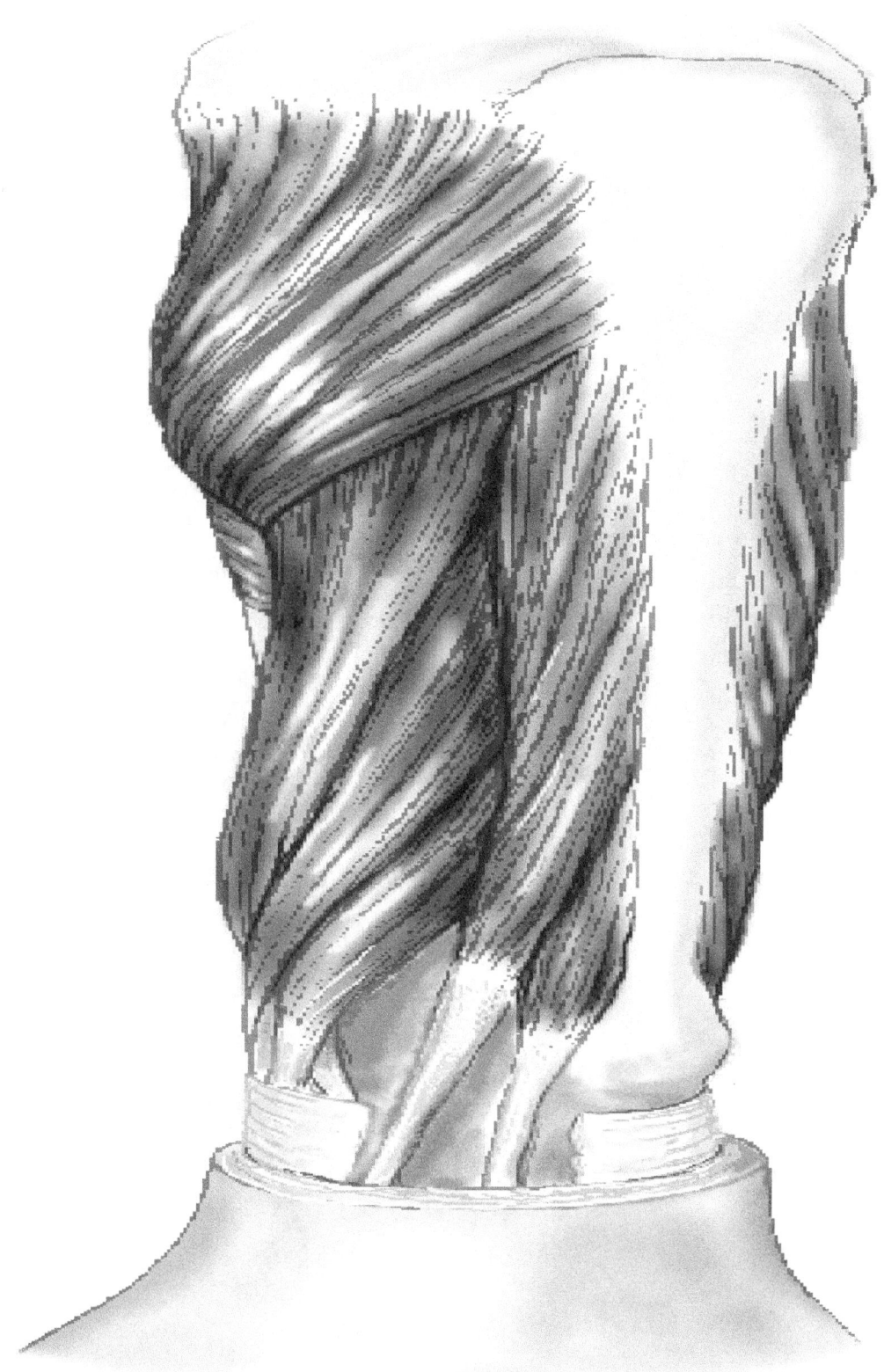

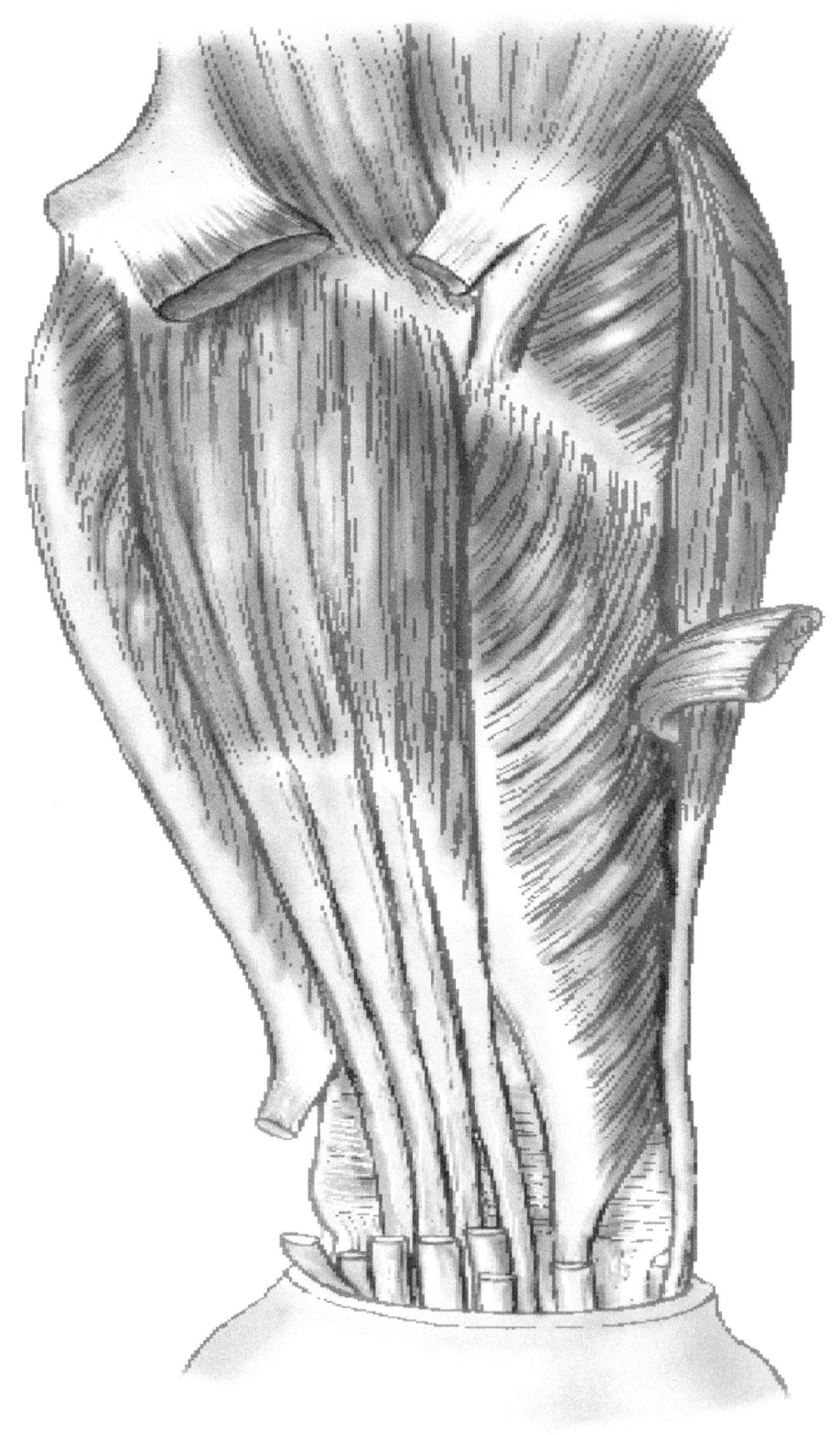

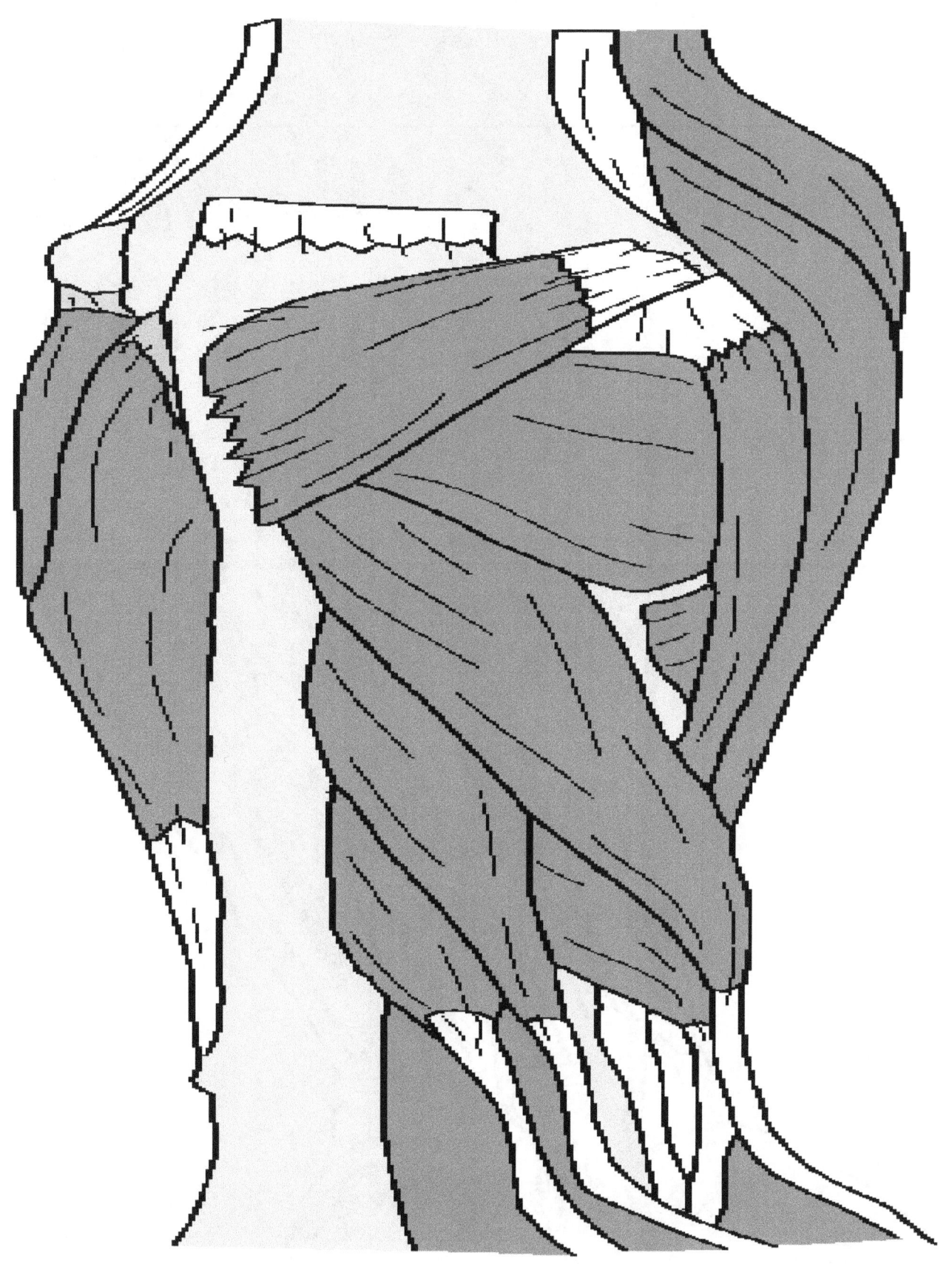

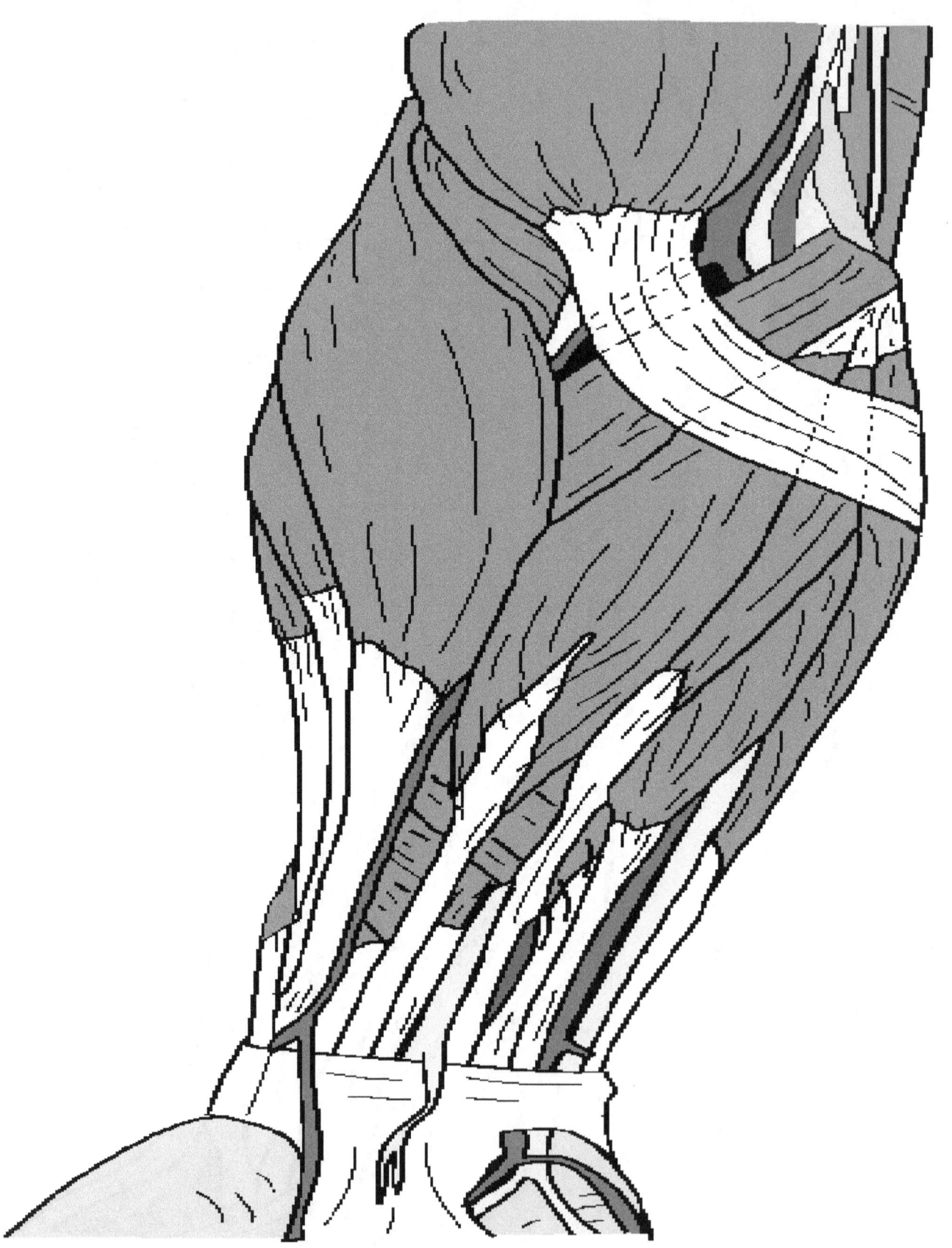

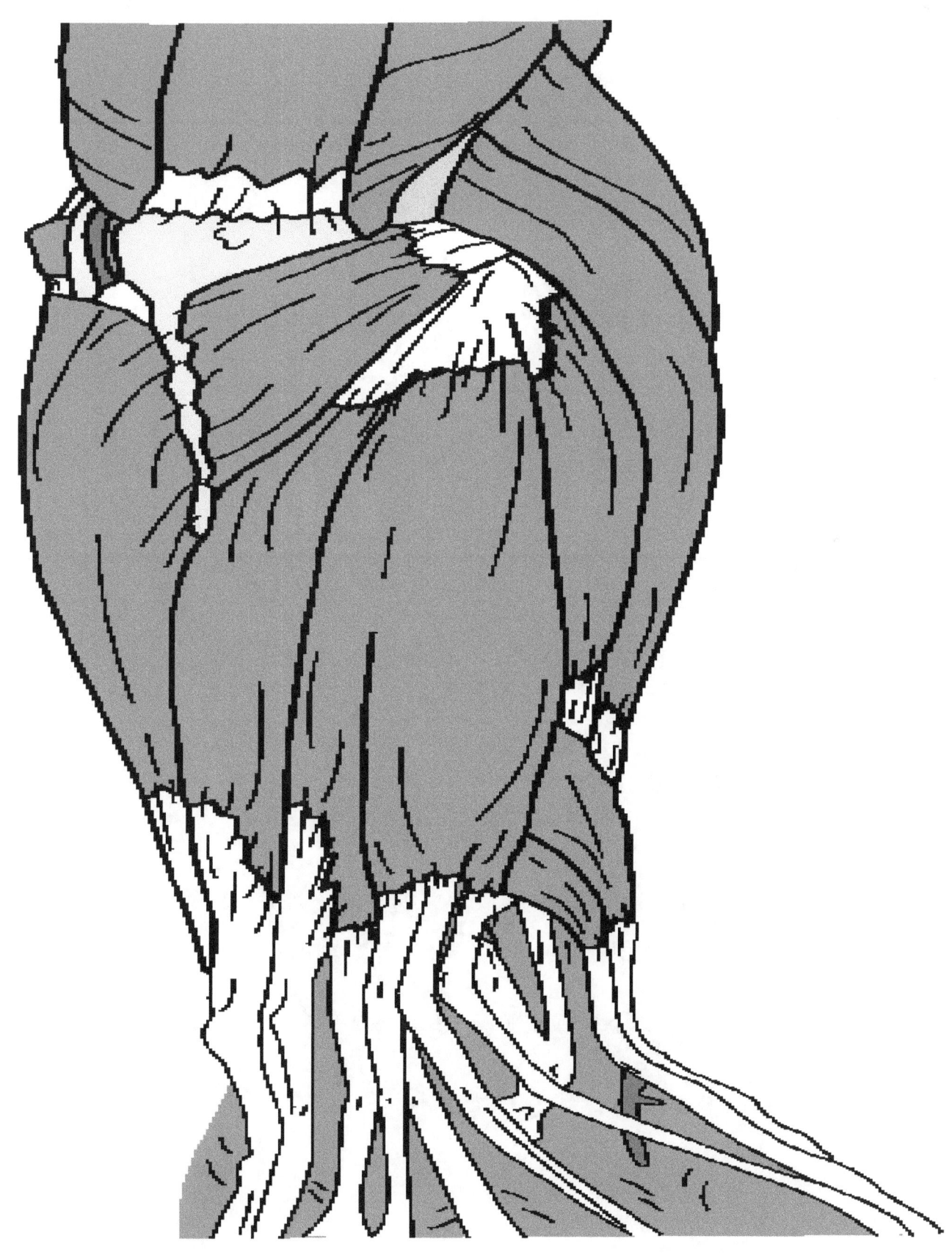

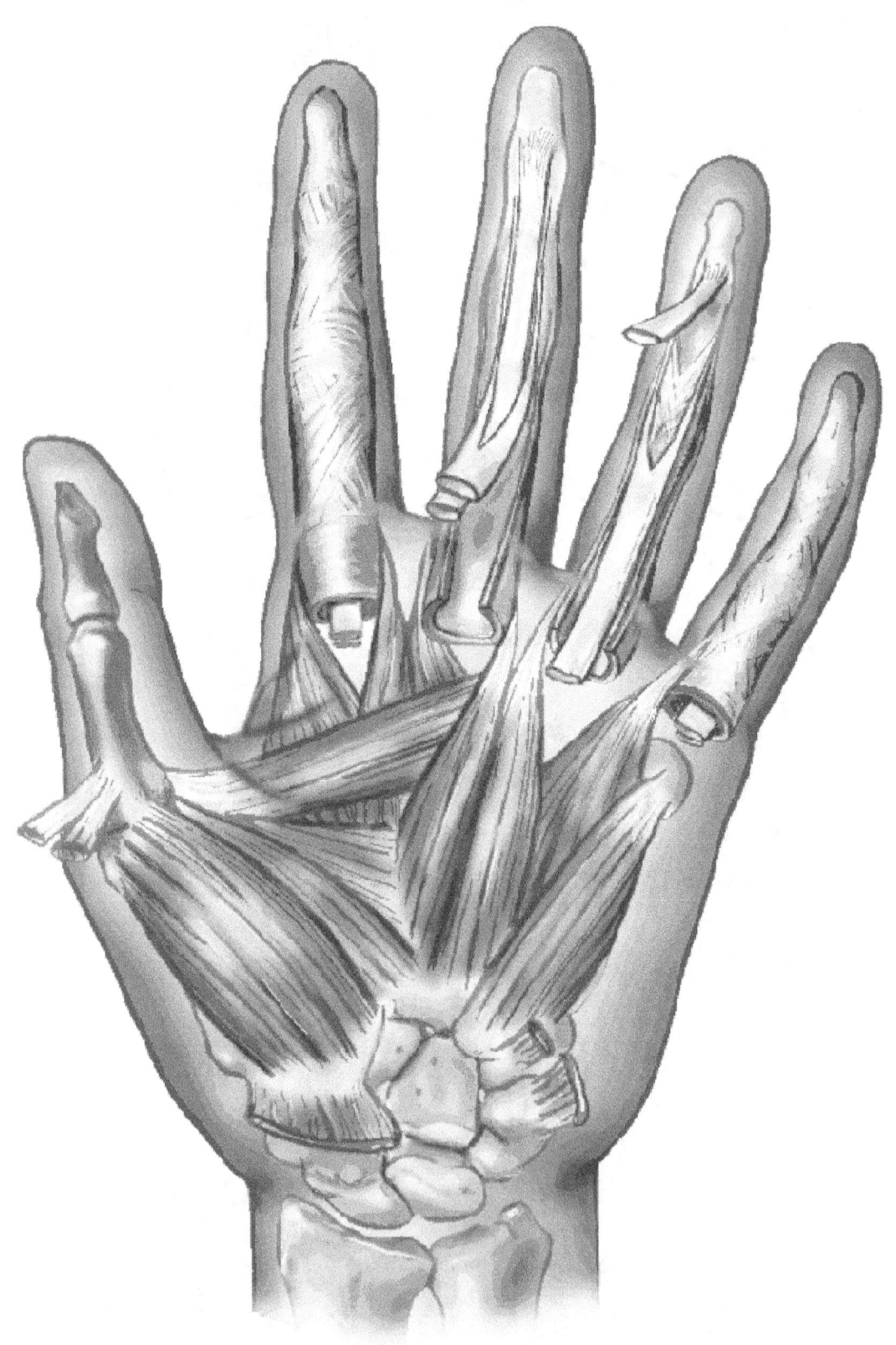

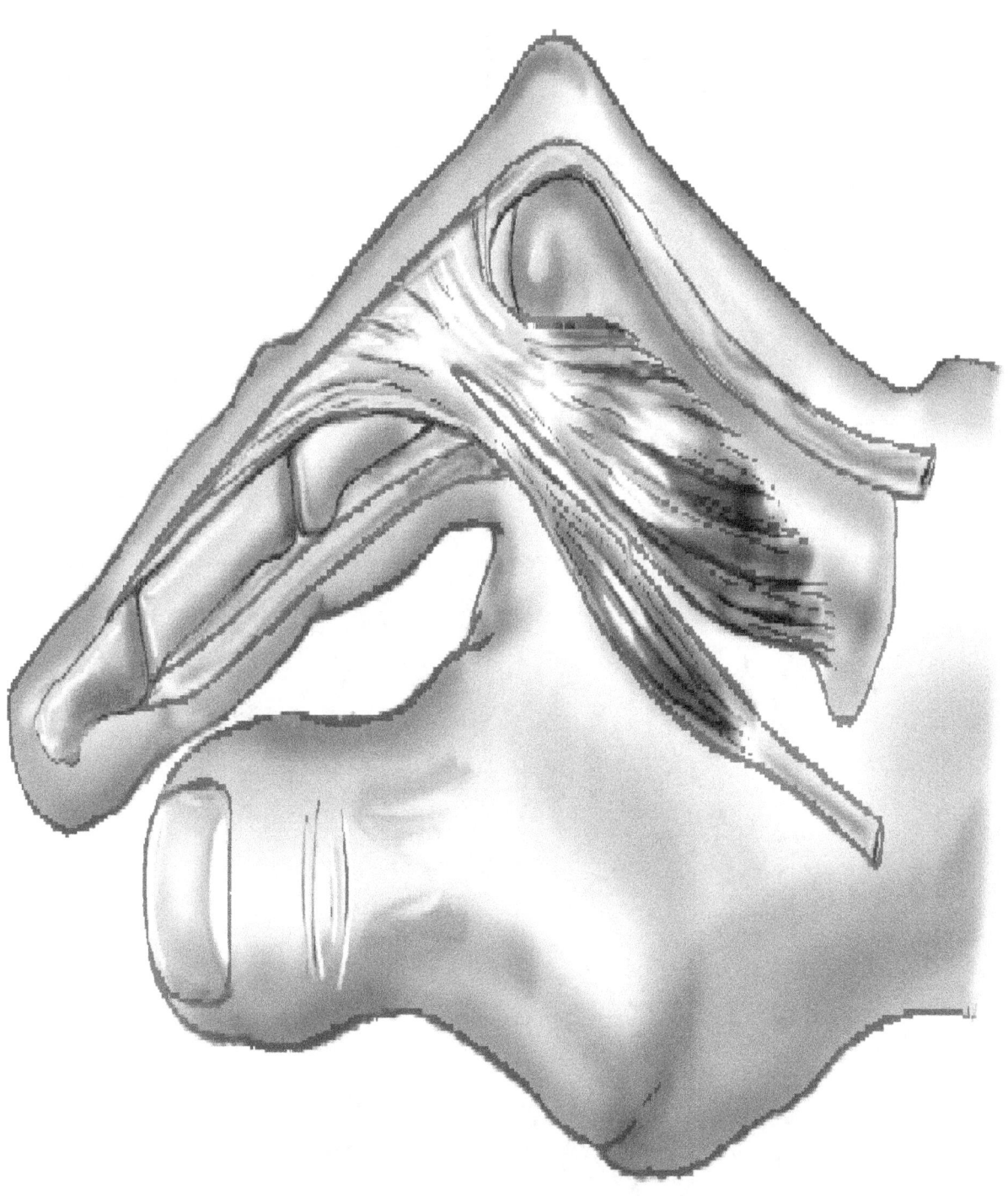

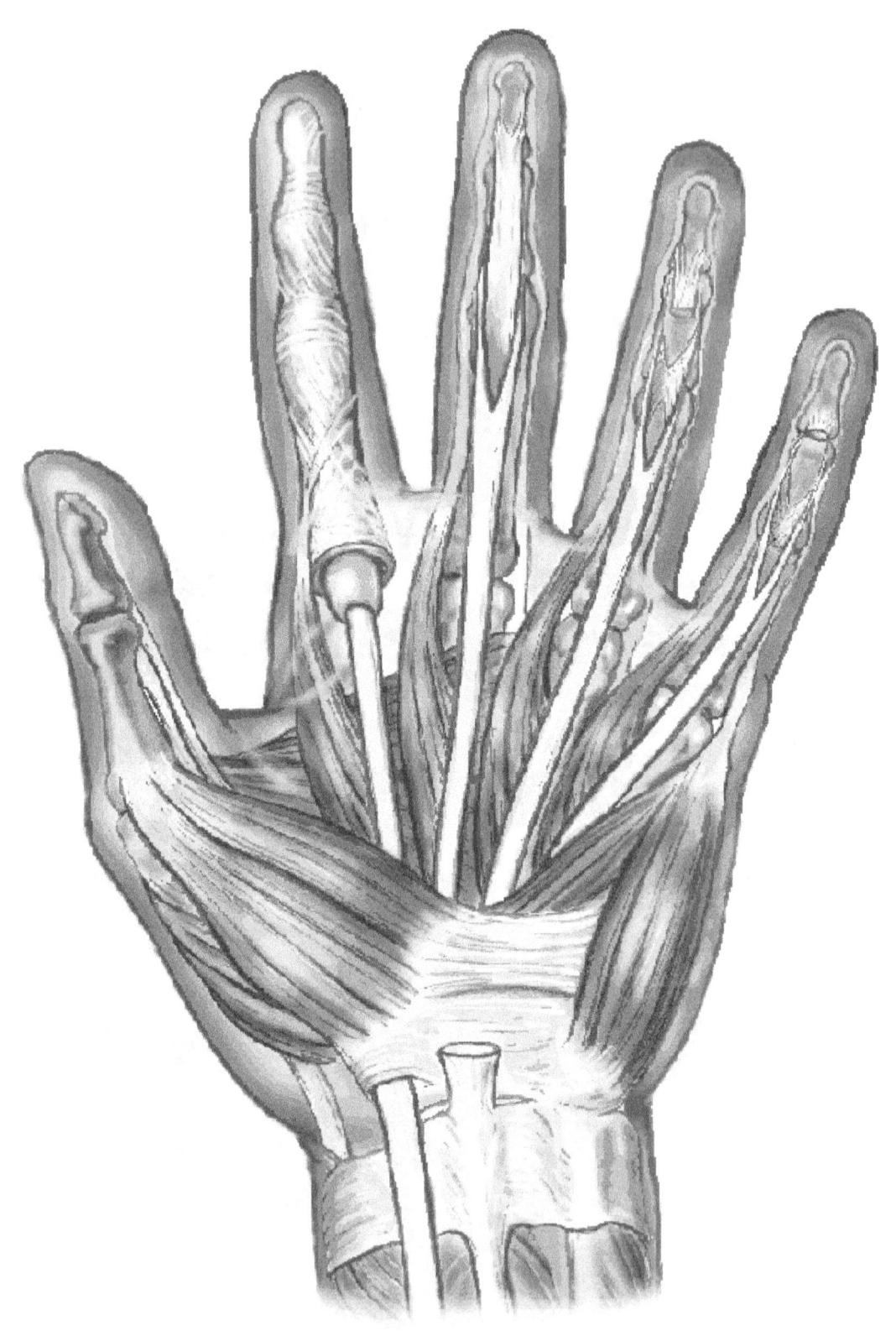

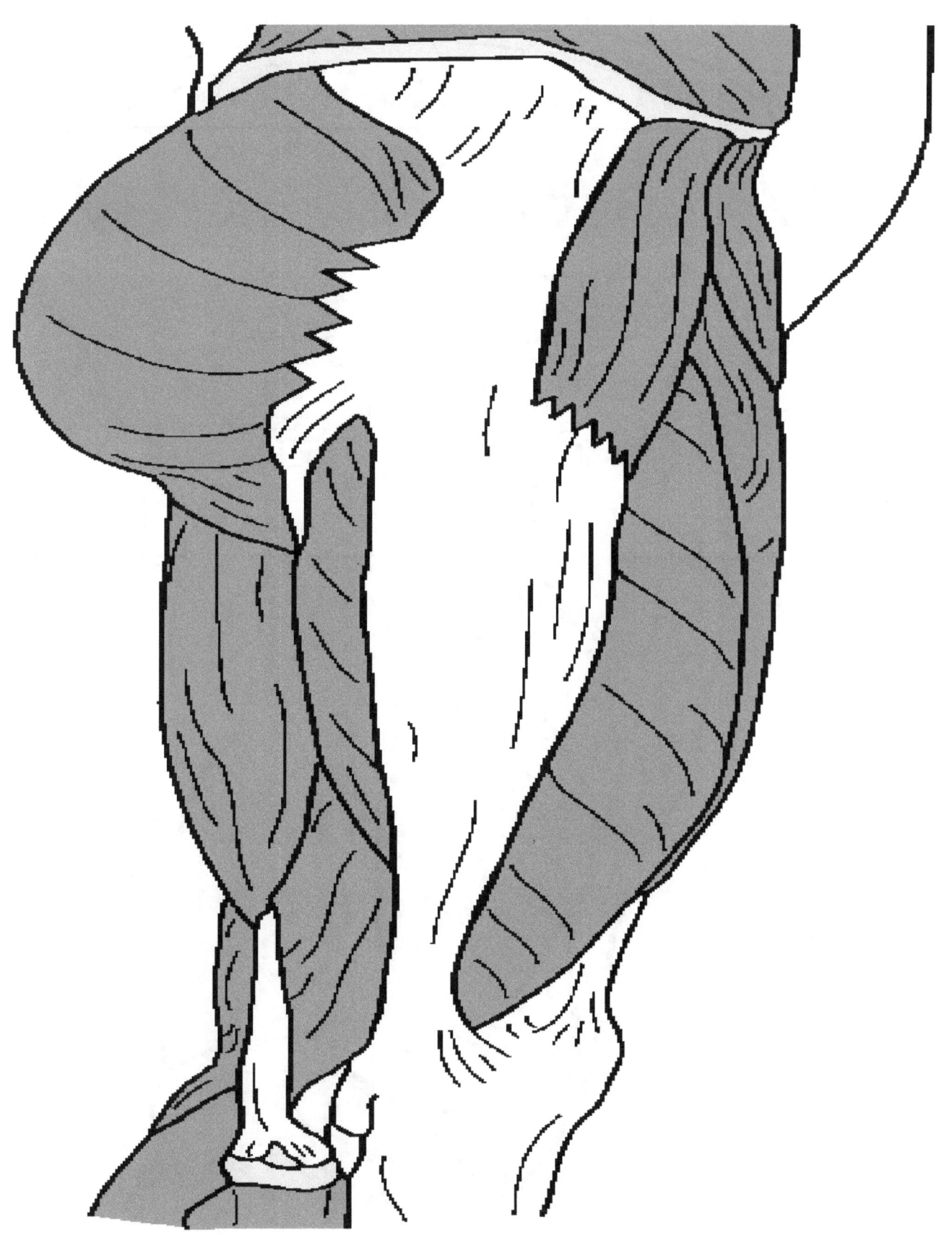

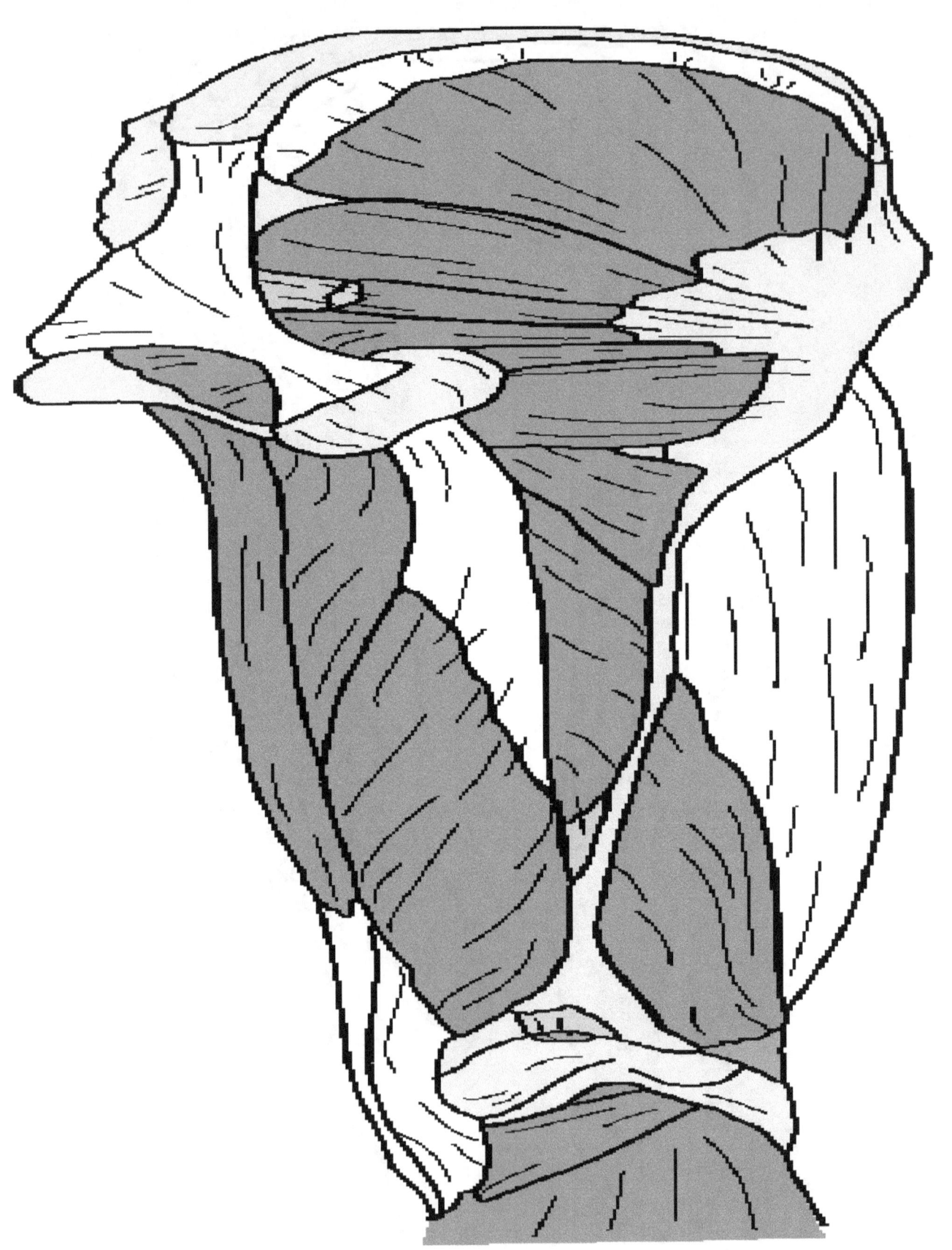

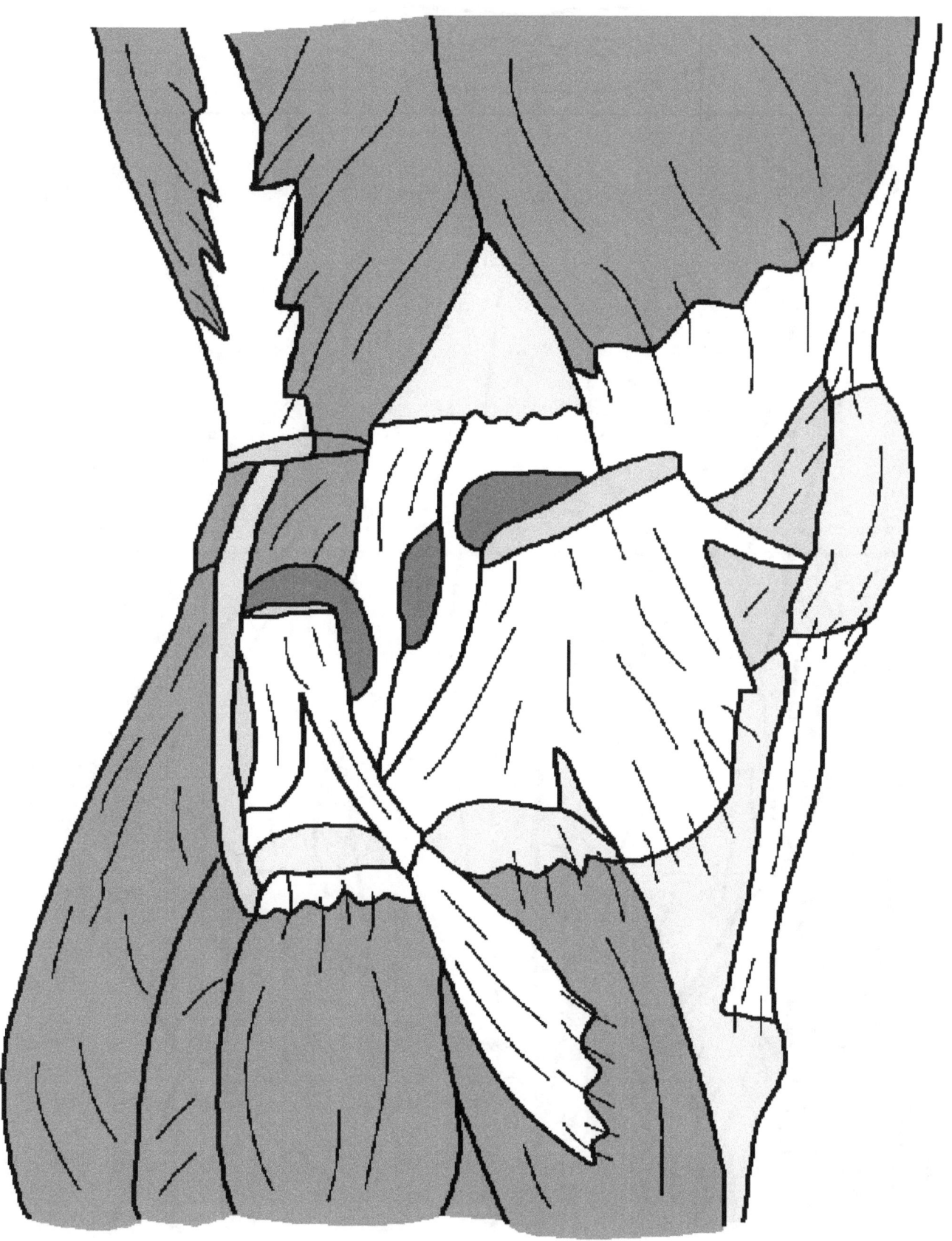

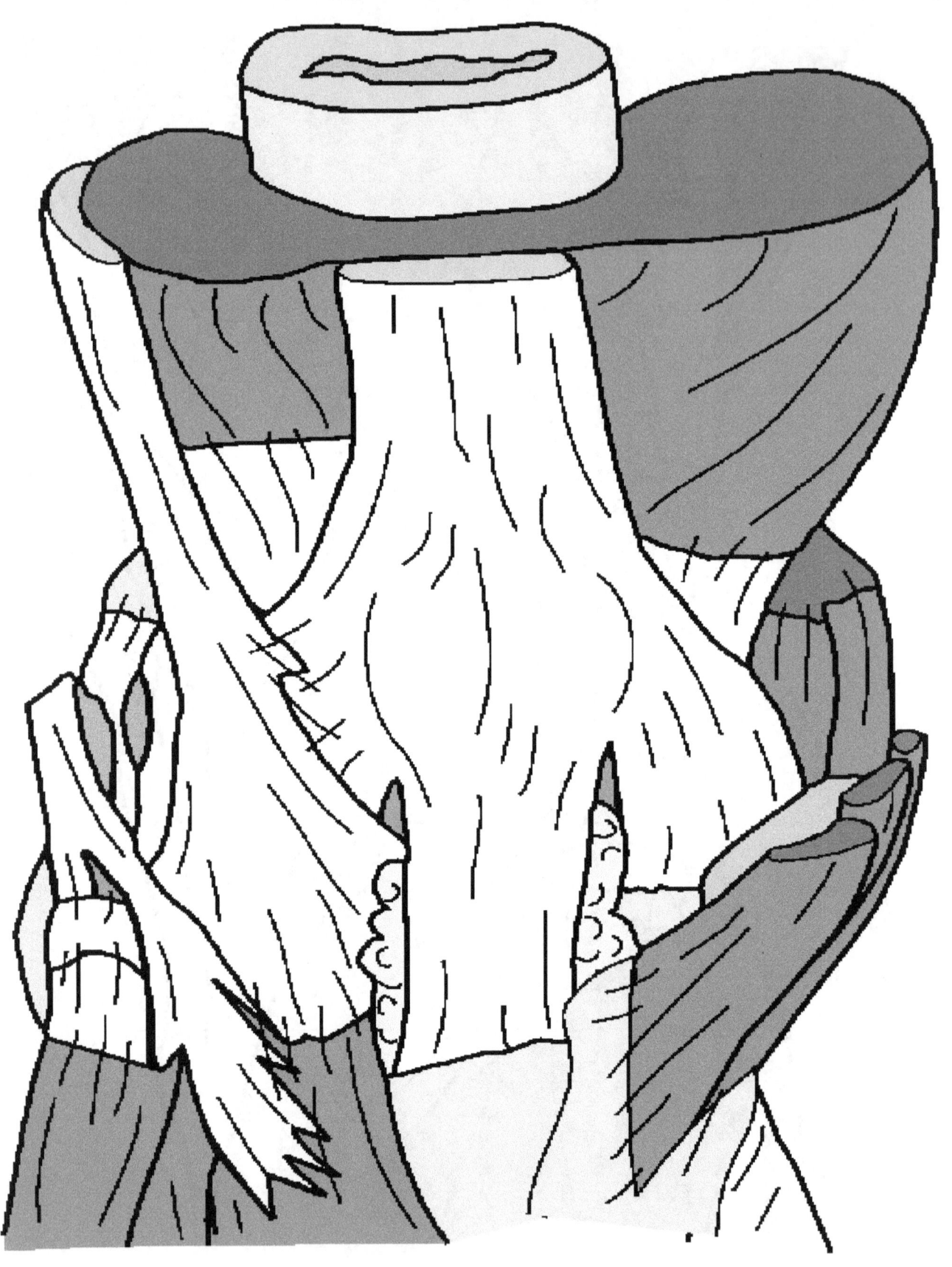

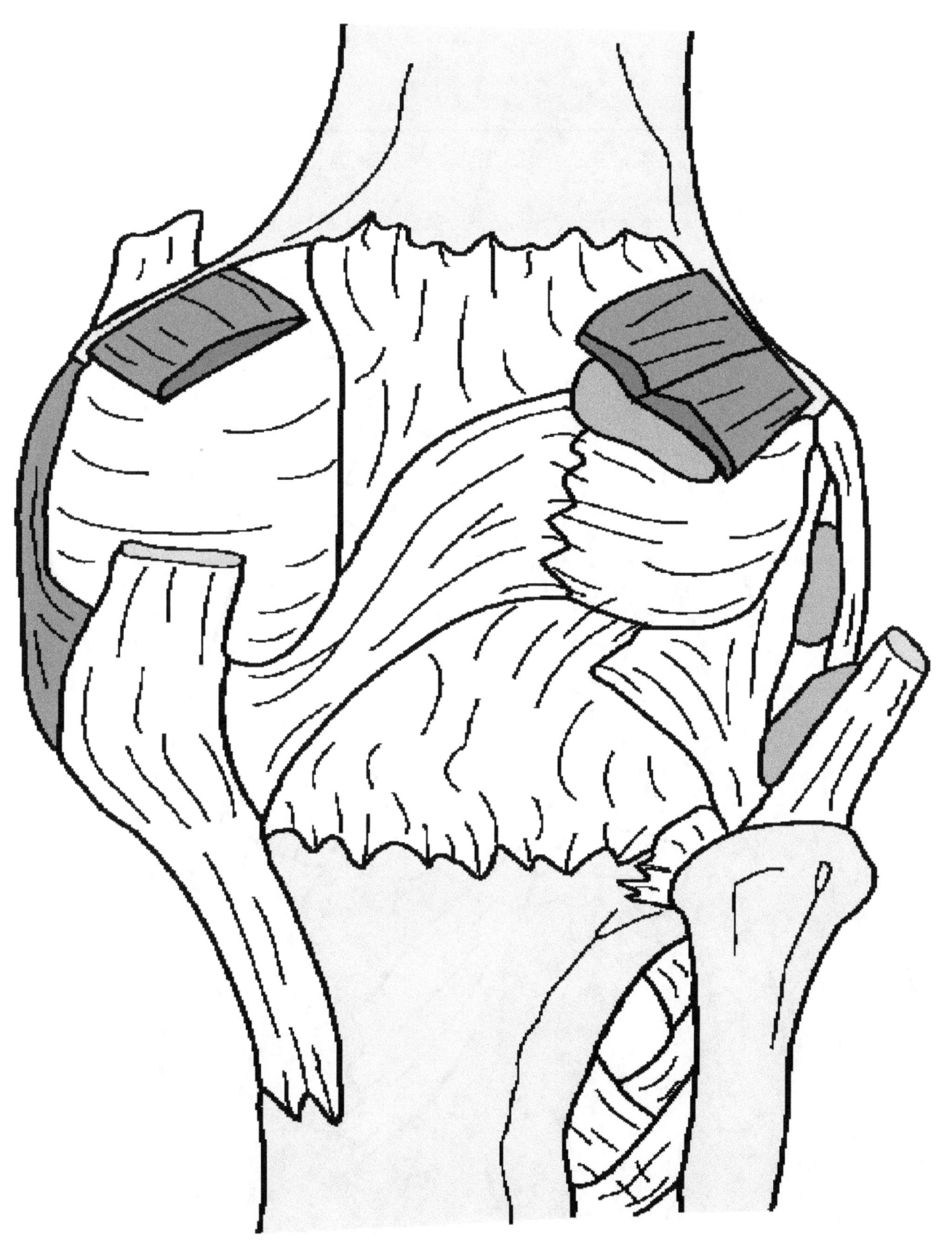

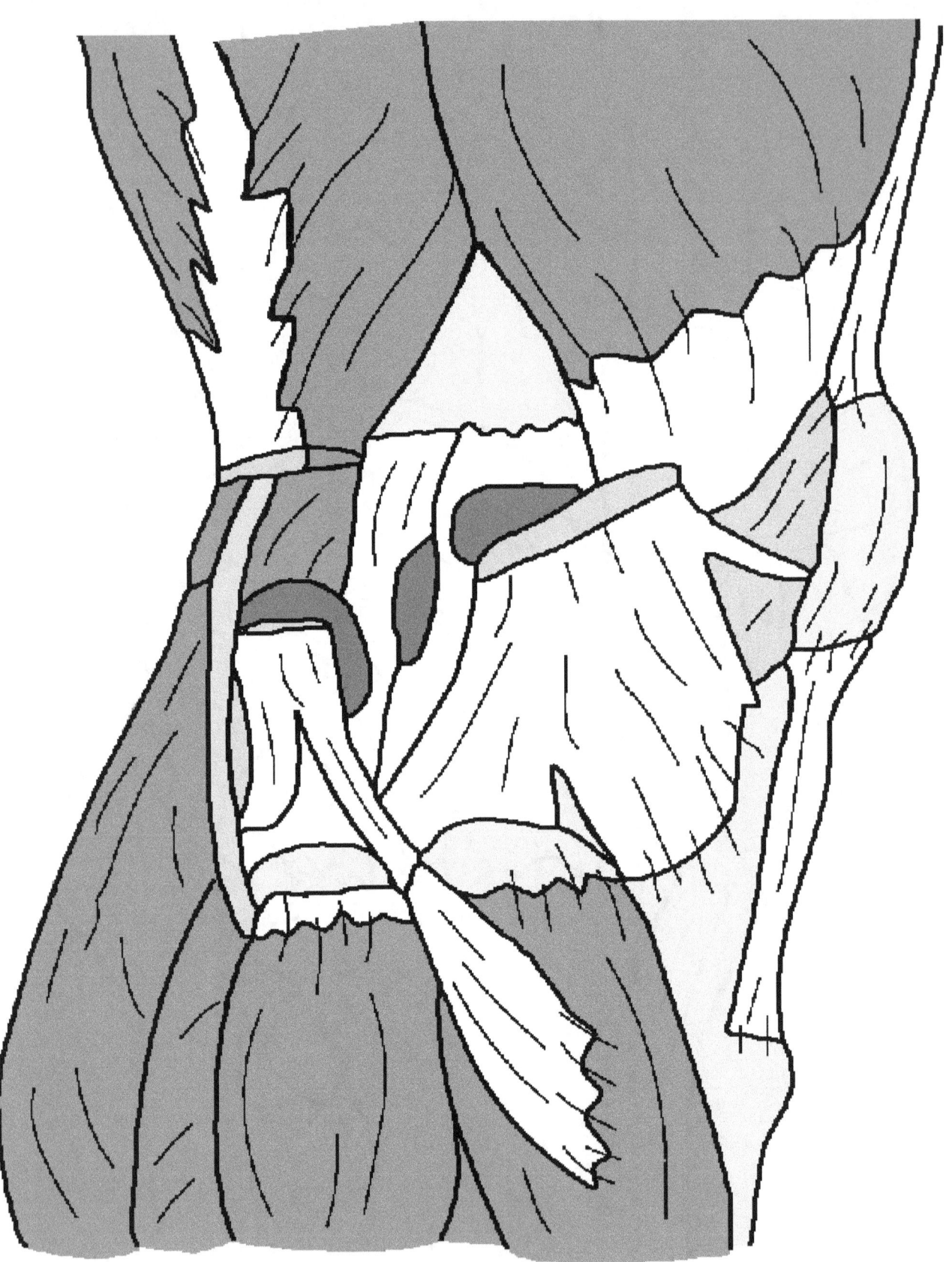

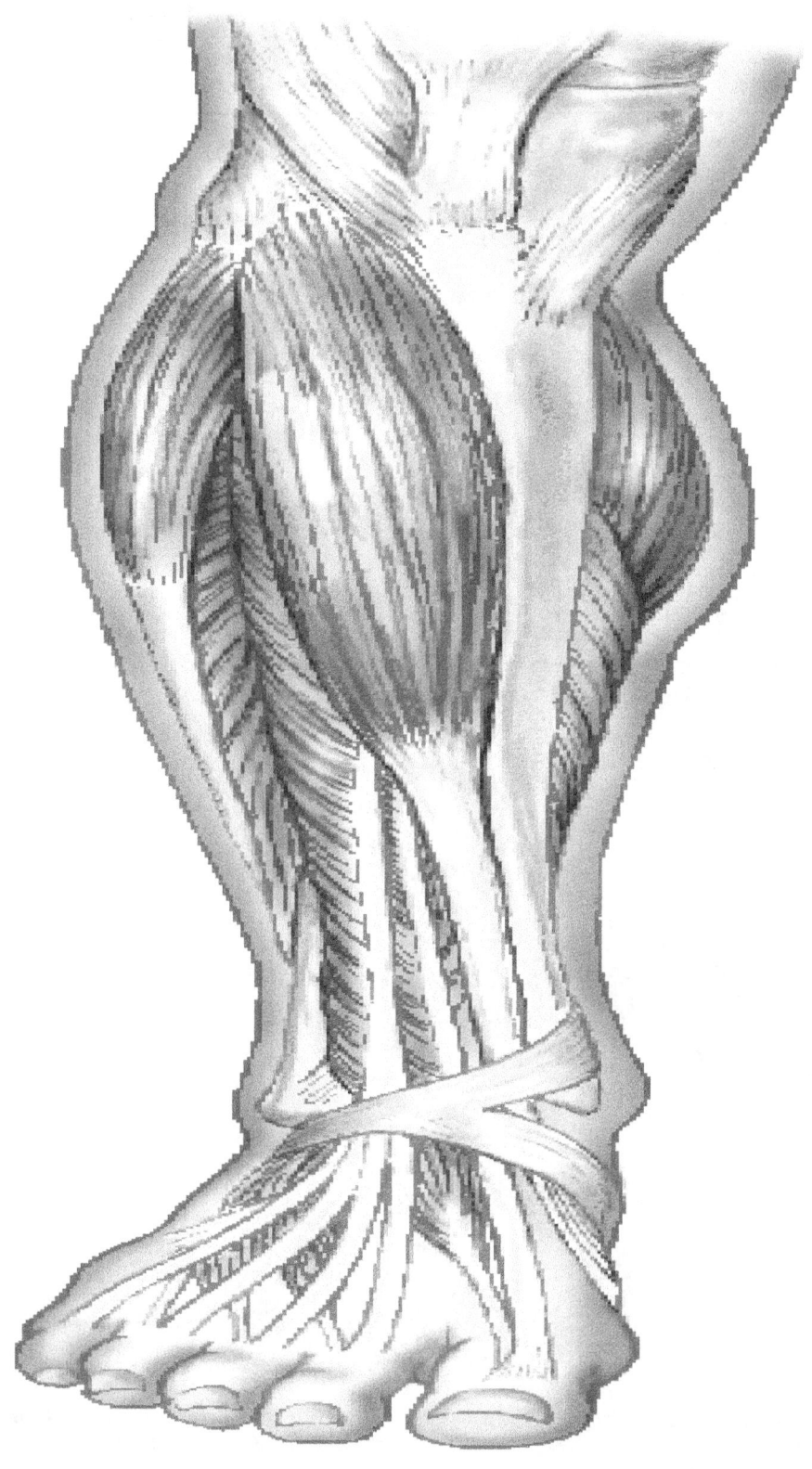

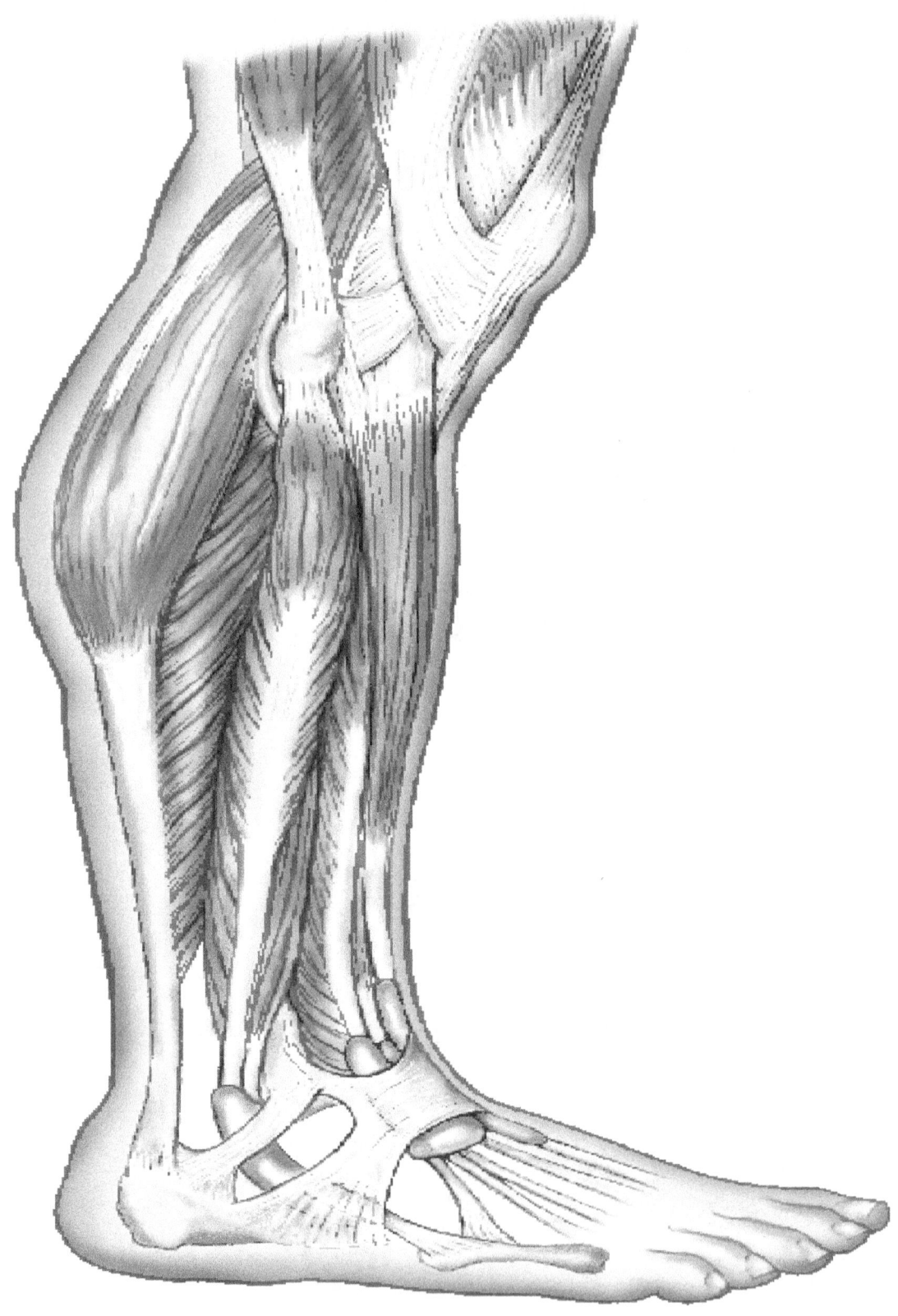

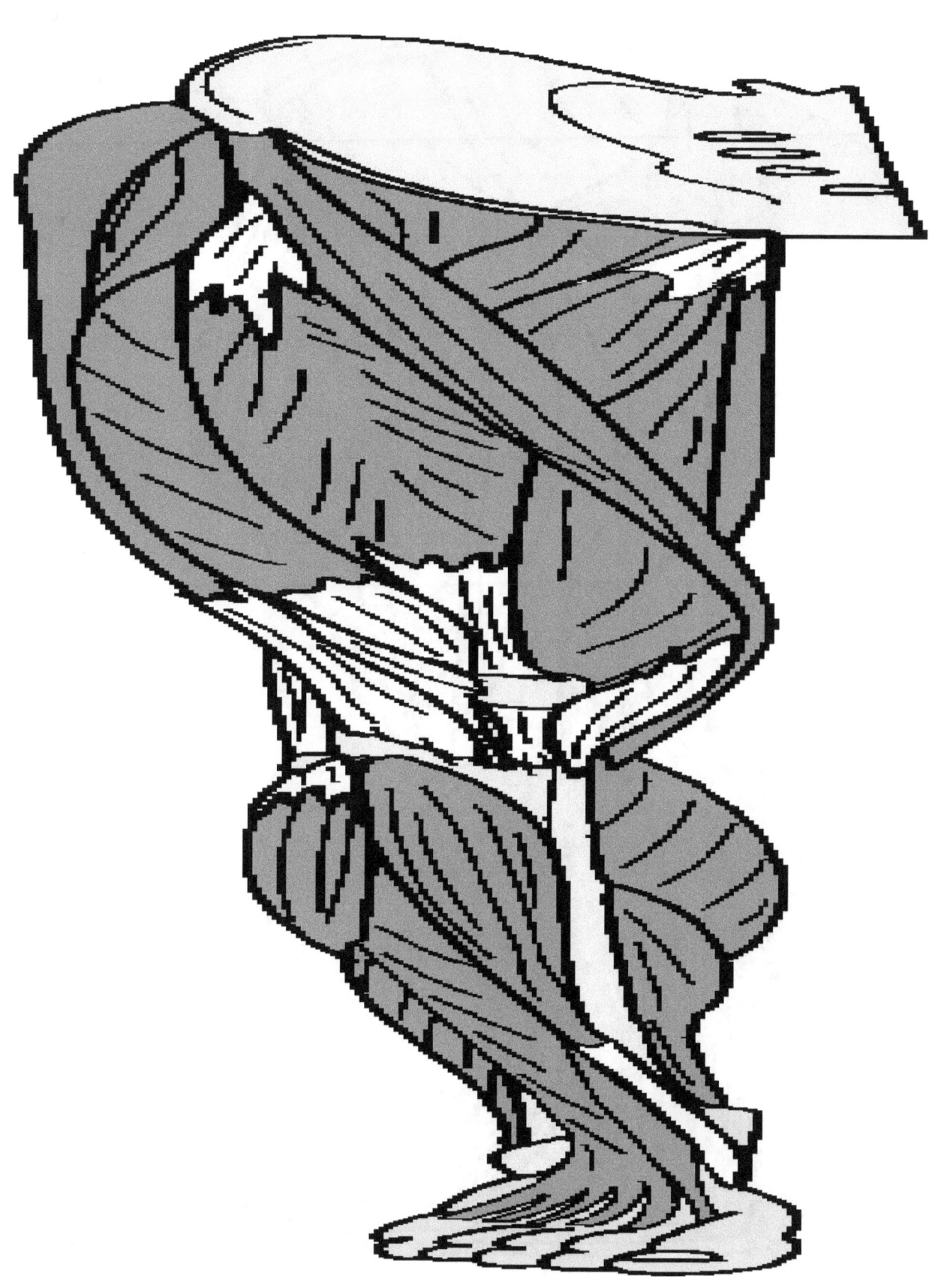

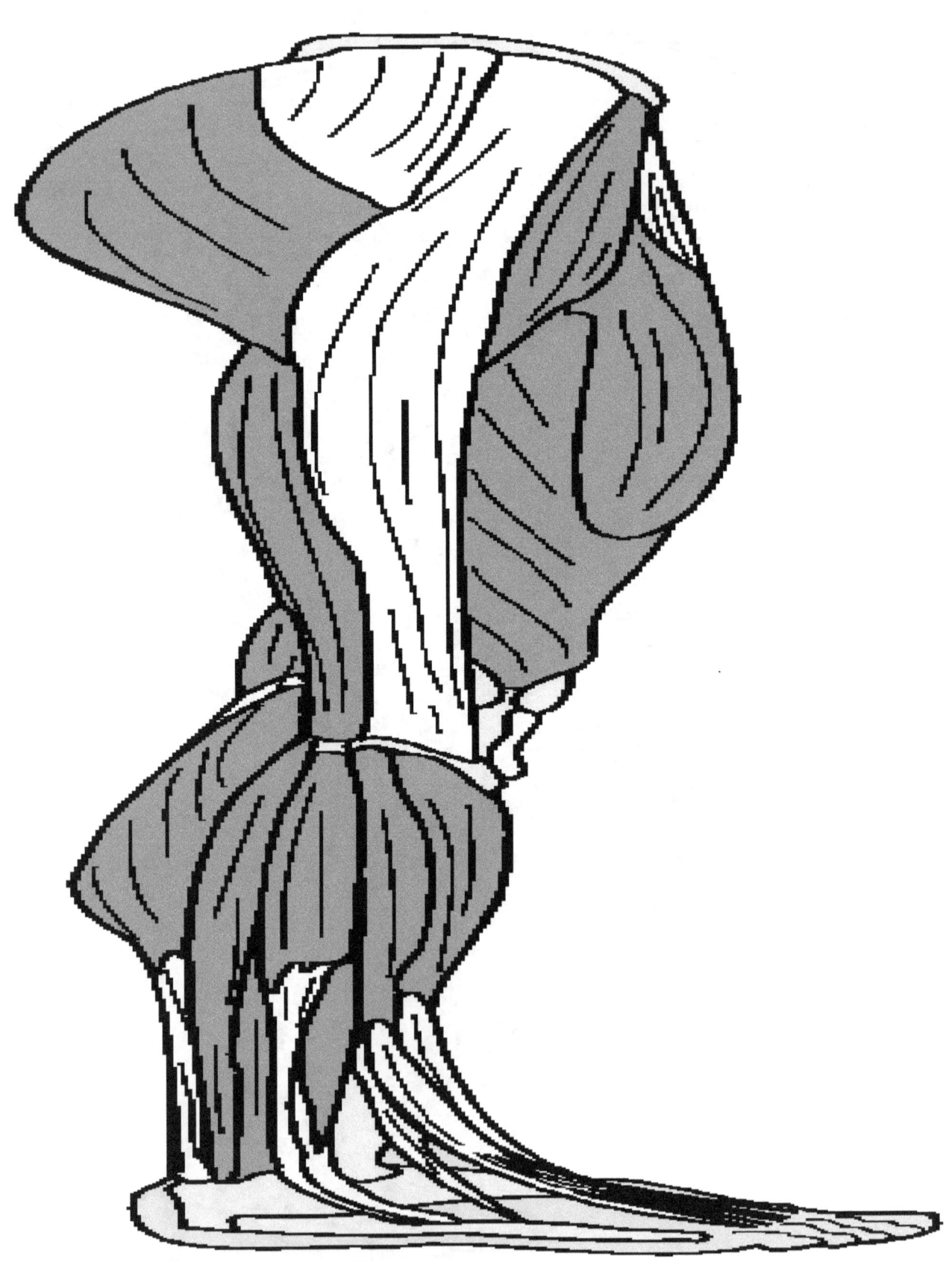

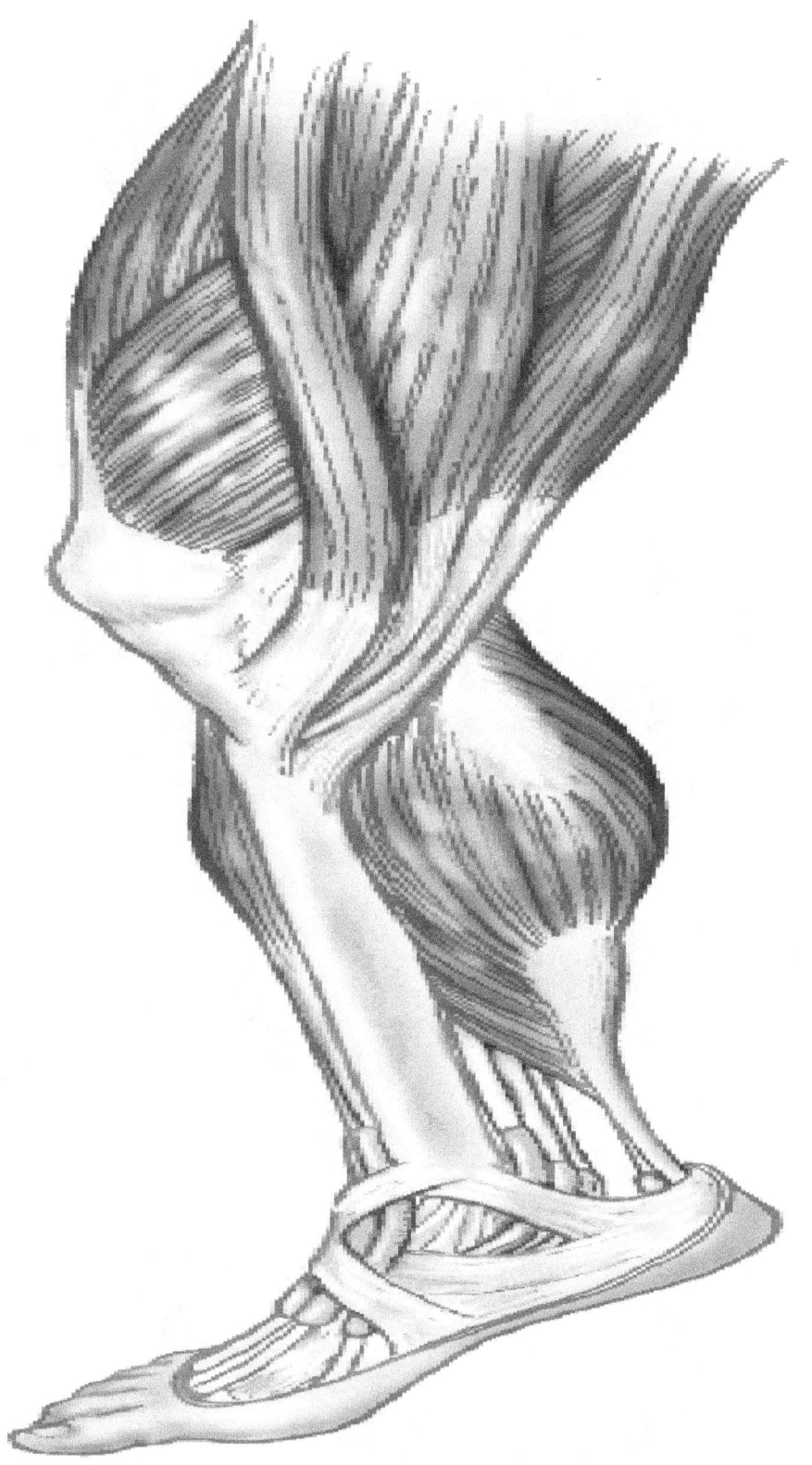

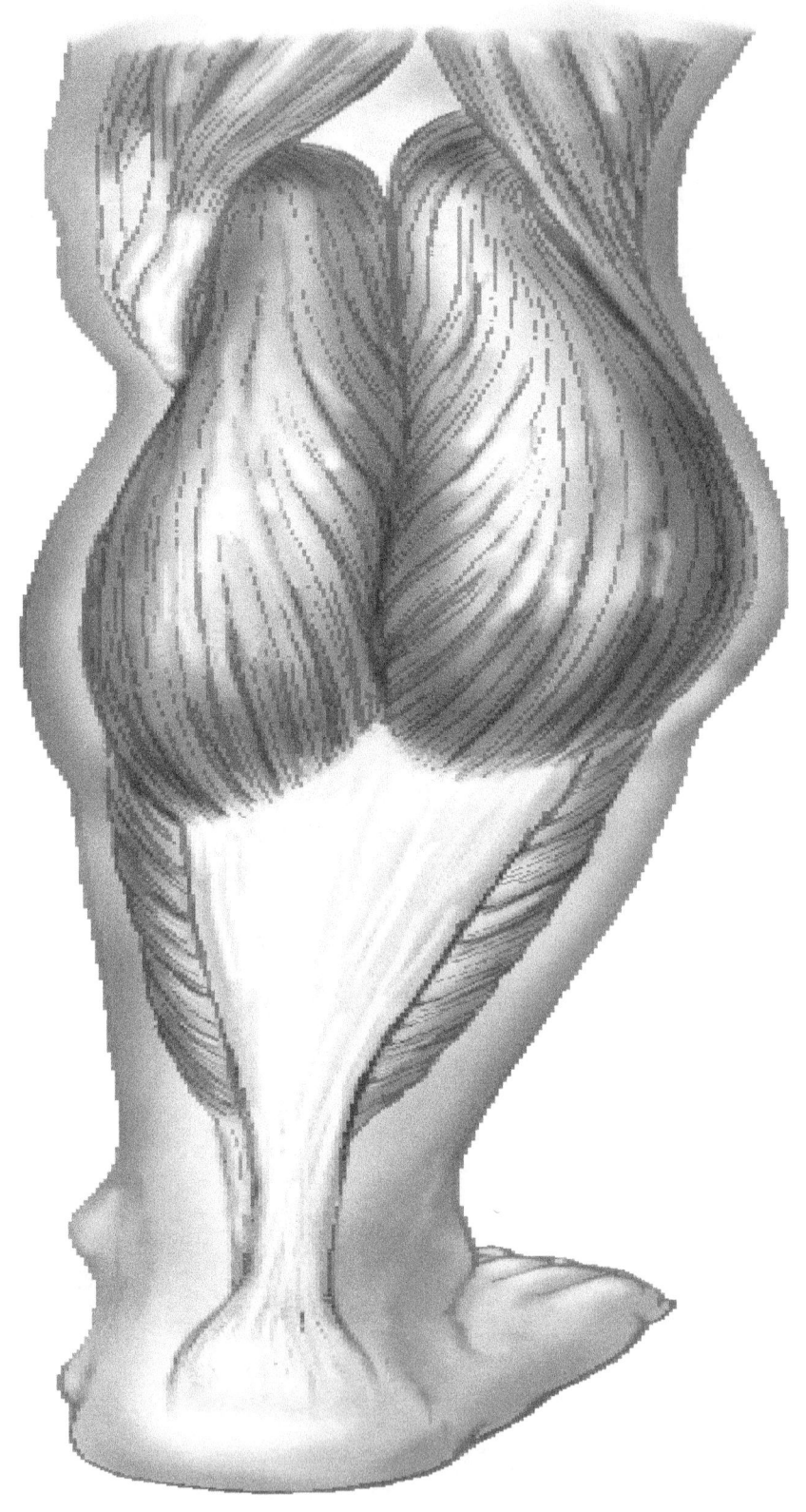

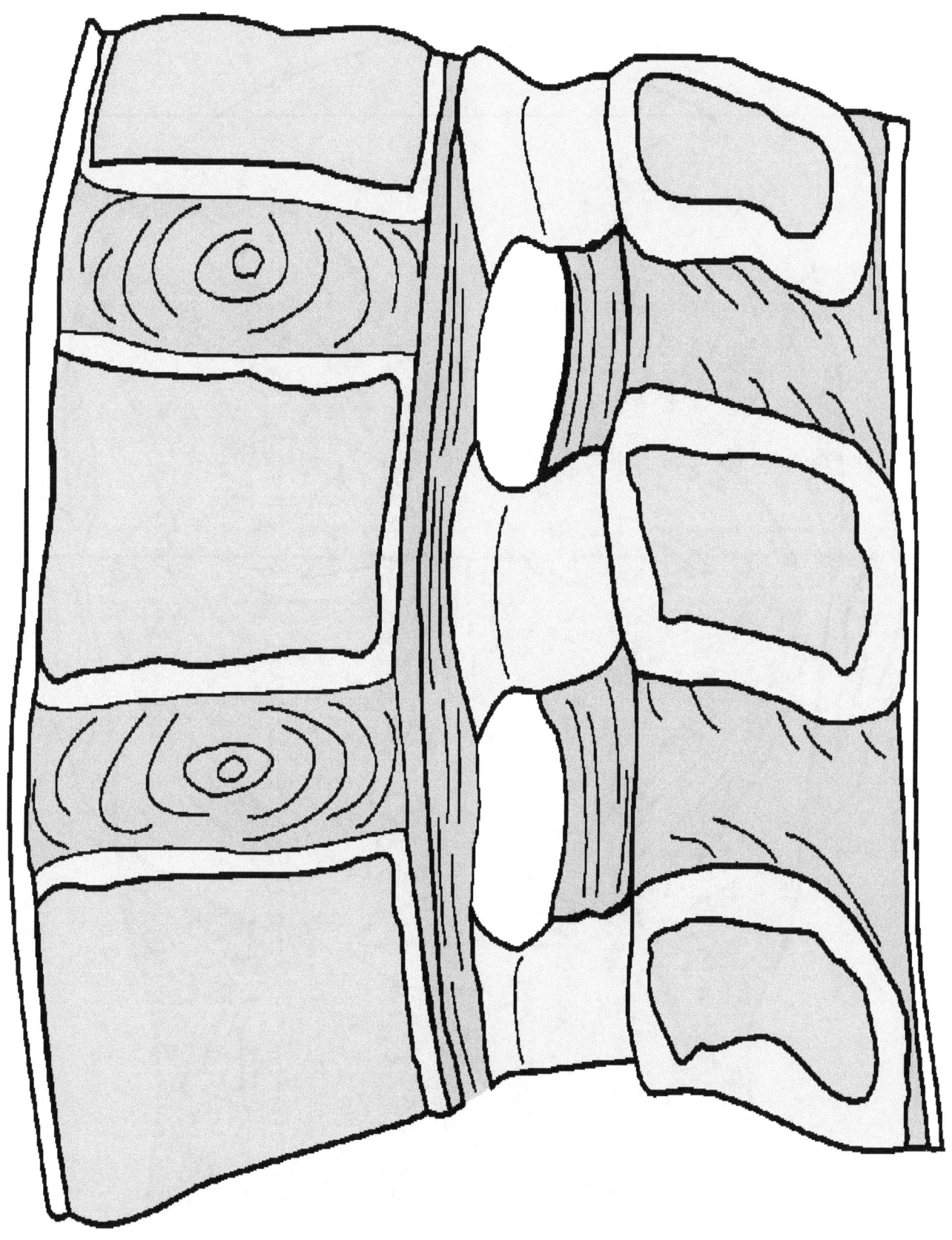

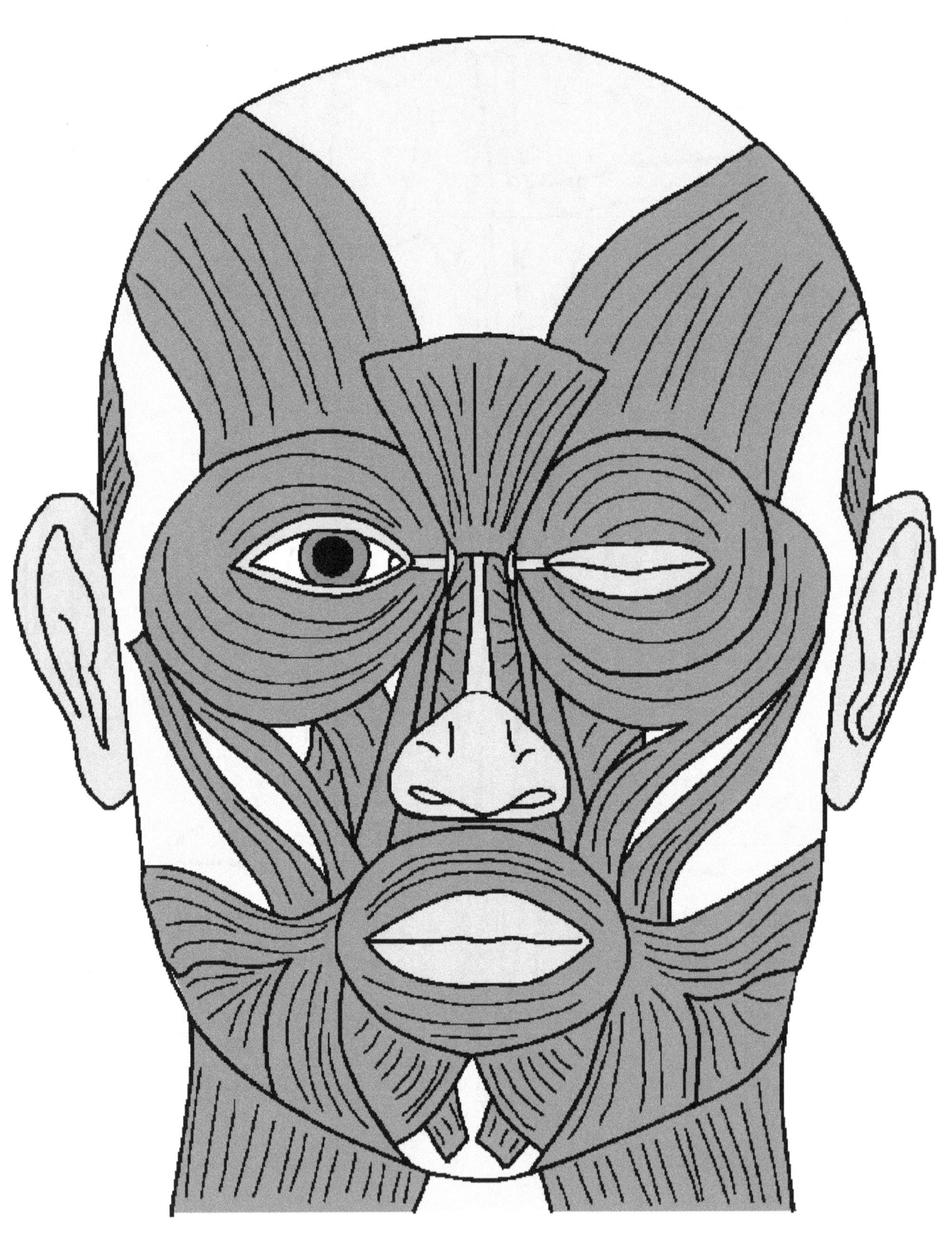

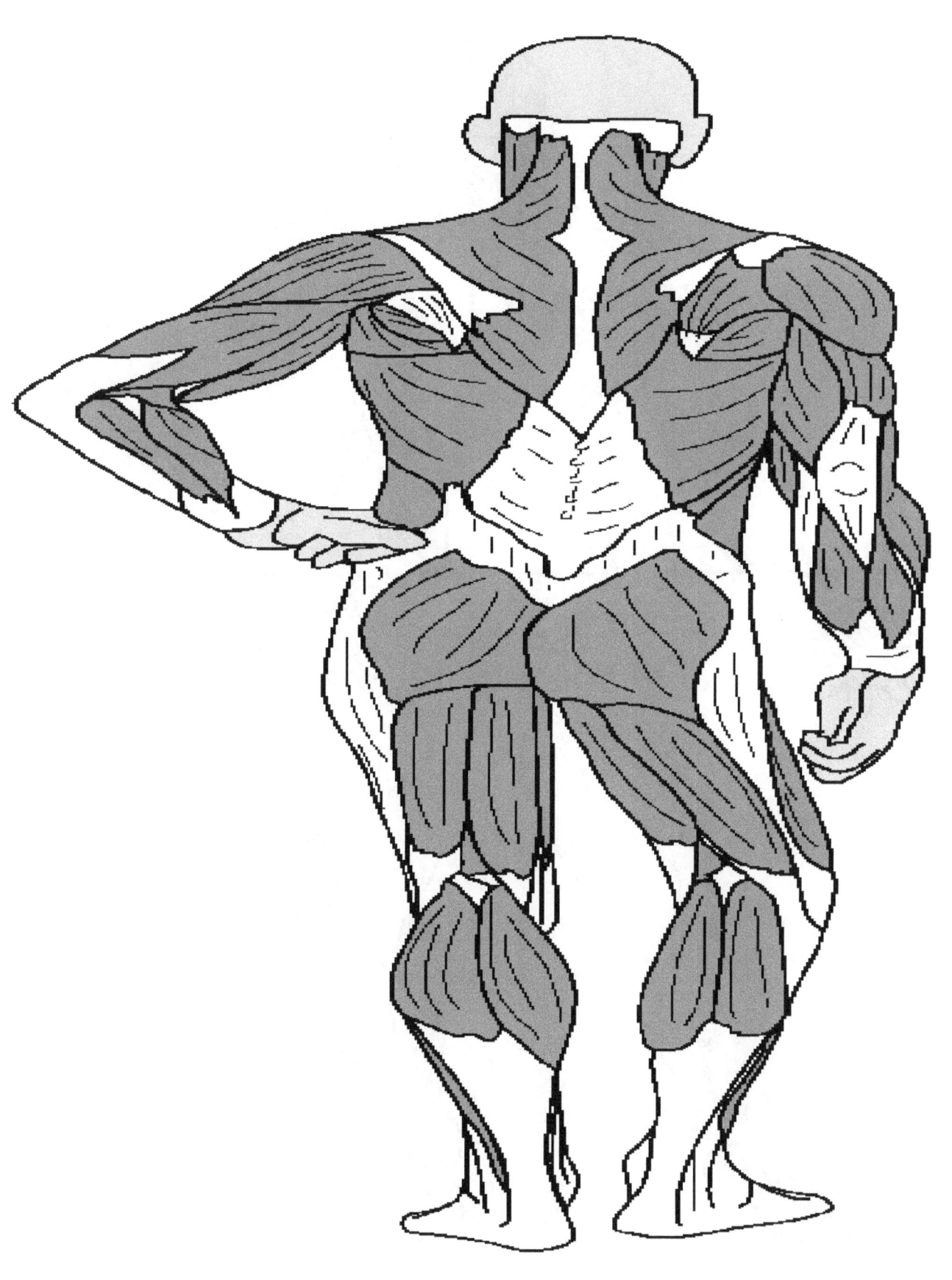

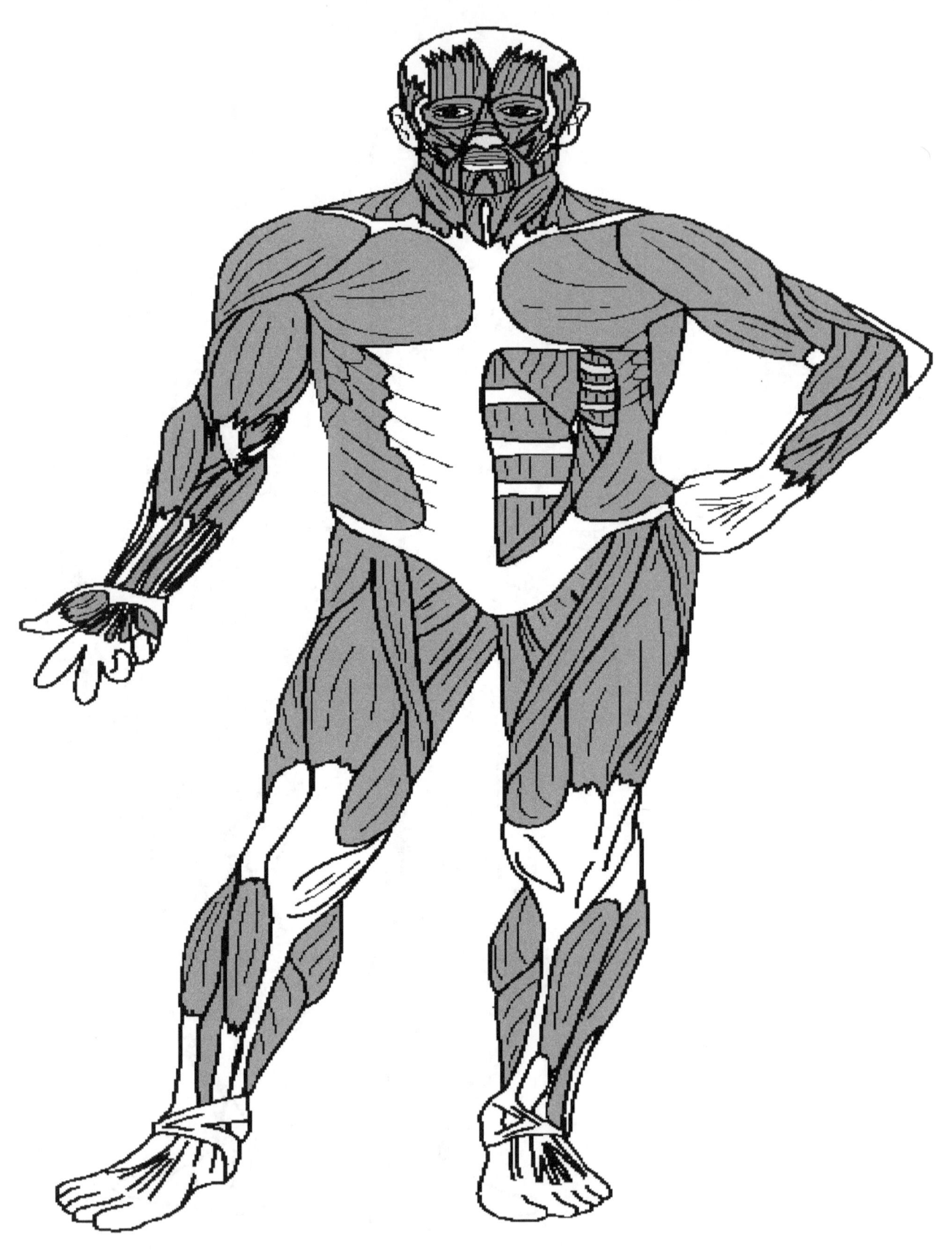

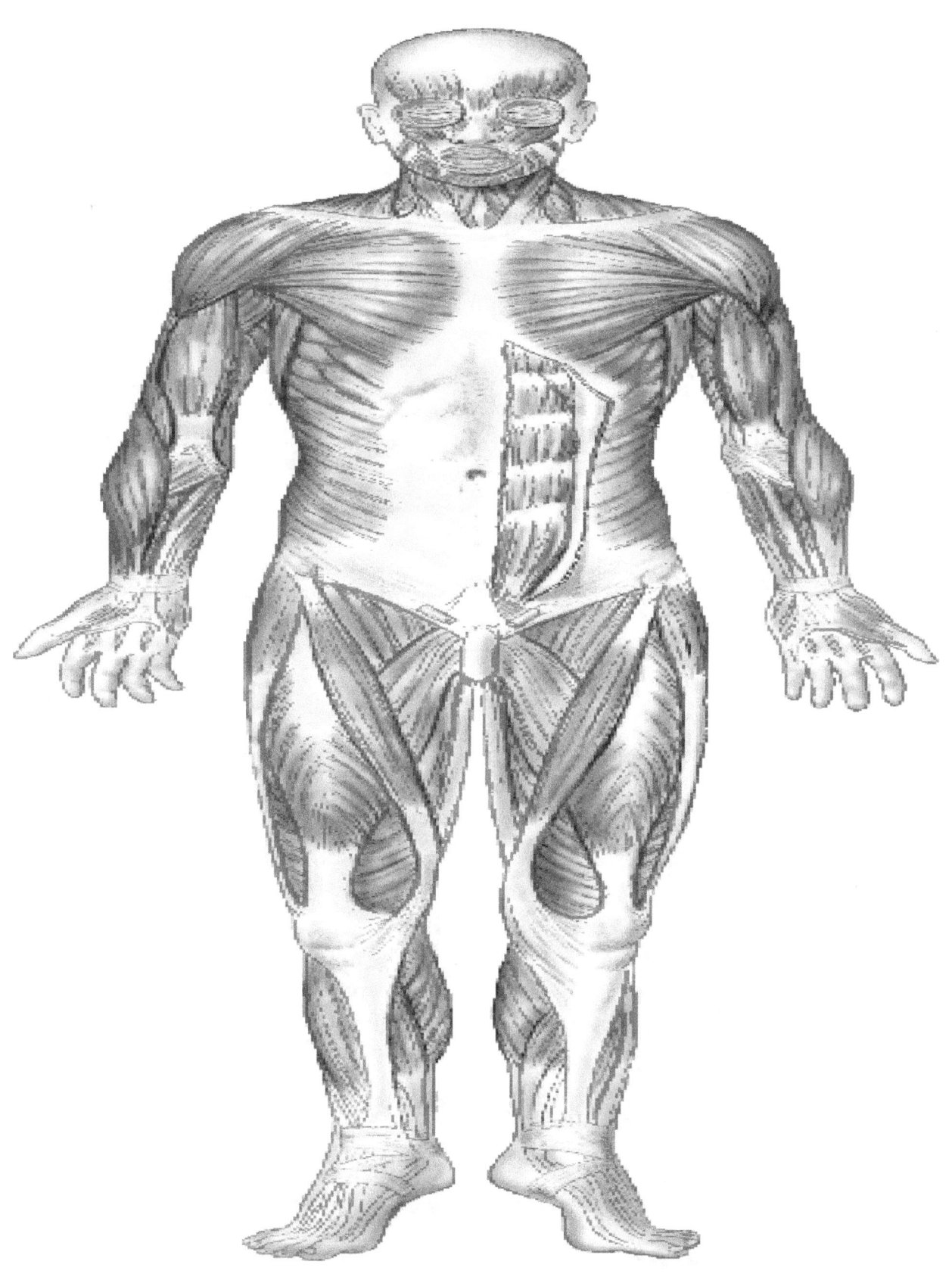

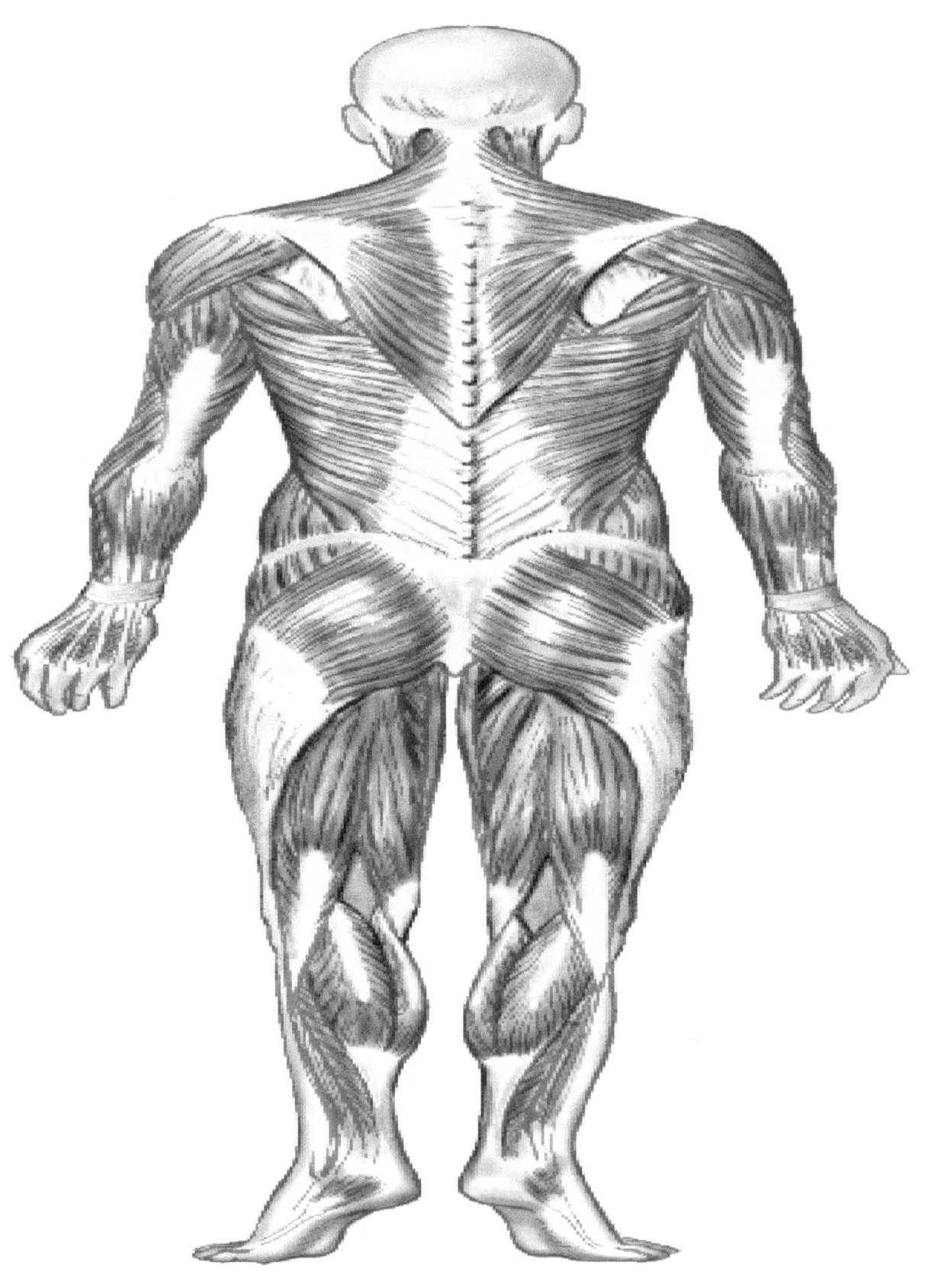

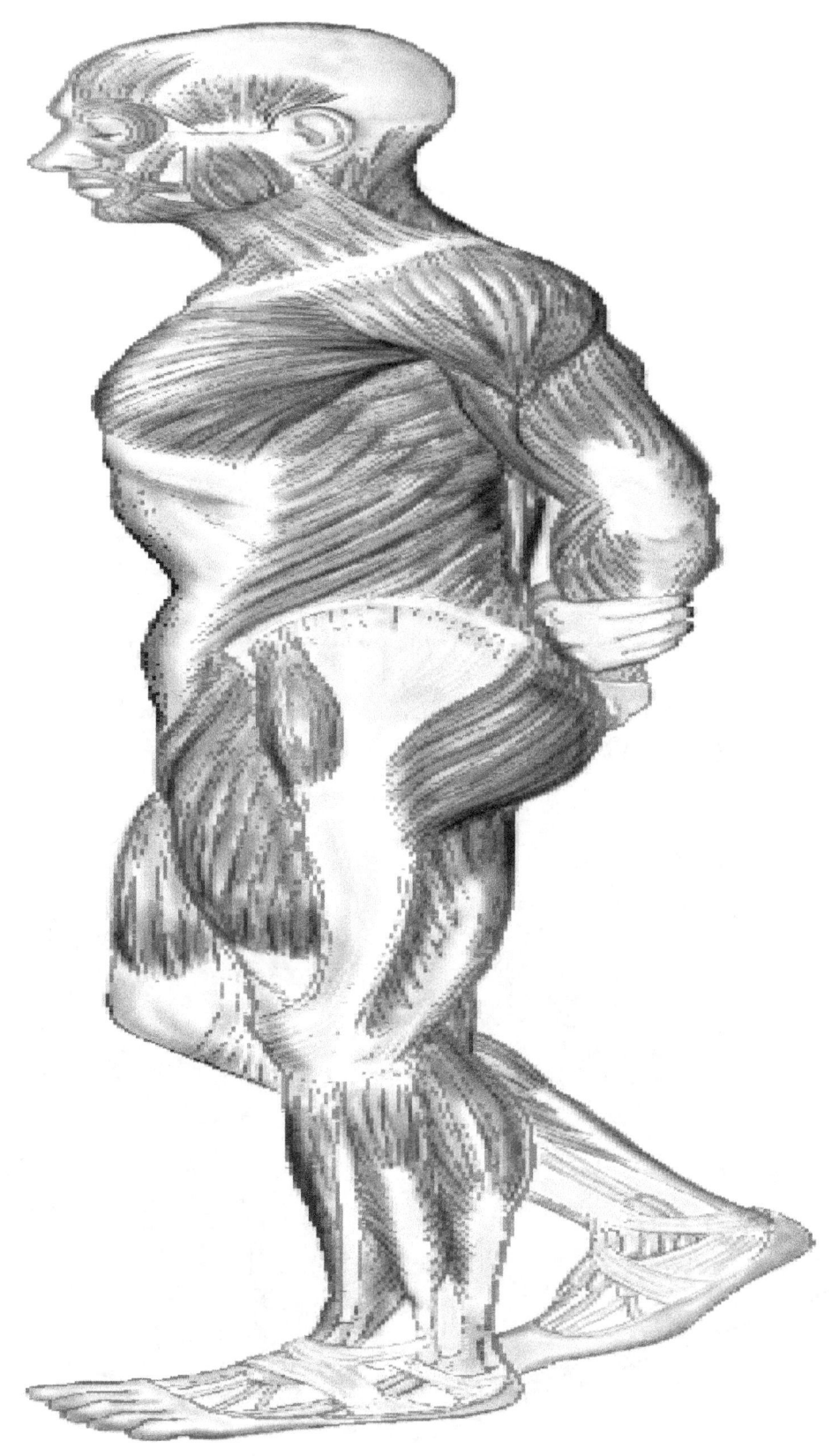

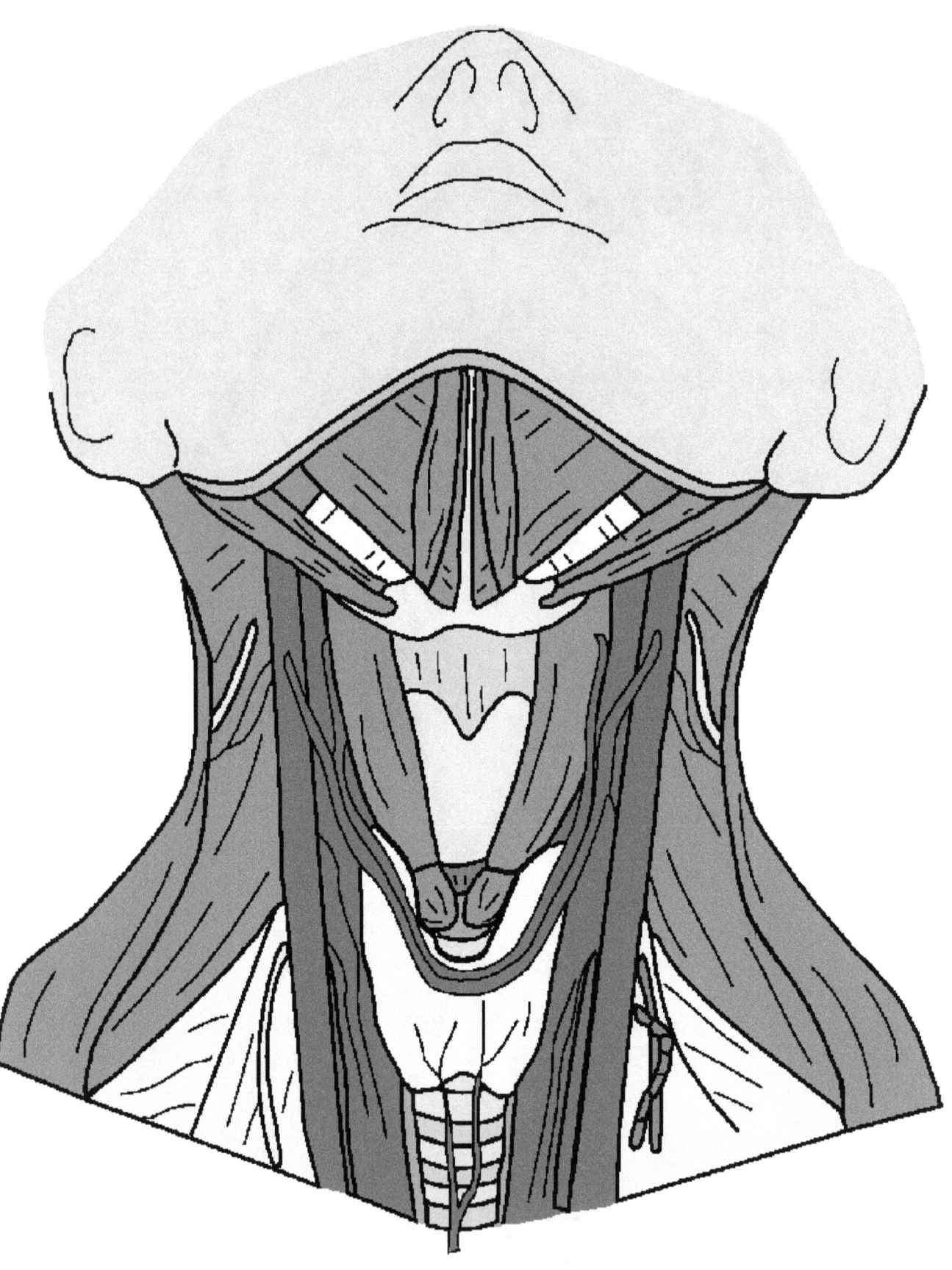

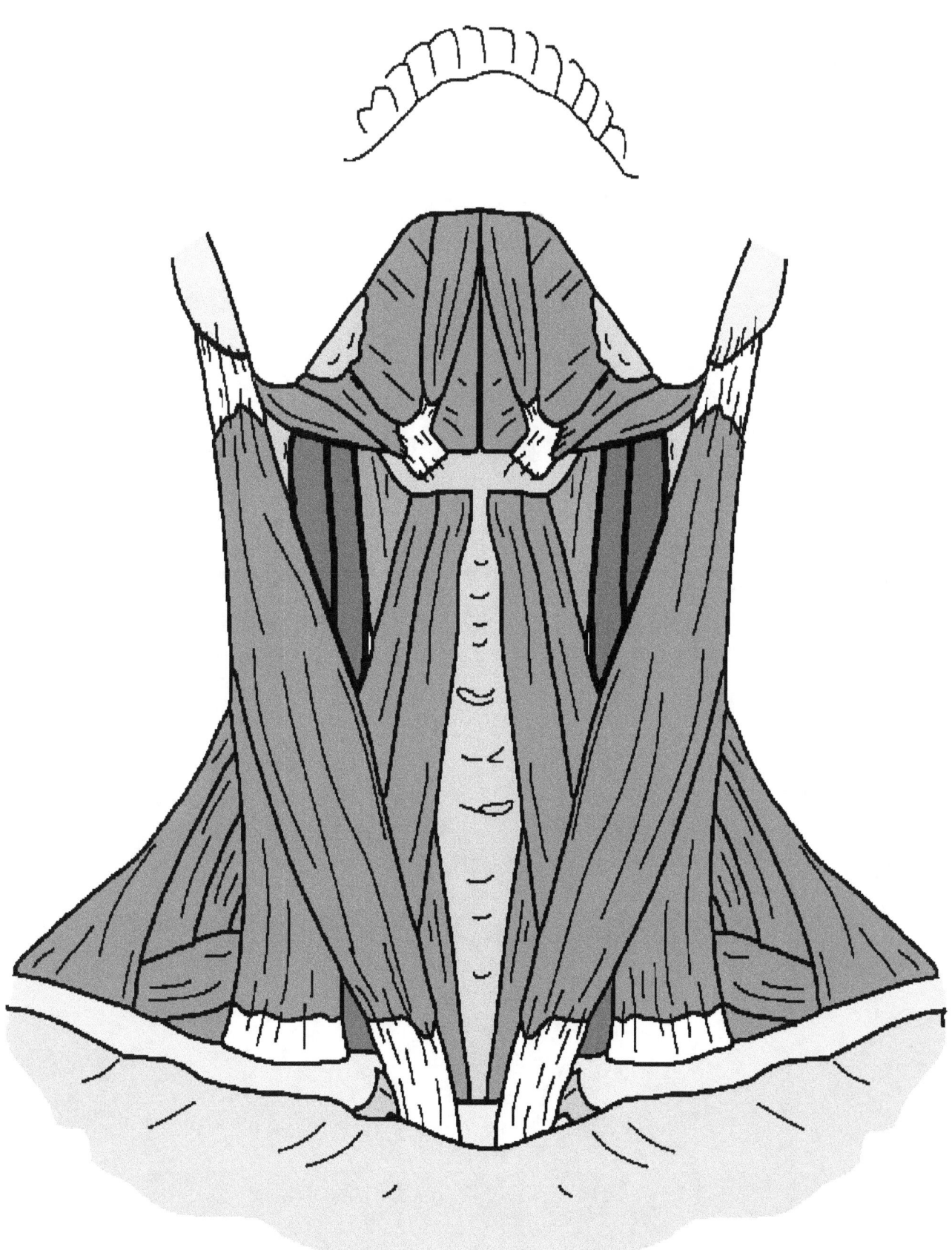

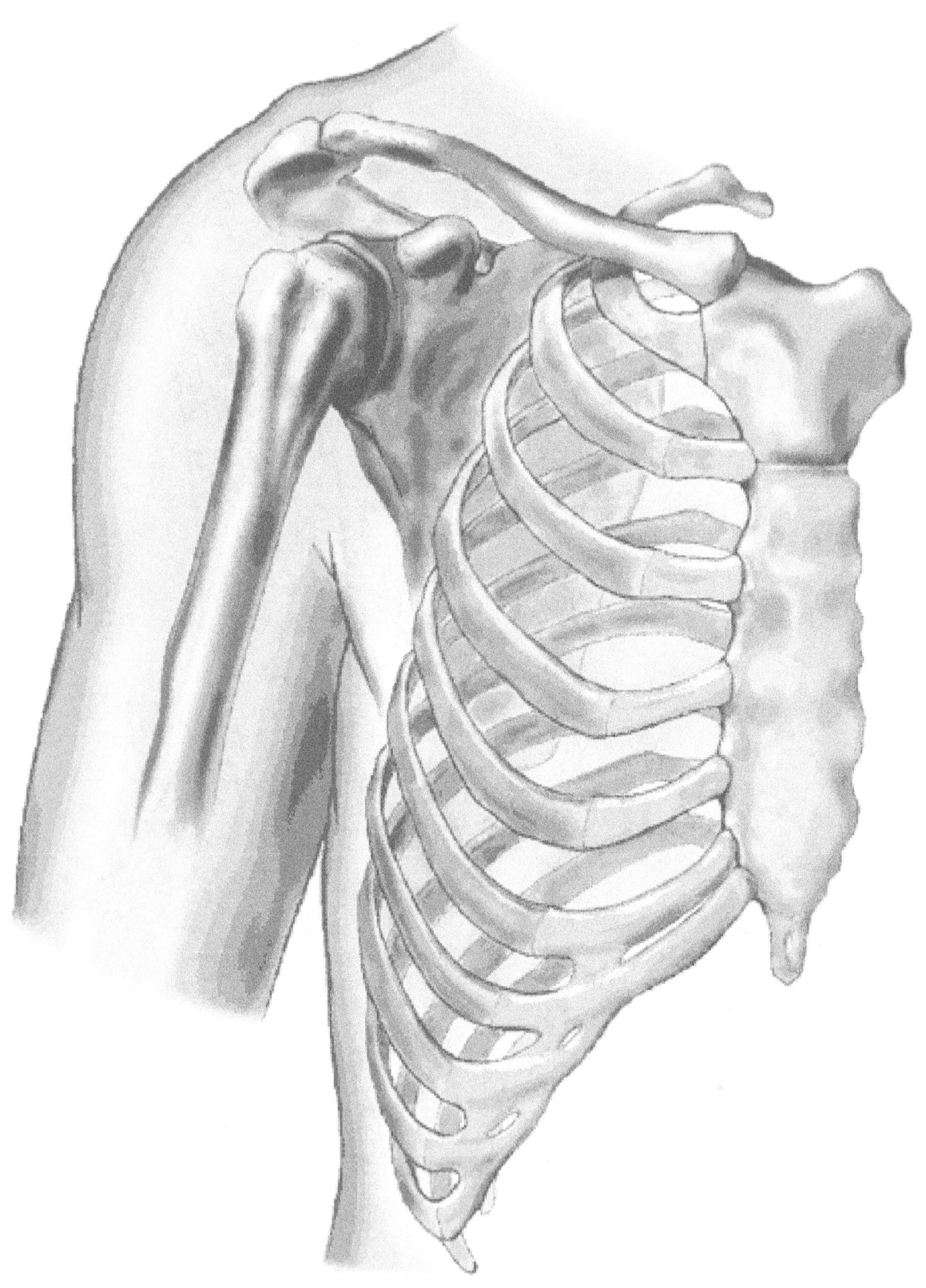

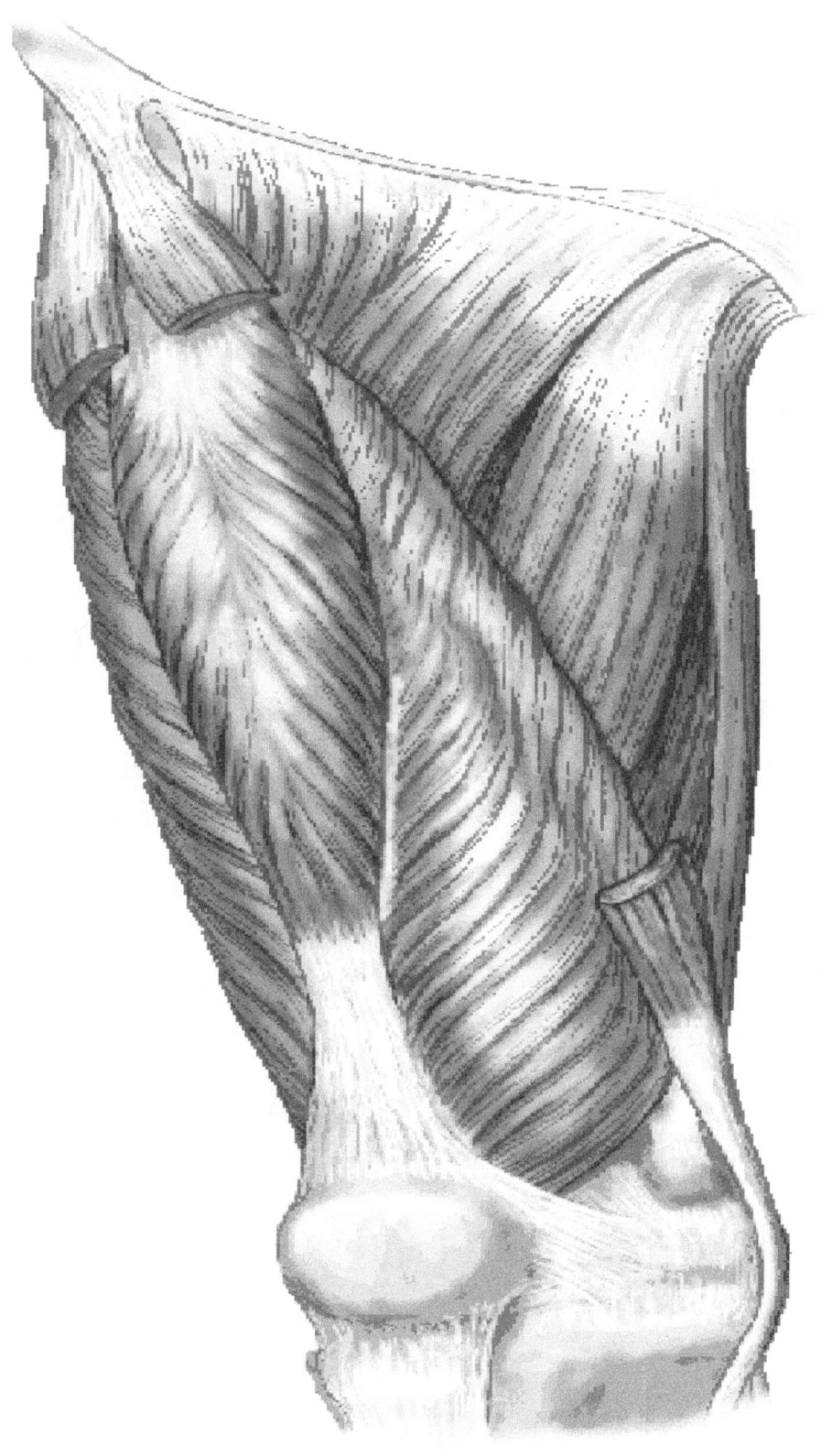

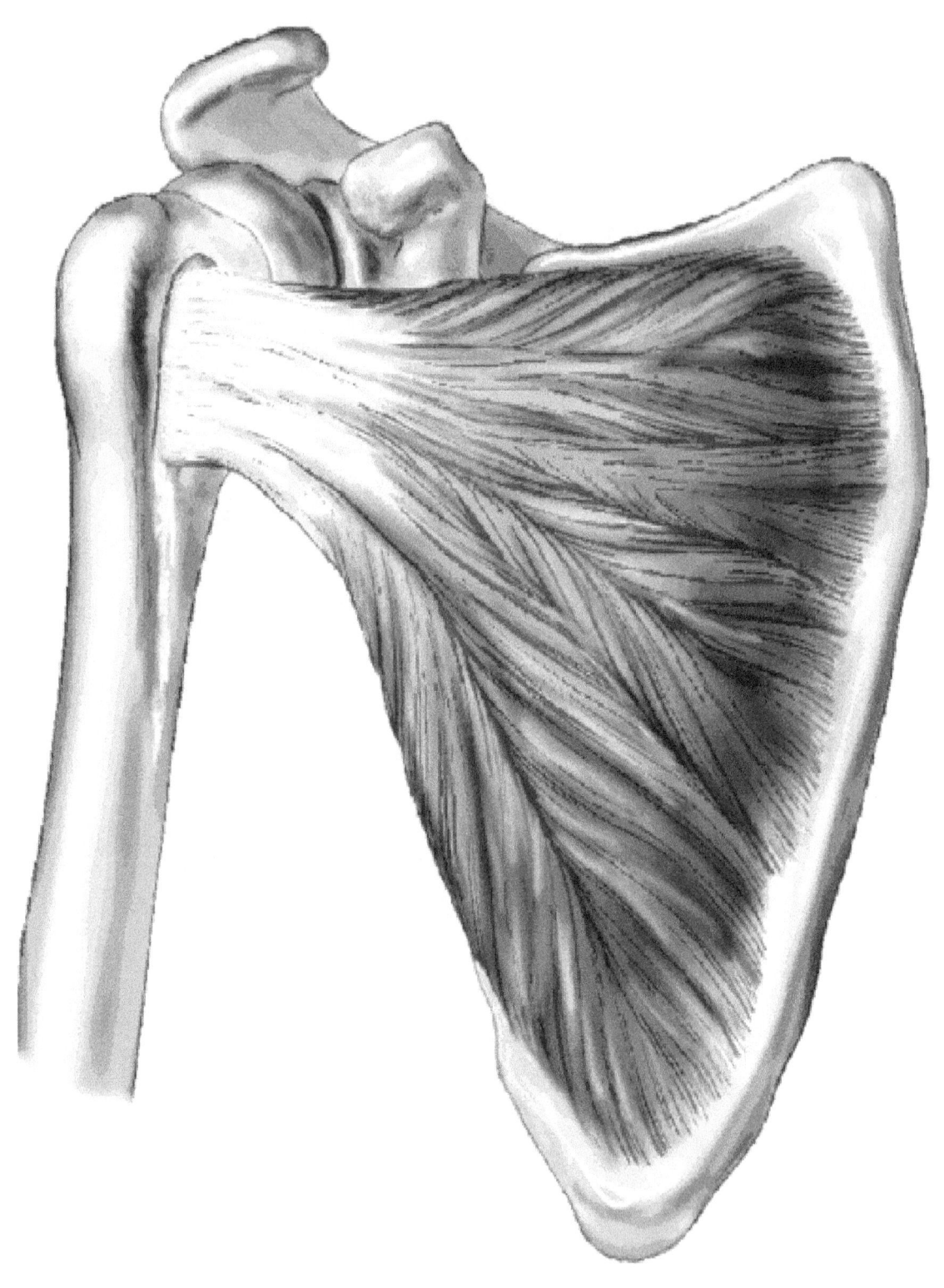

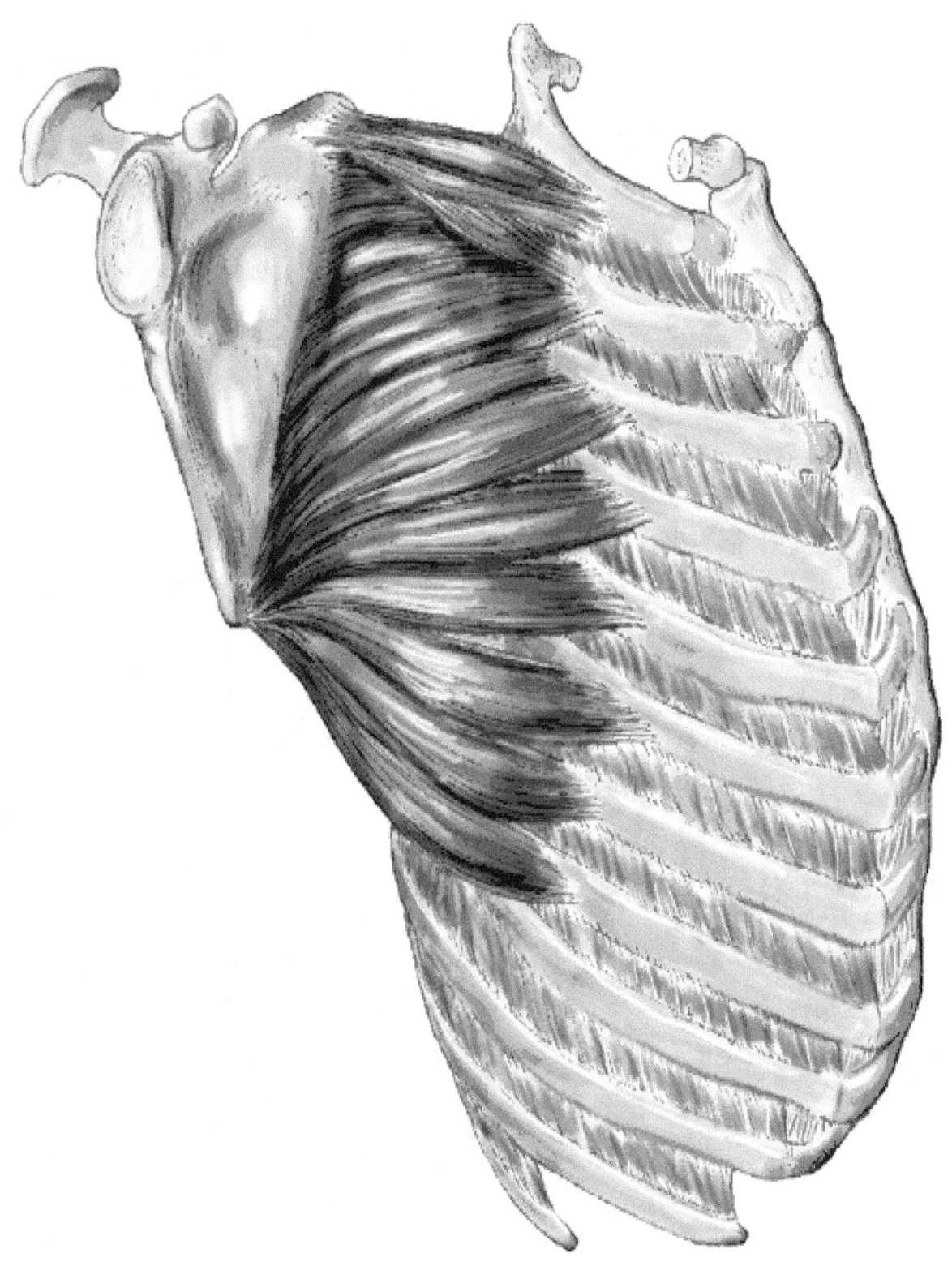

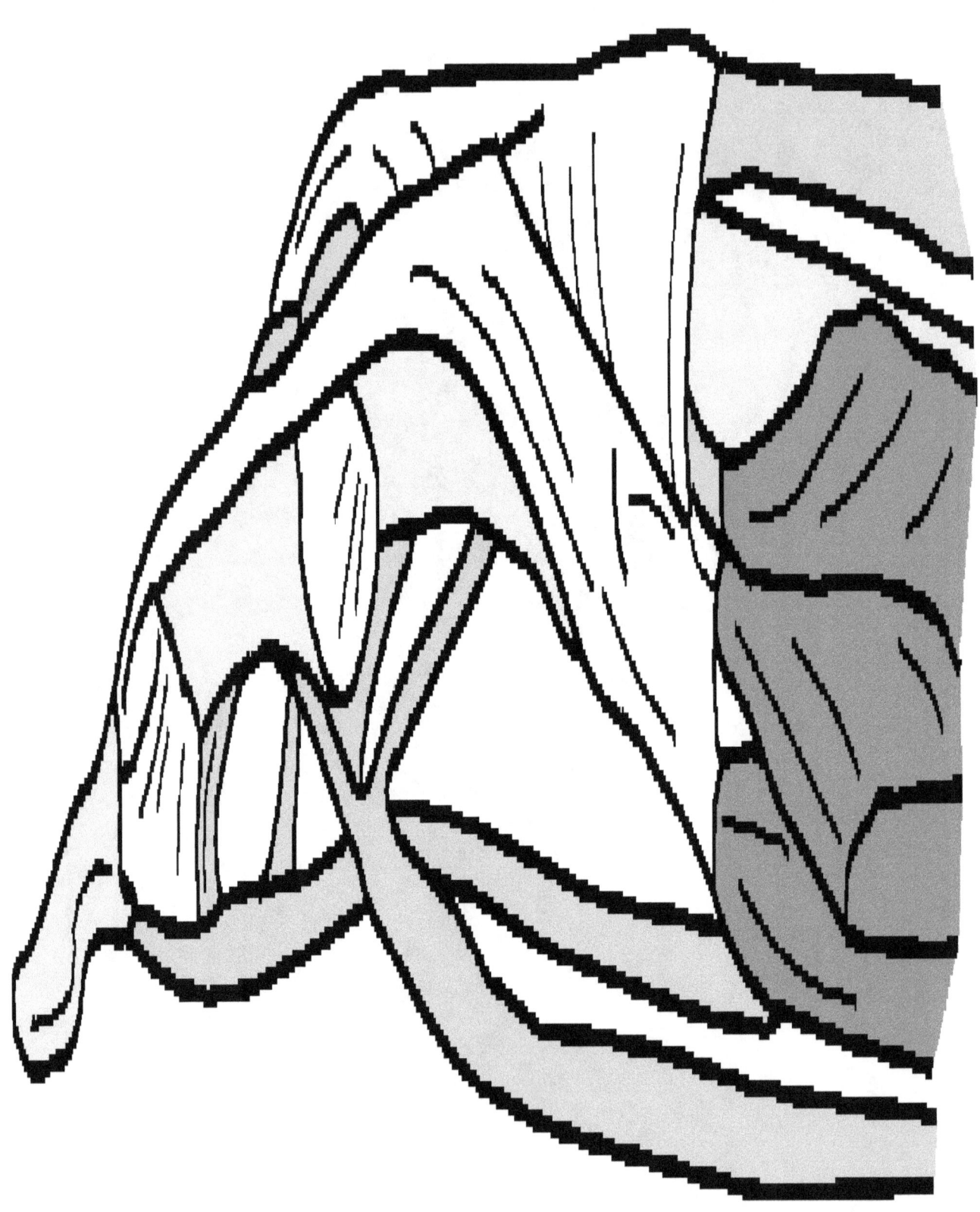

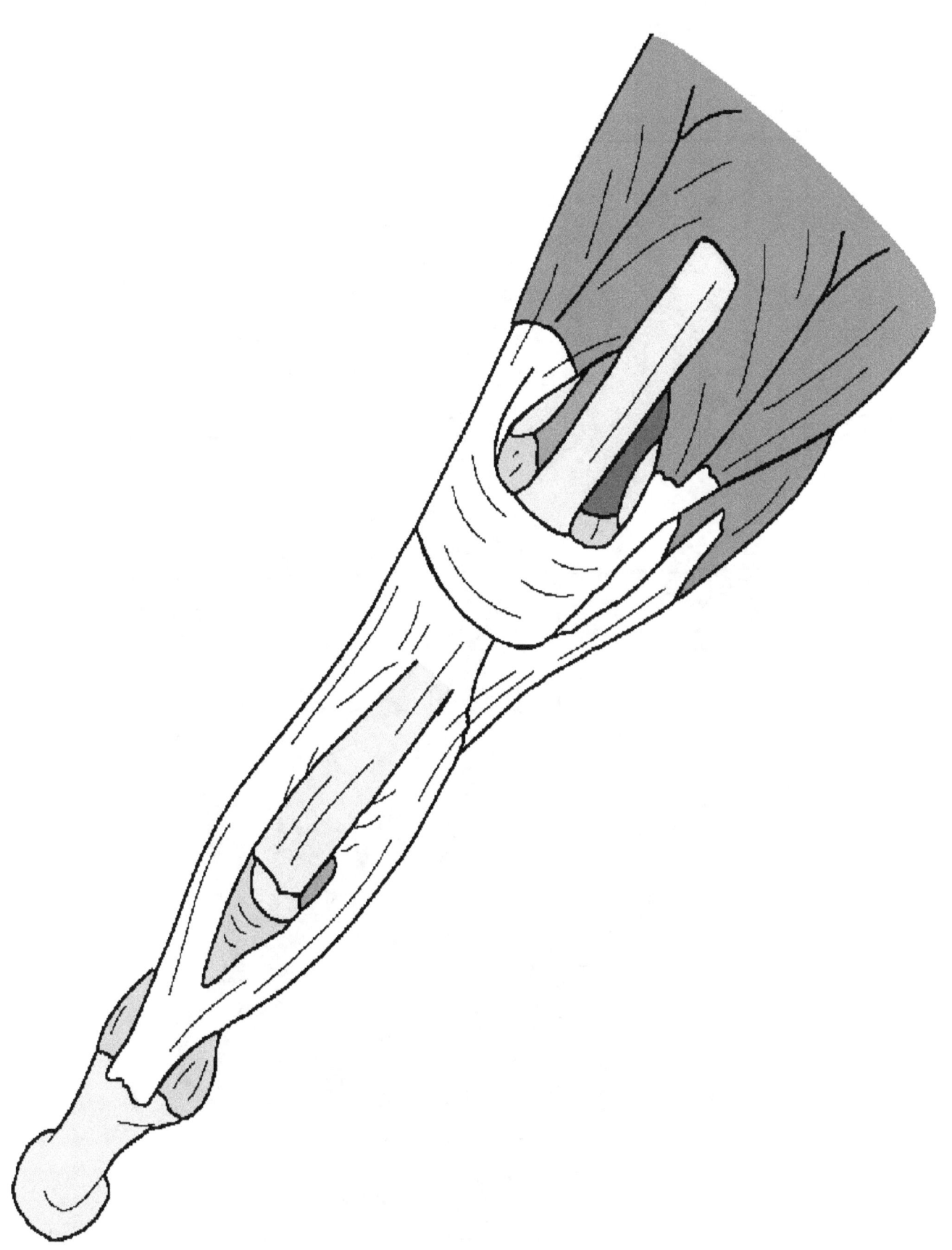

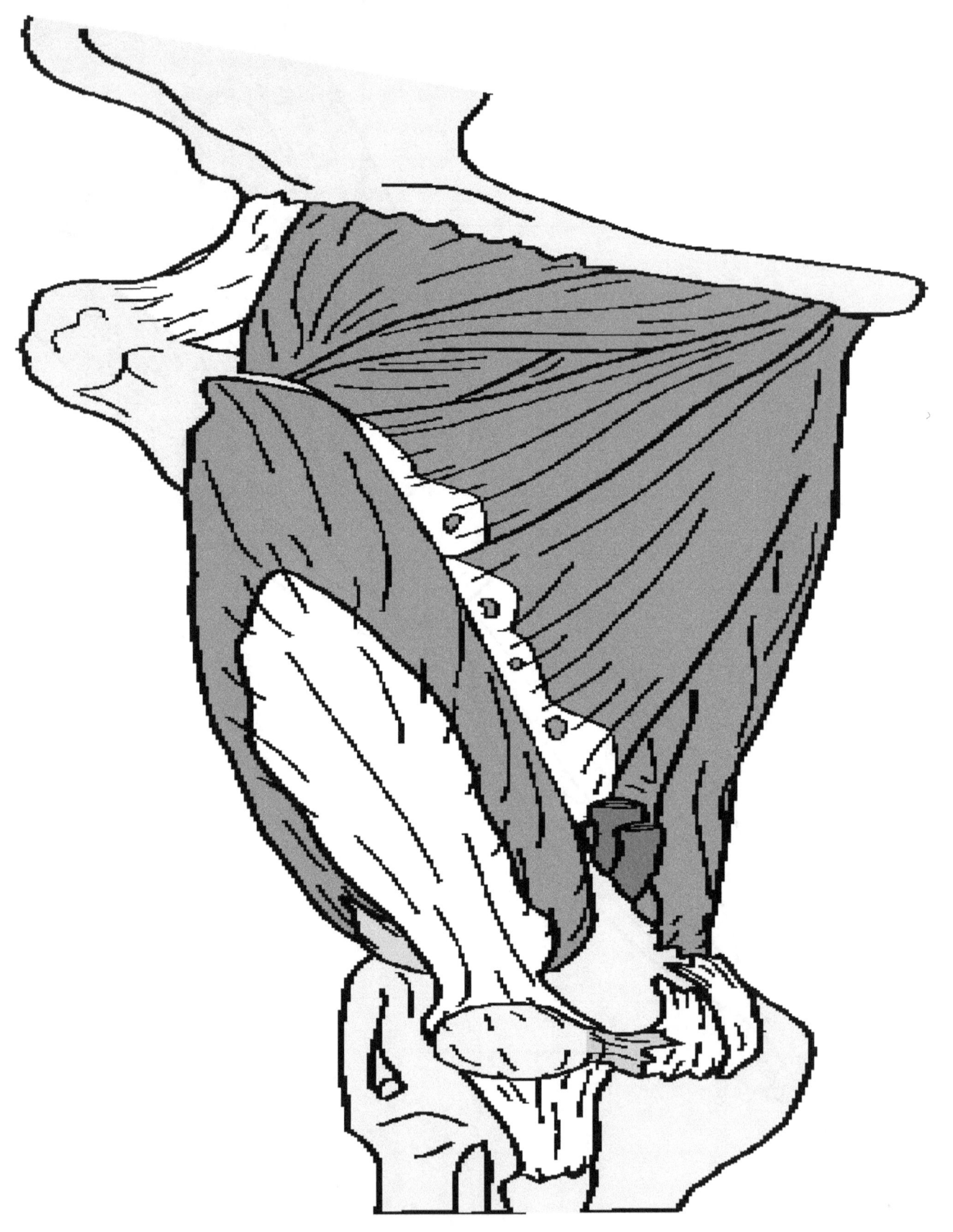

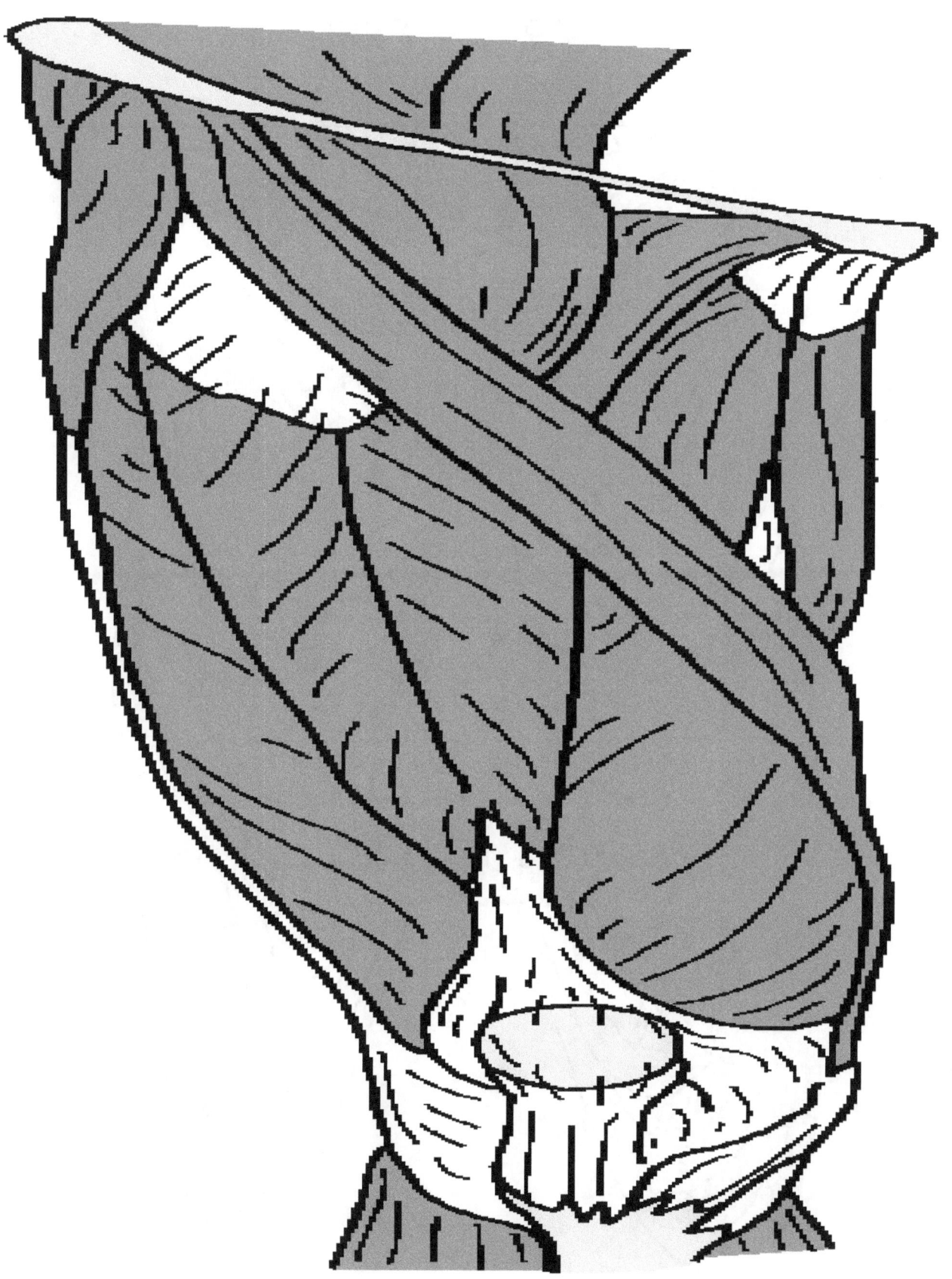

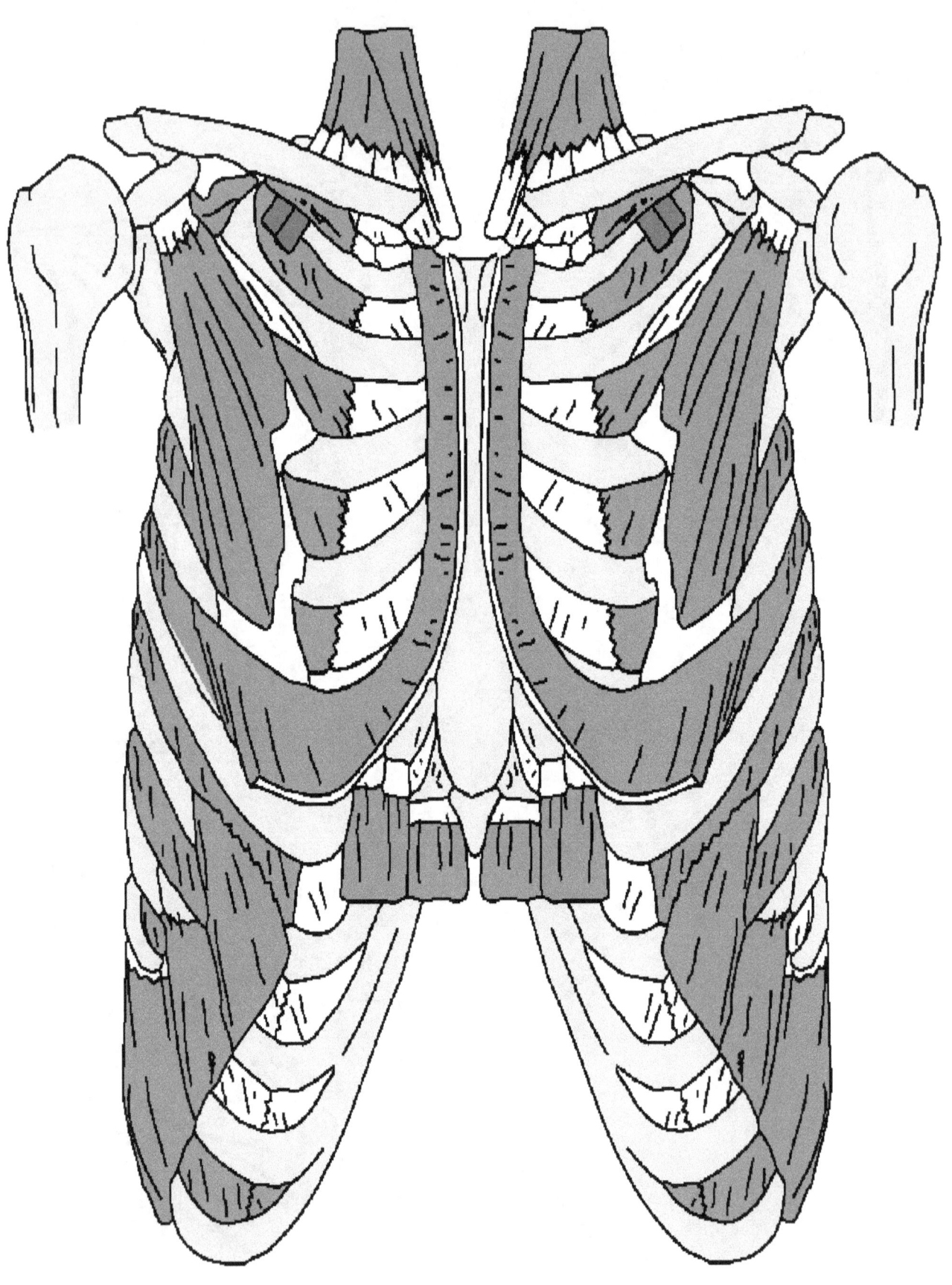

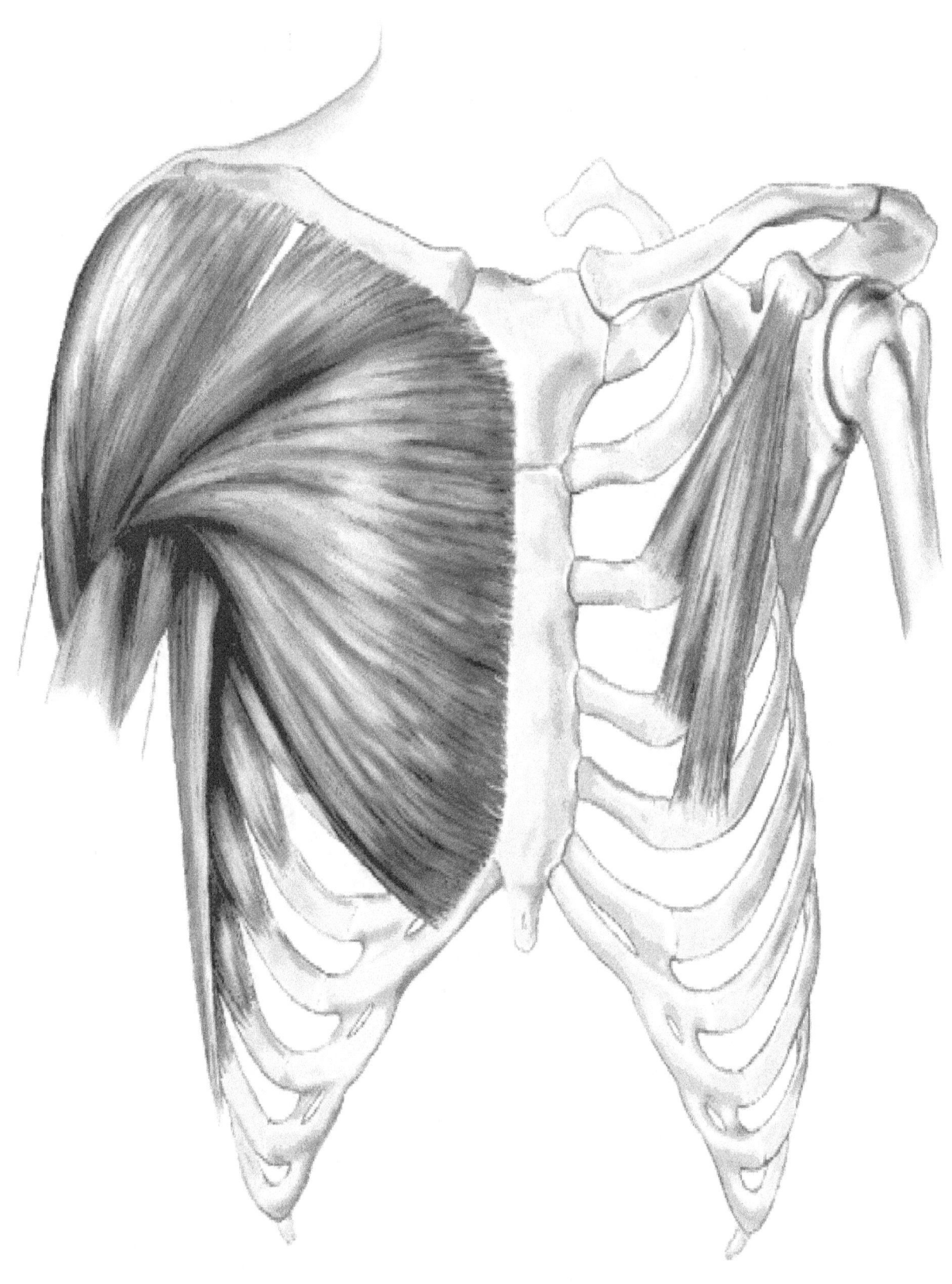

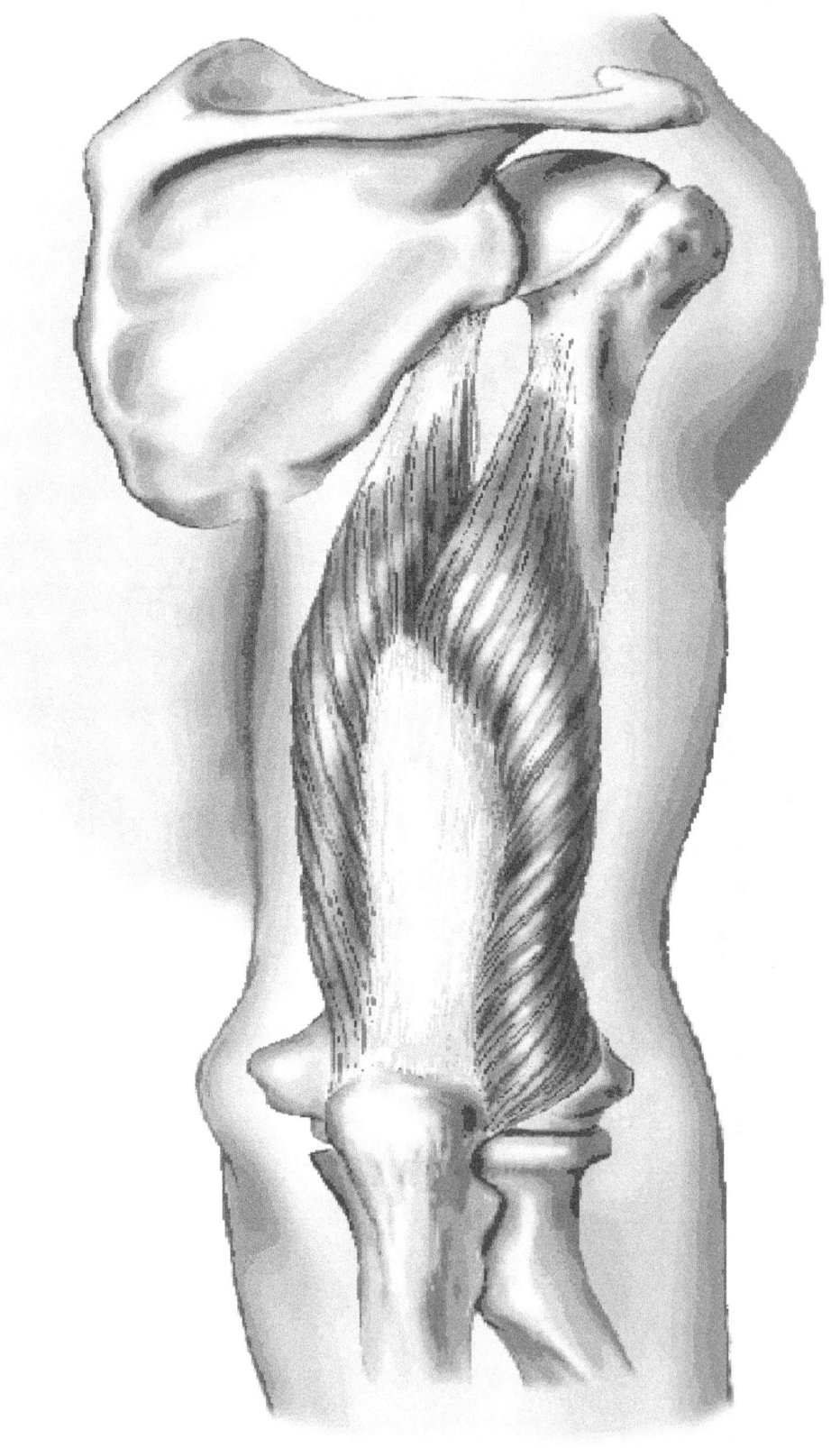

SKELETAL SYSTEM - PAGE 72 - 161

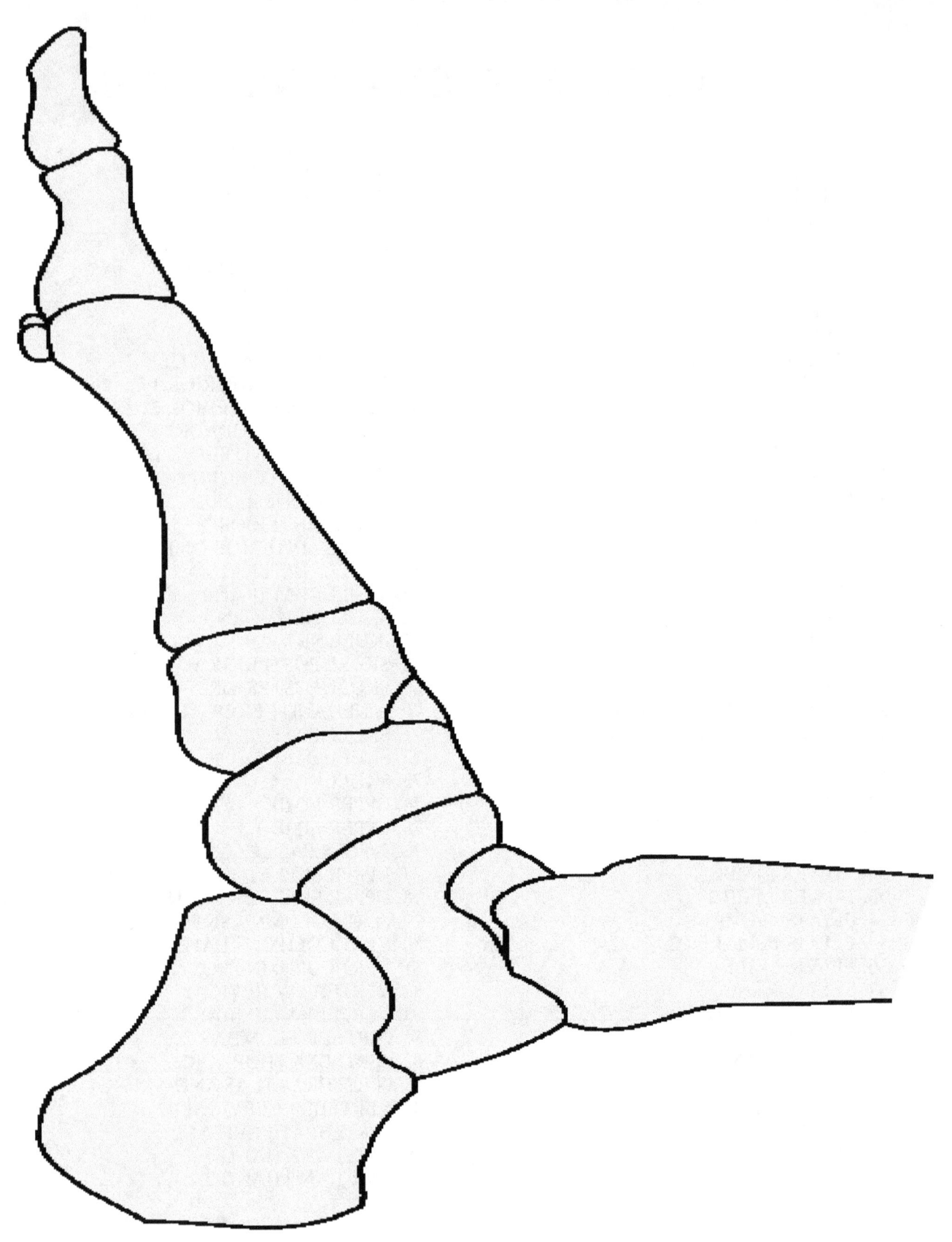

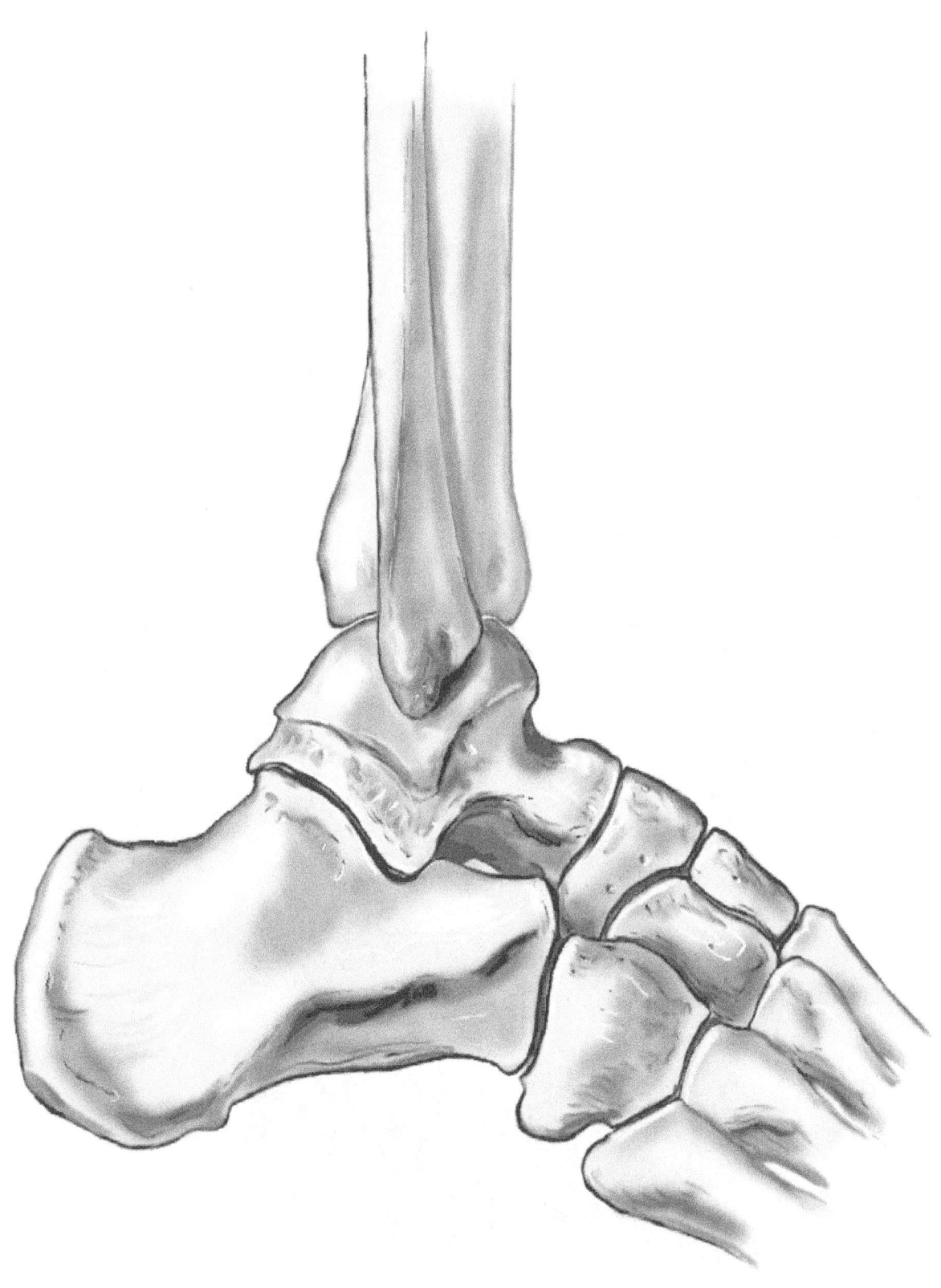

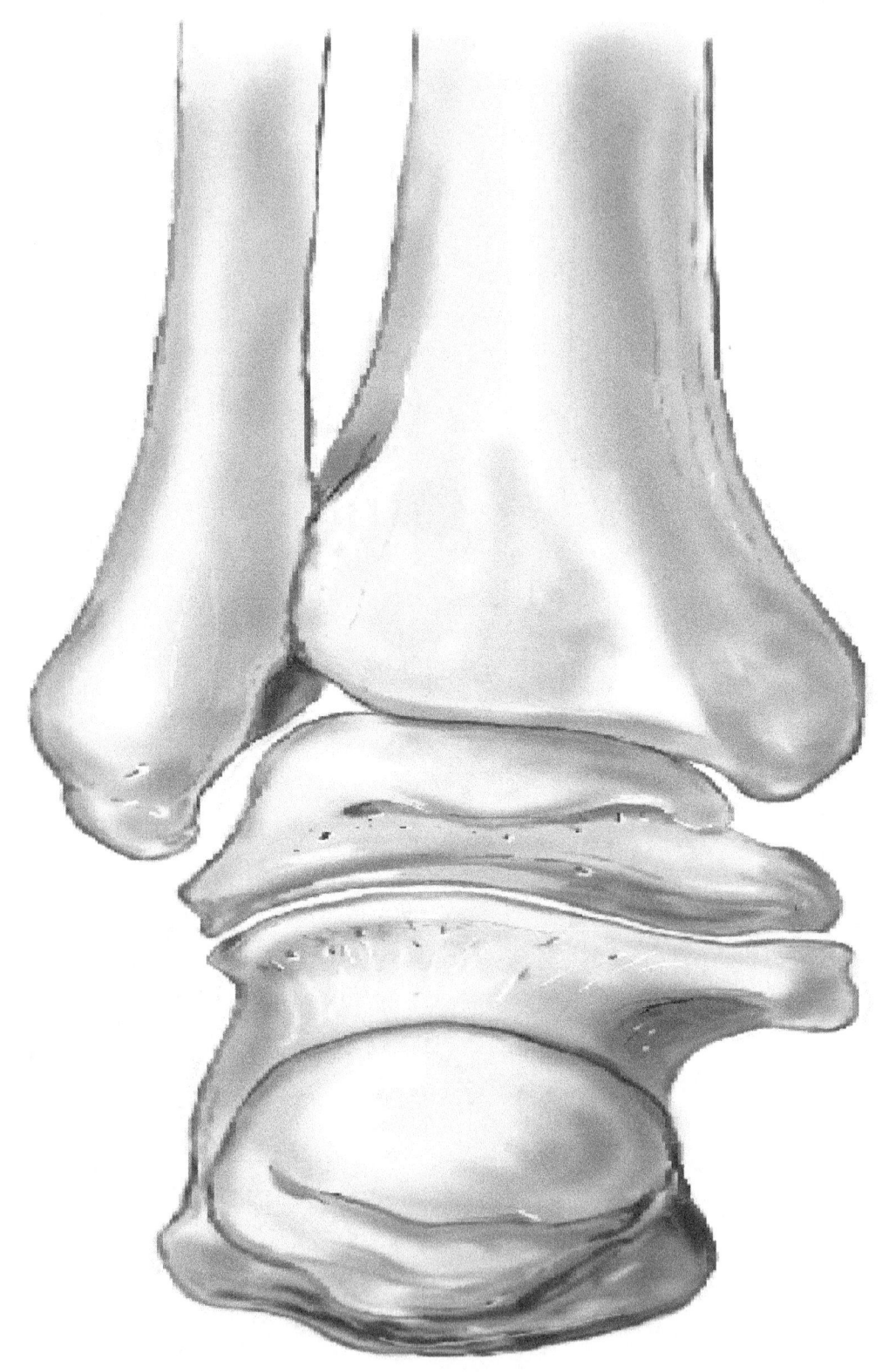

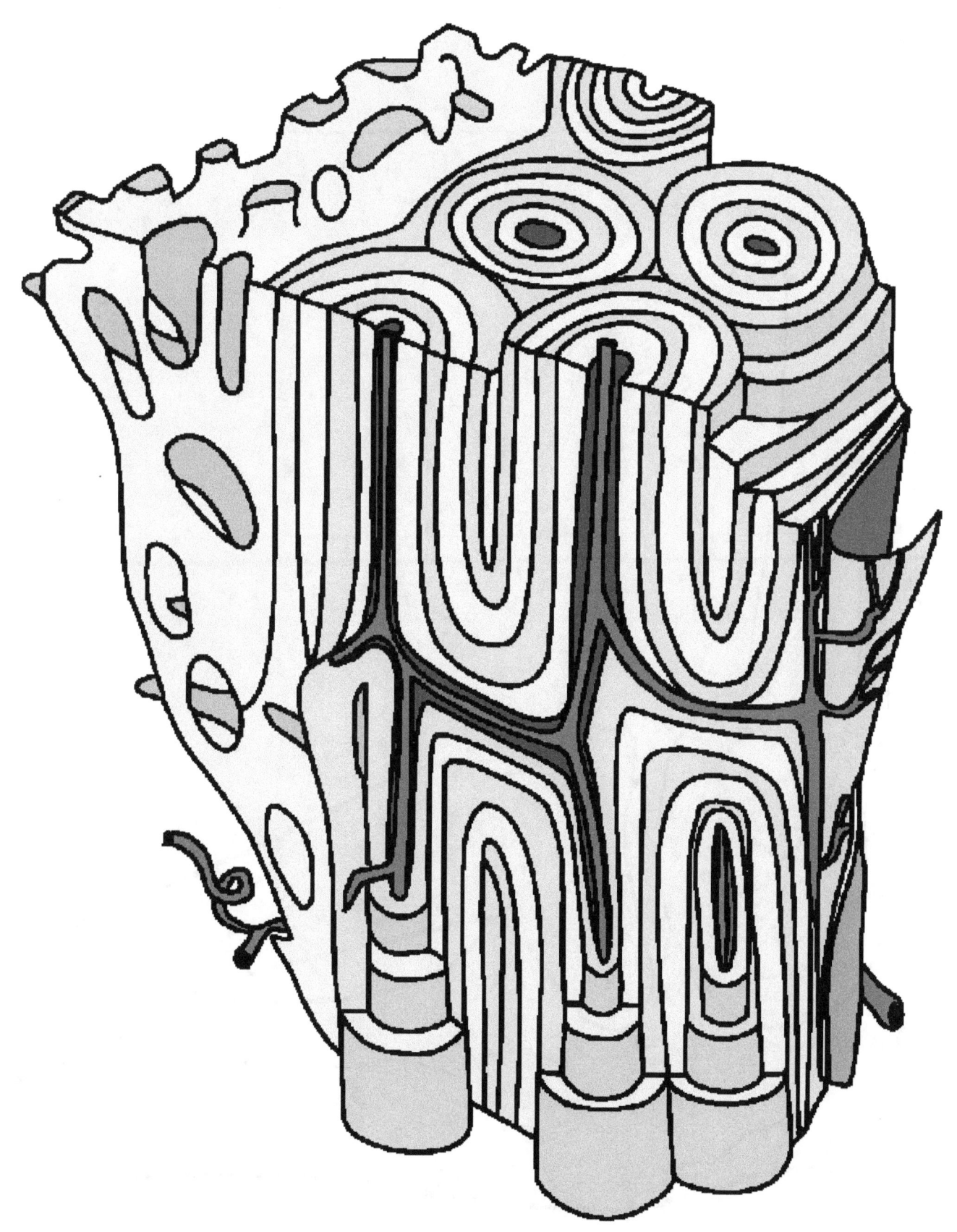

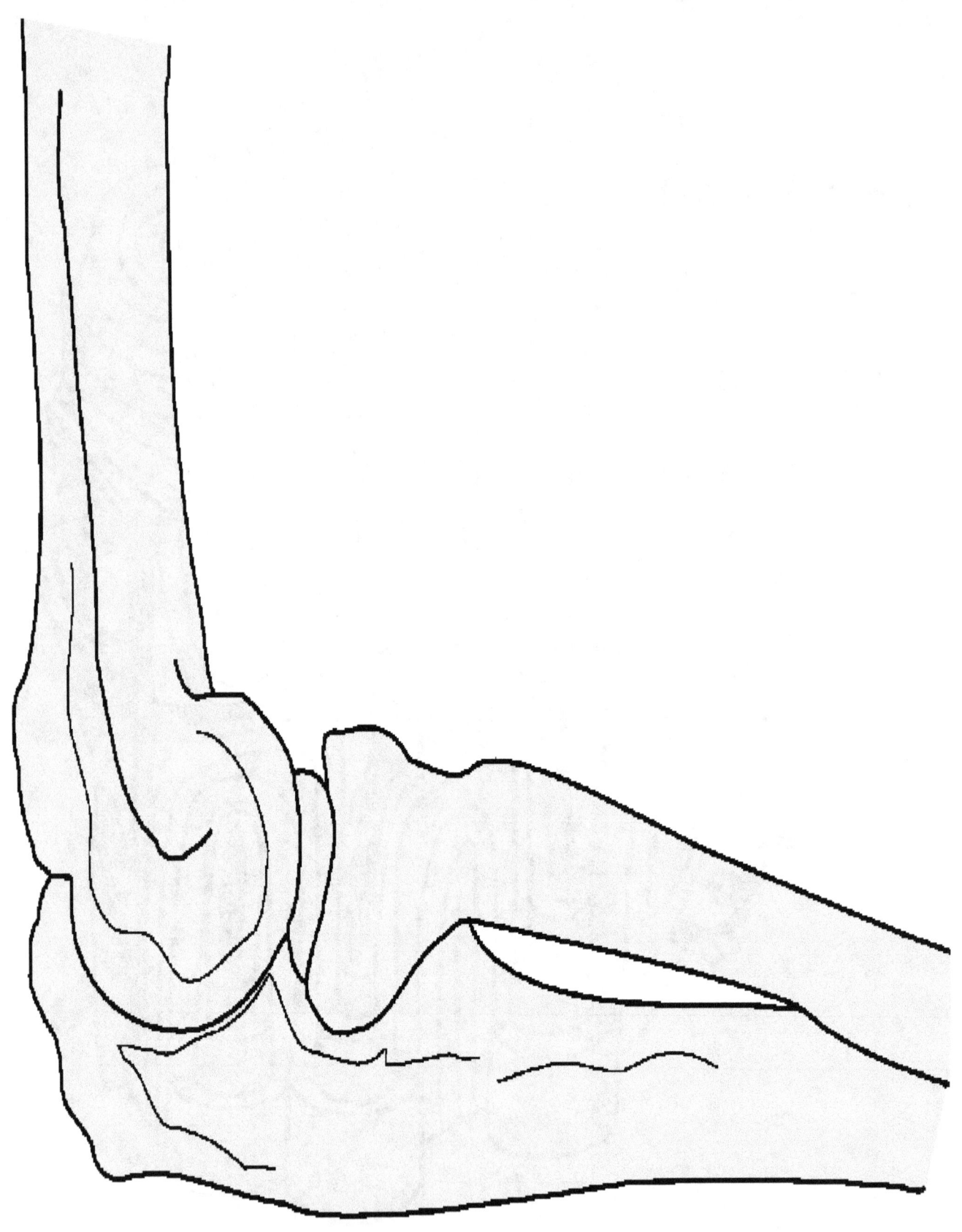

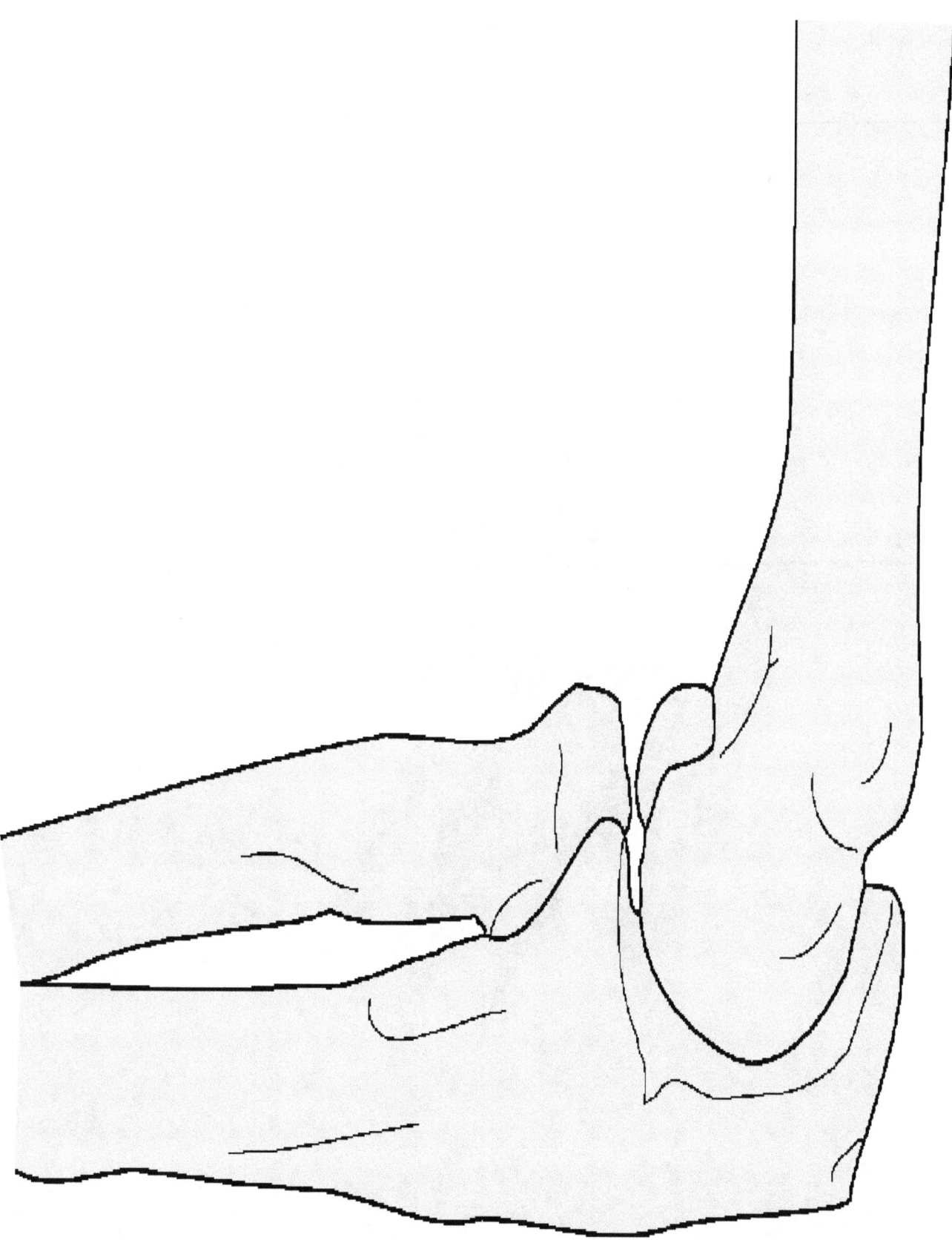

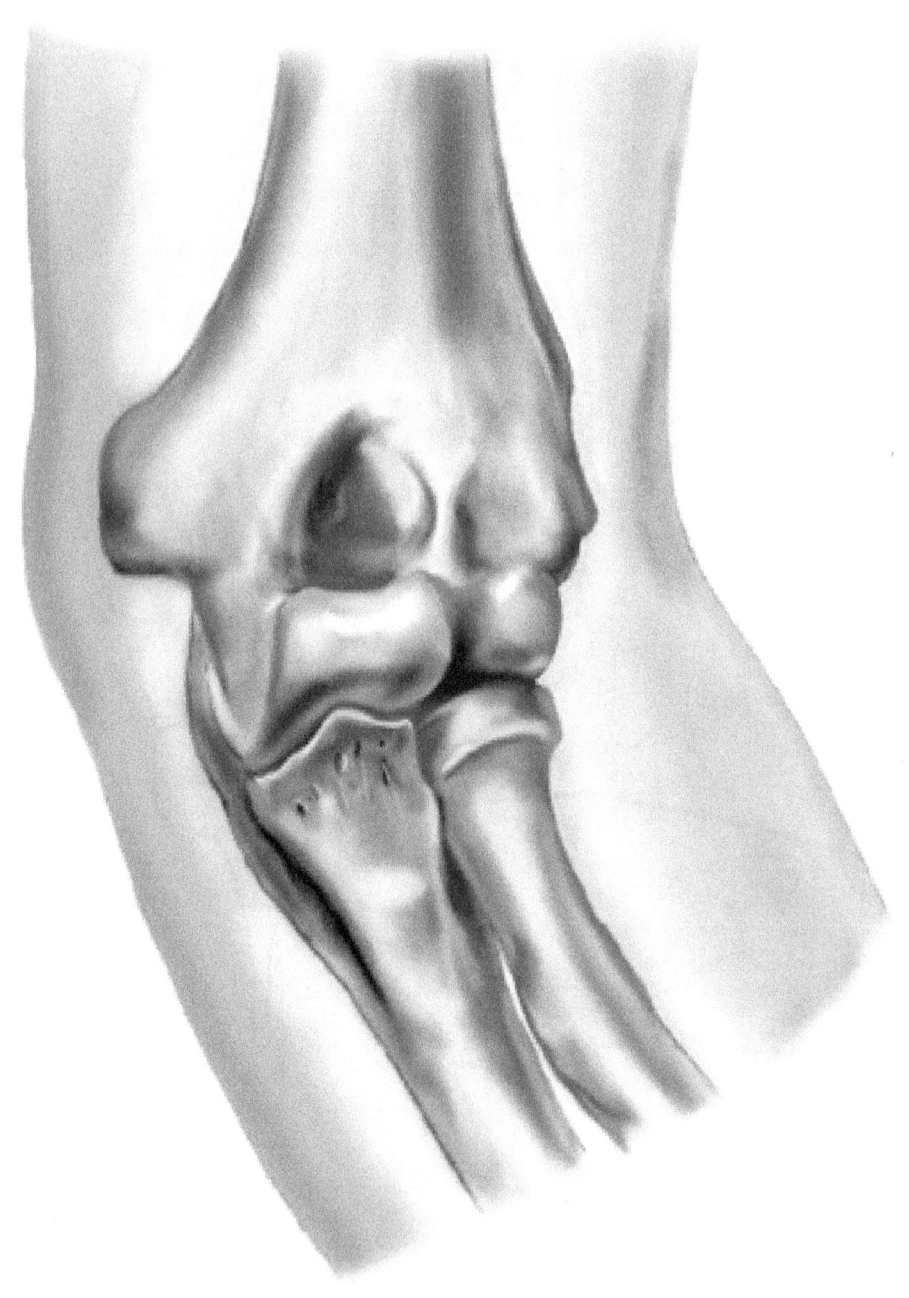

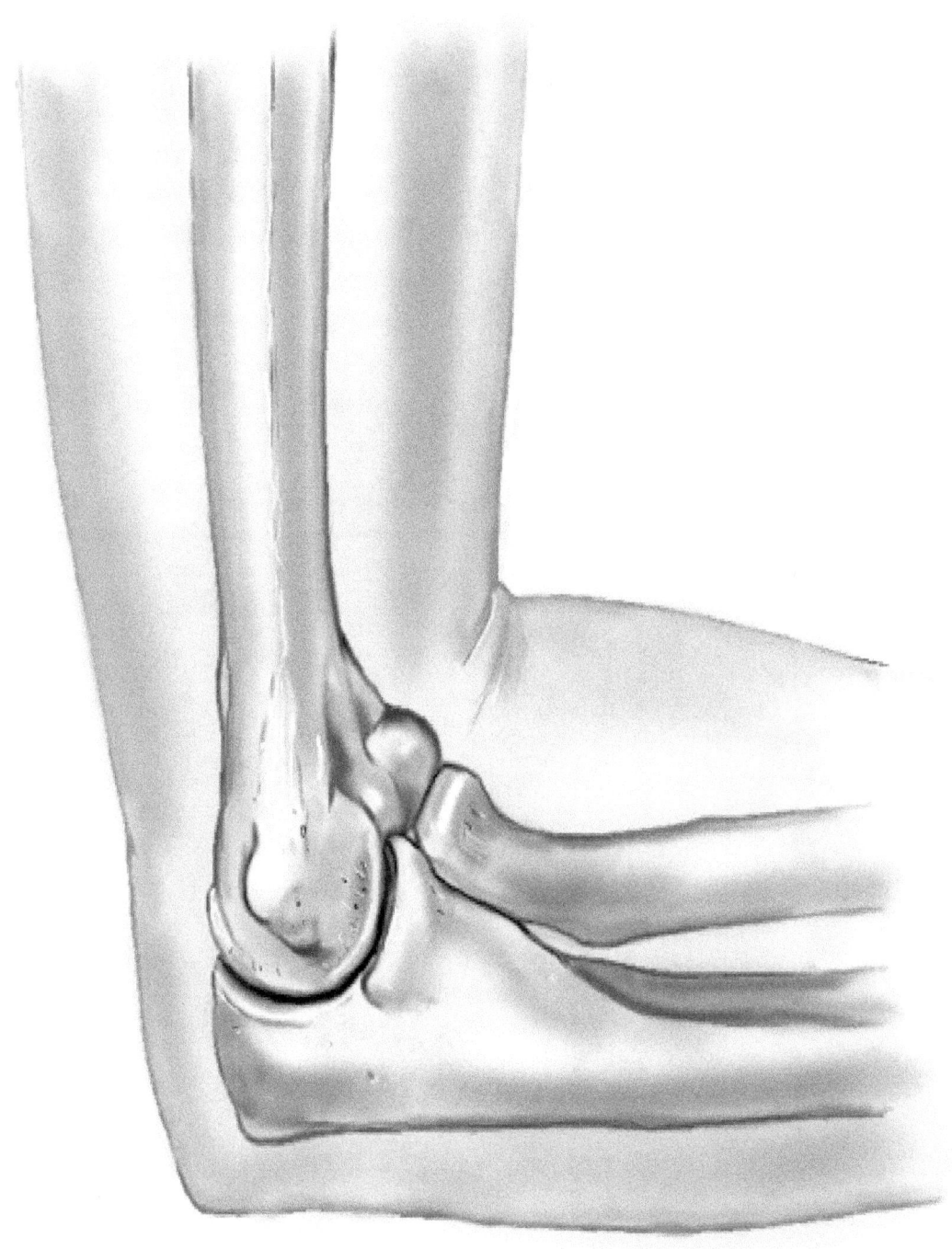

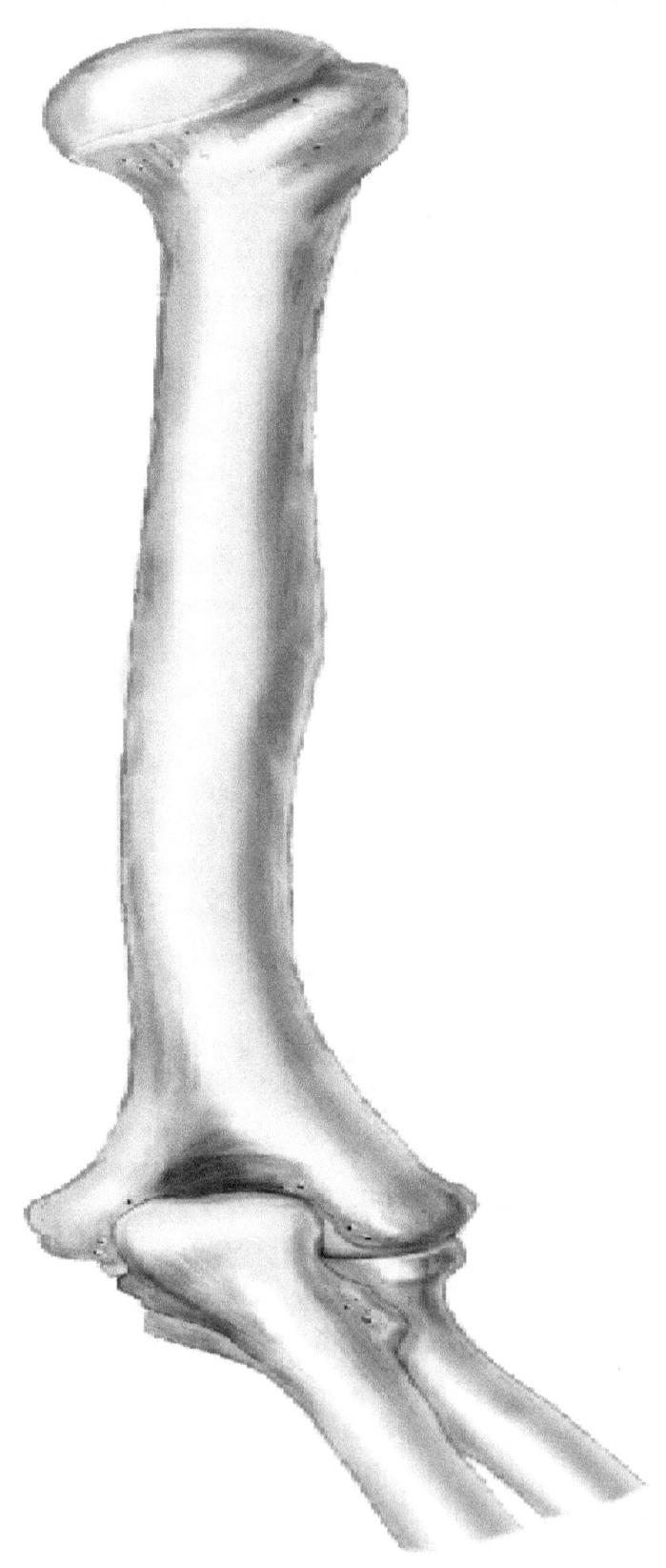

80

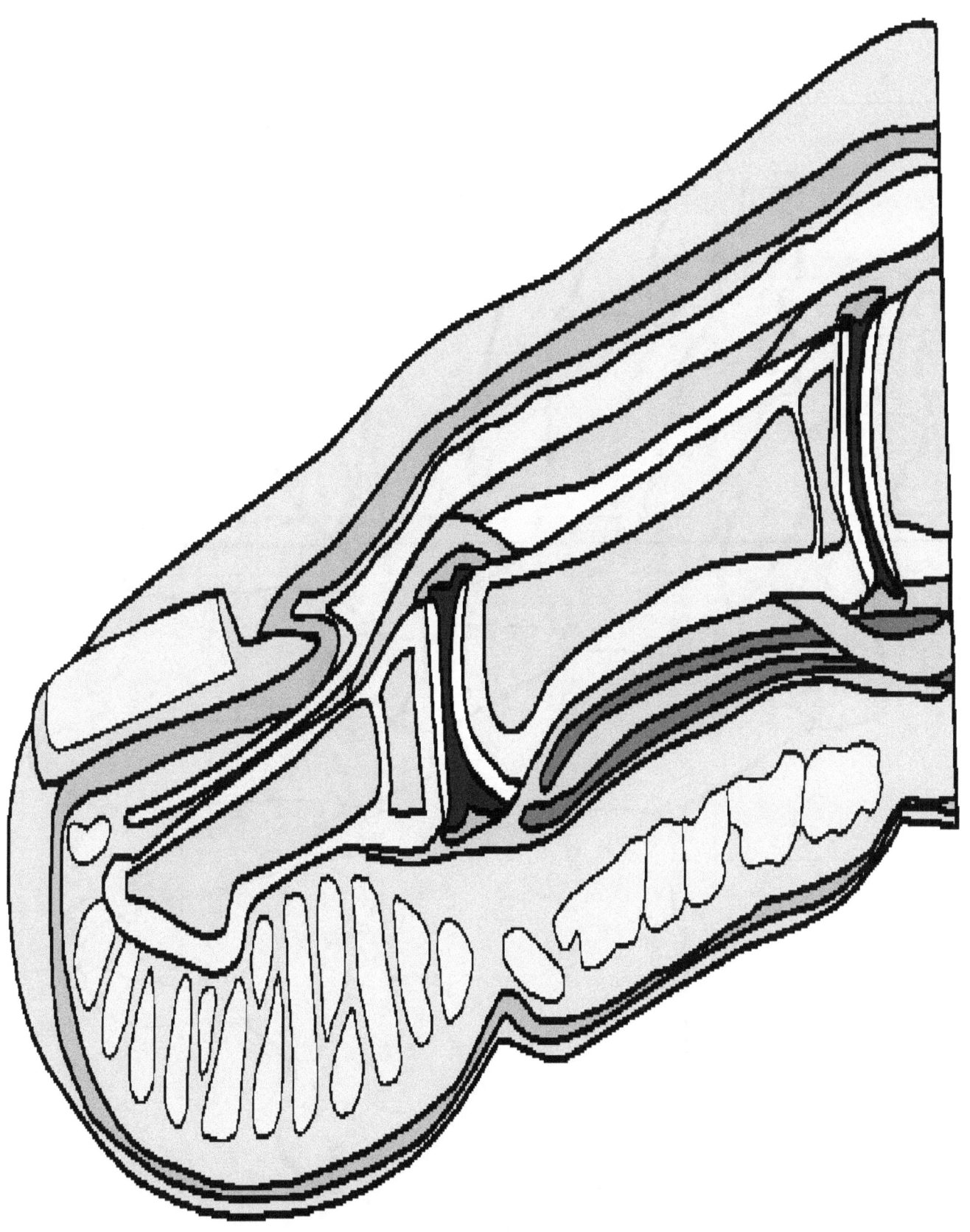

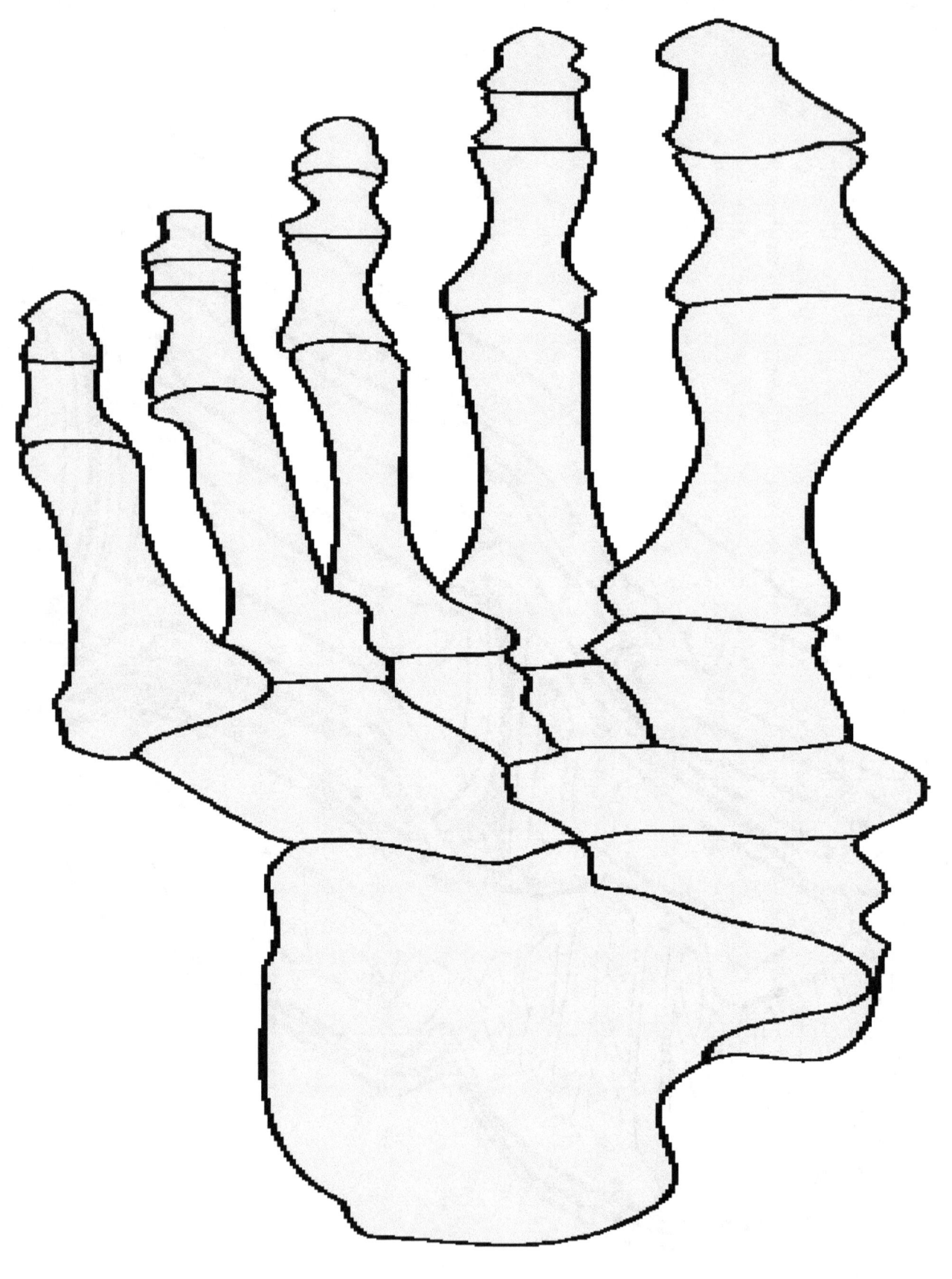

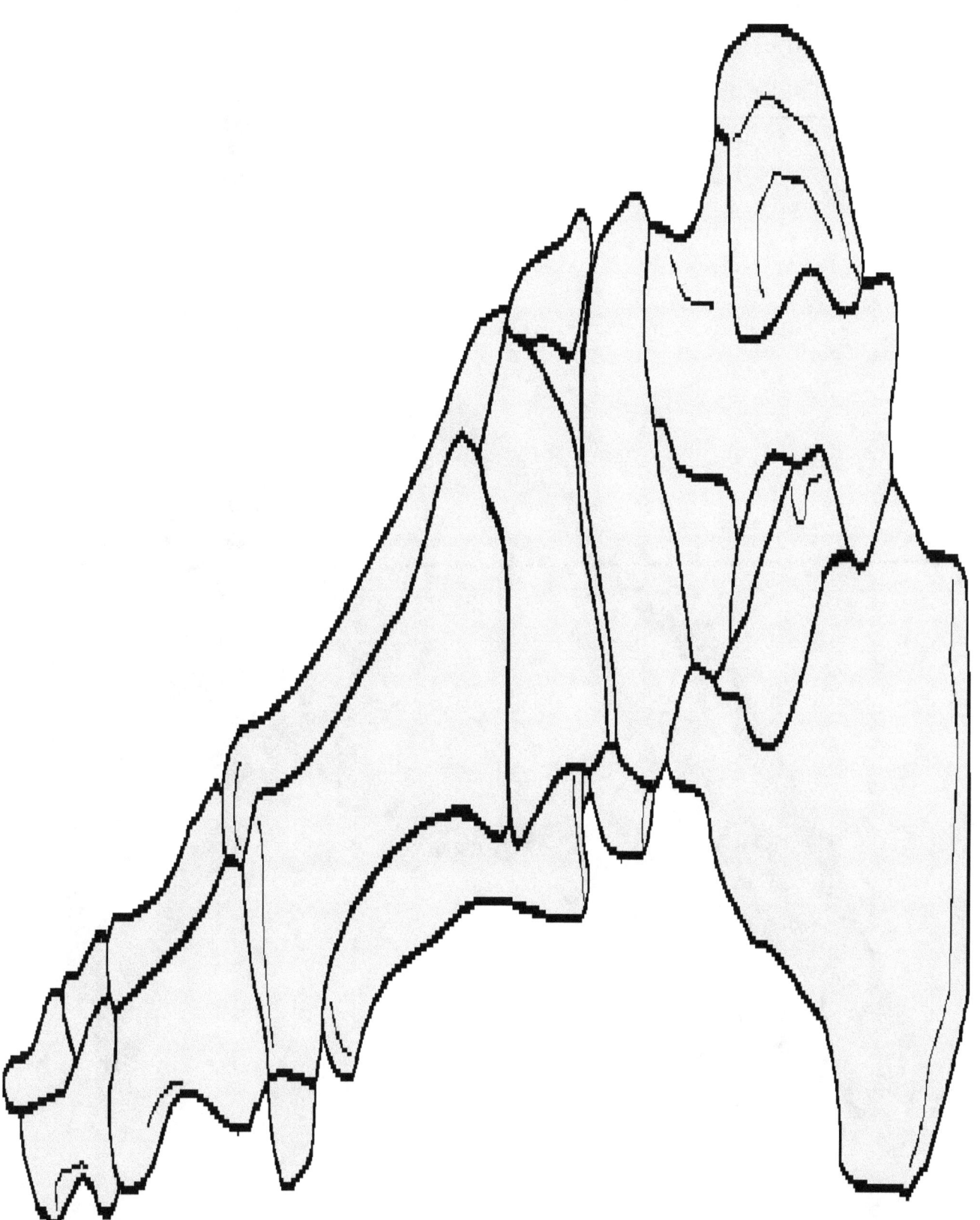

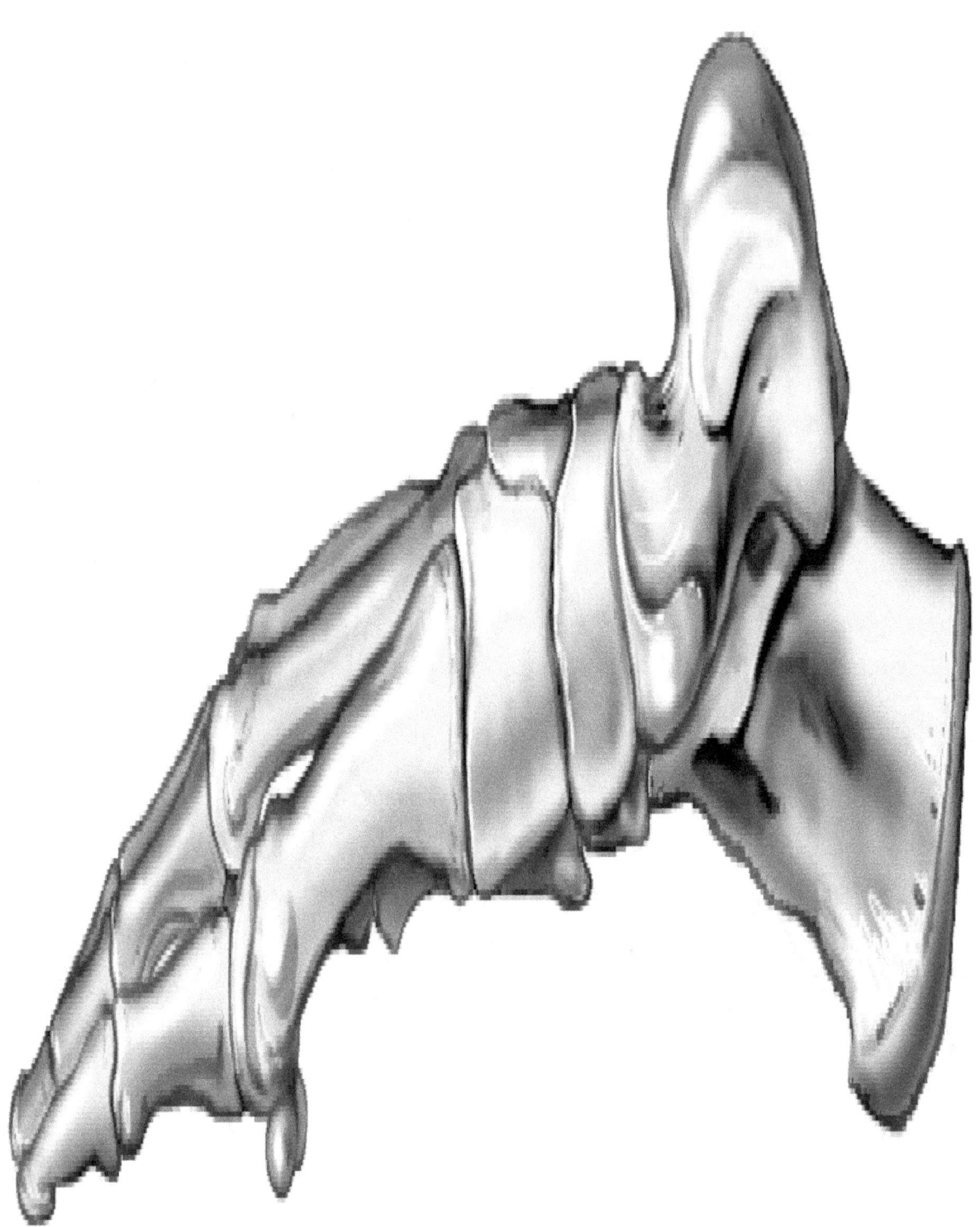

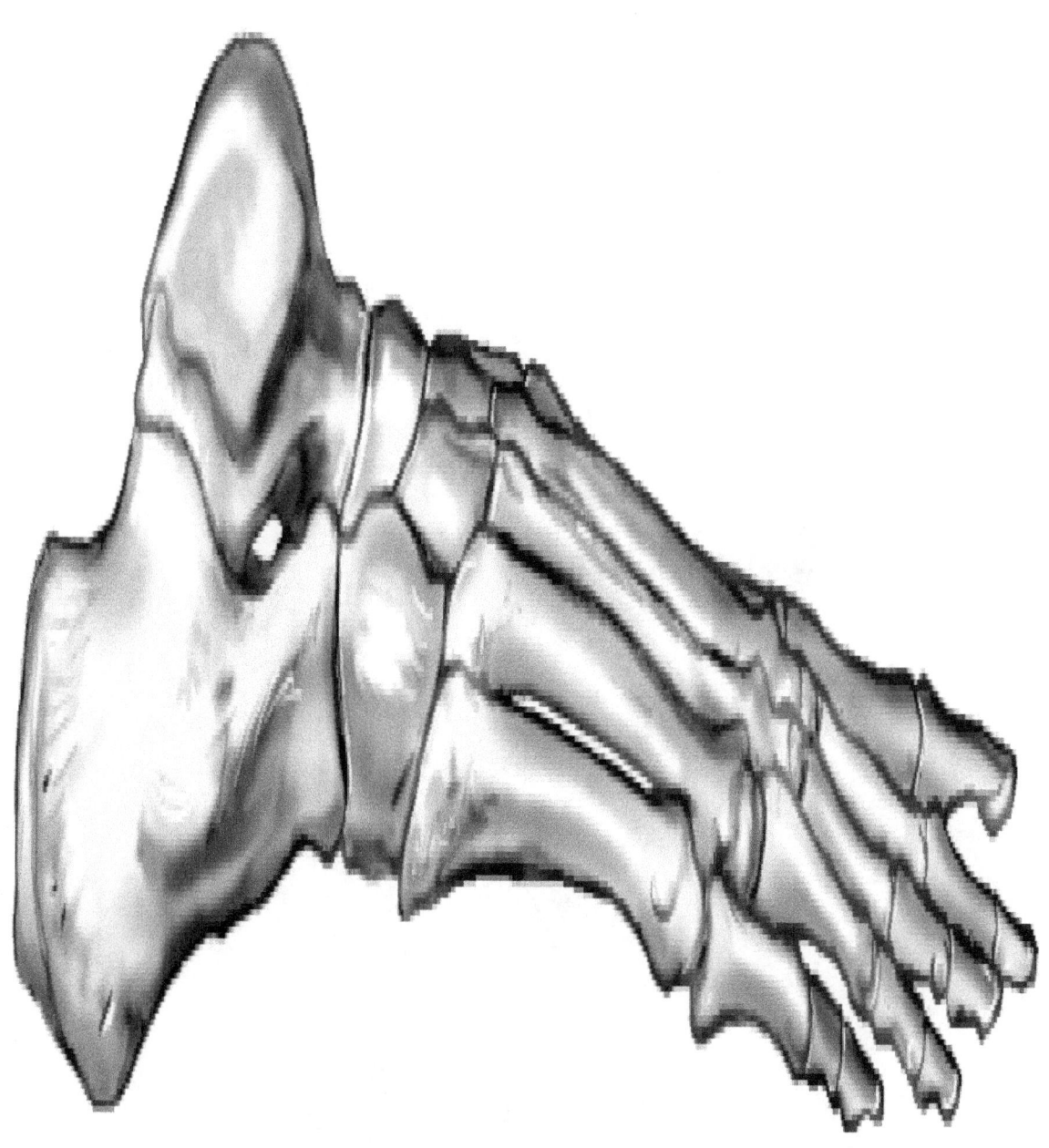

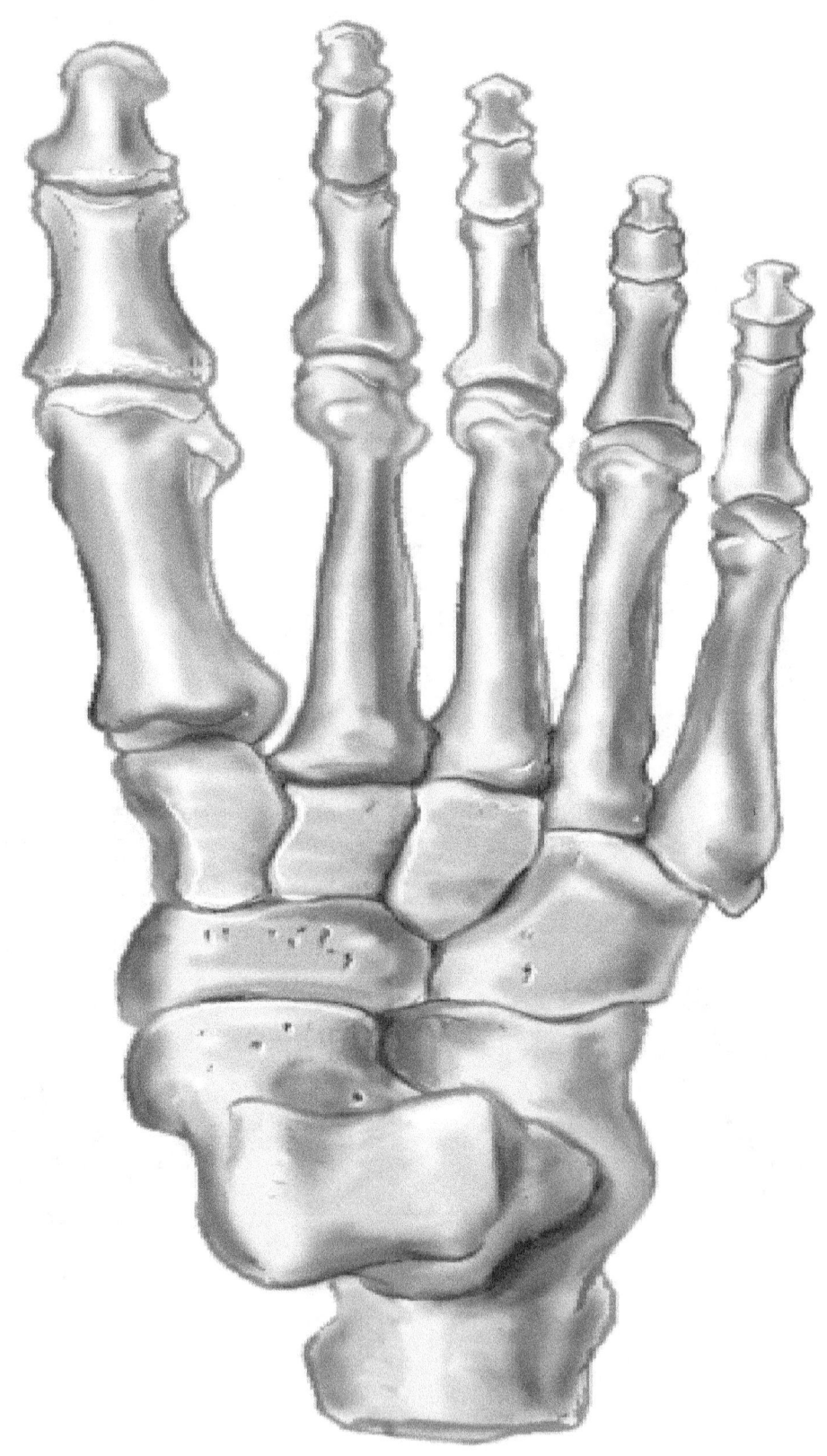

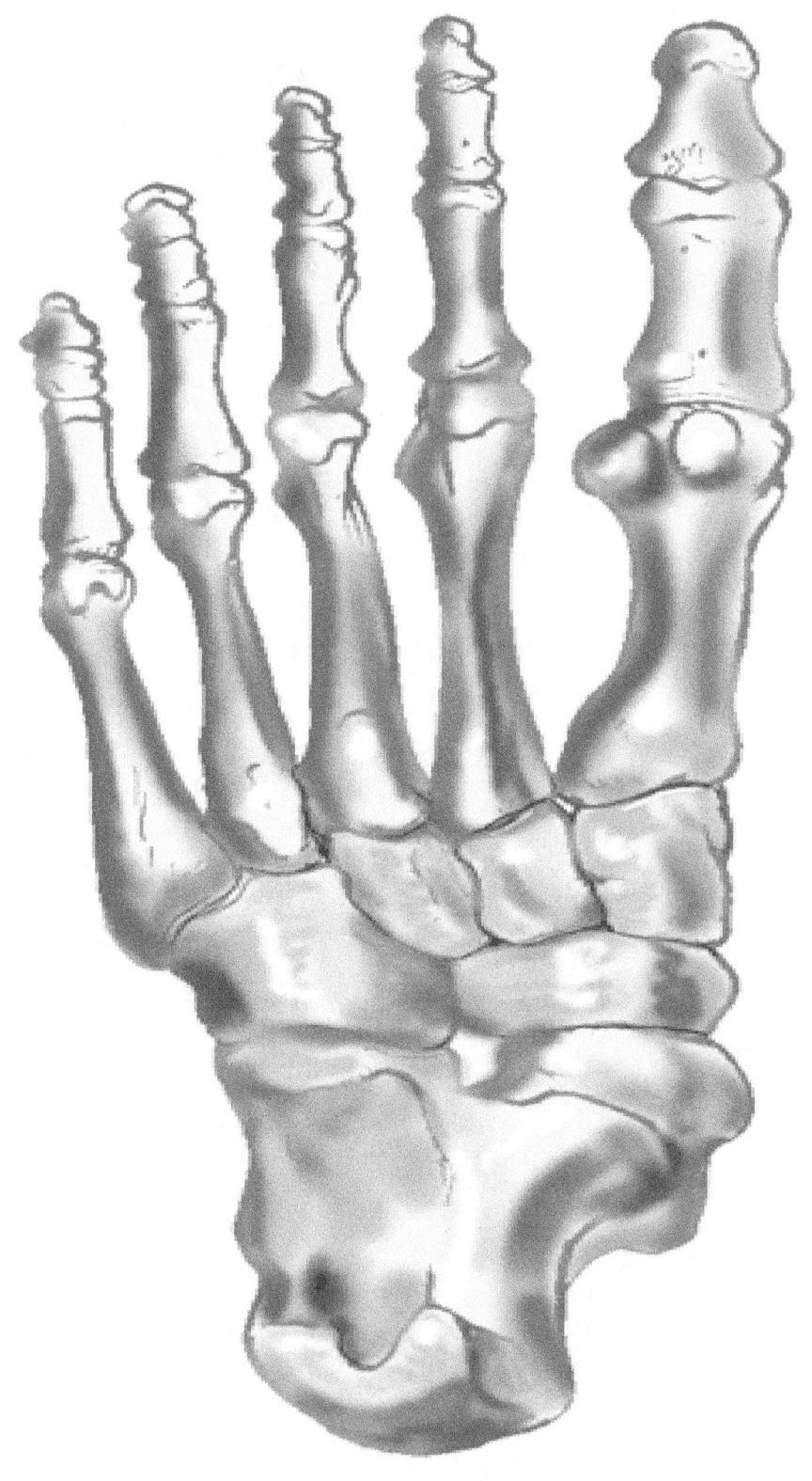

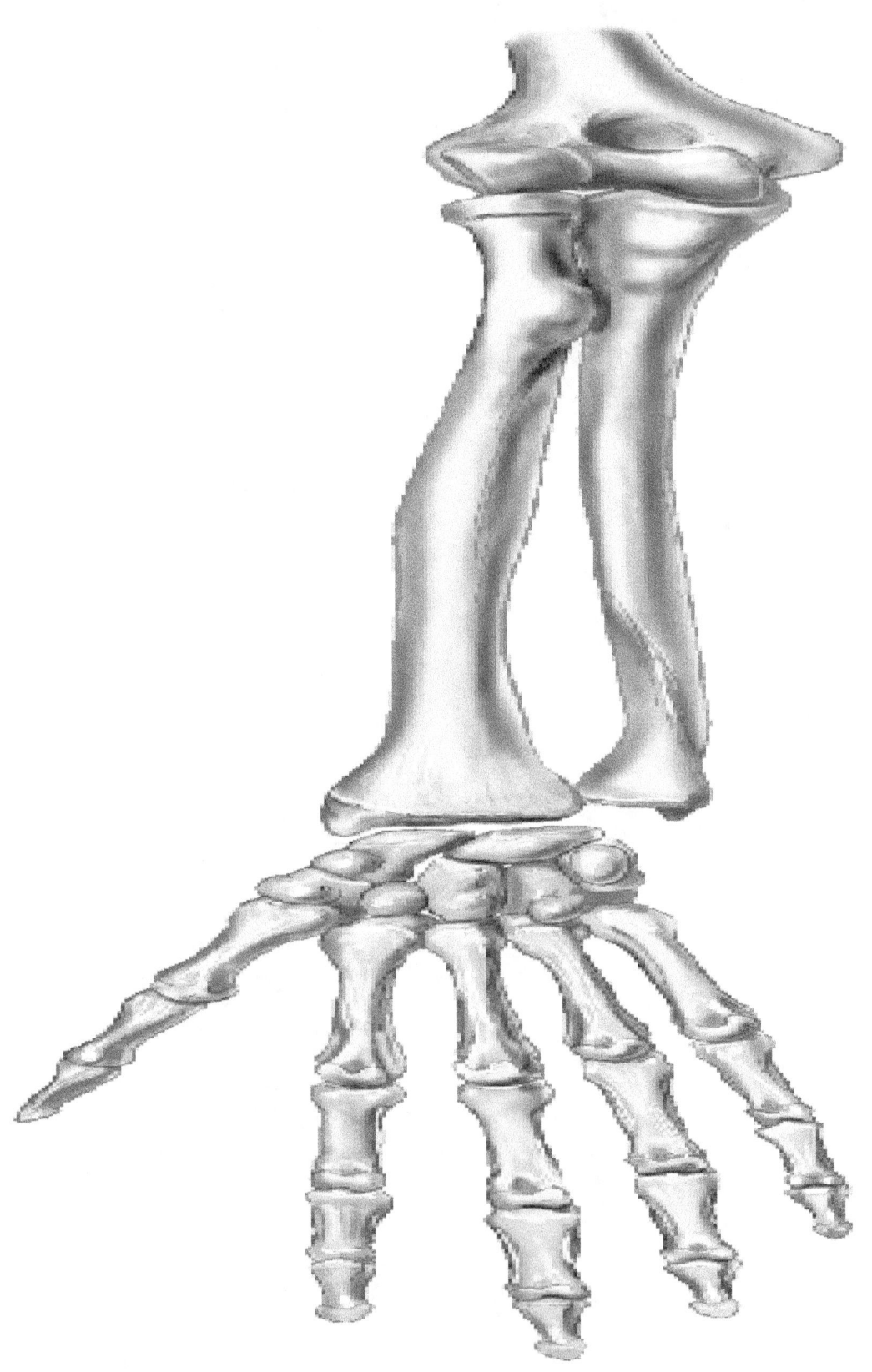

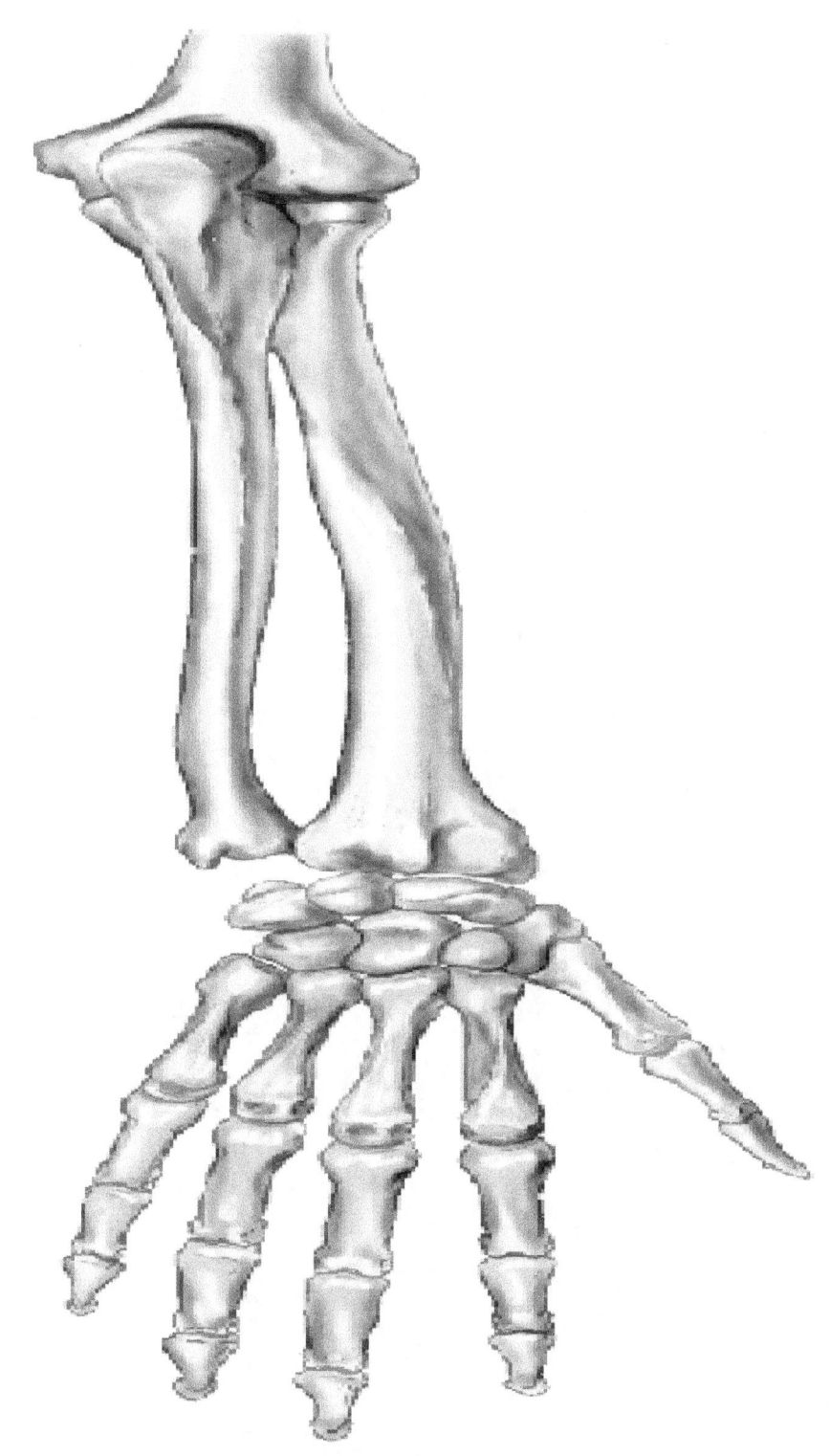

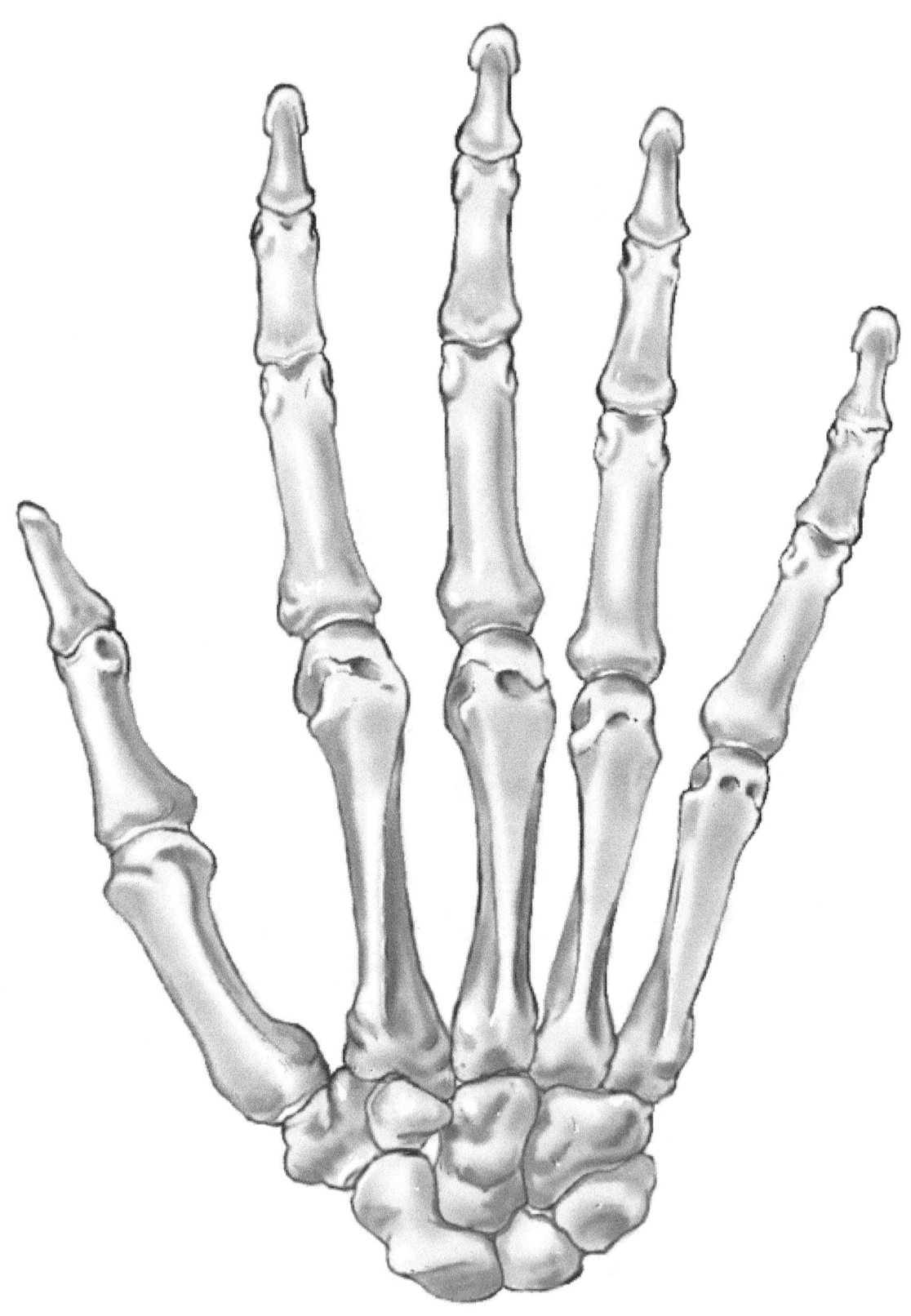

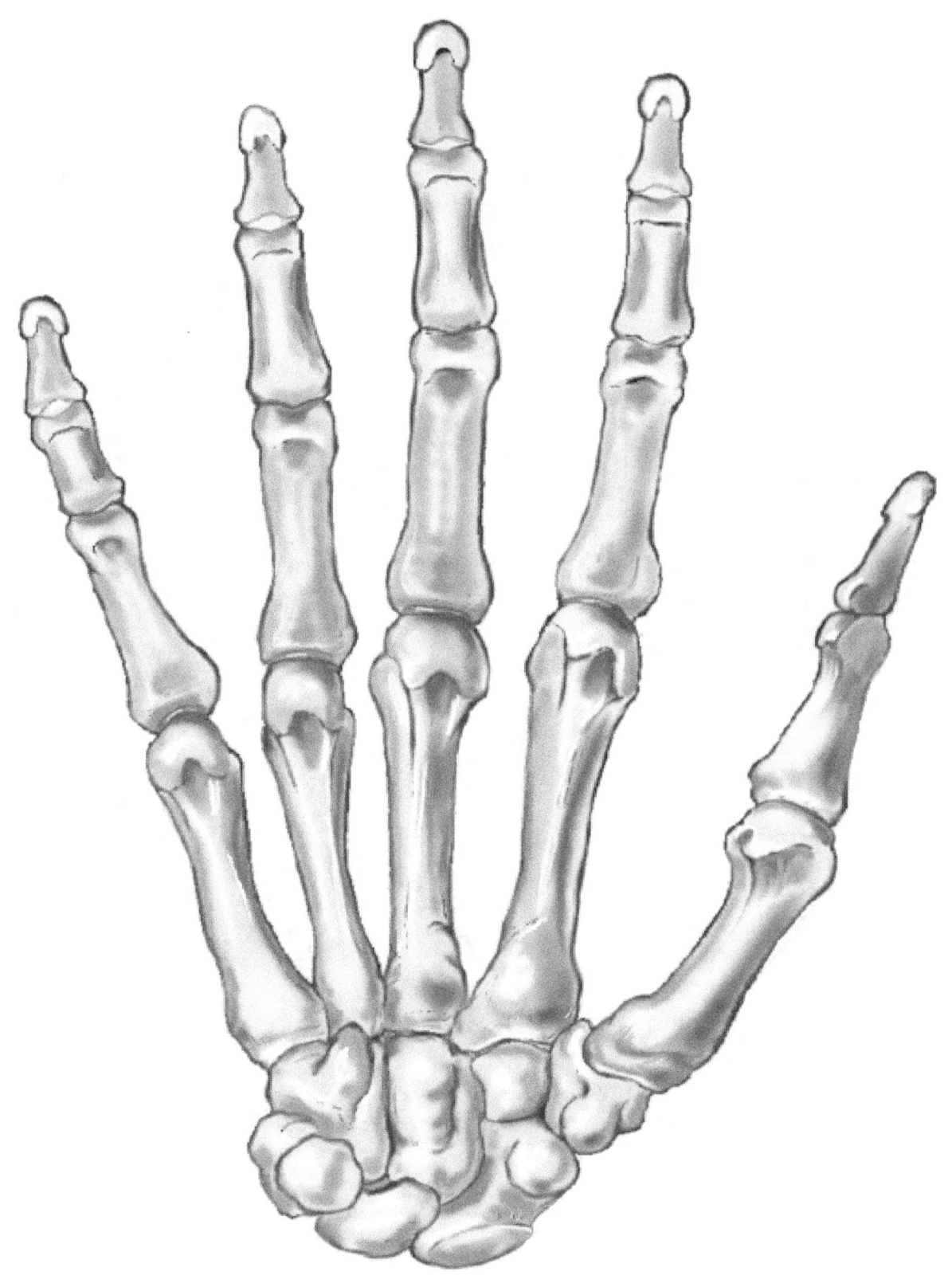

91

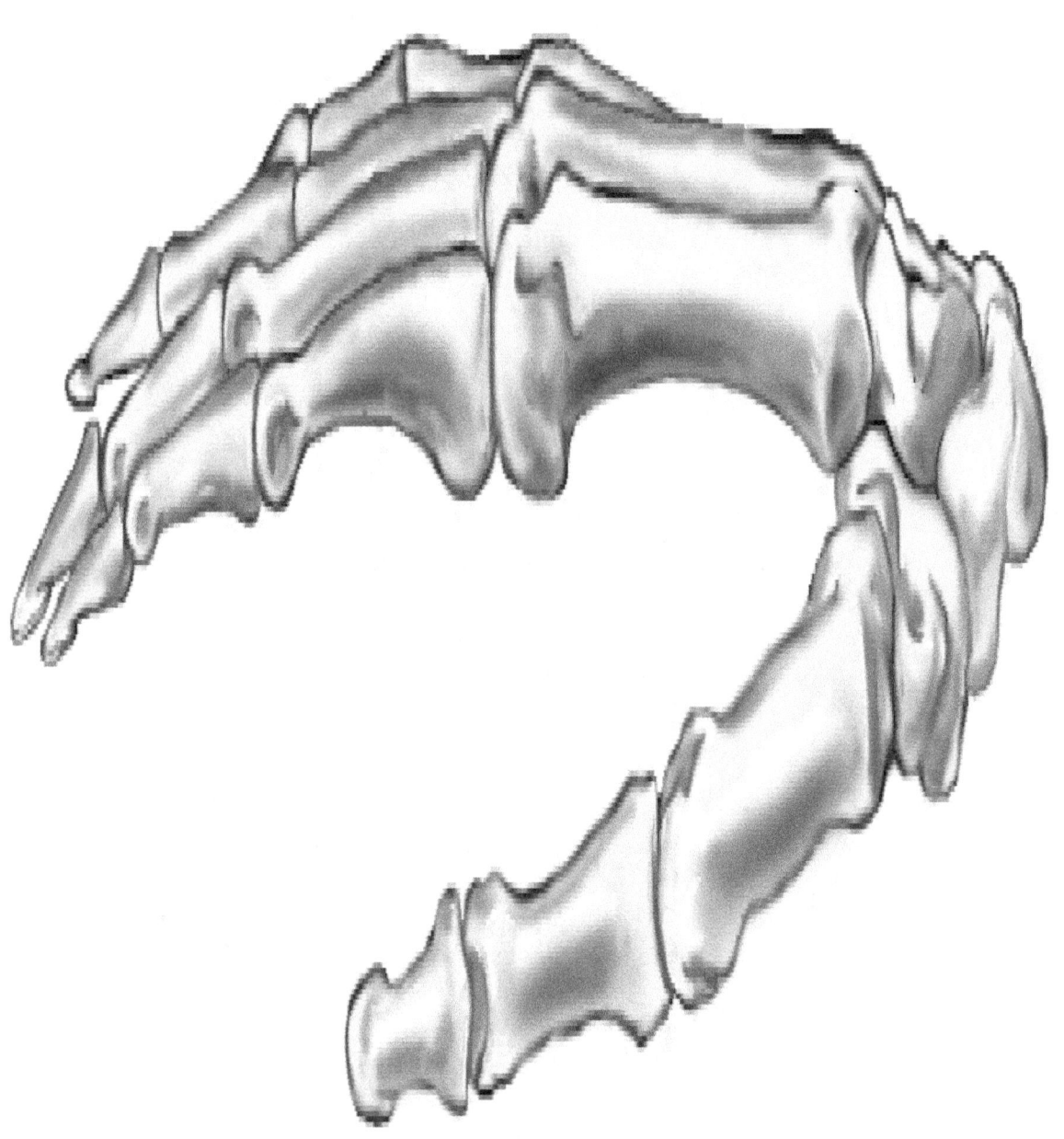

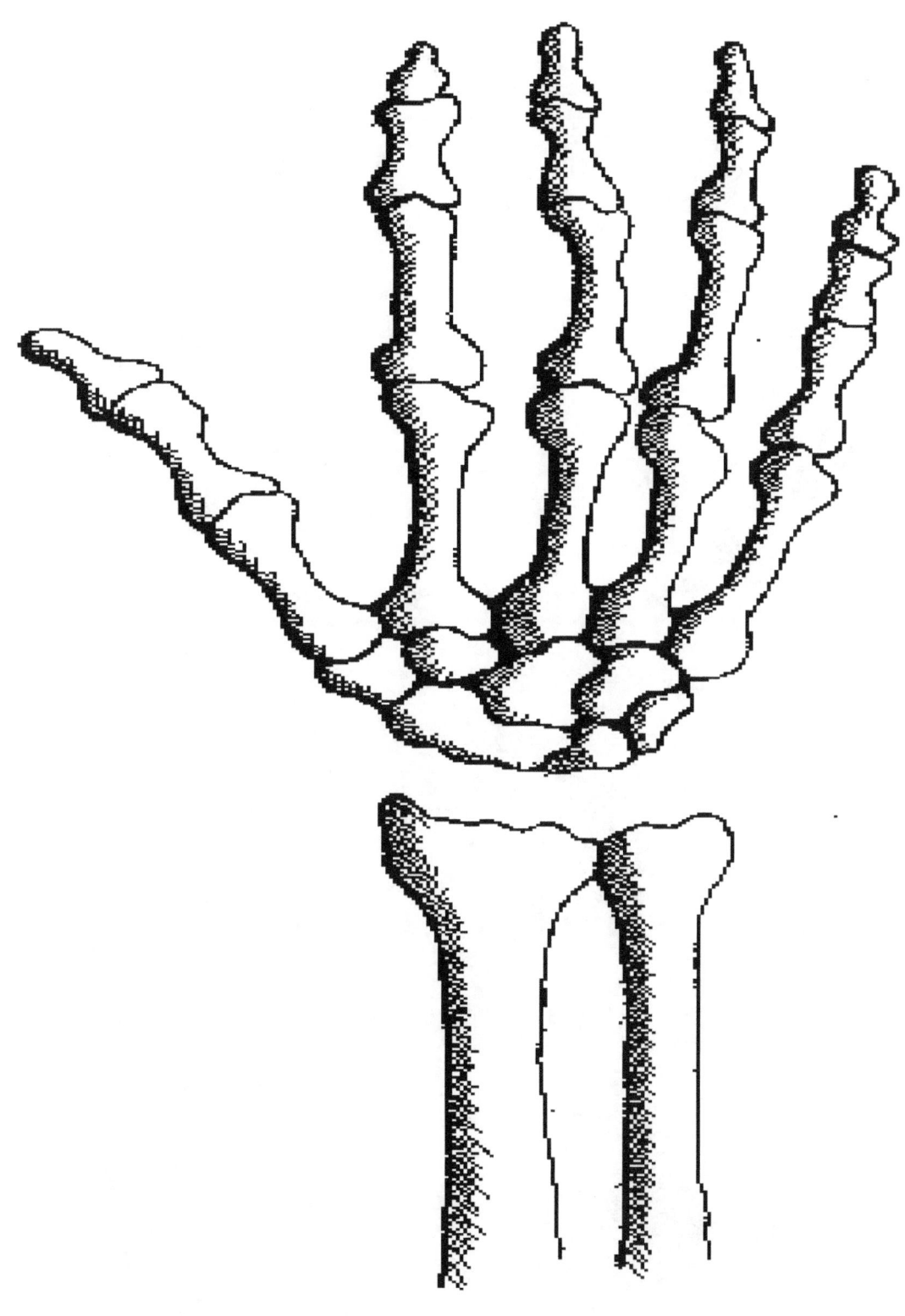

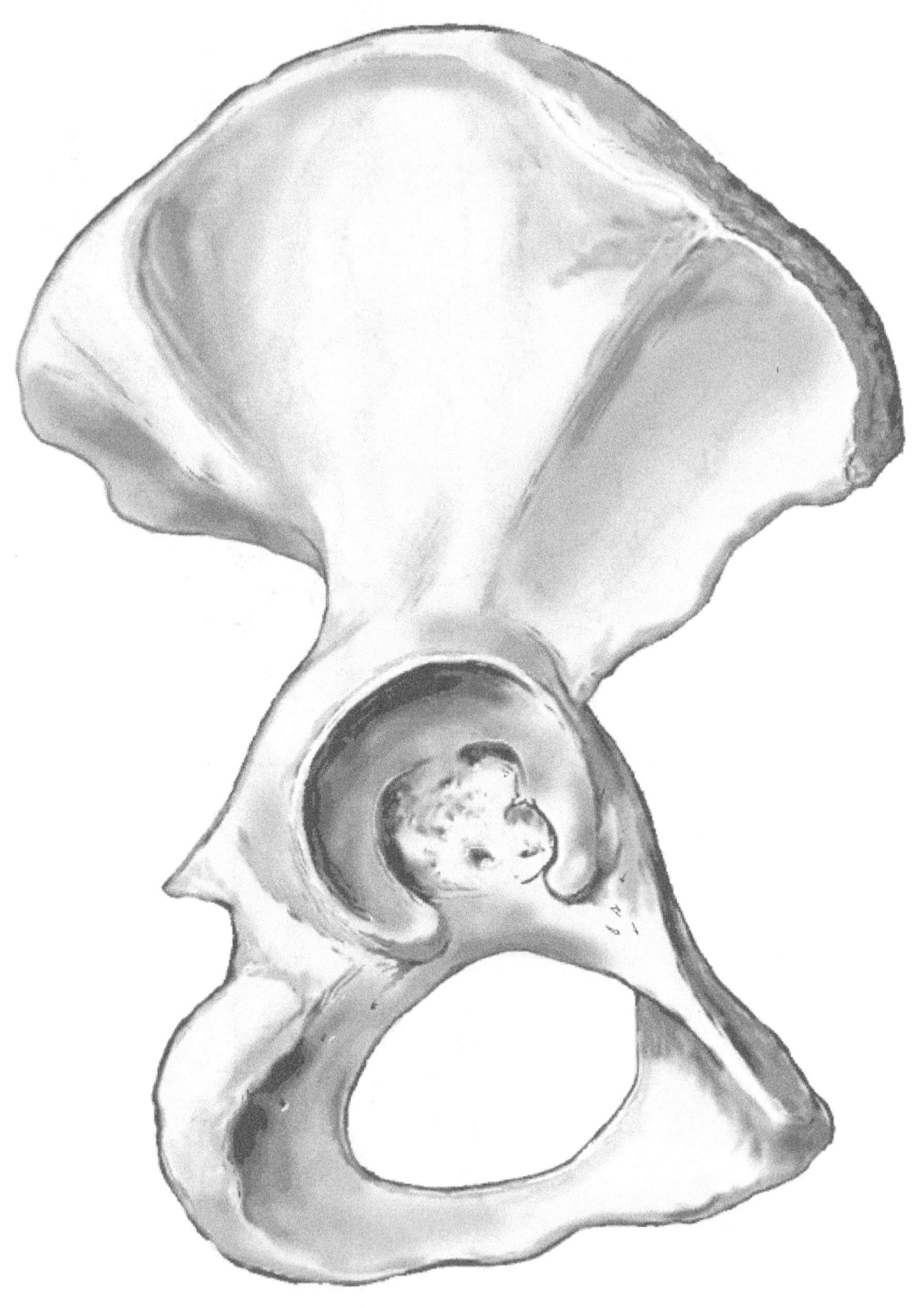

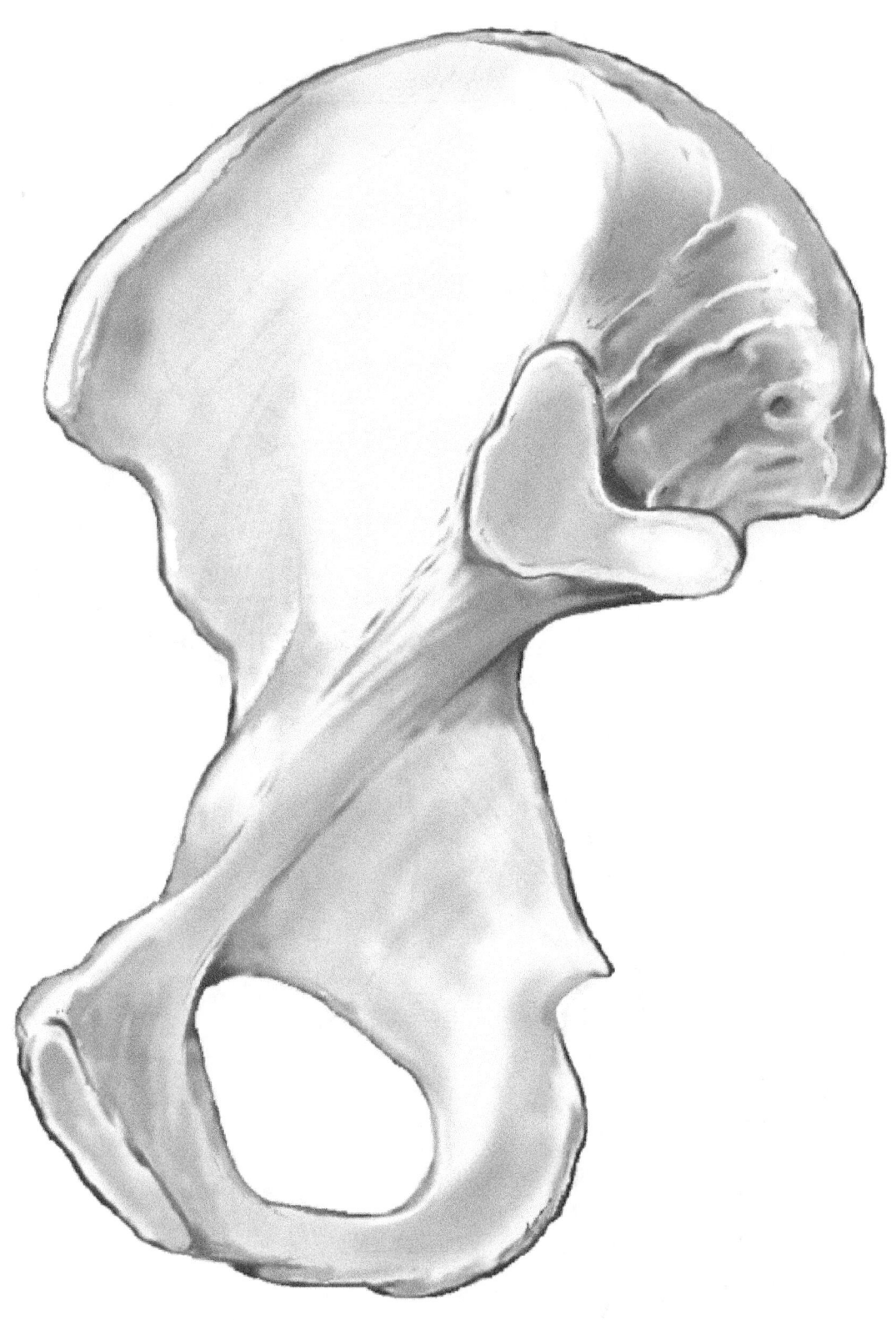

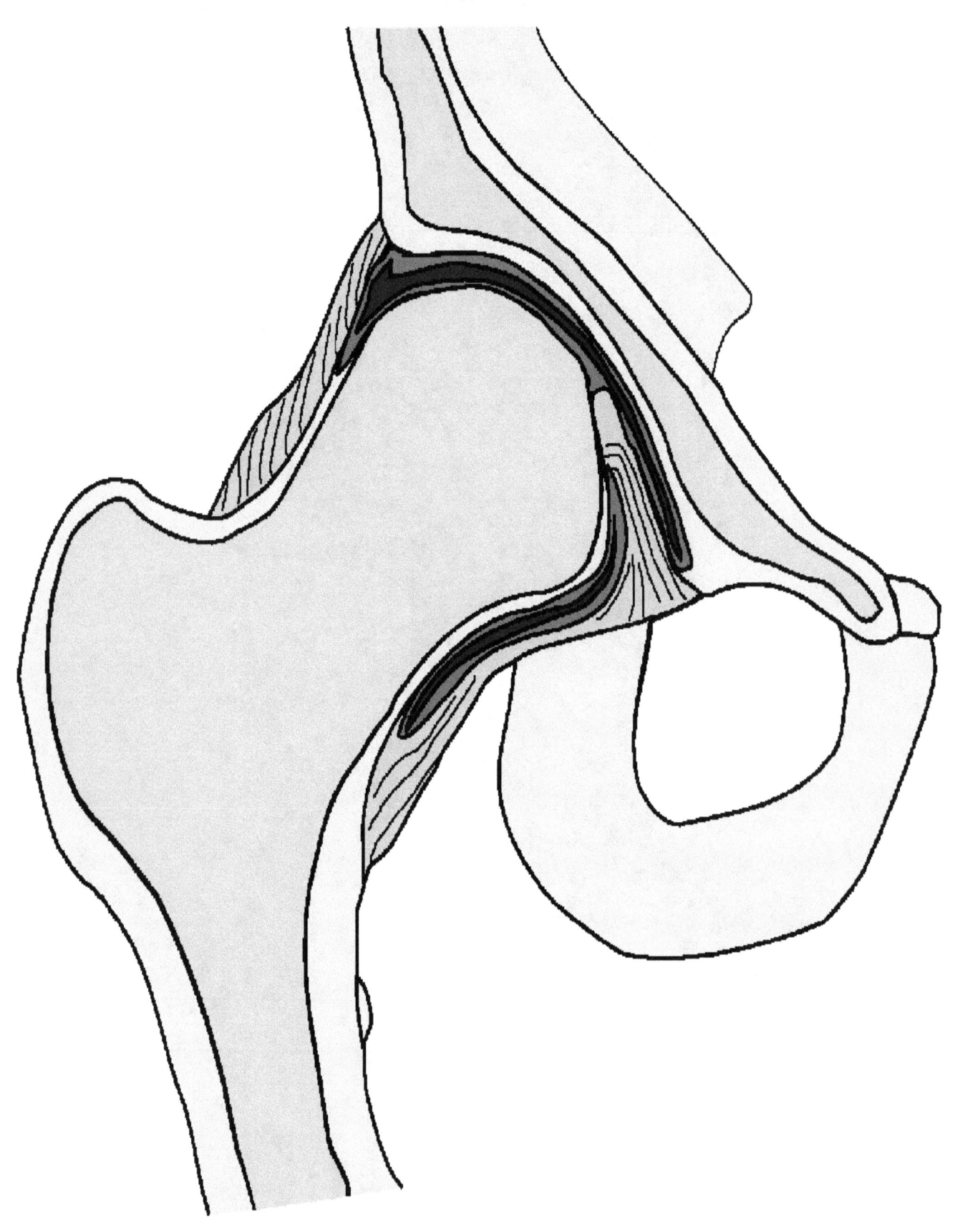

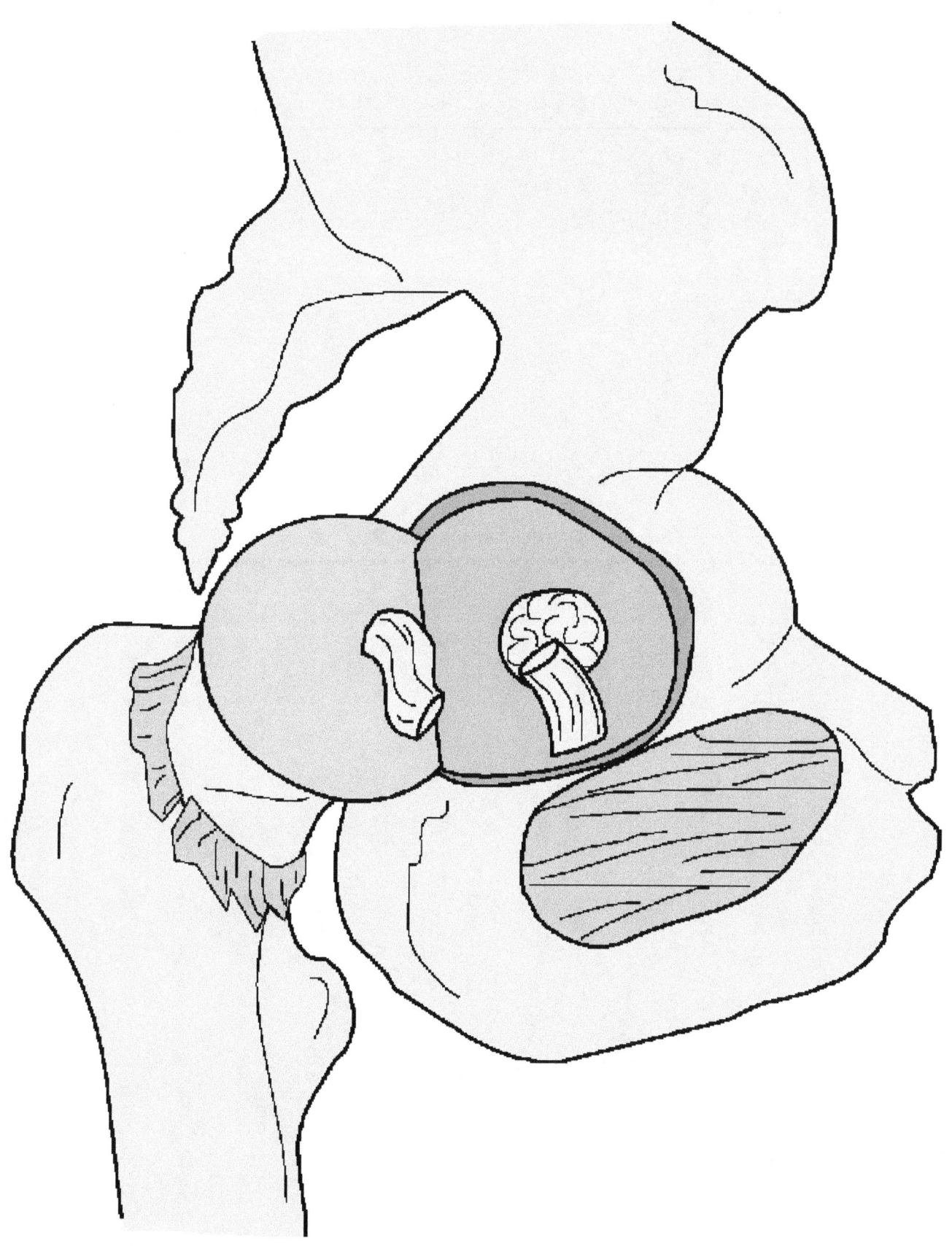

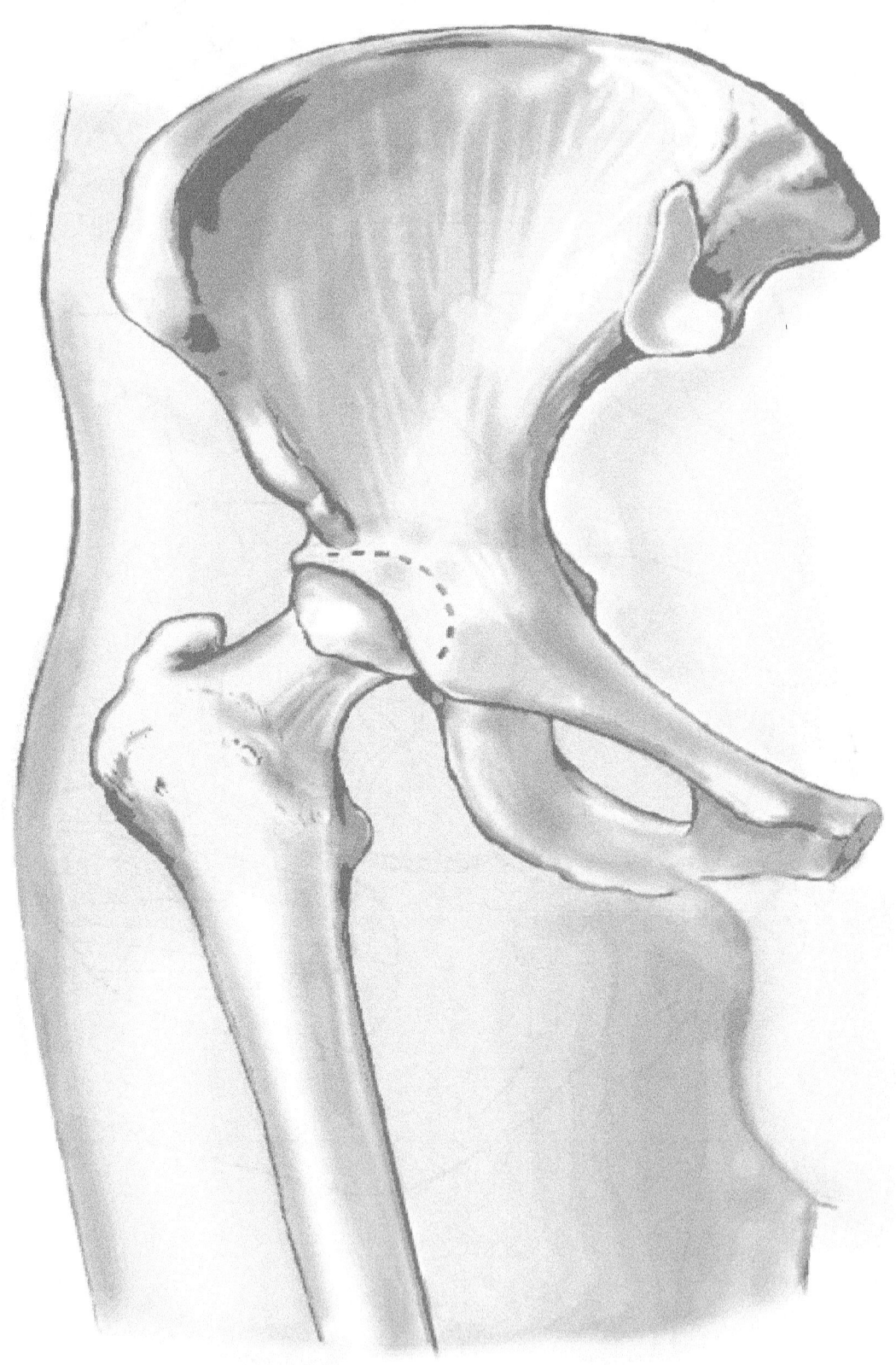

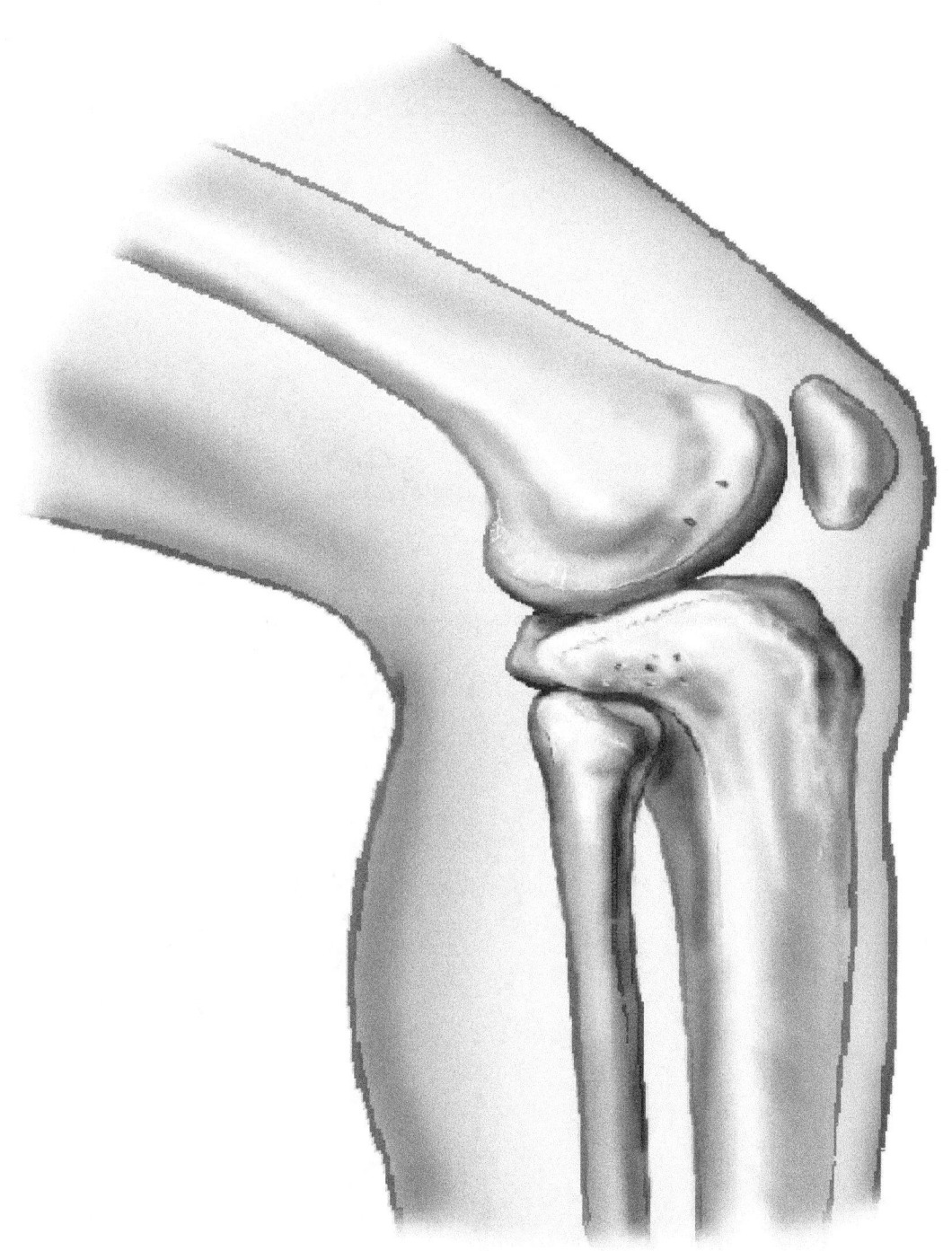

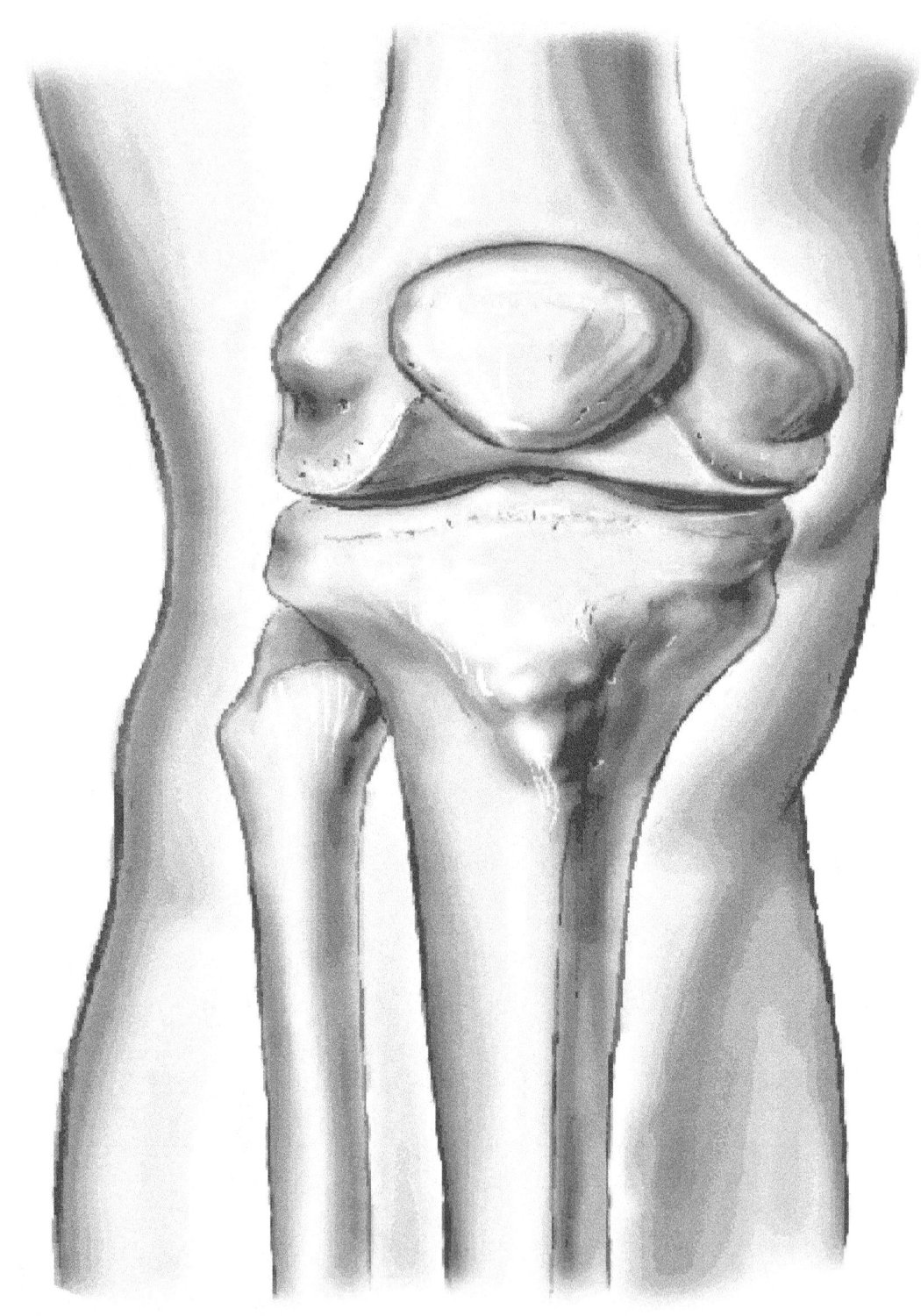

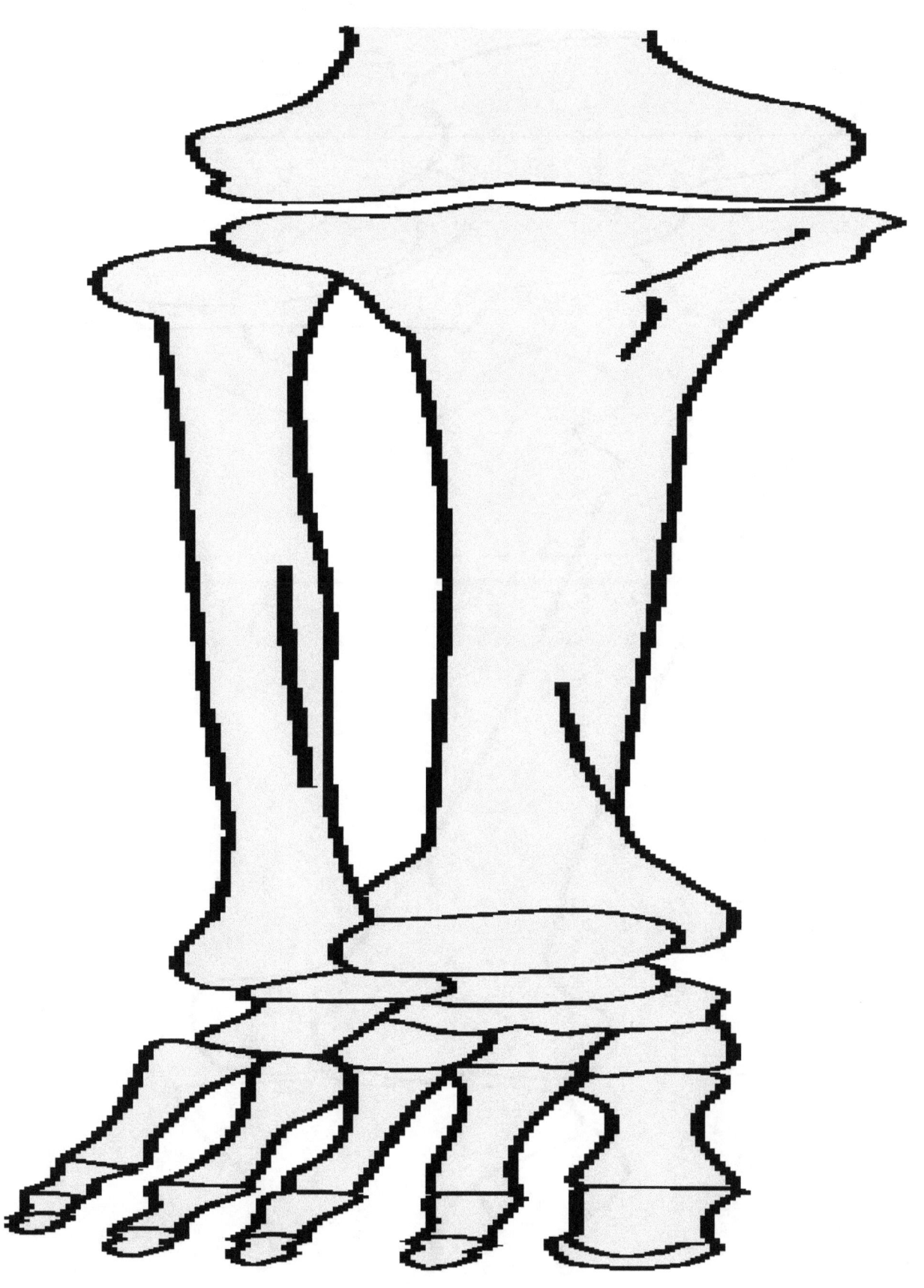

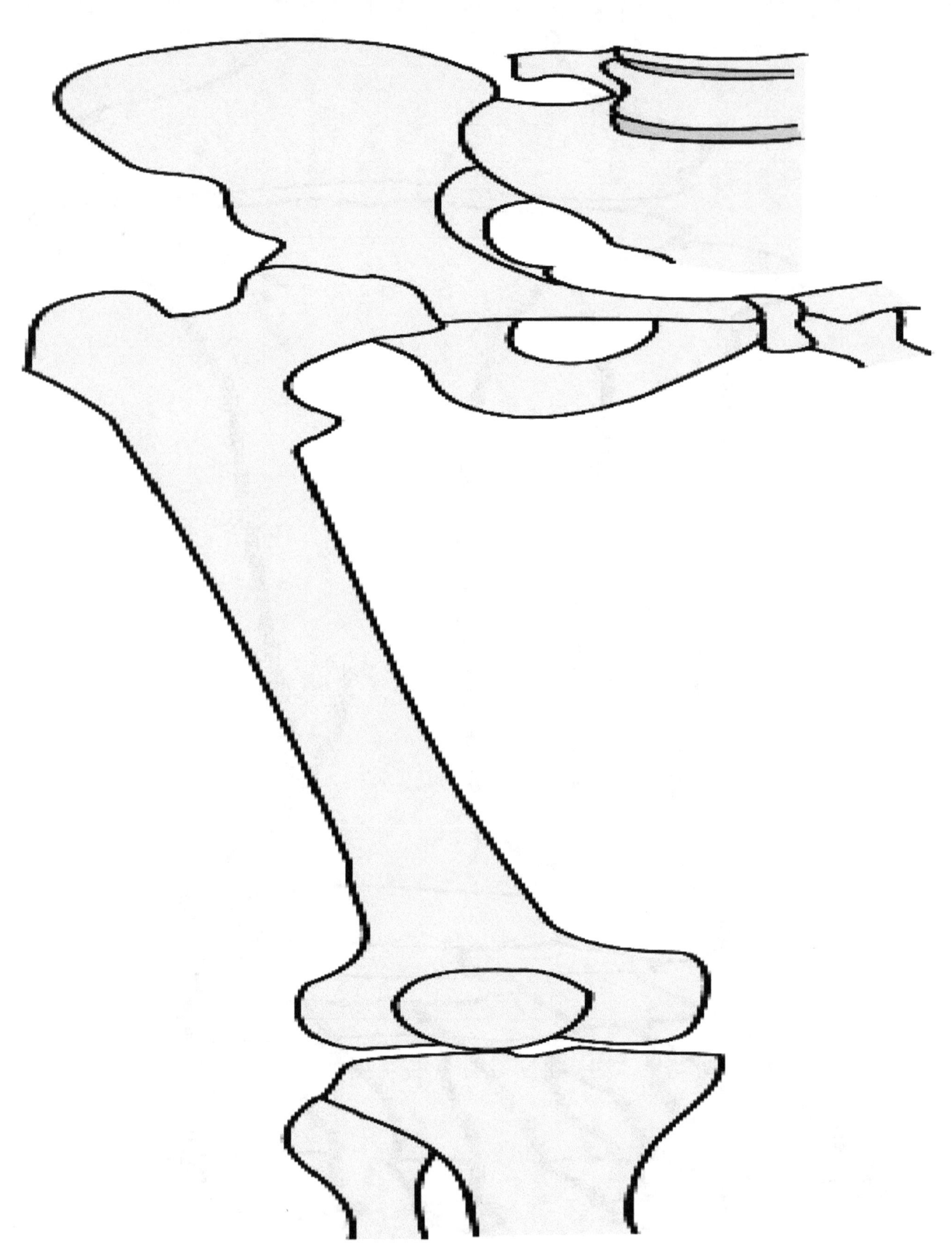

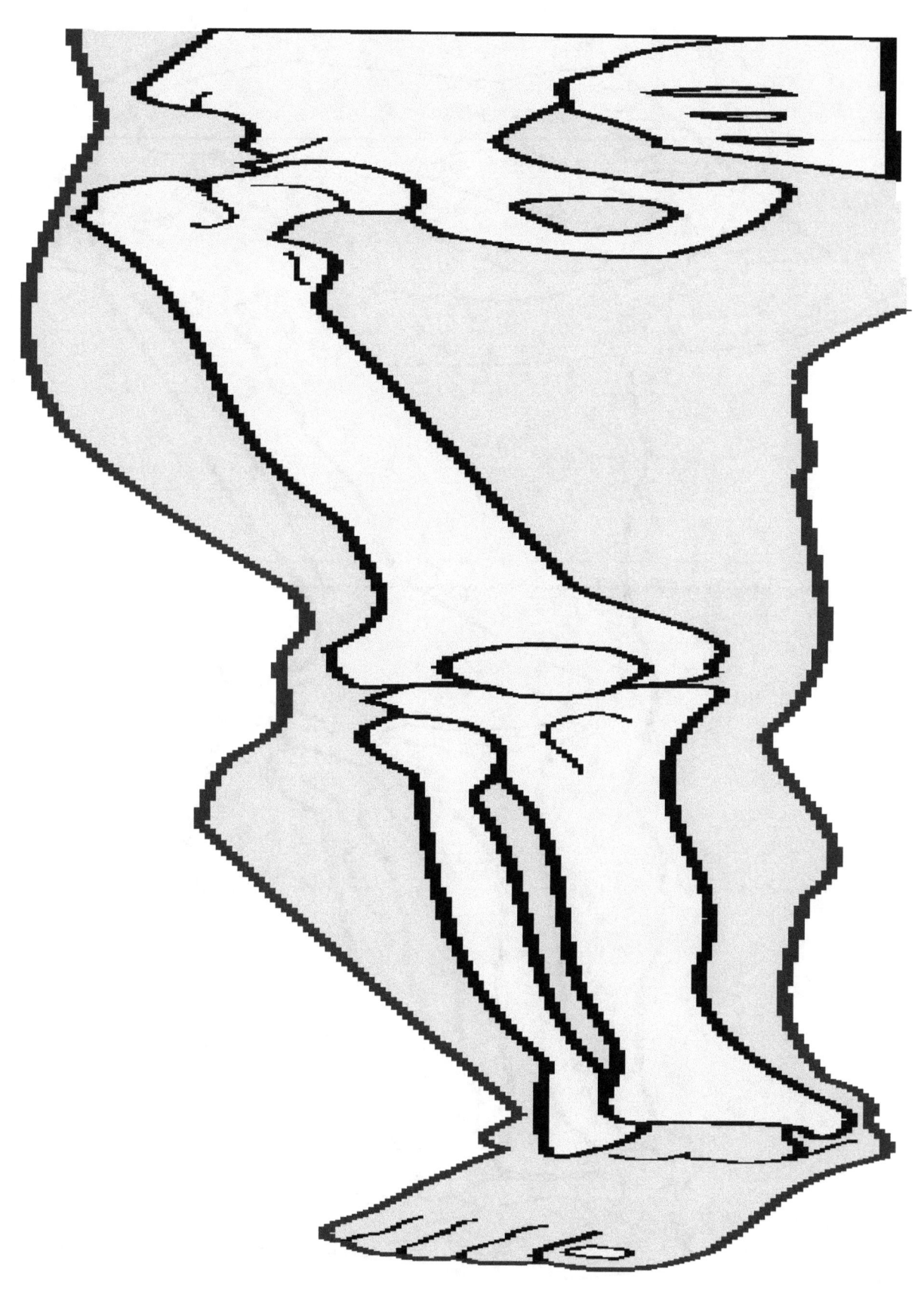

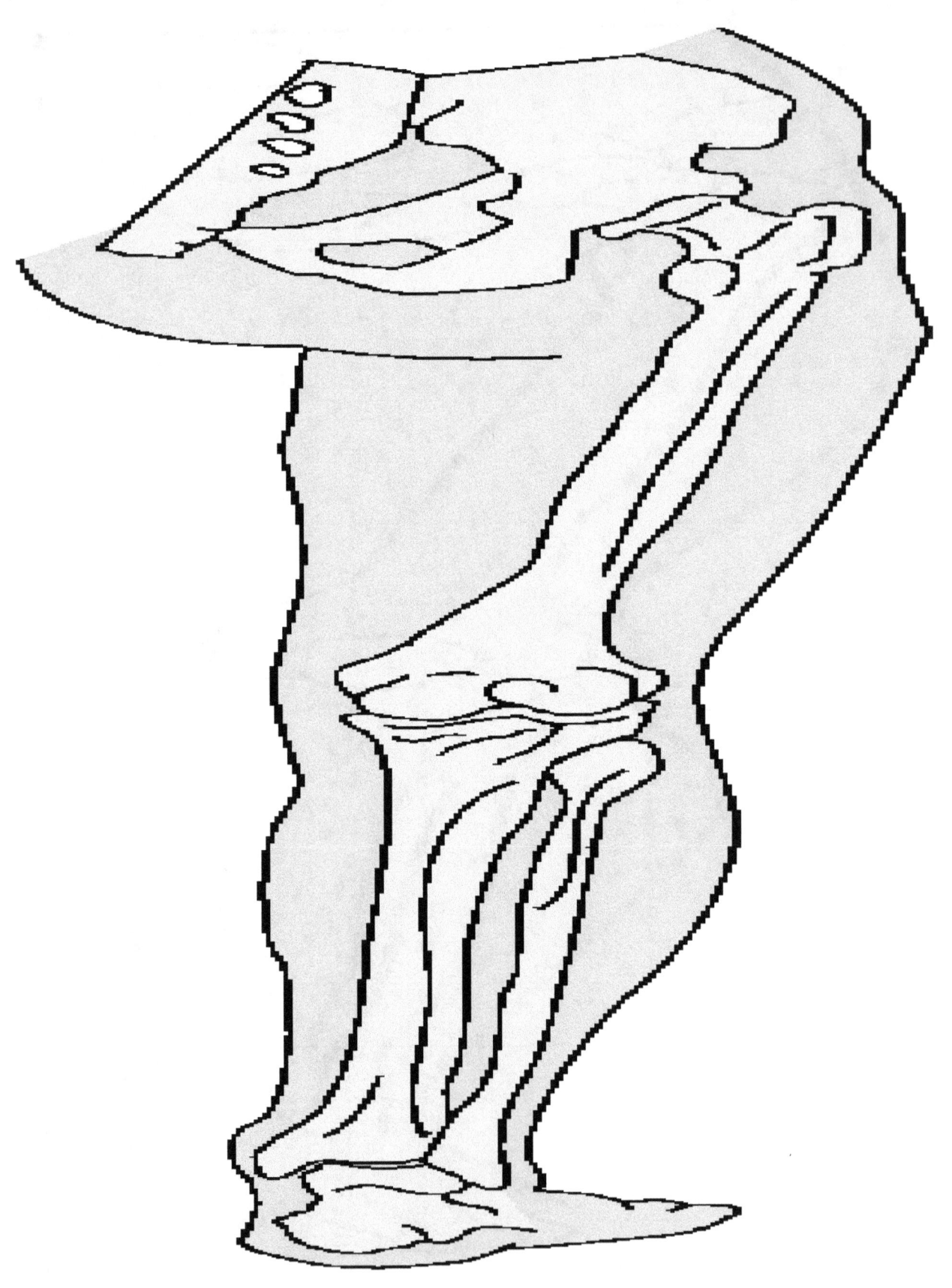

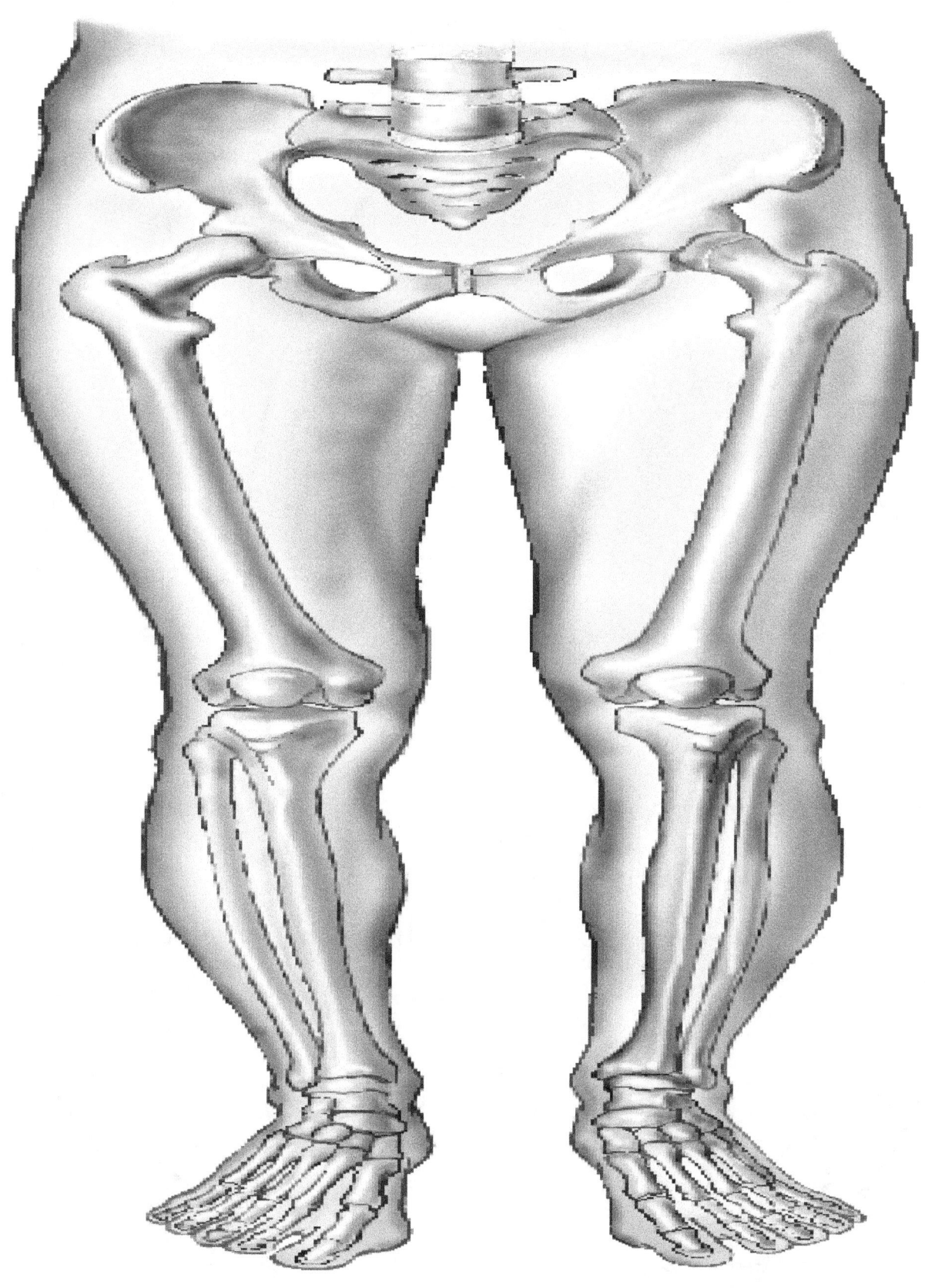

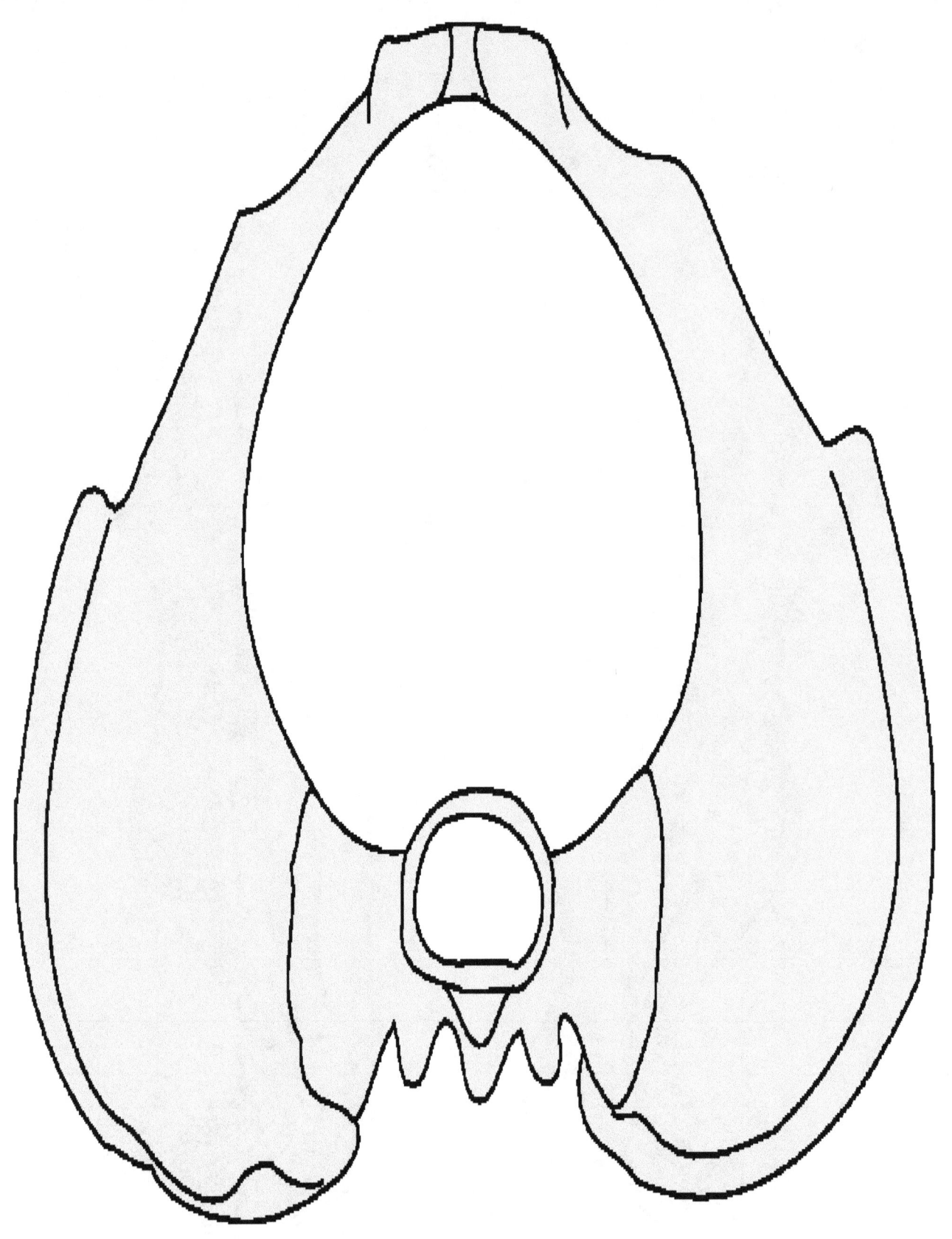

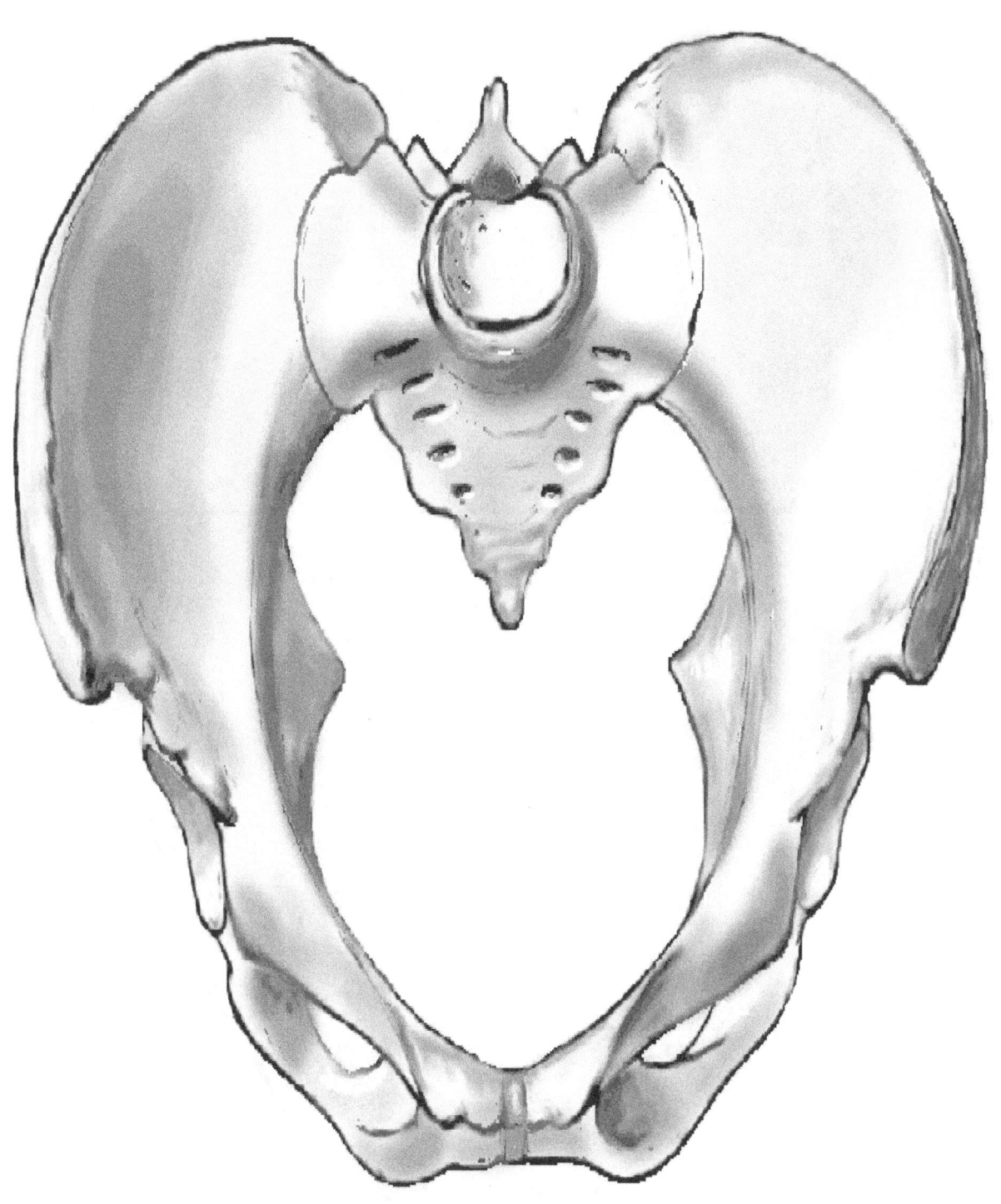

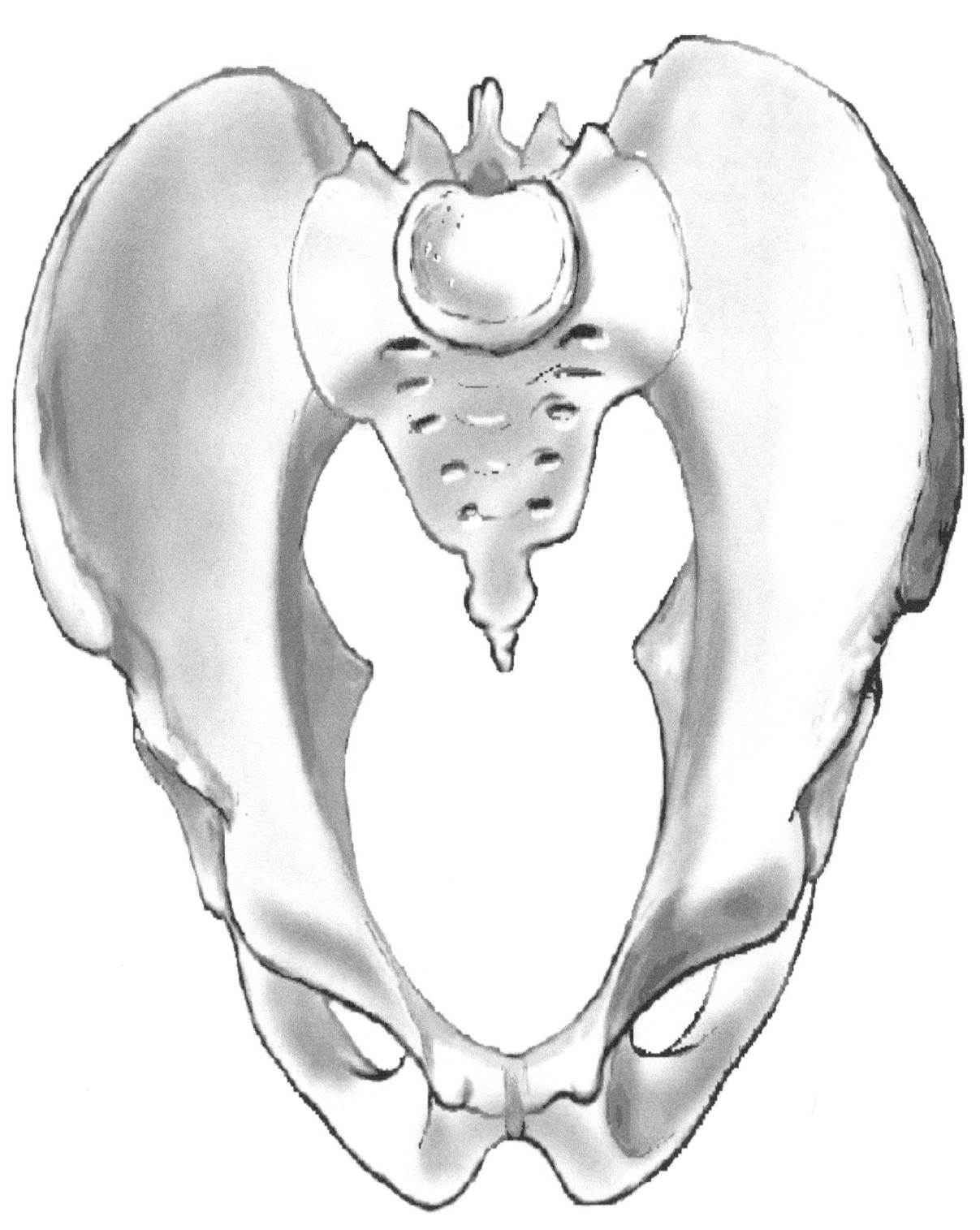

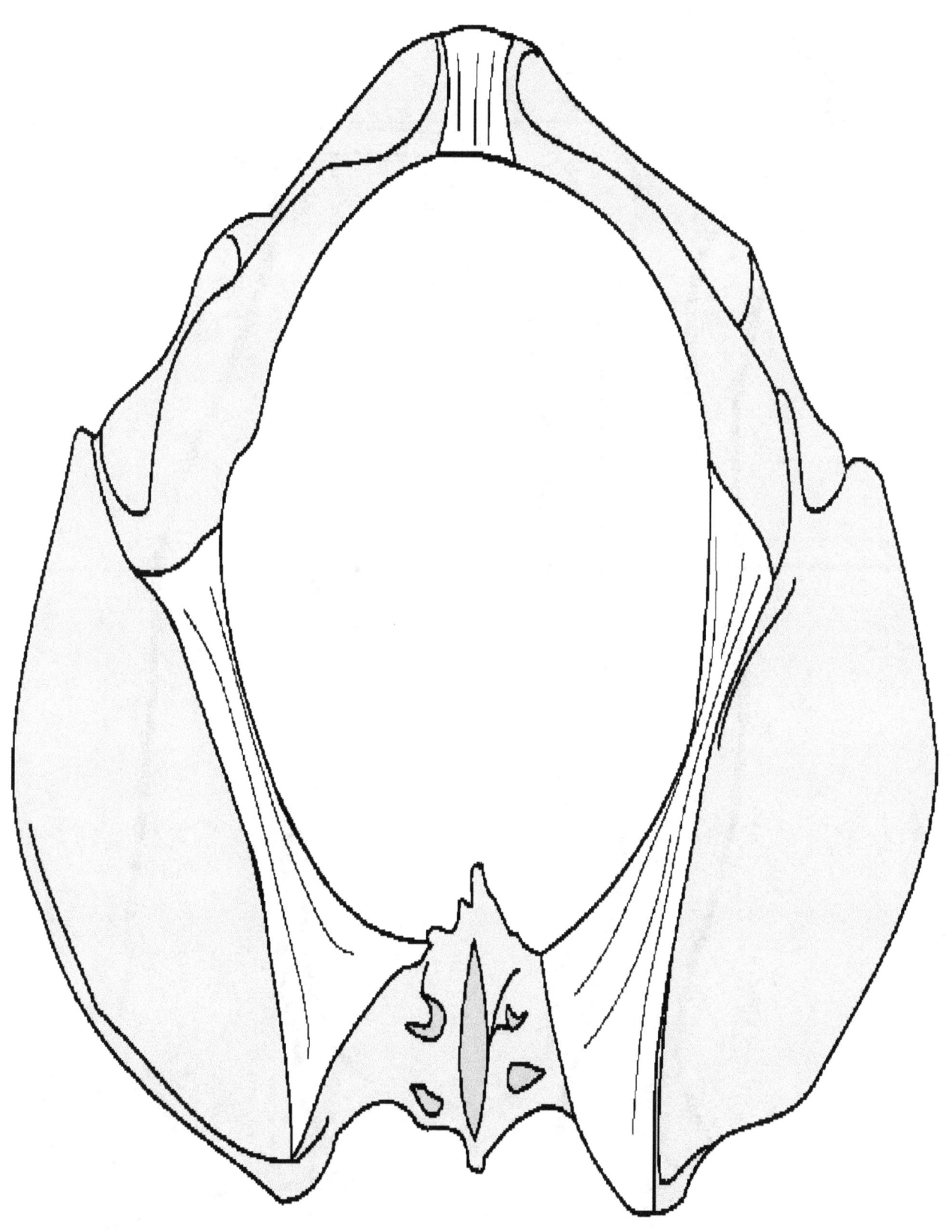

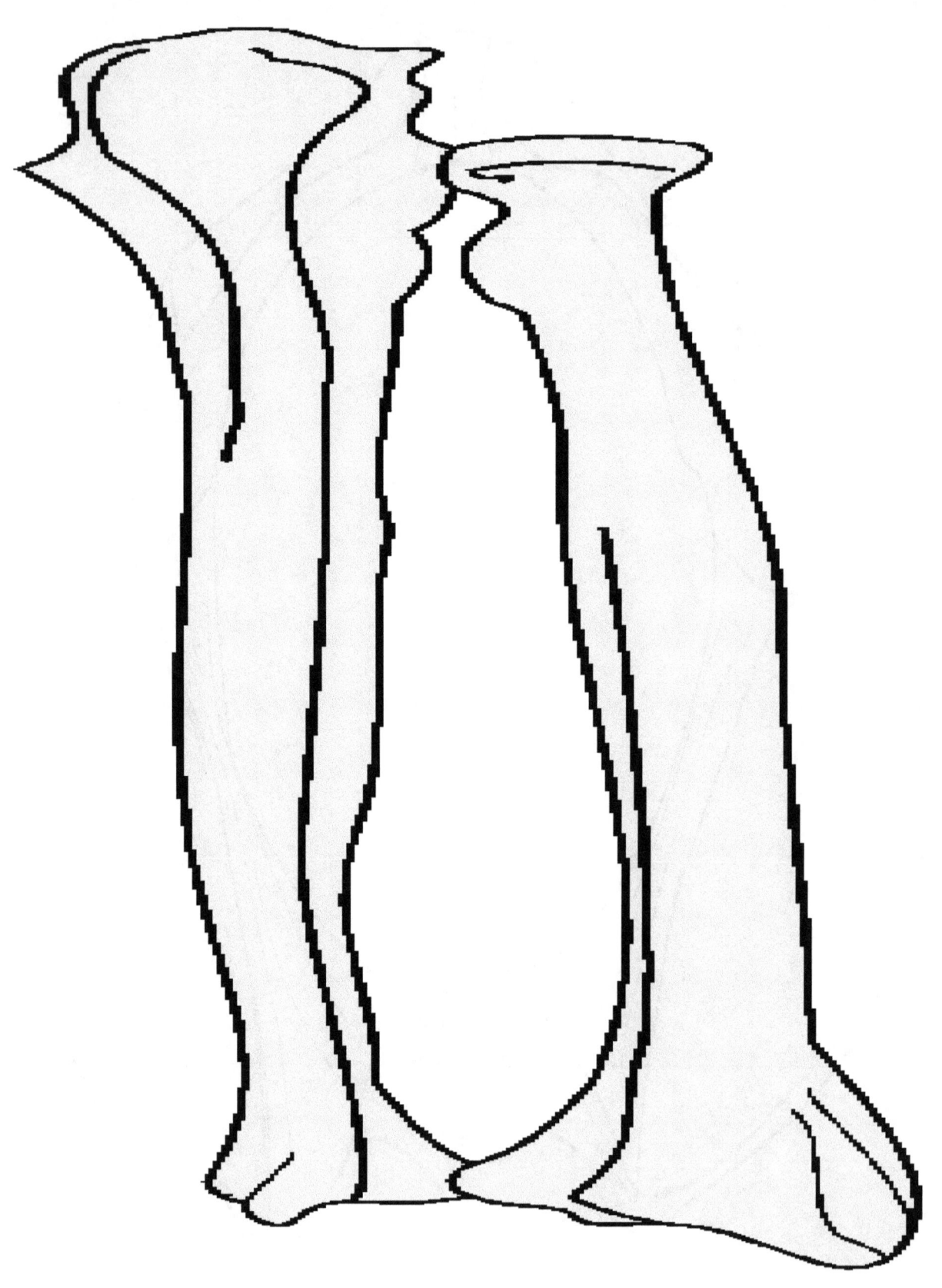

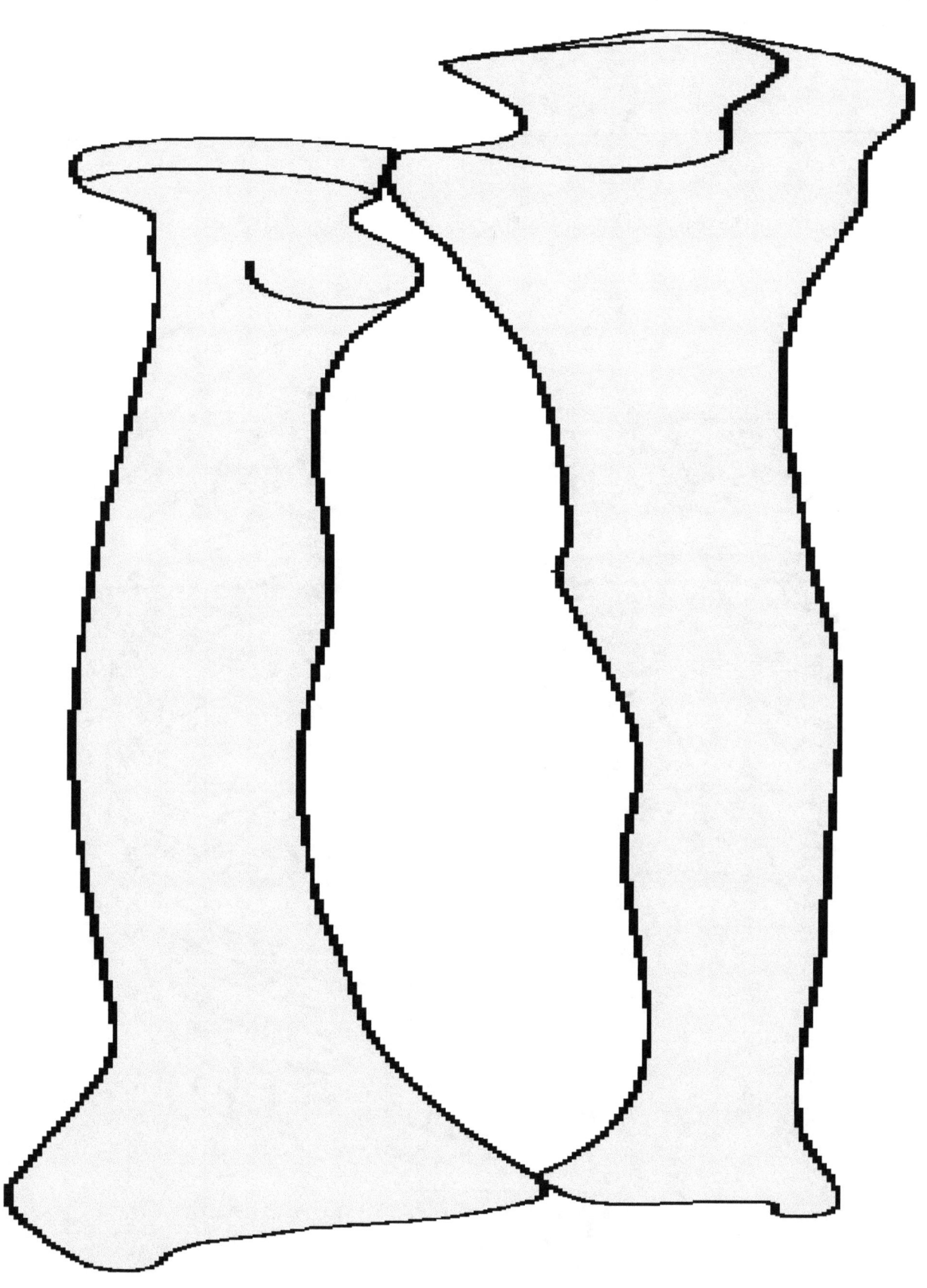

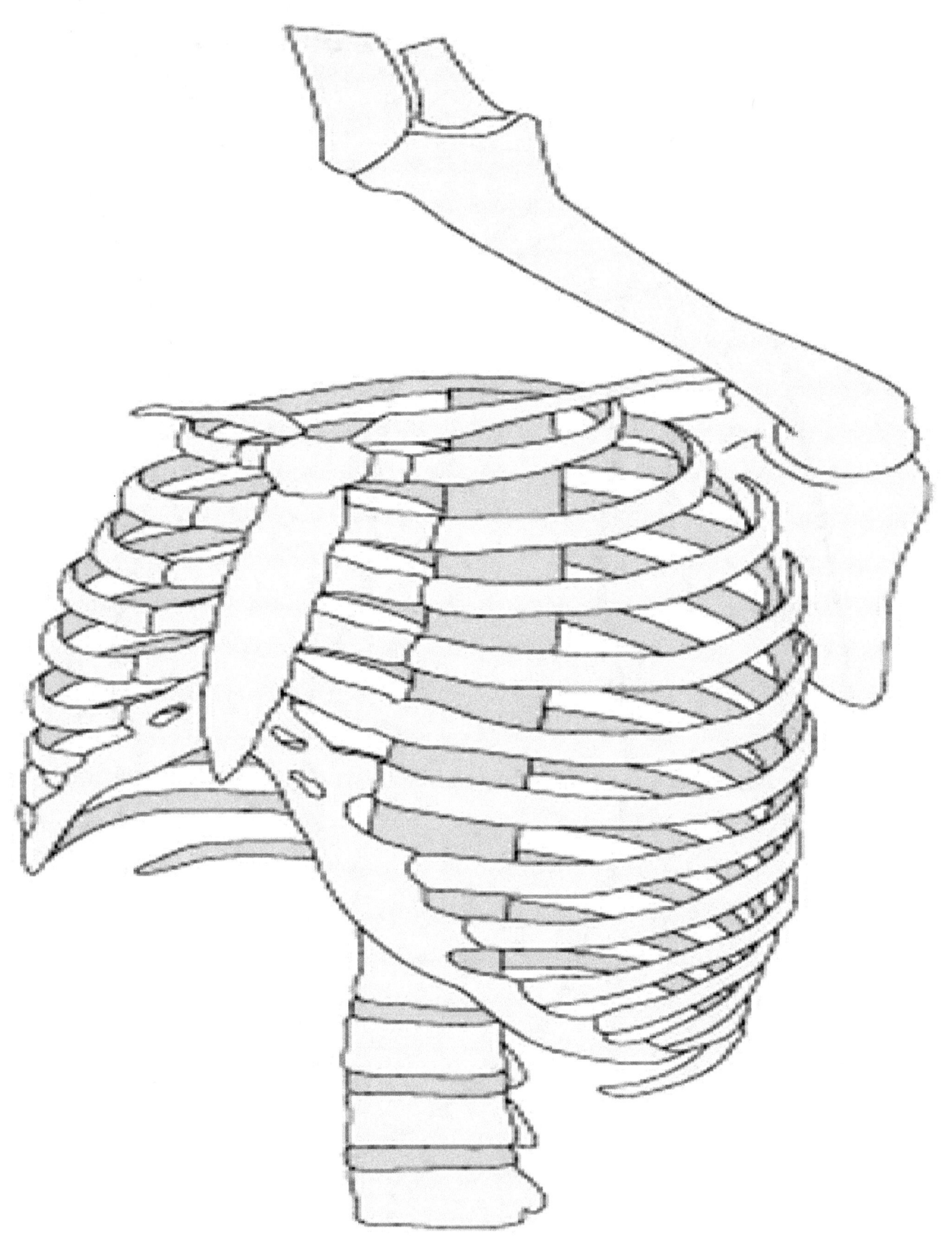

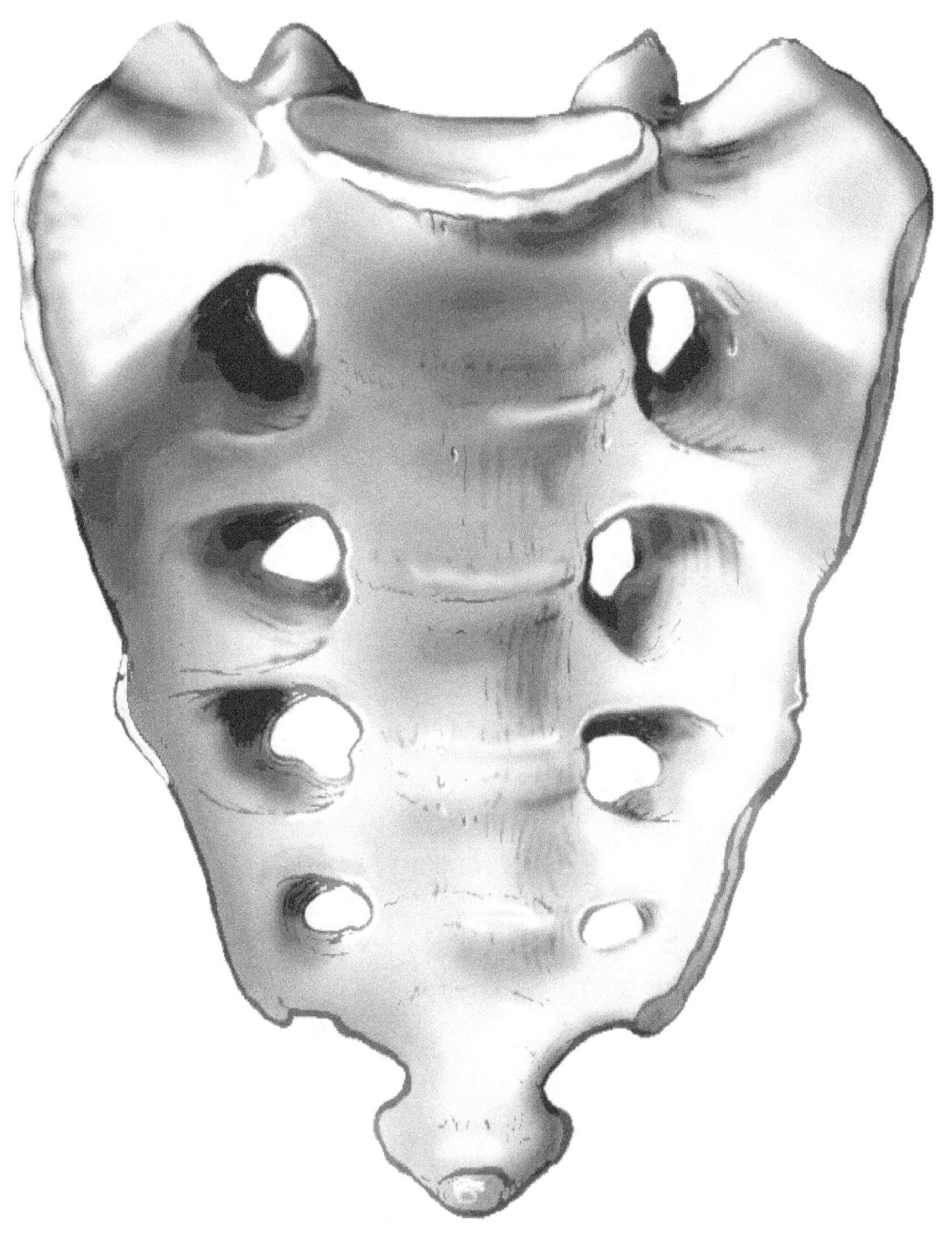

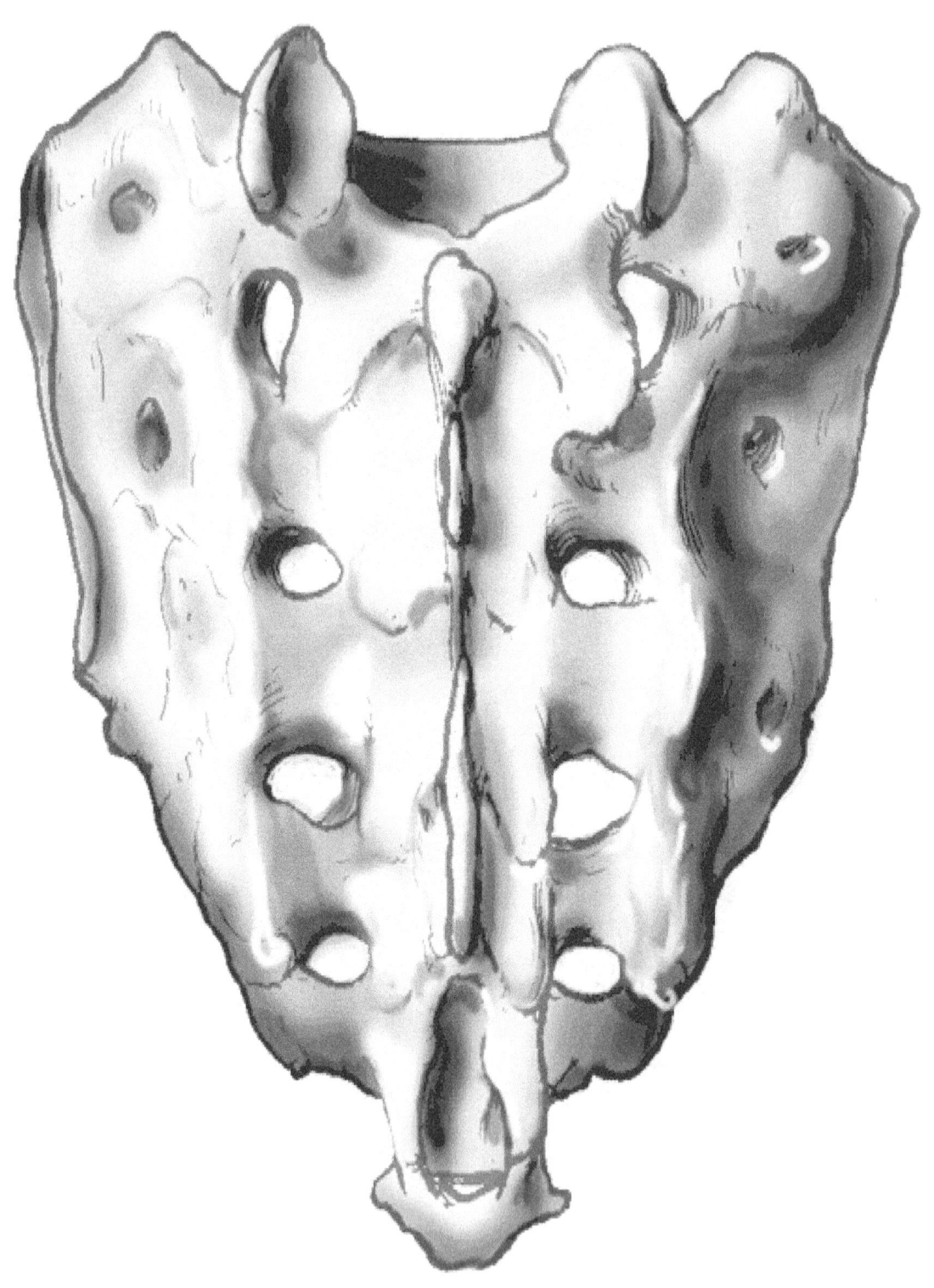

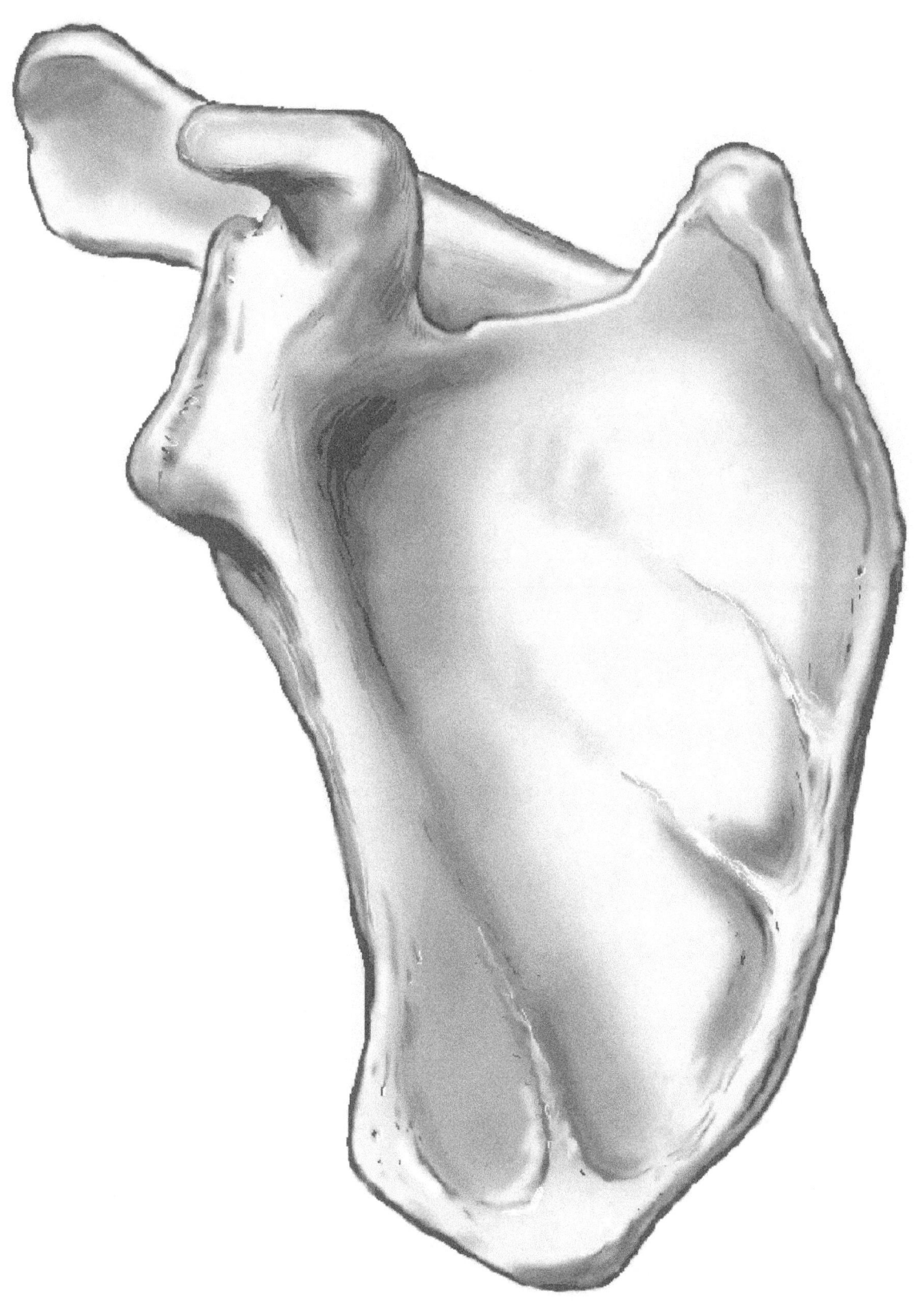

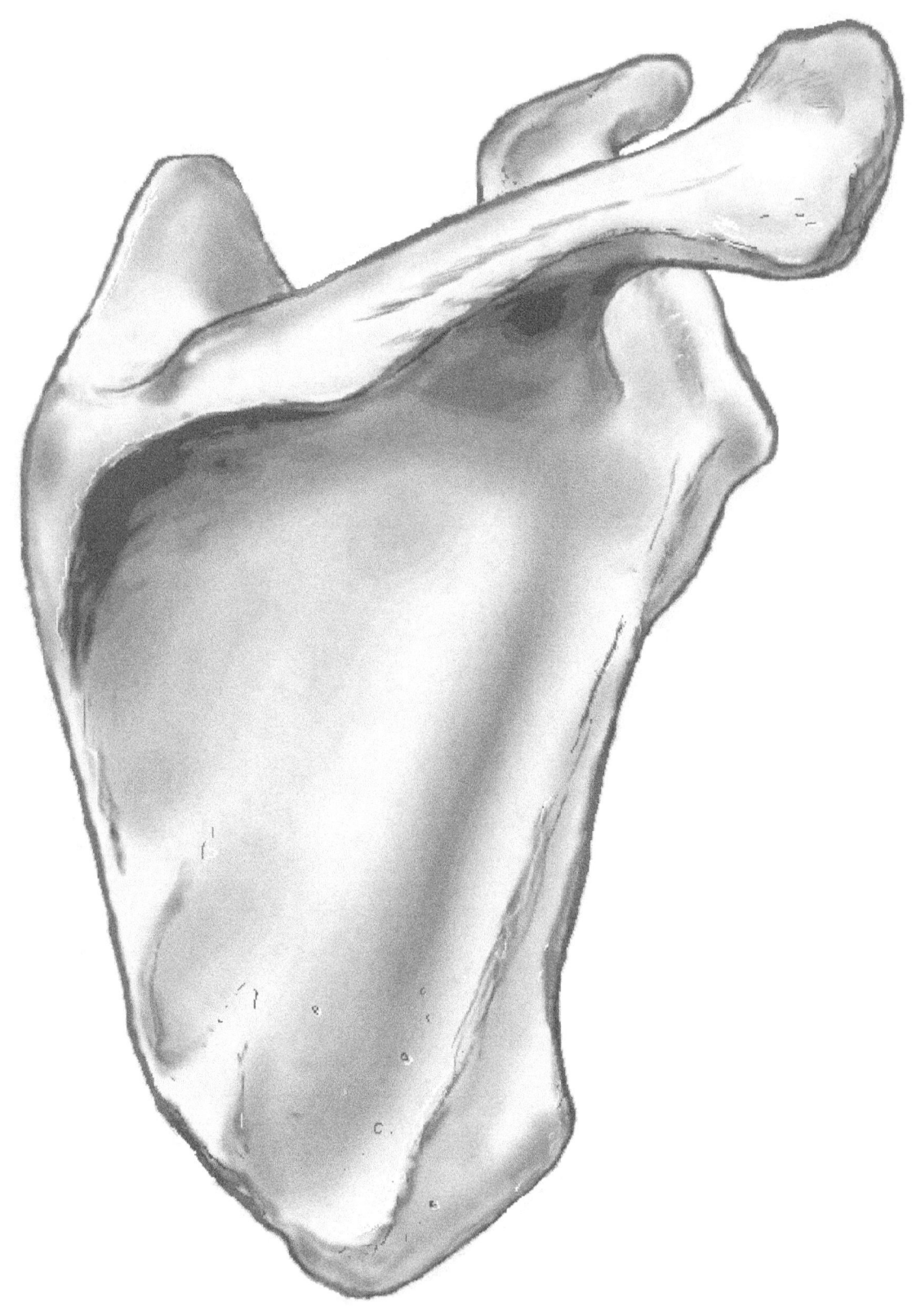

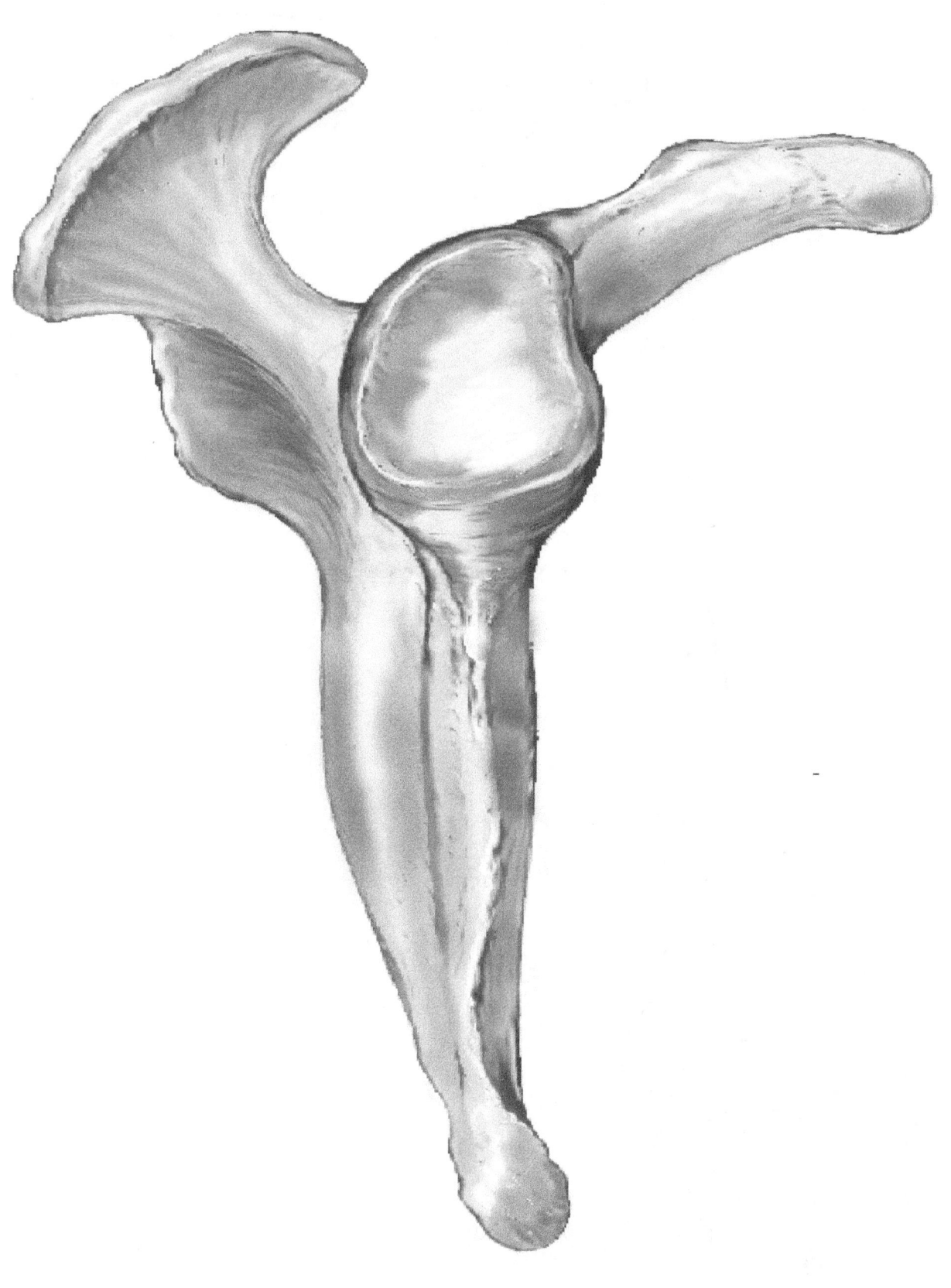

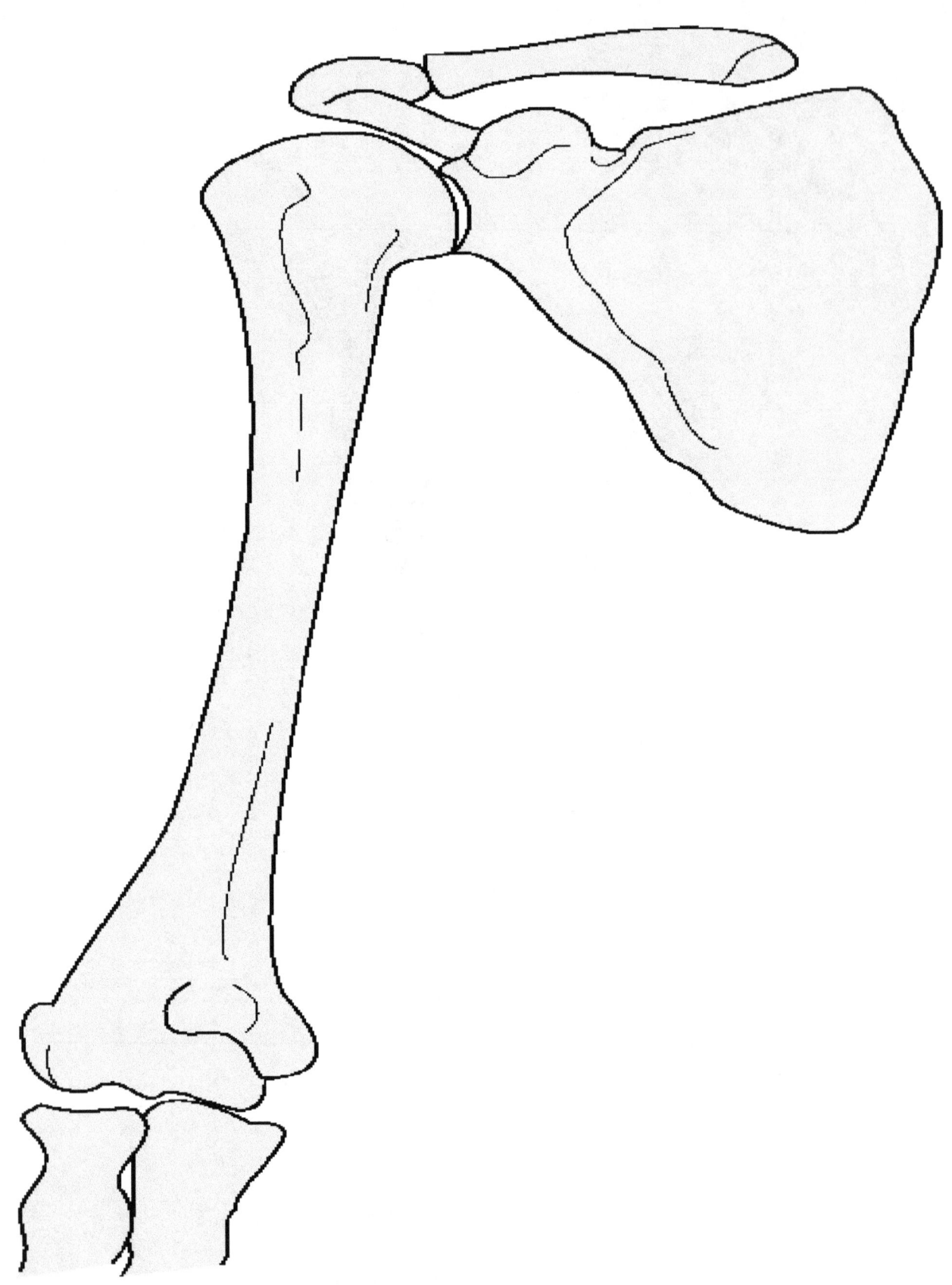

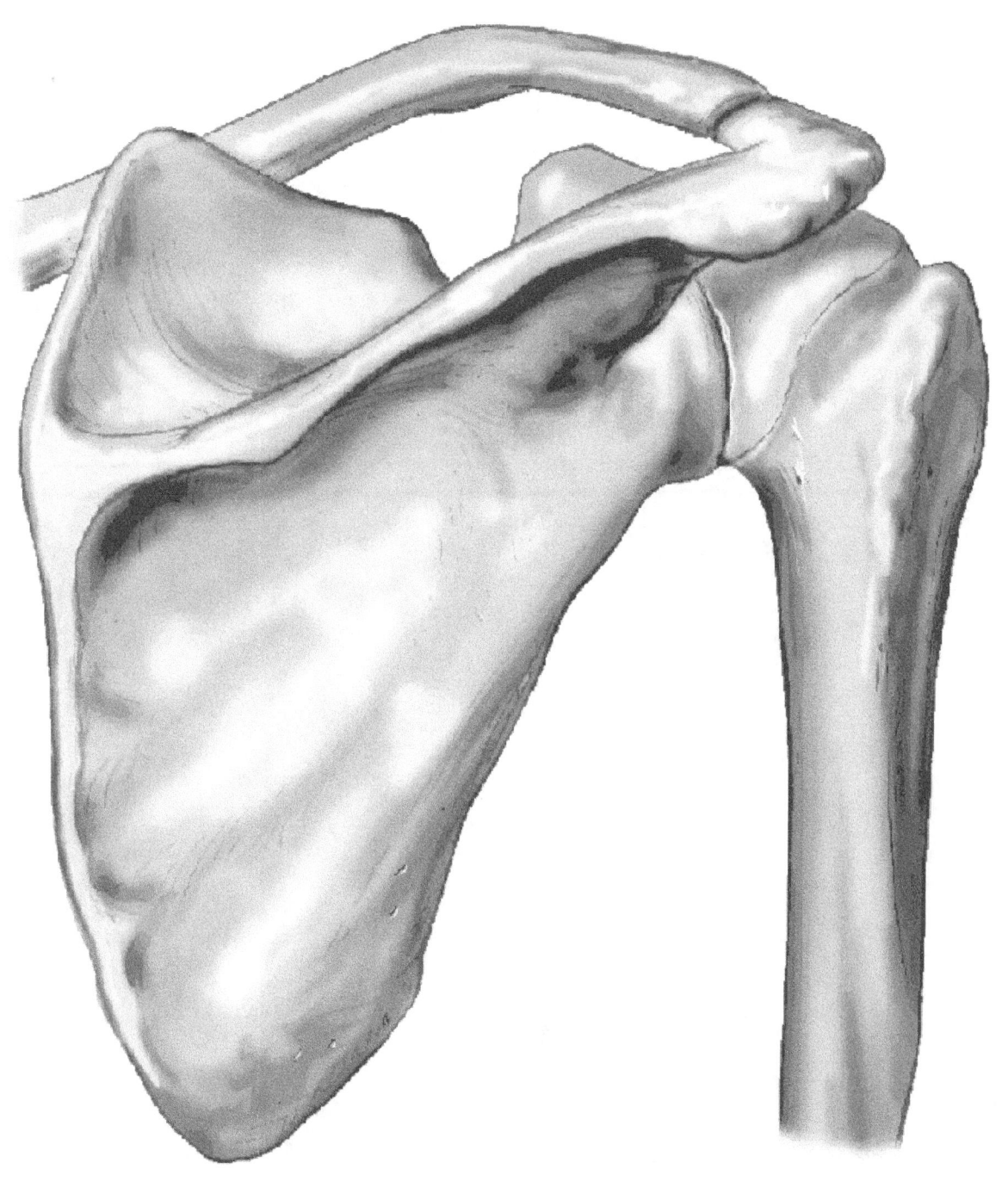

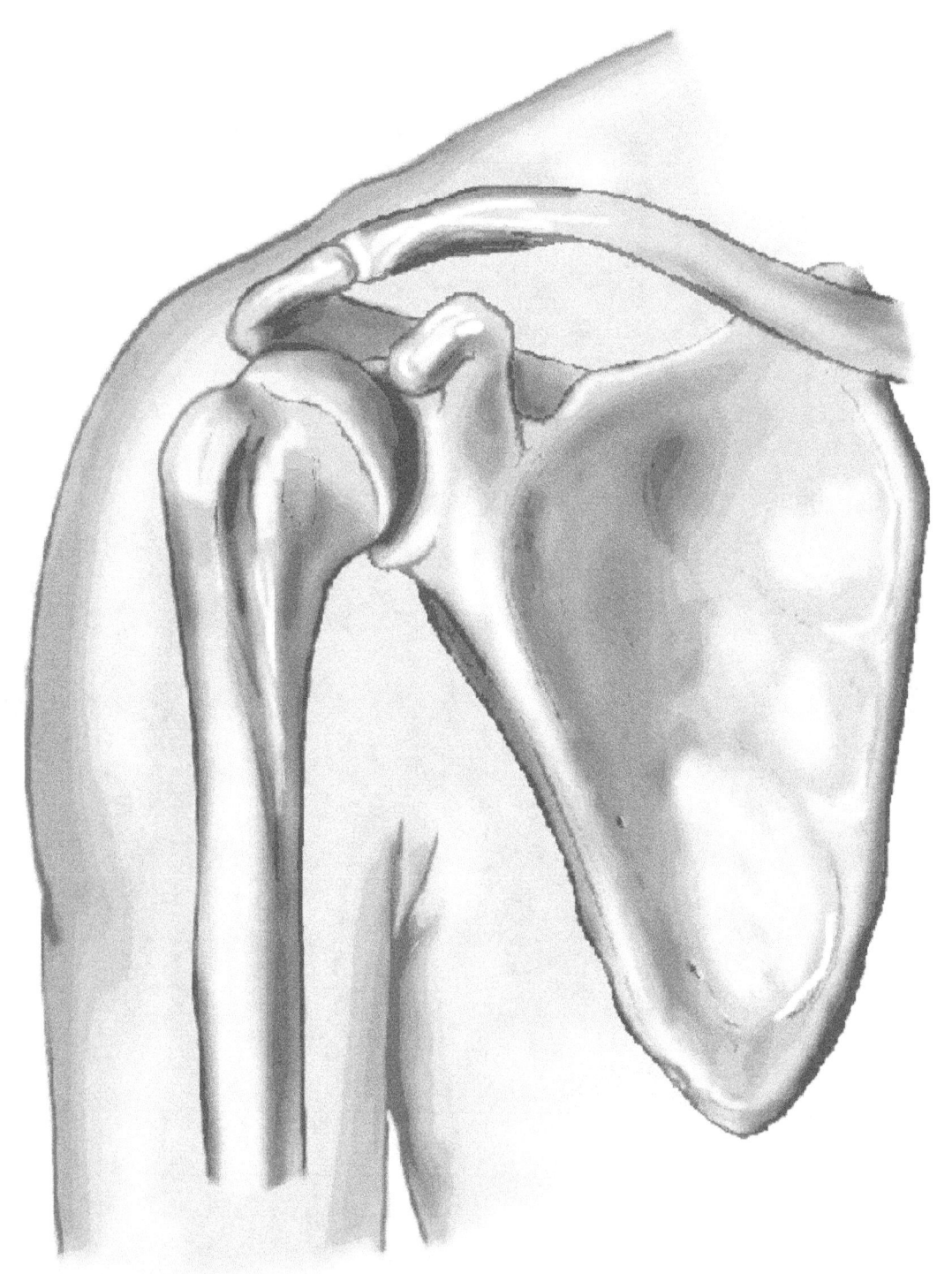

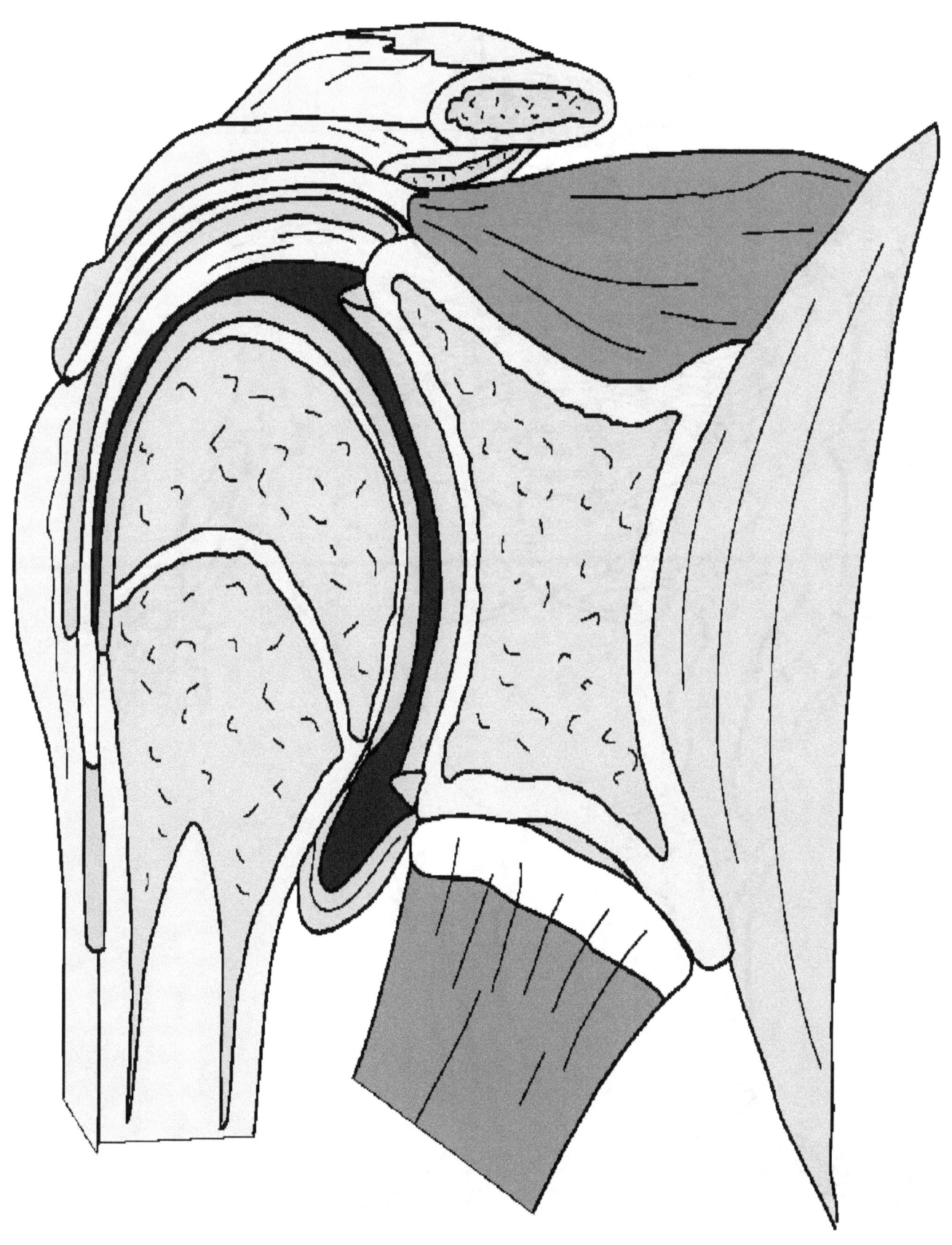

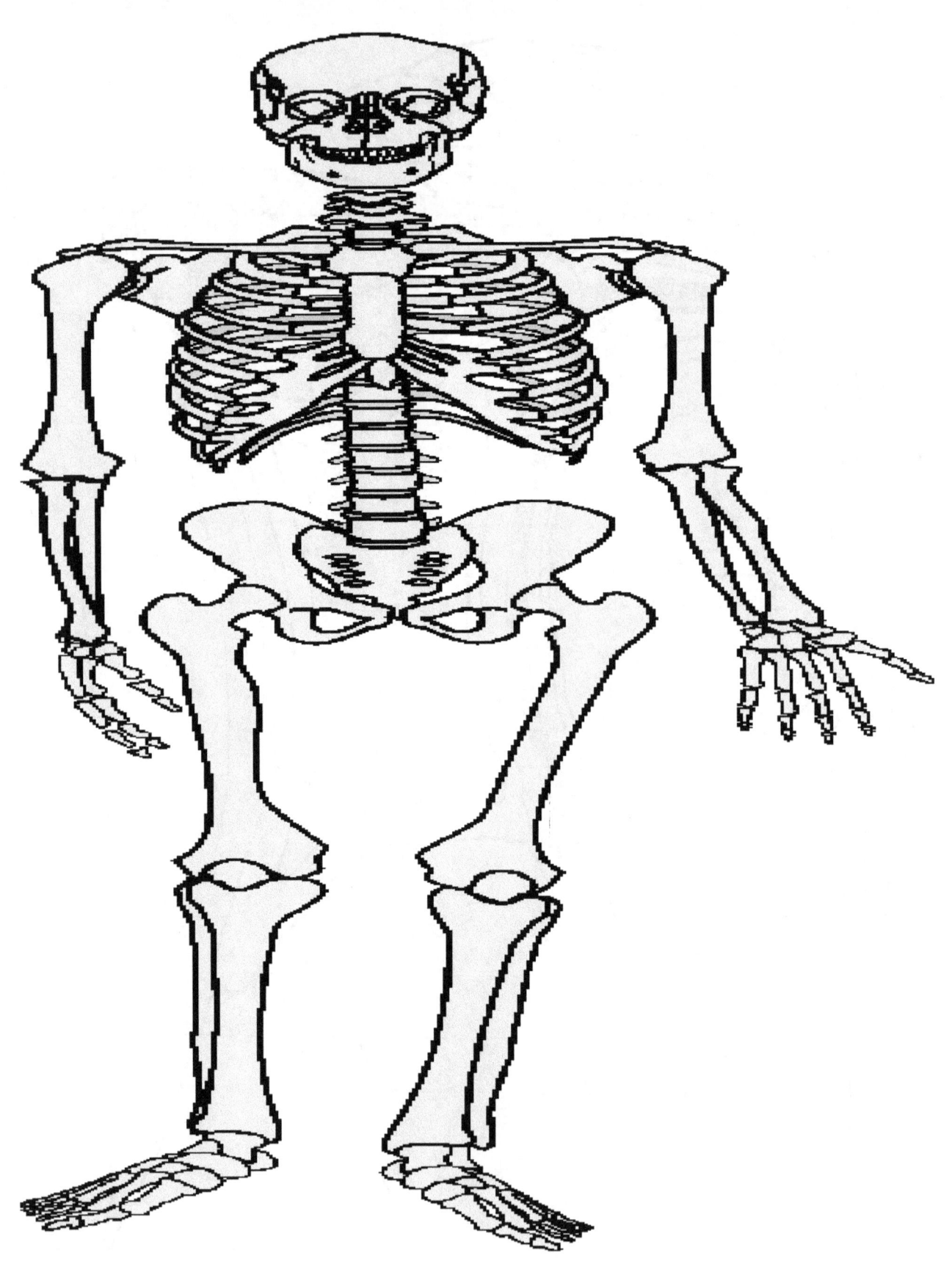

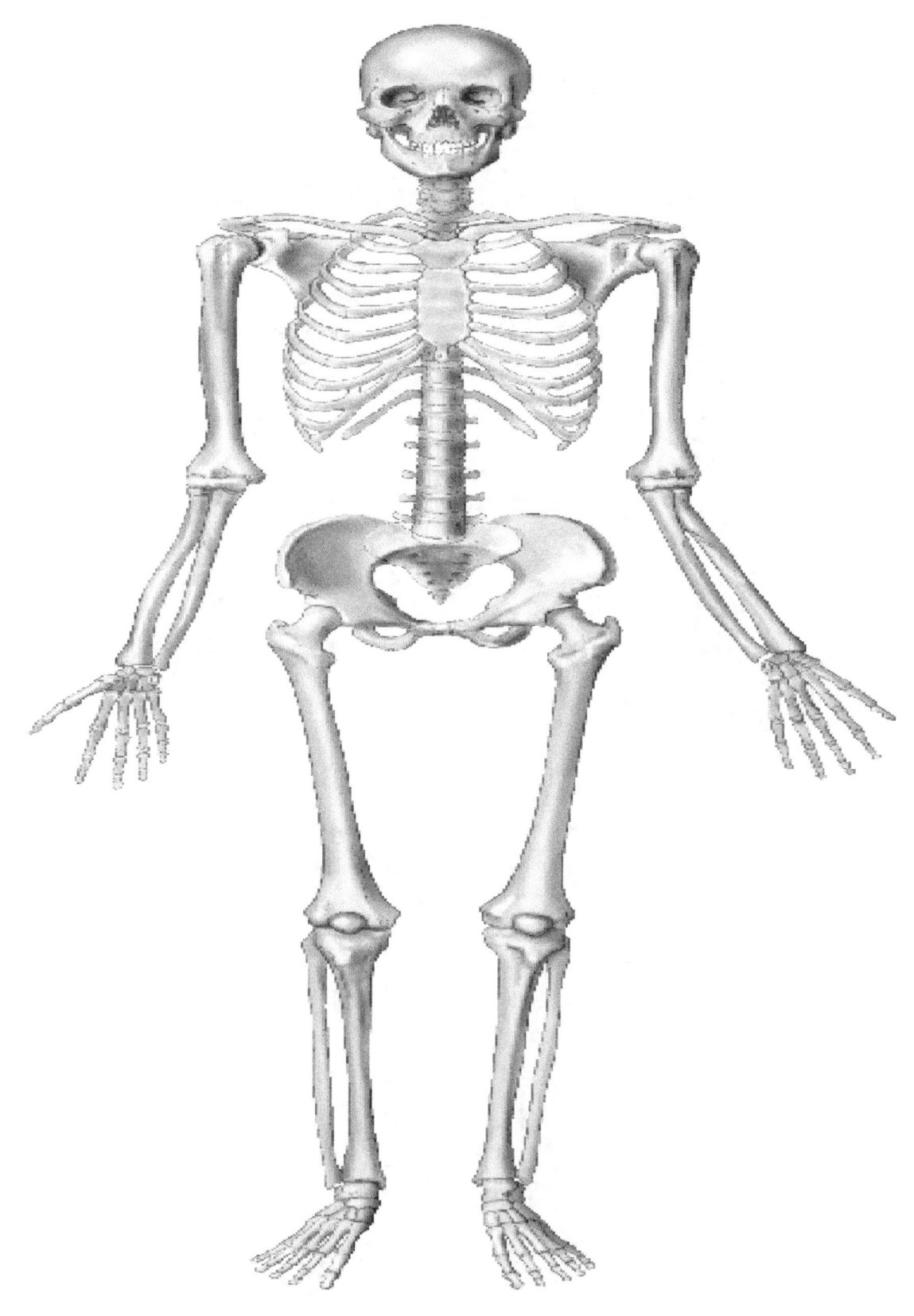

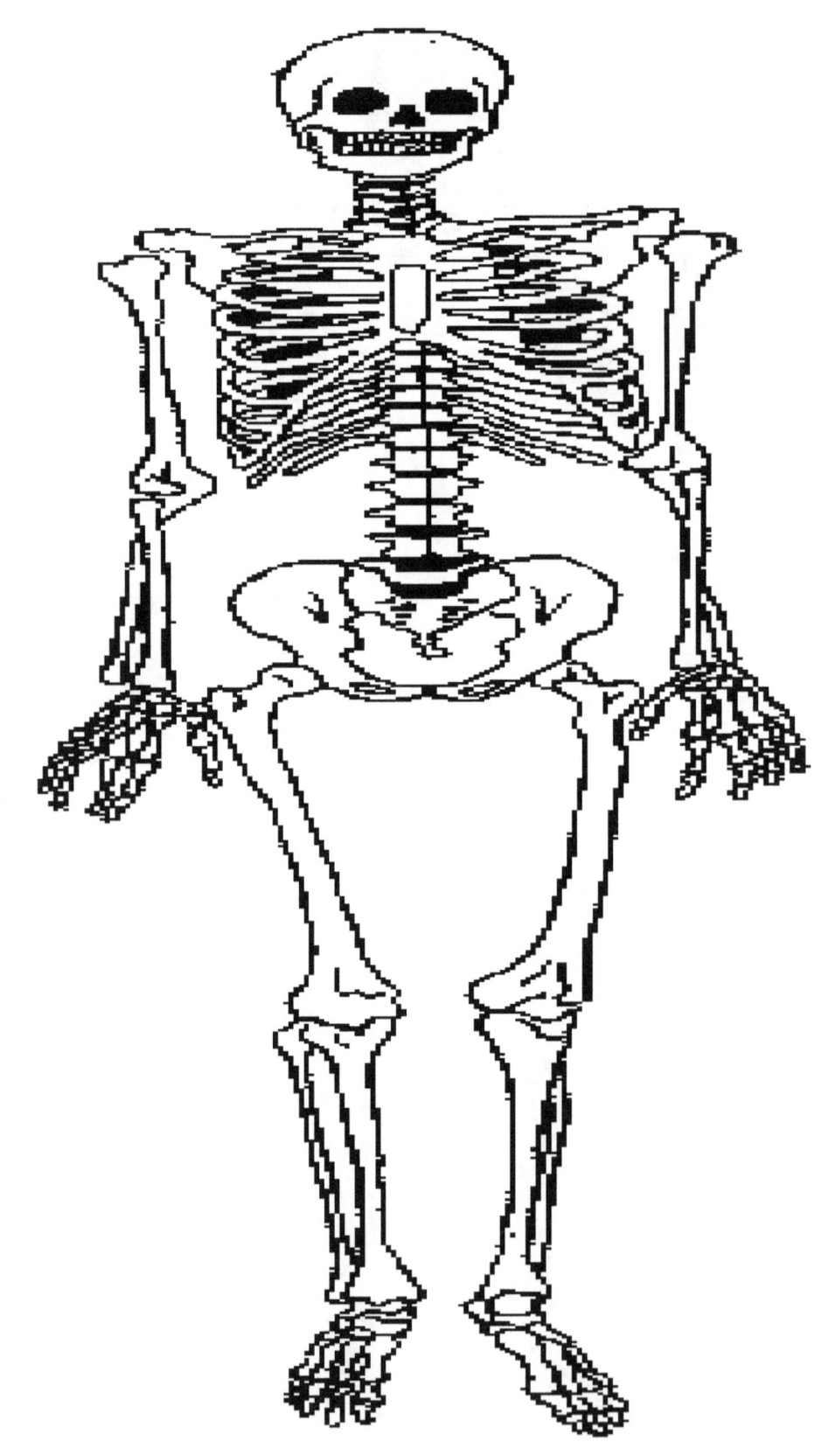

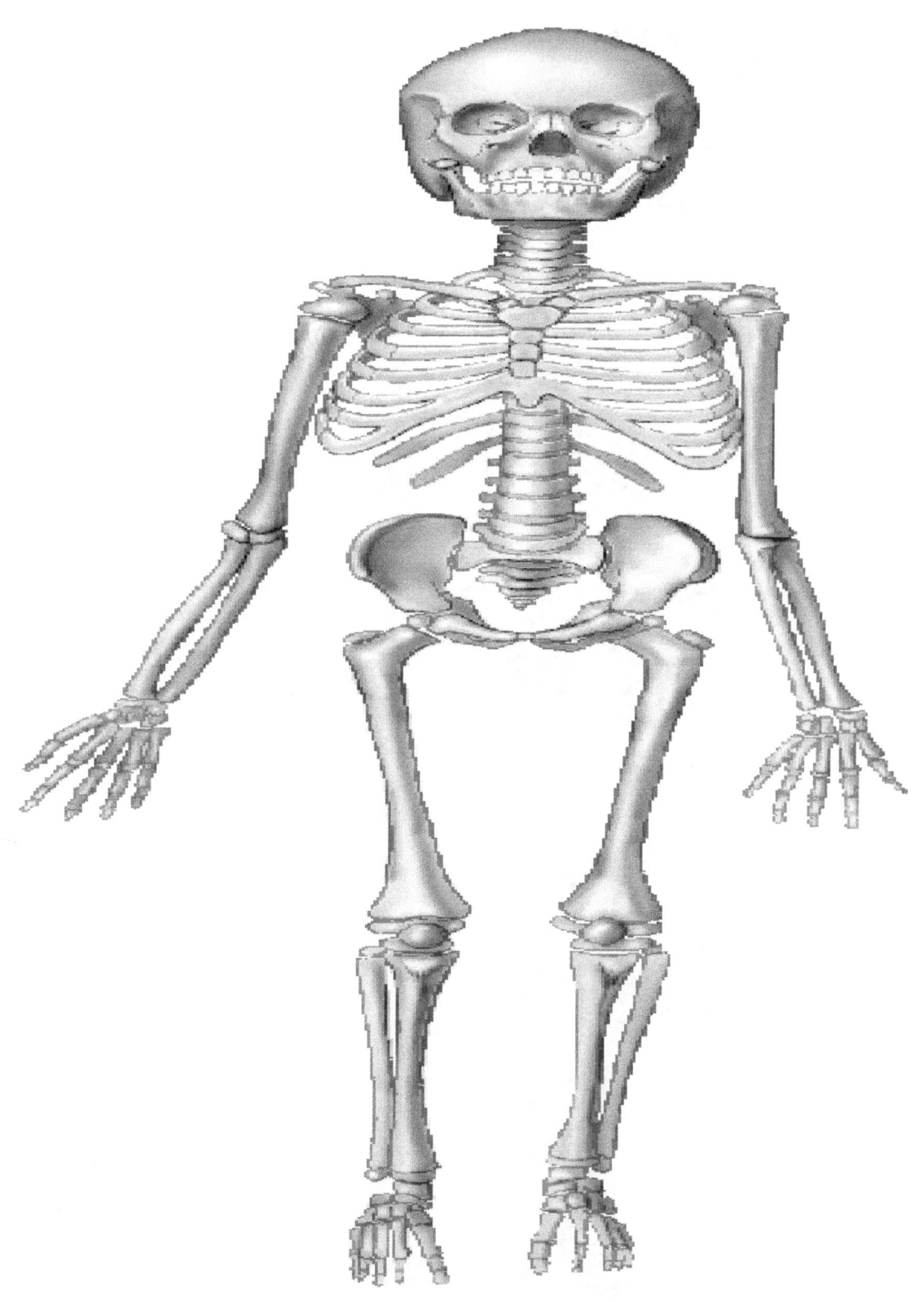

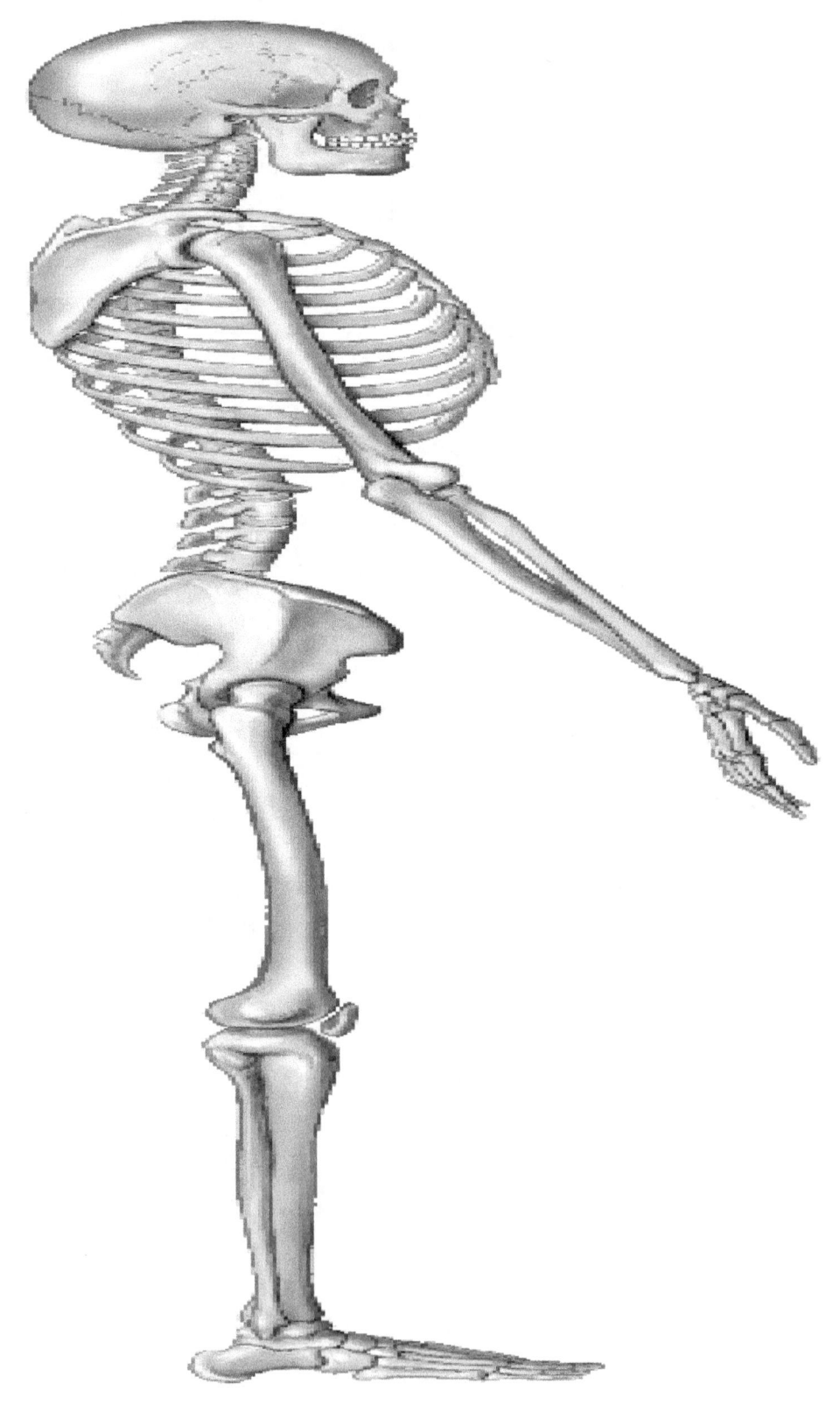

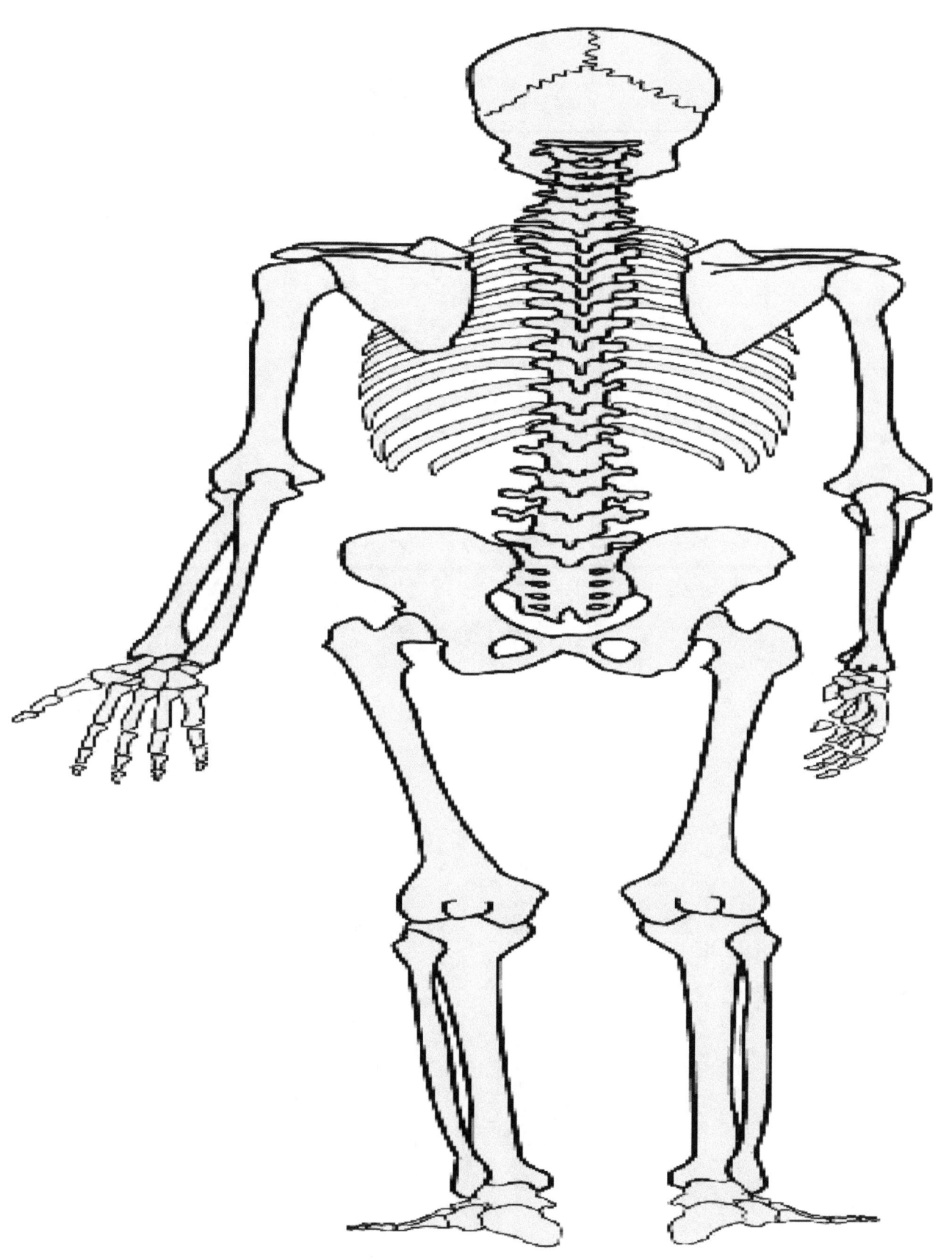

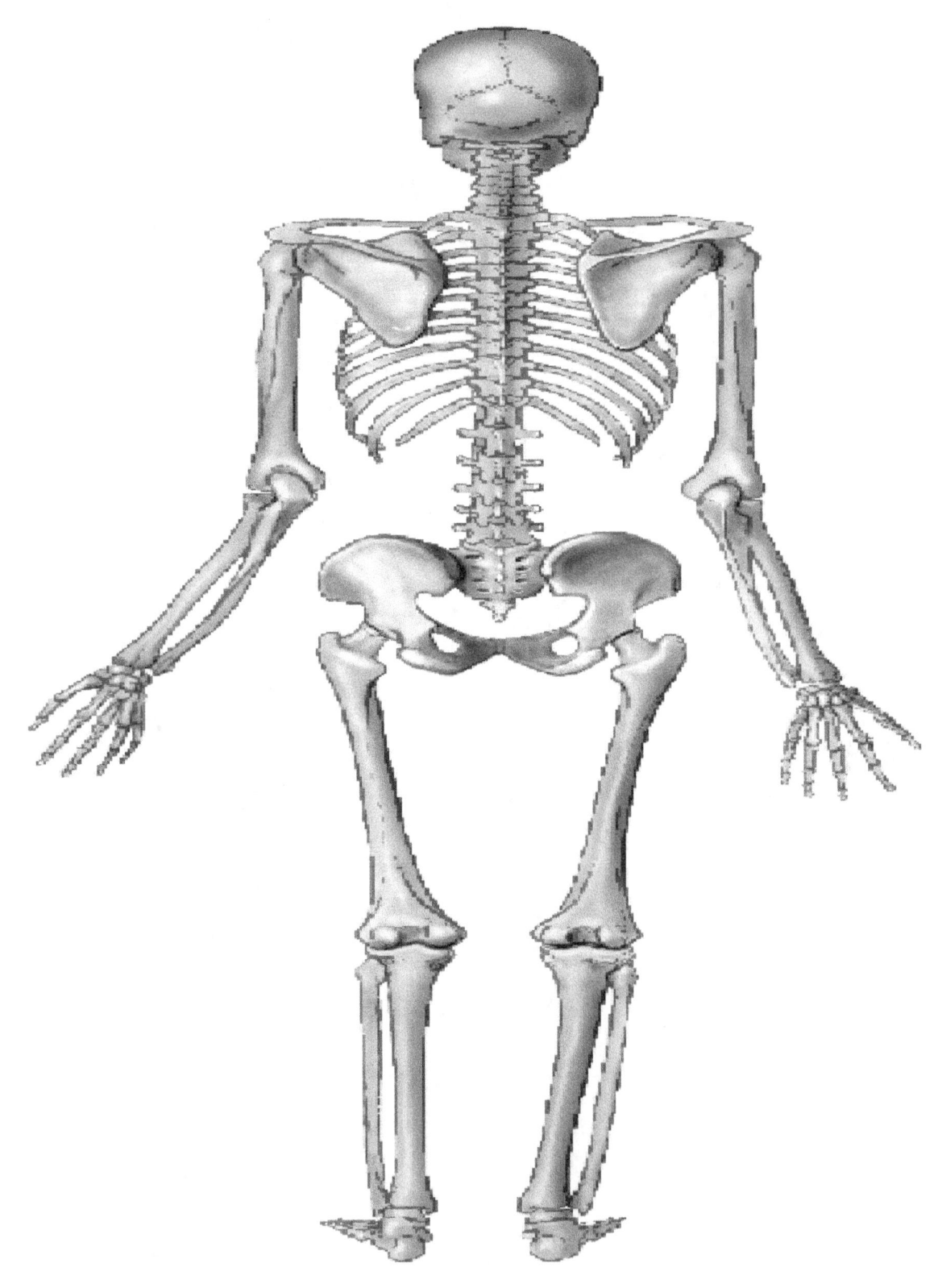

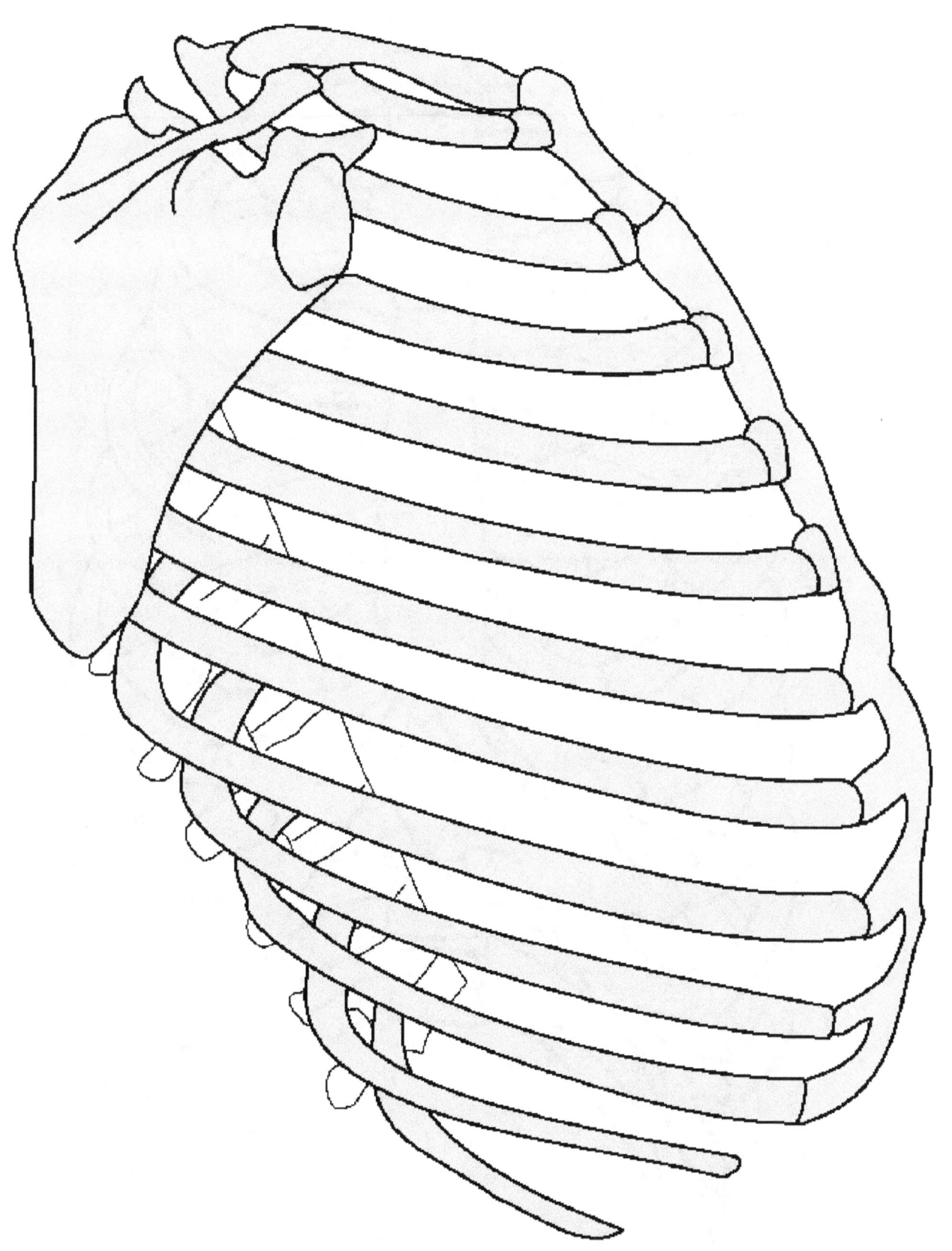

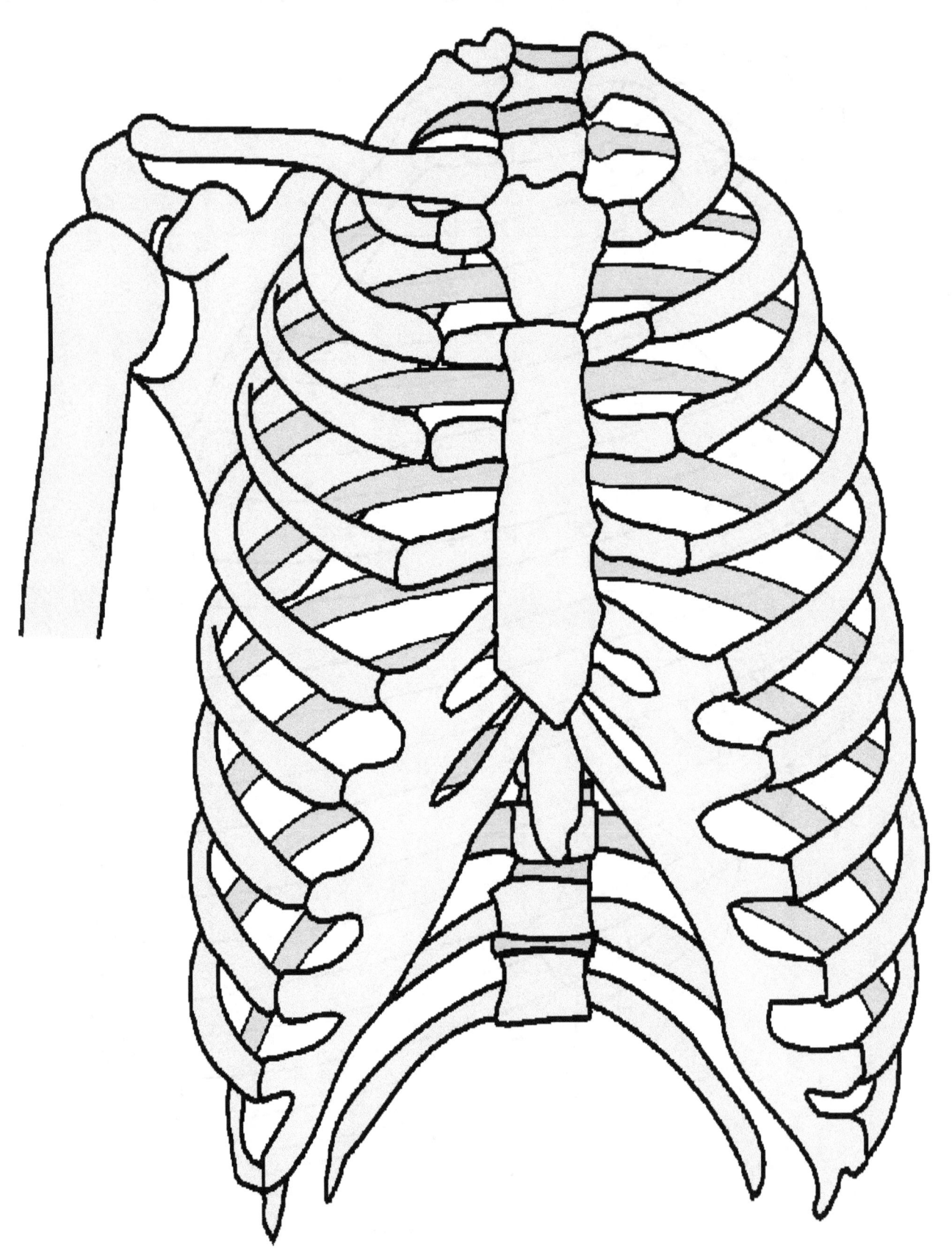

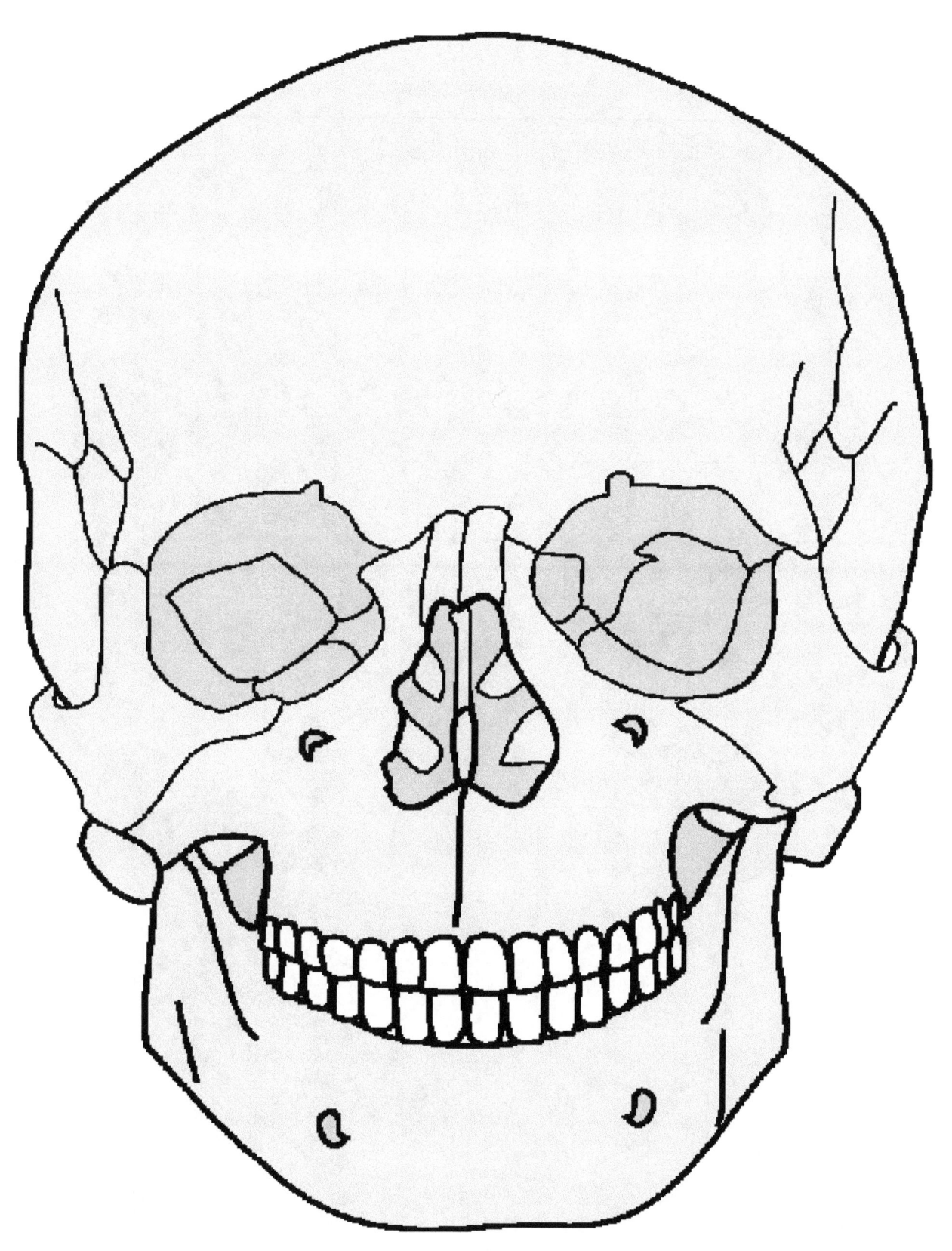

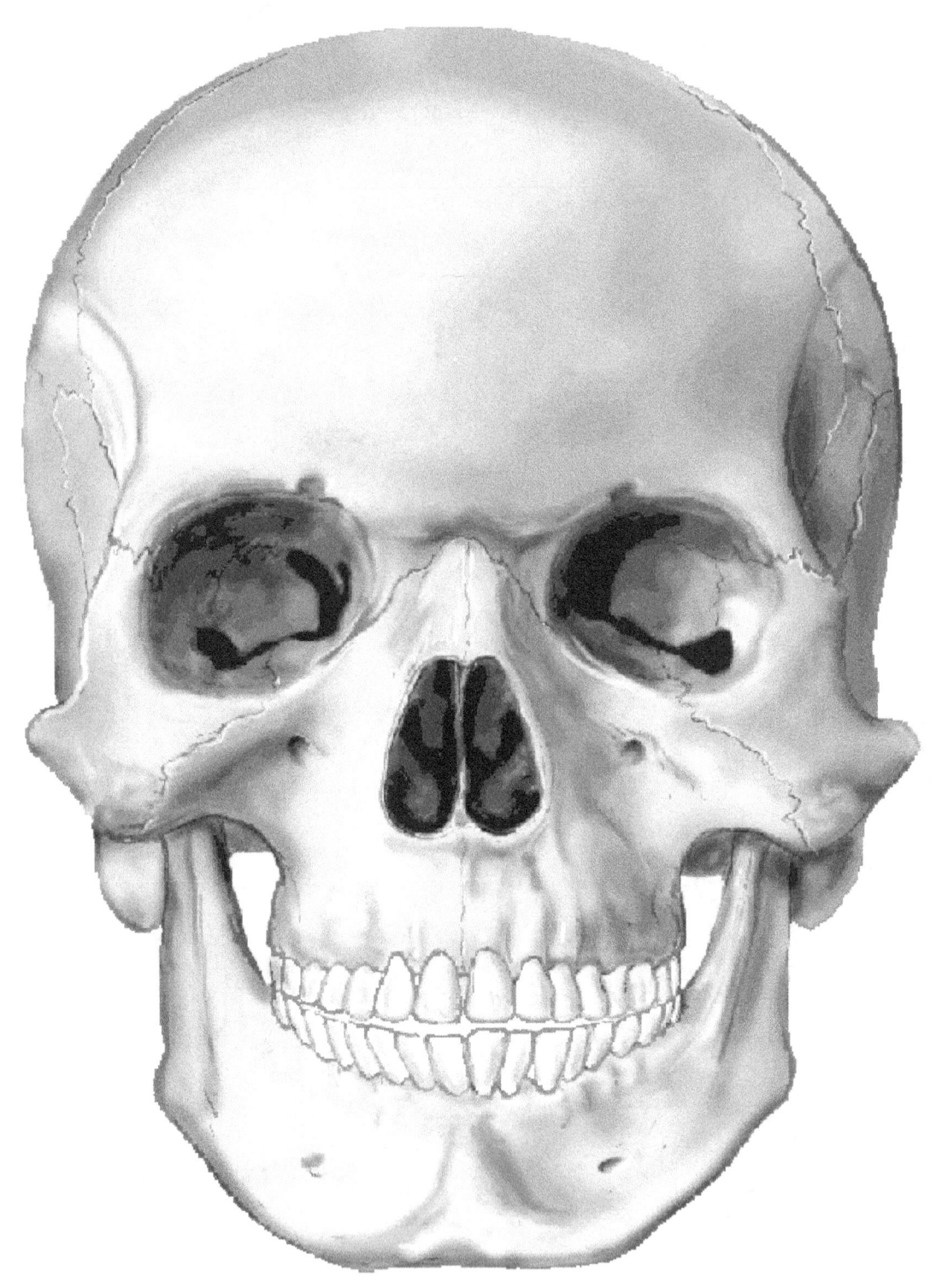

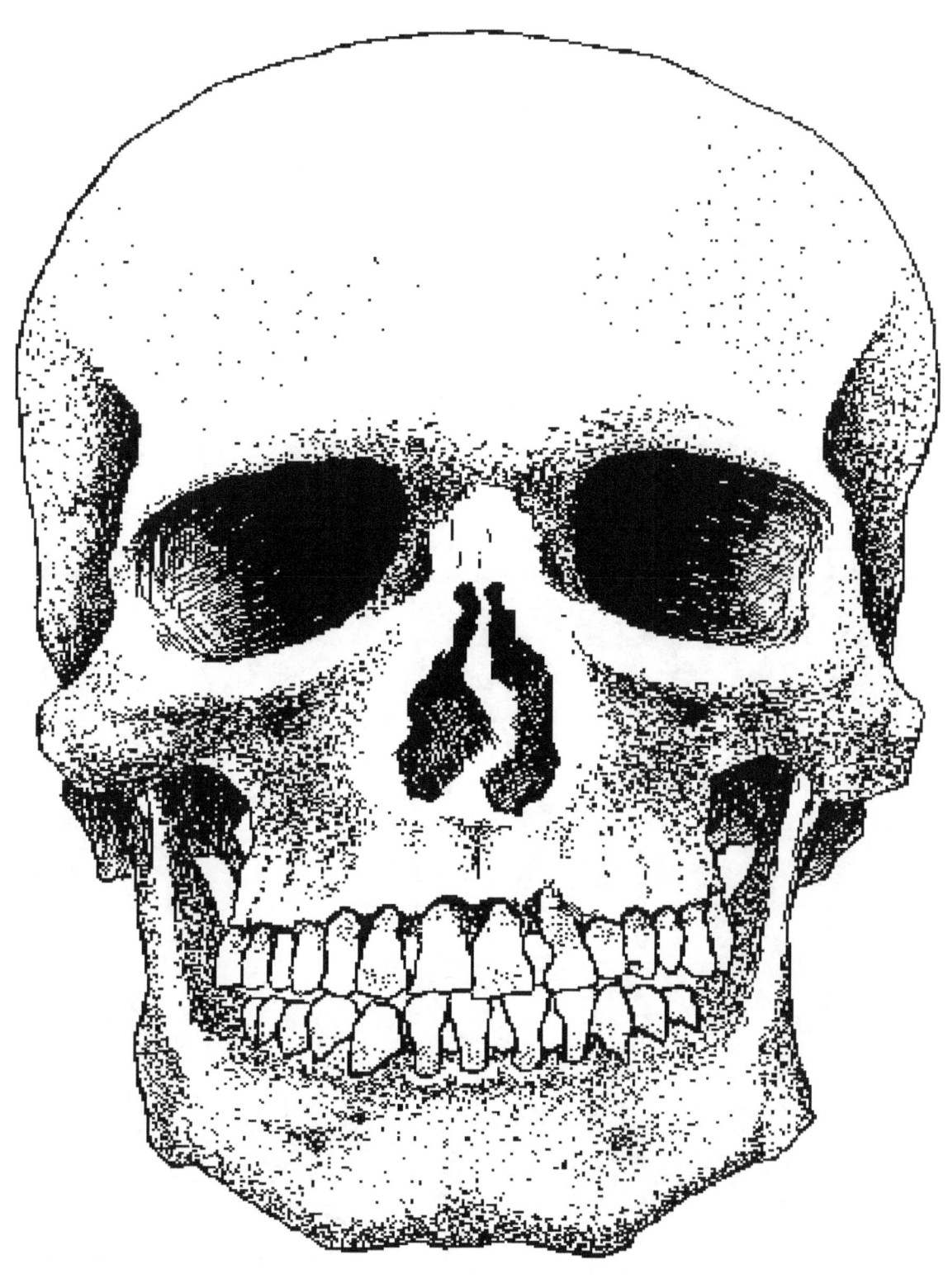

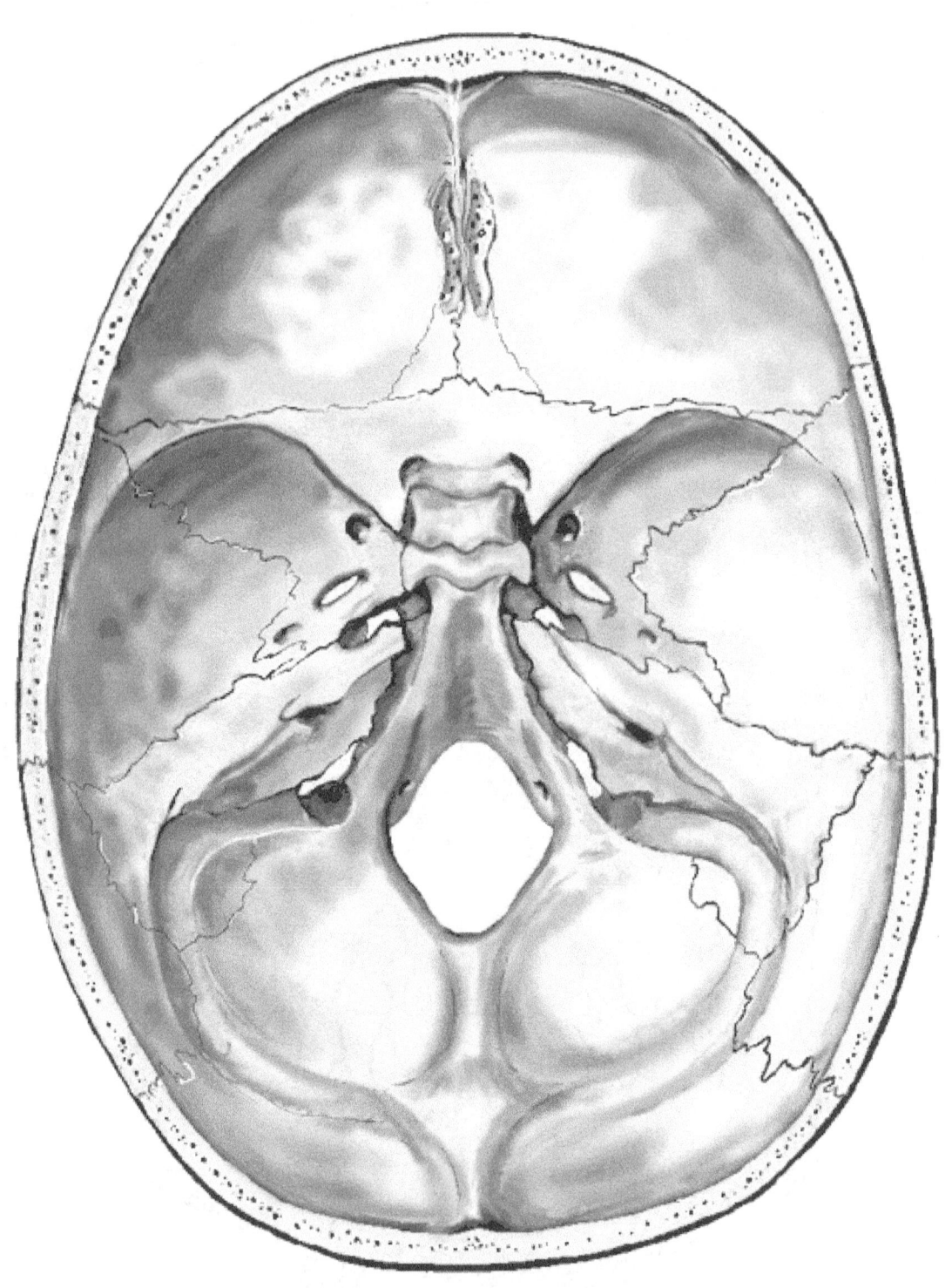

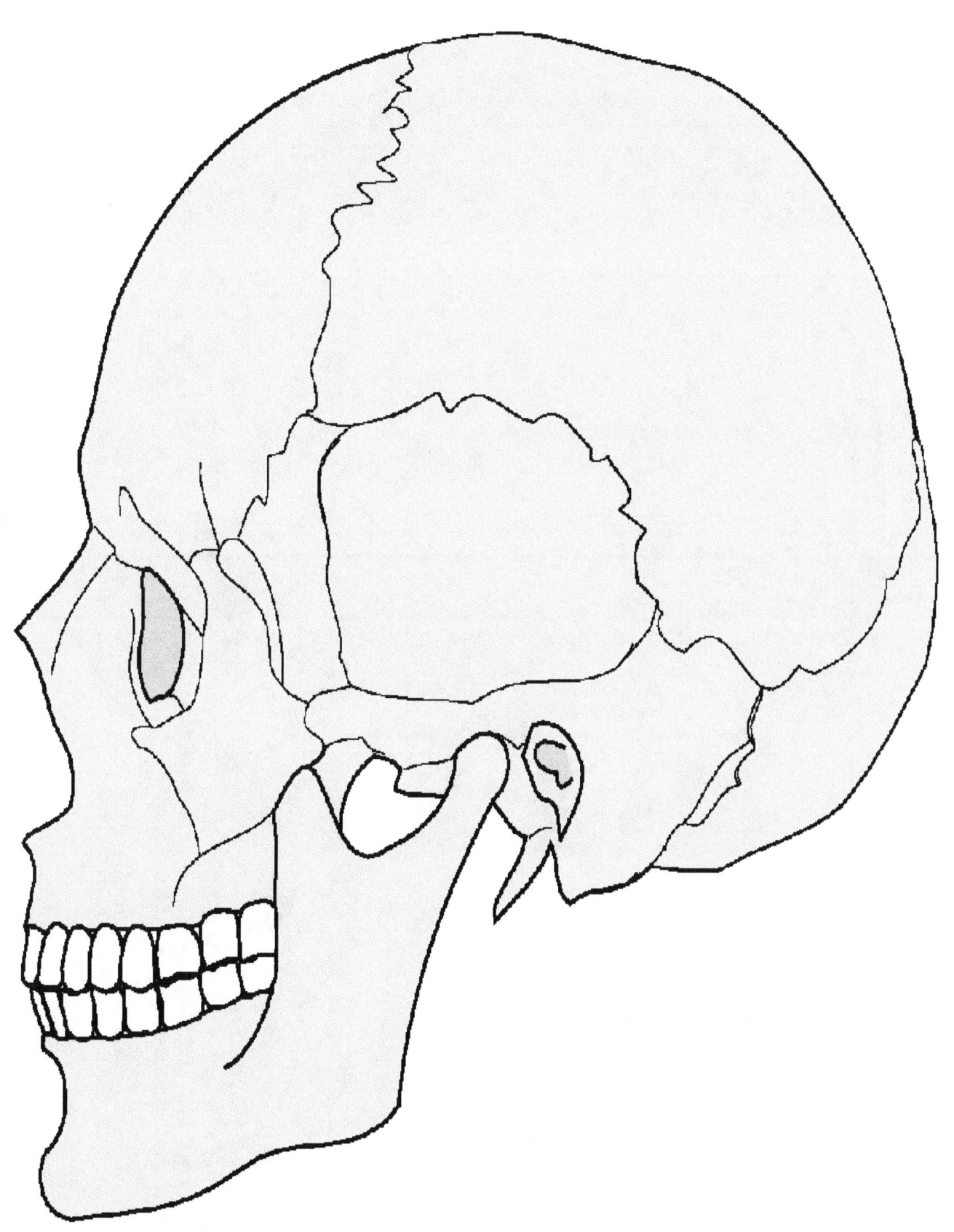

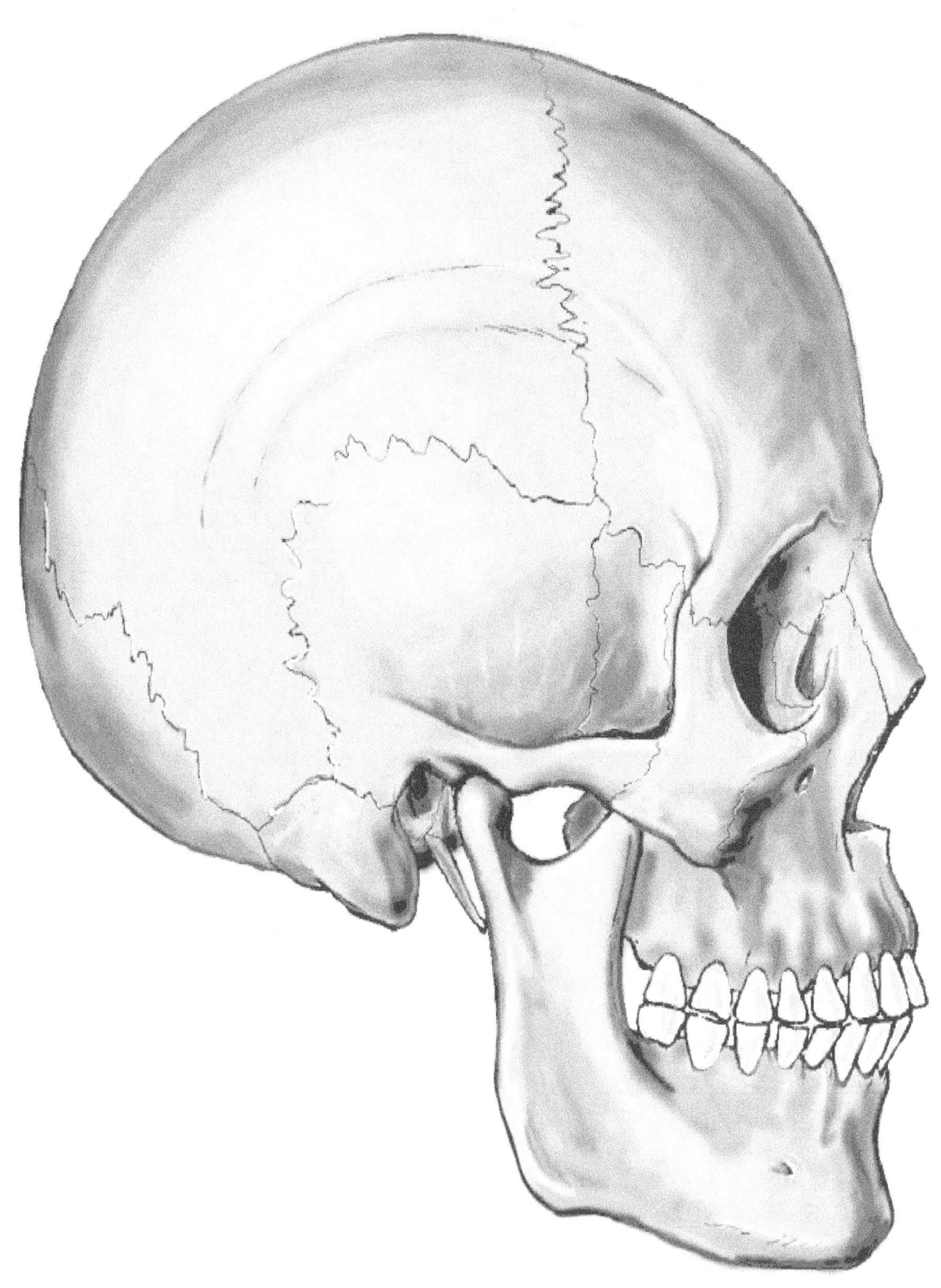

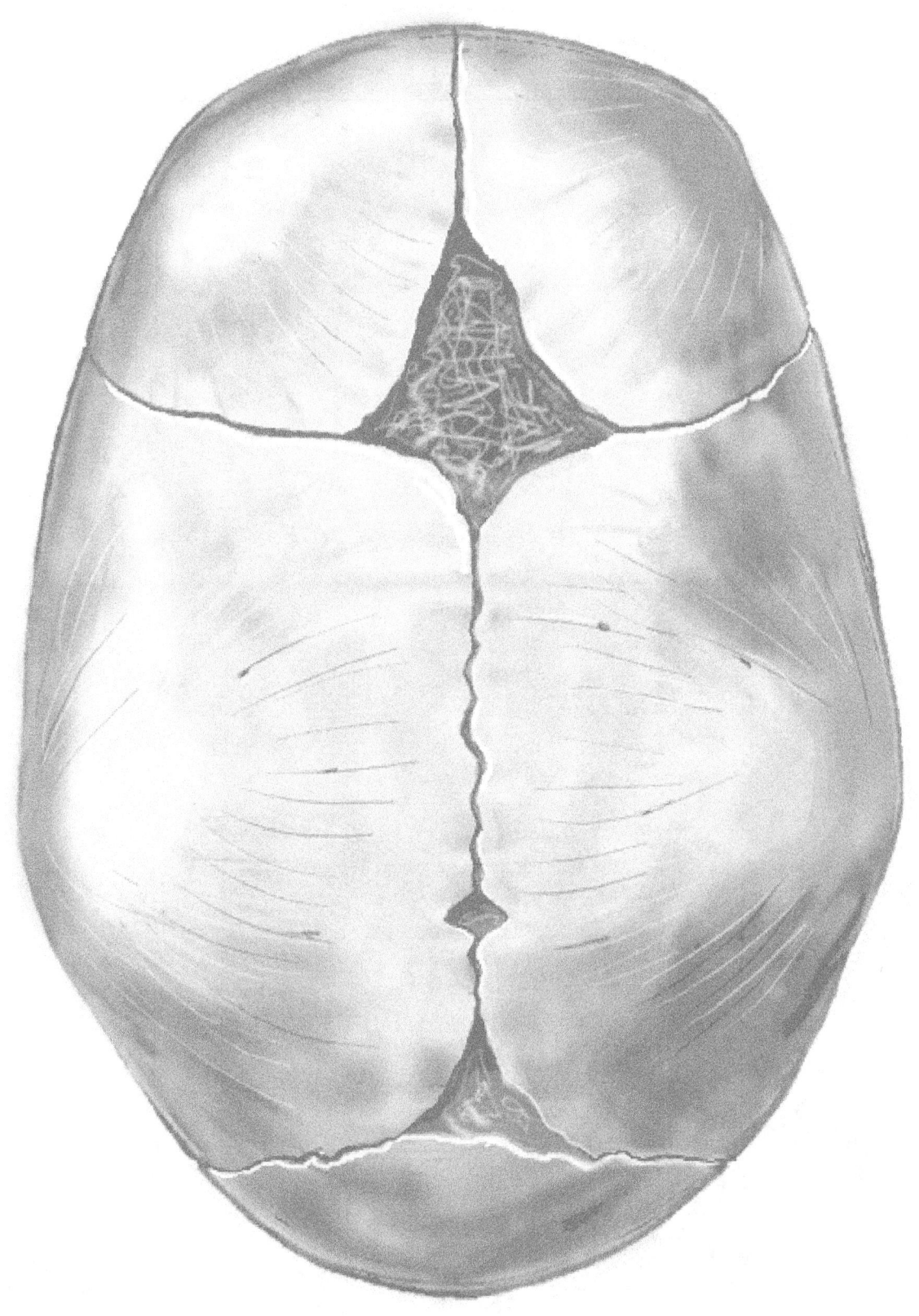

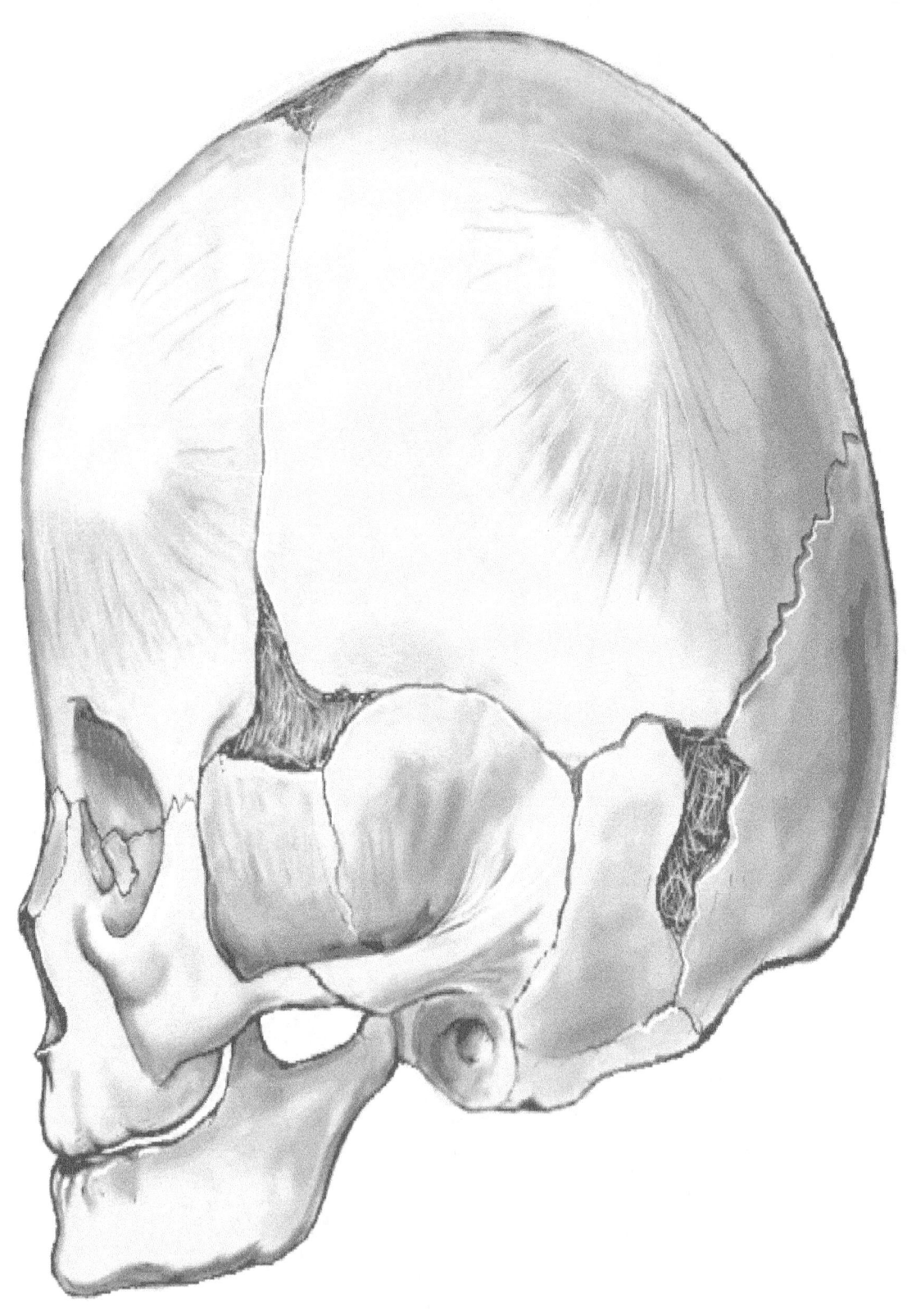

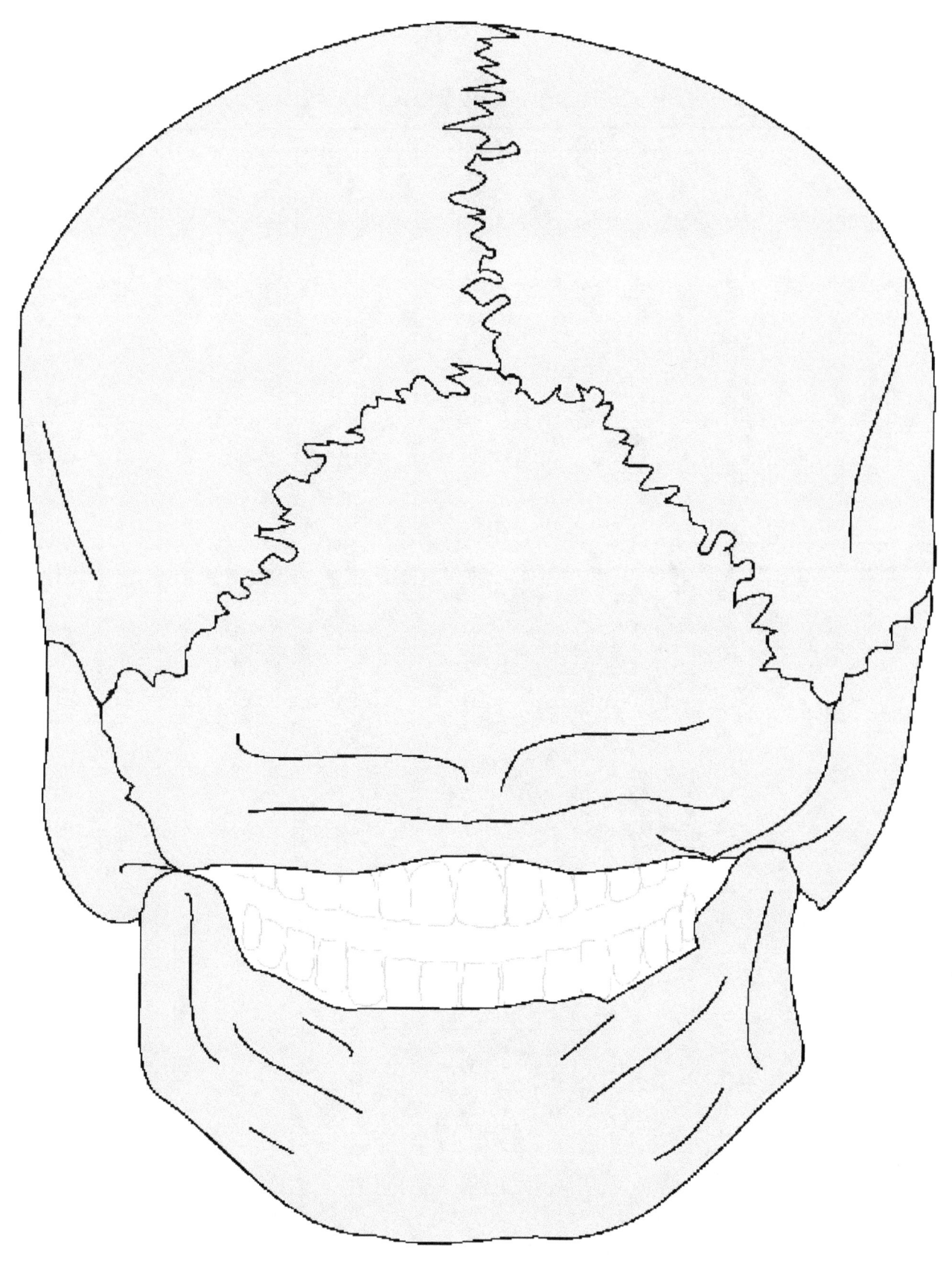

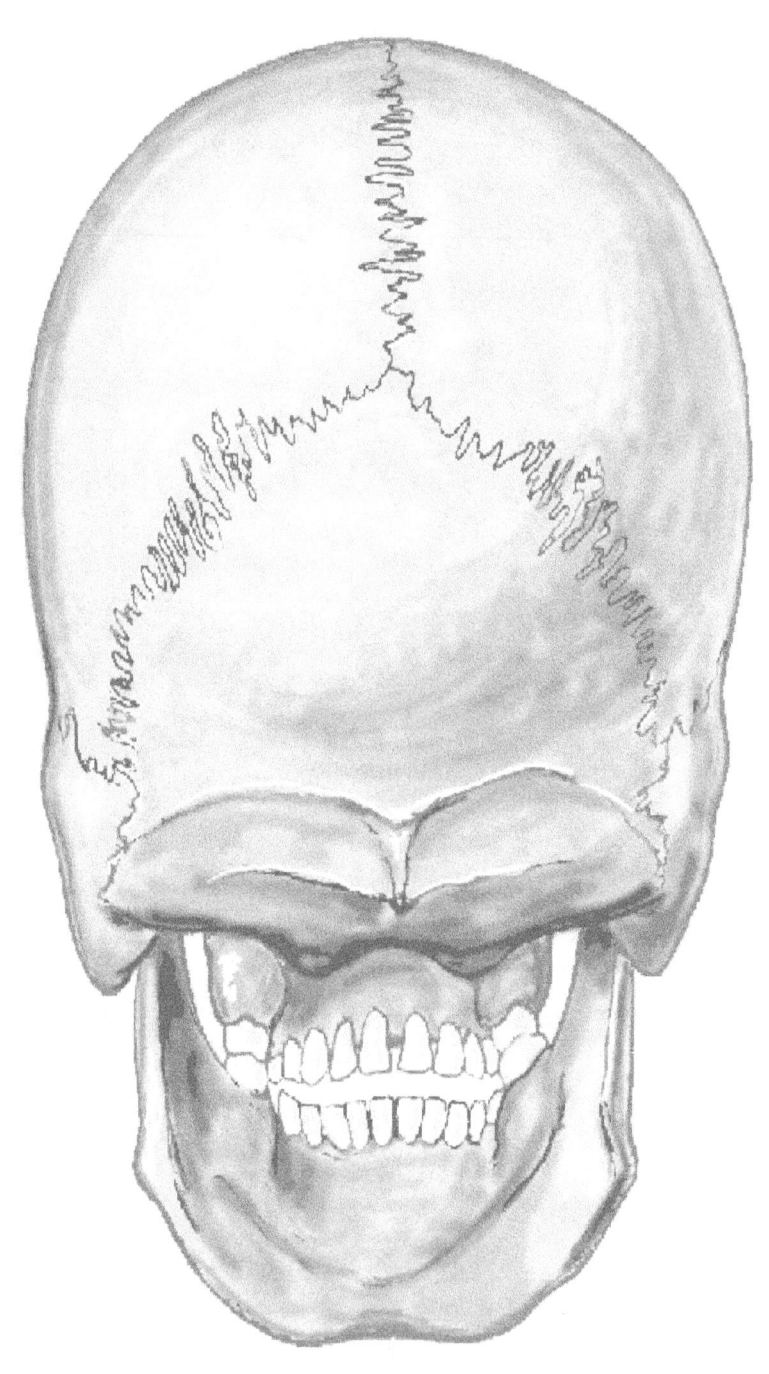

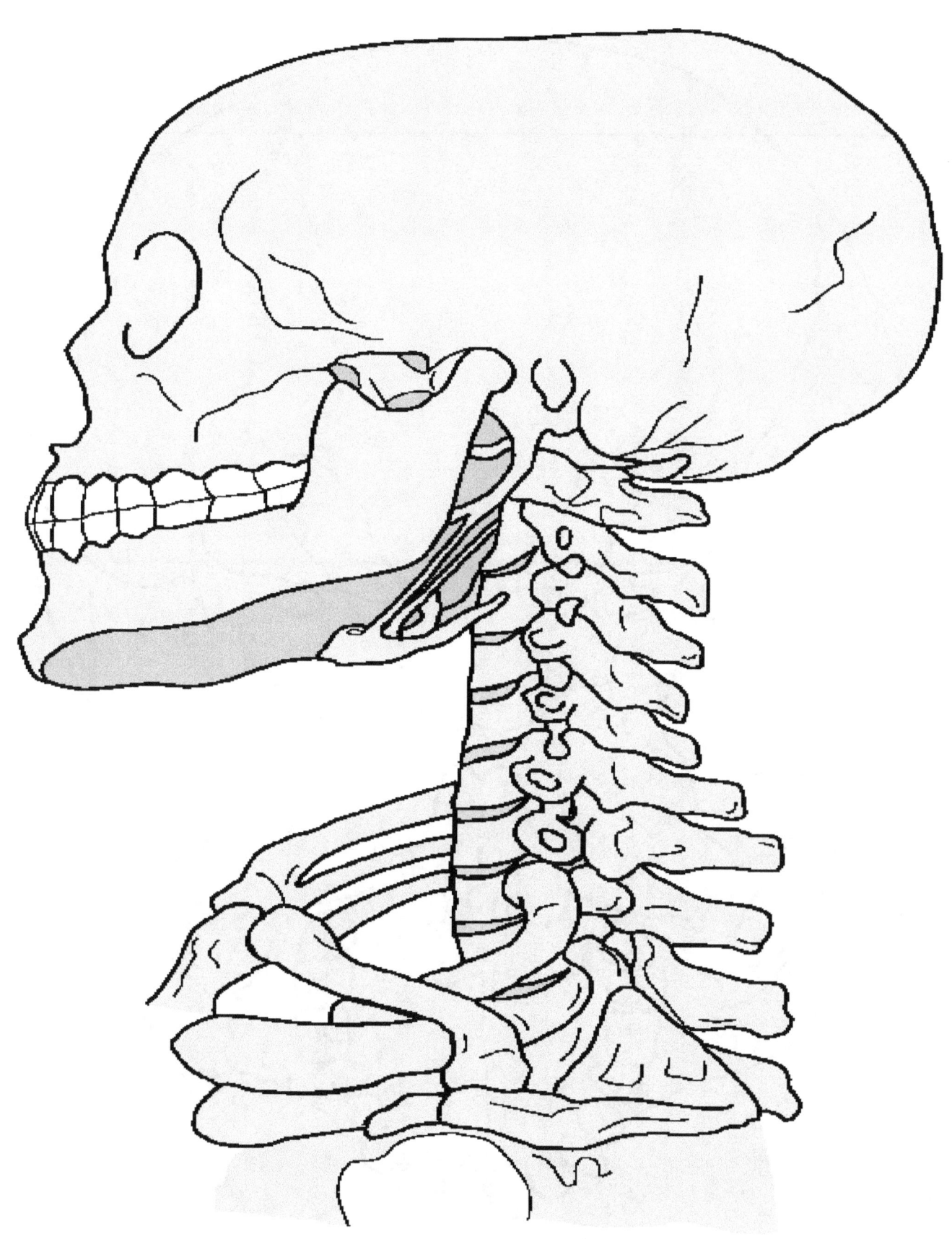

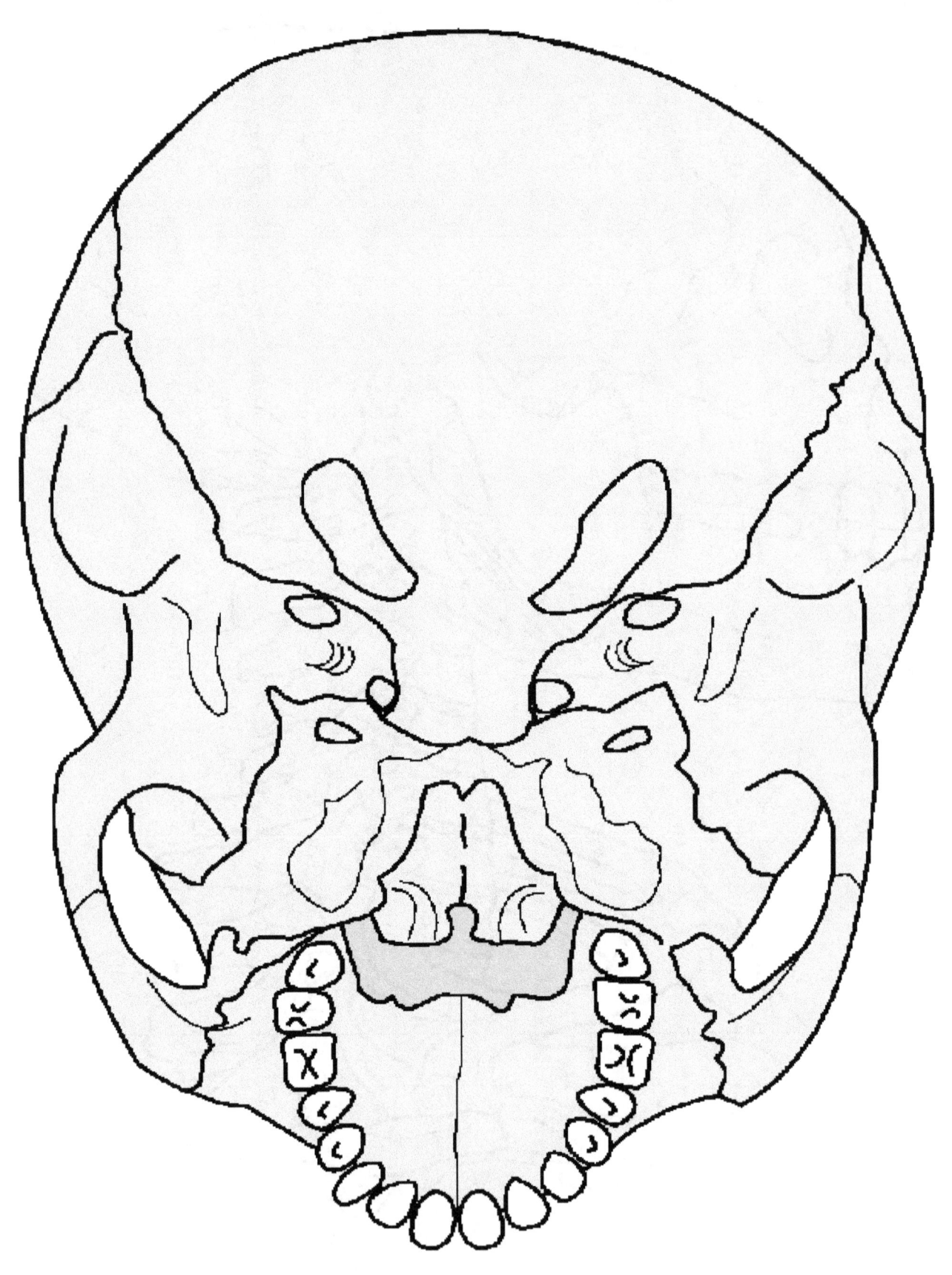

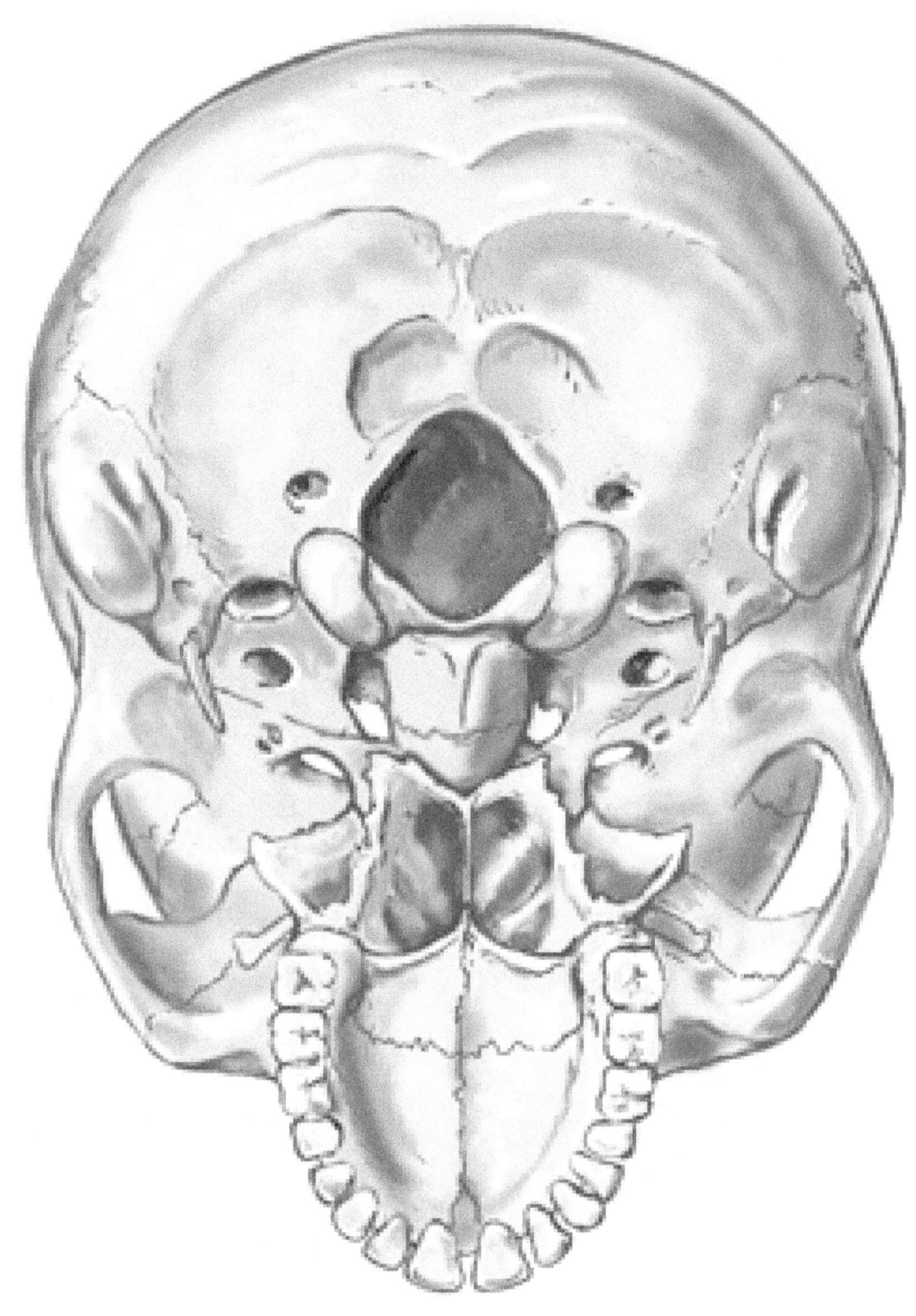

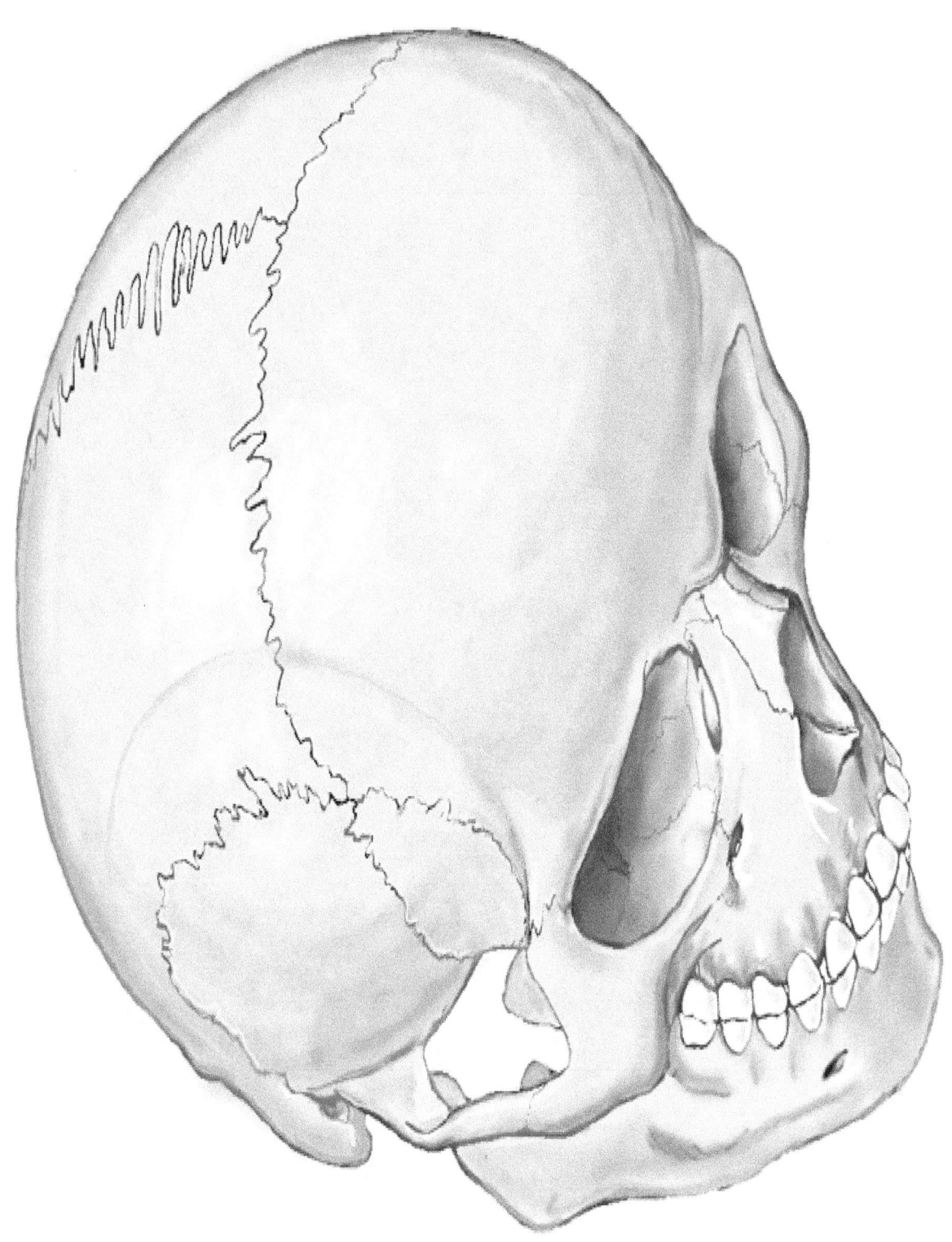

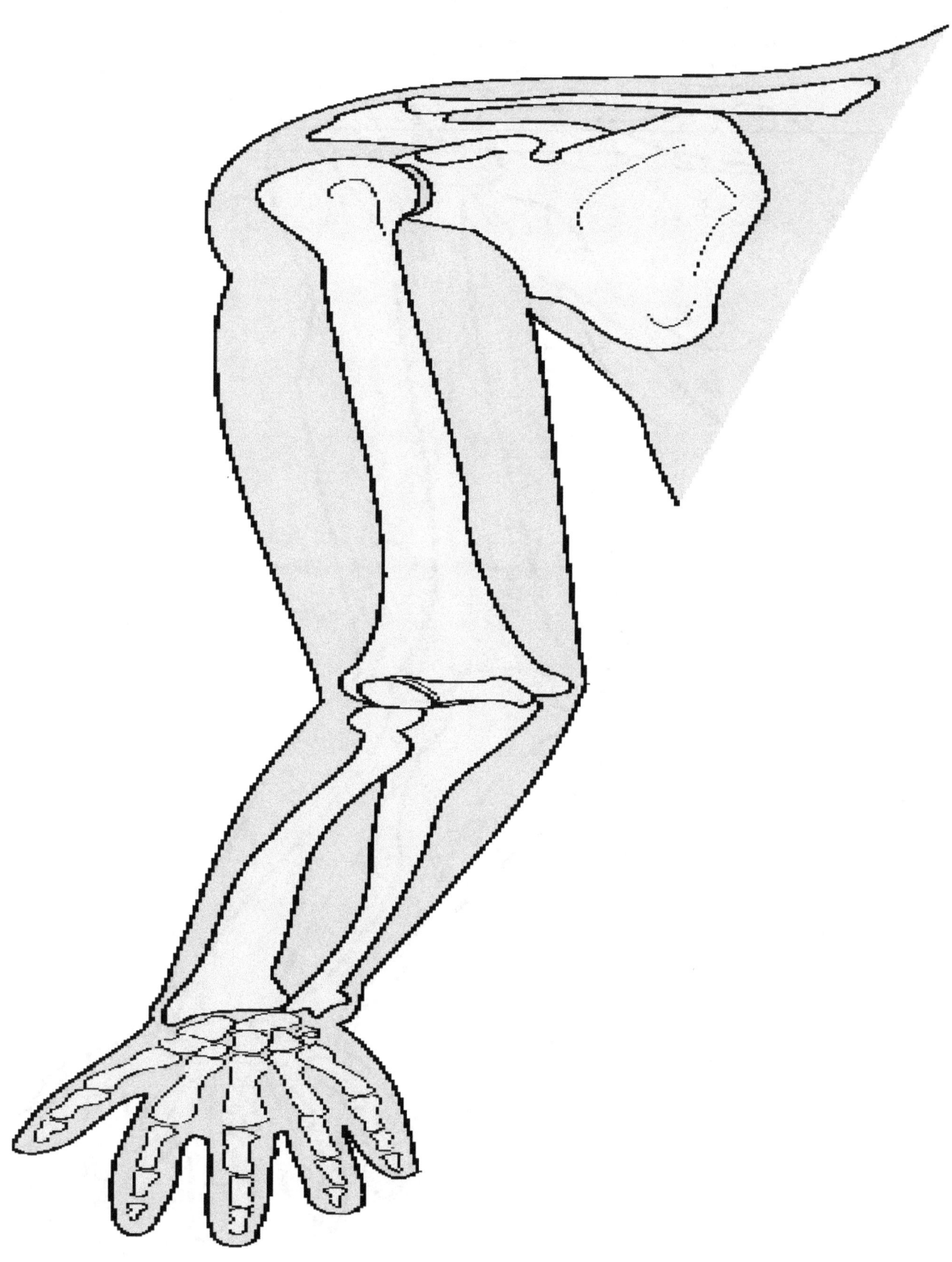

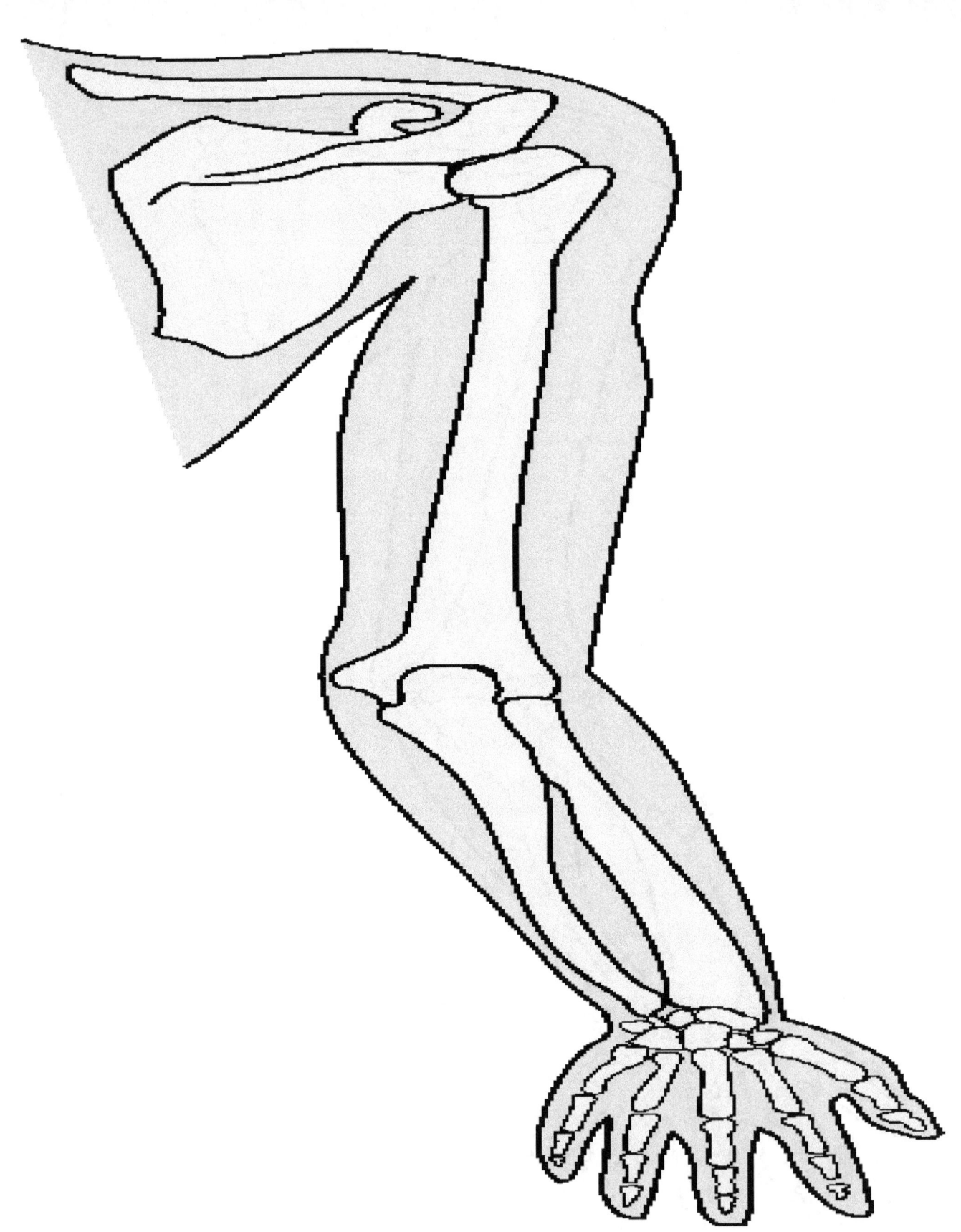

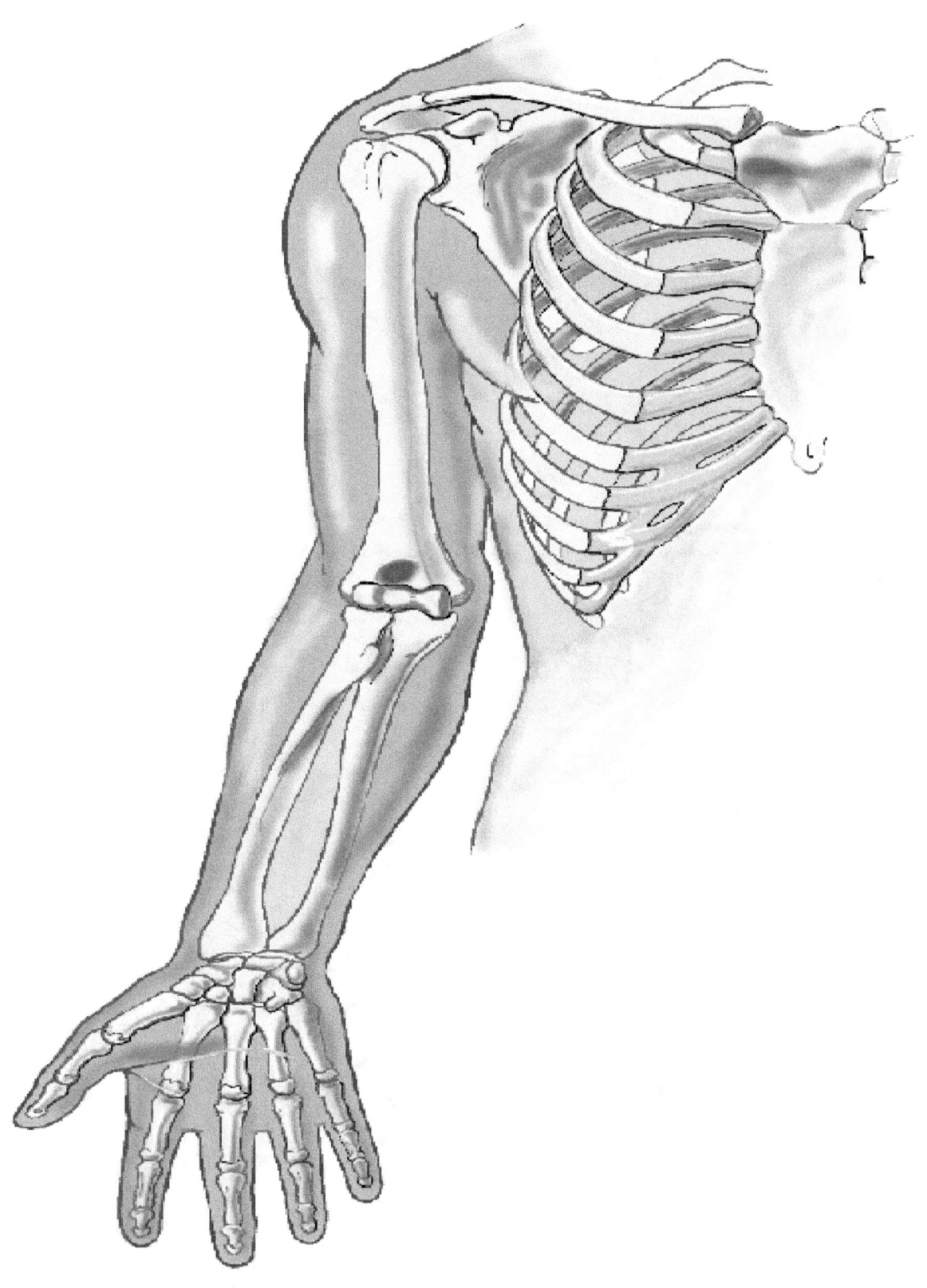

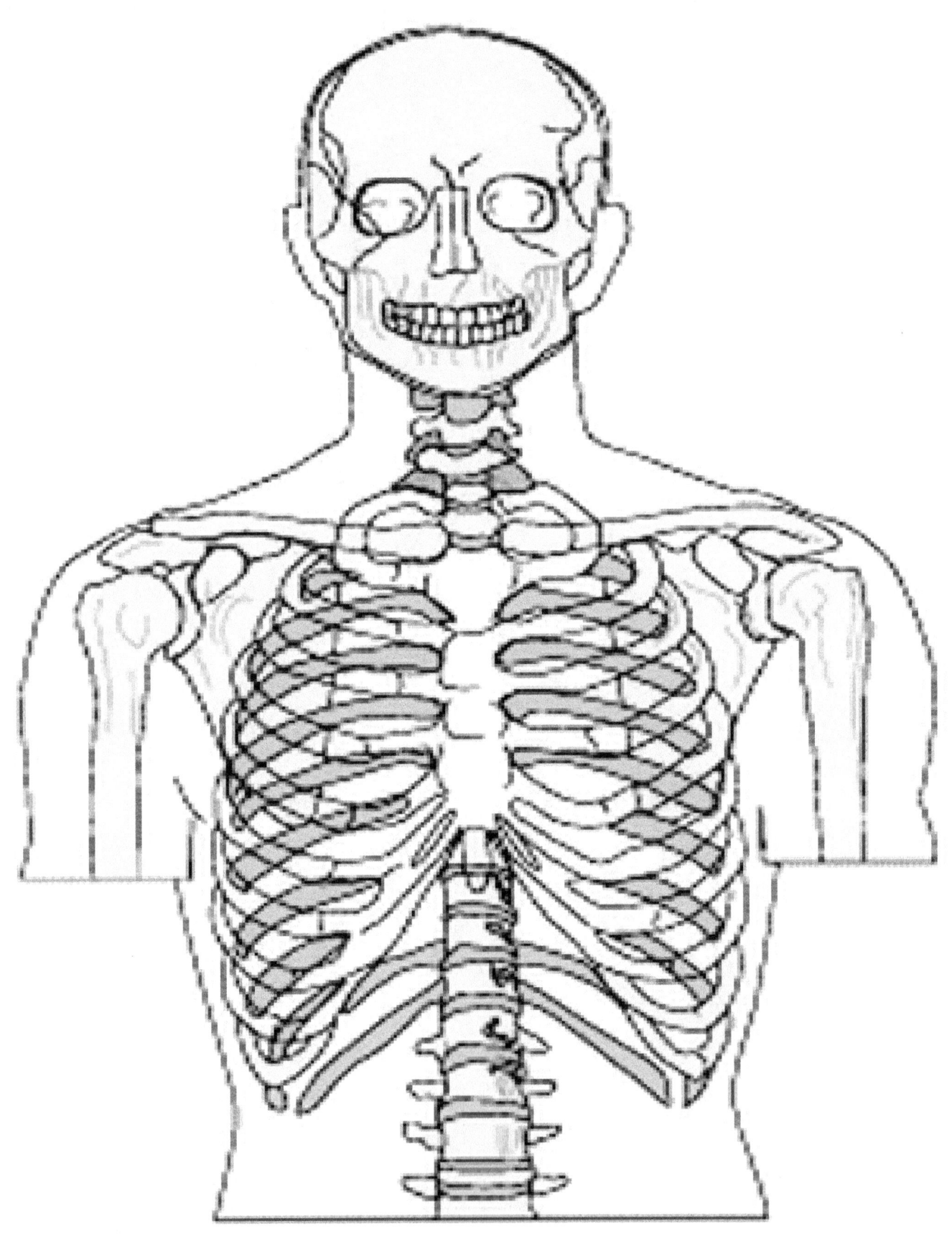

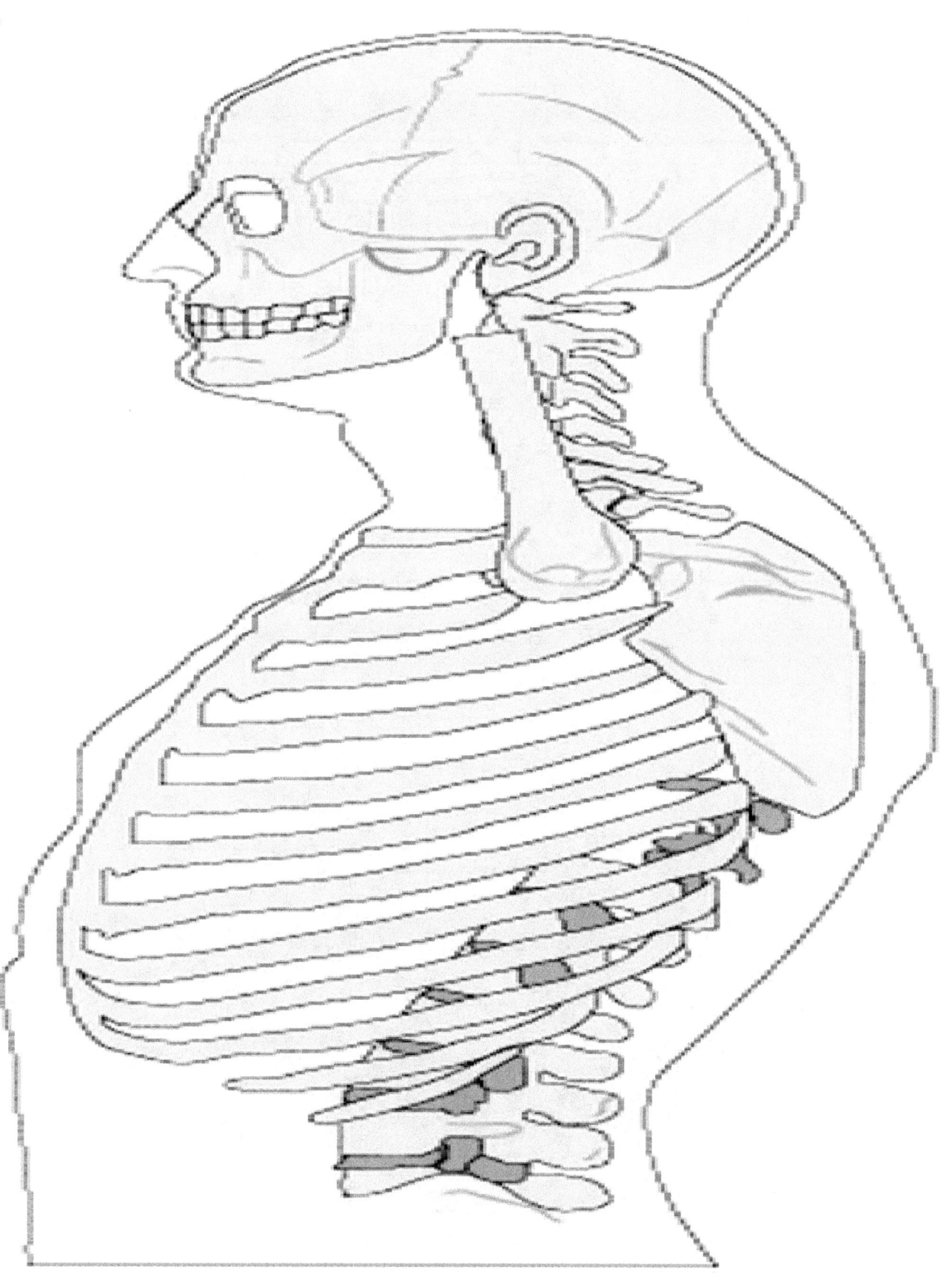

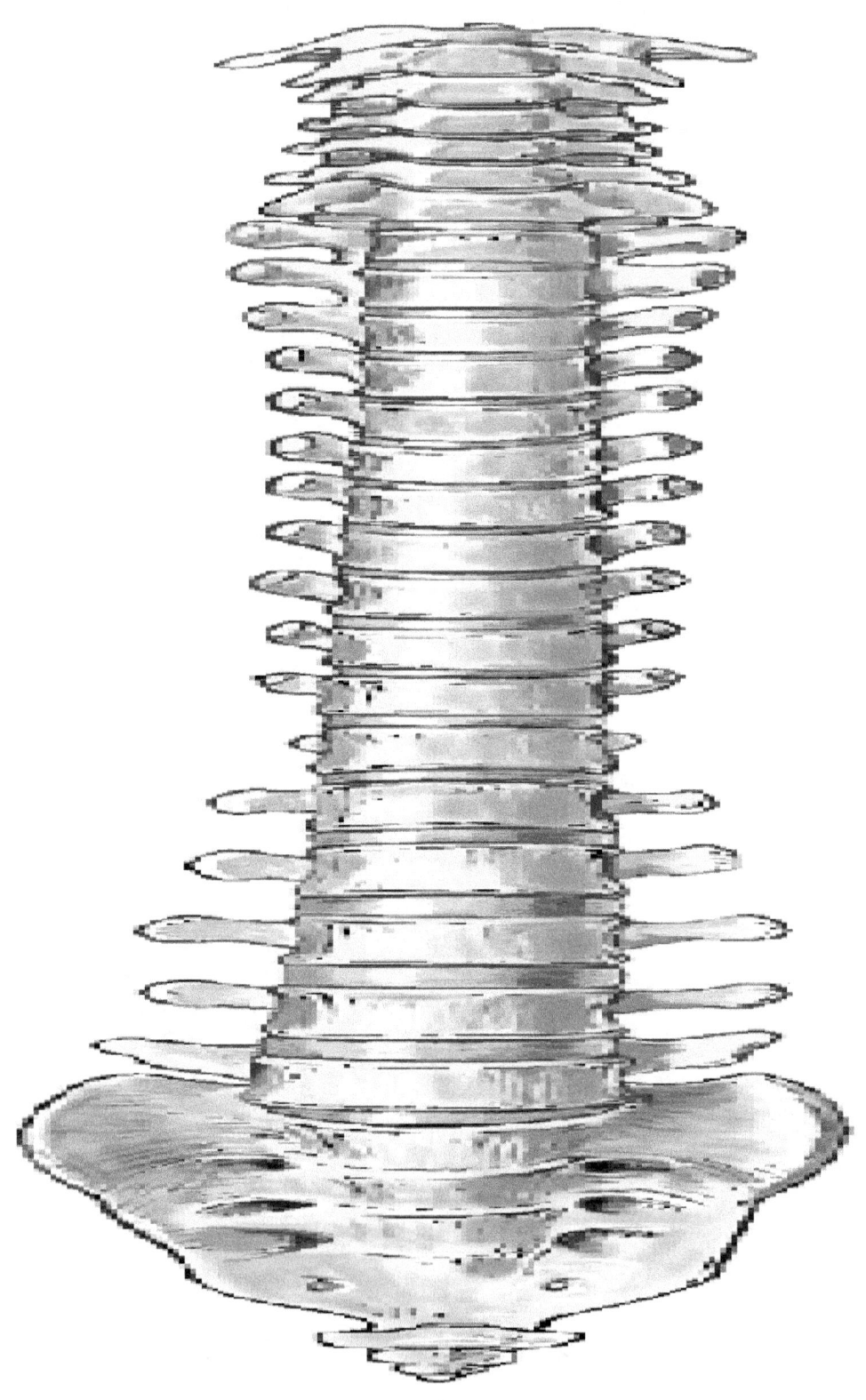

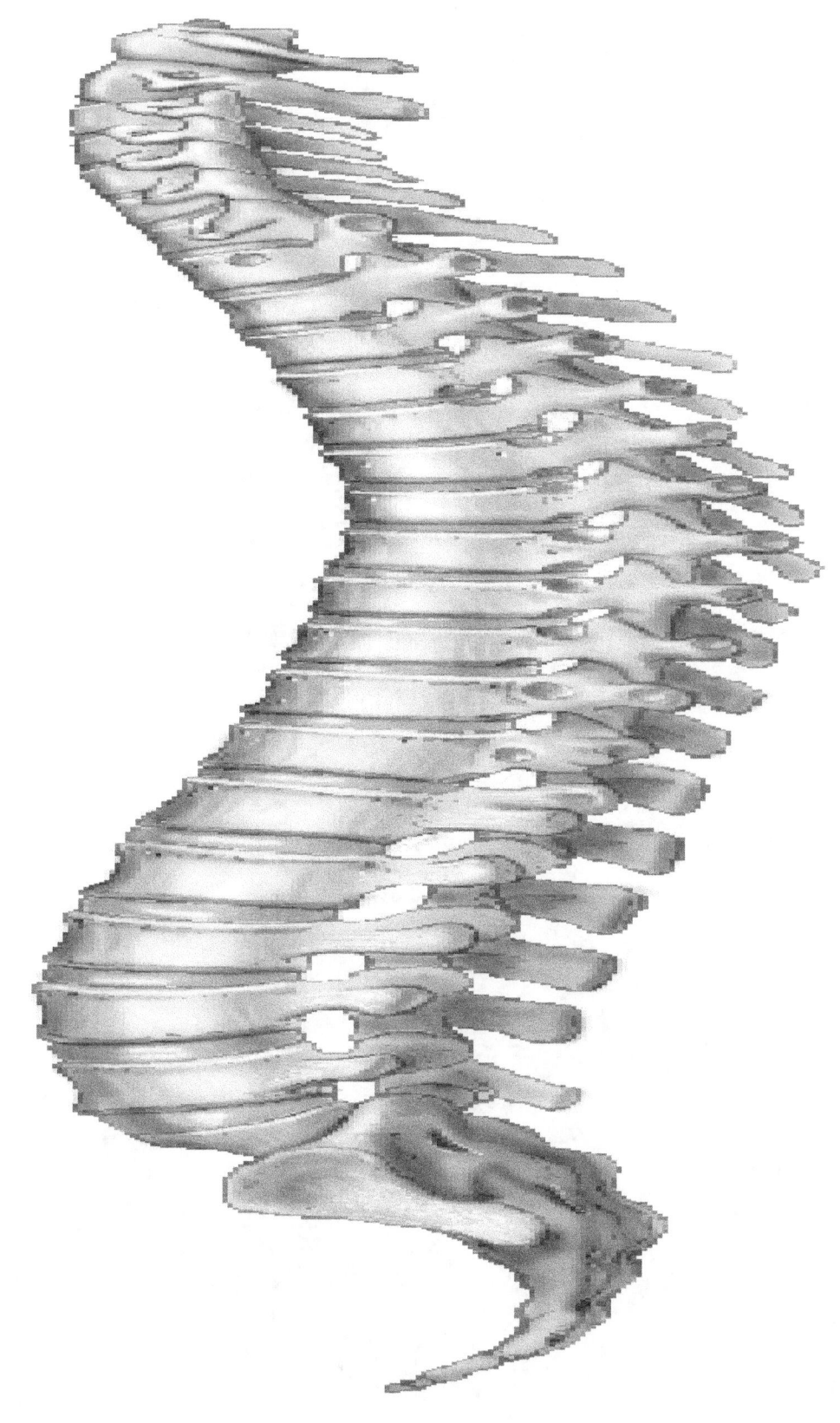

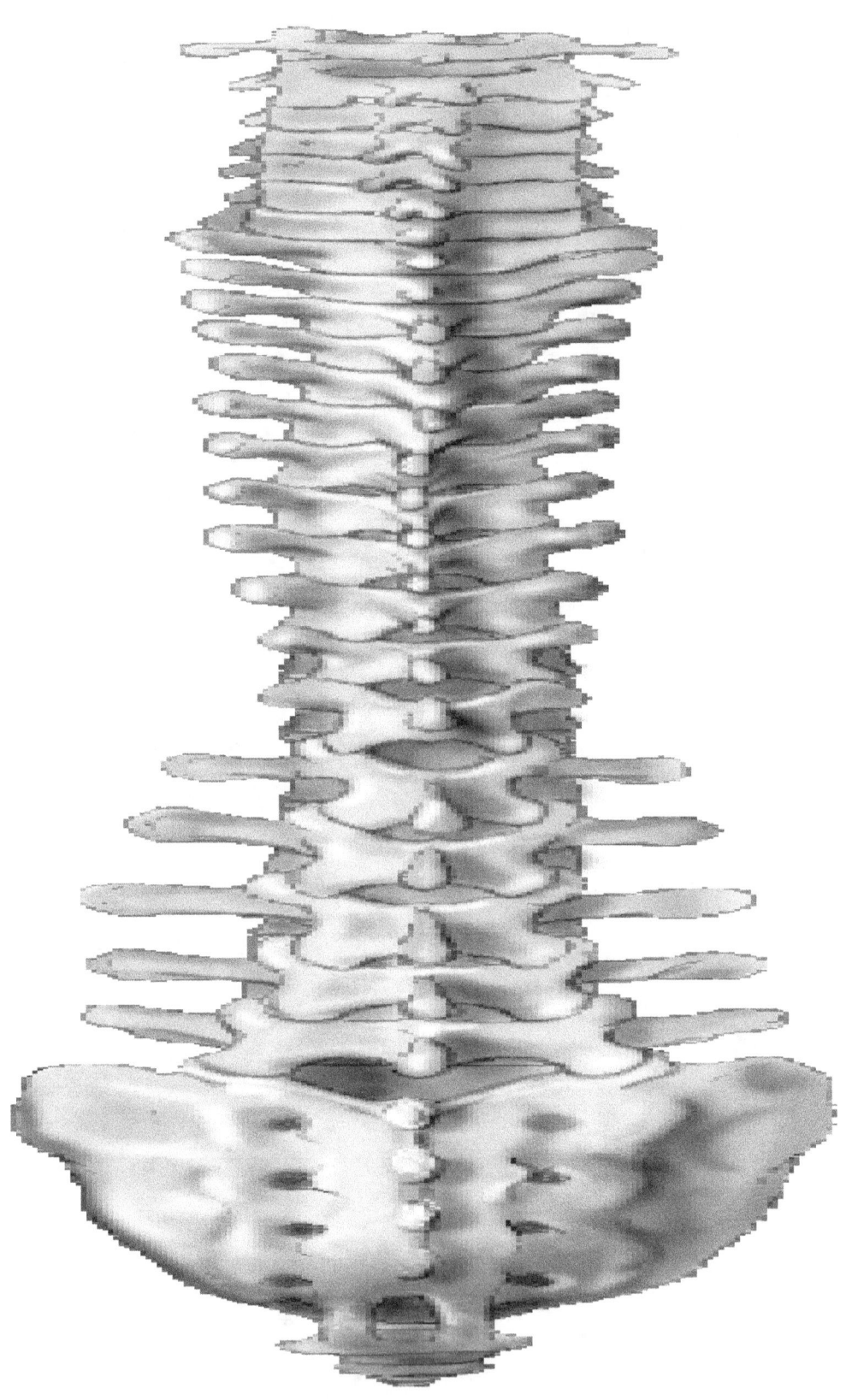

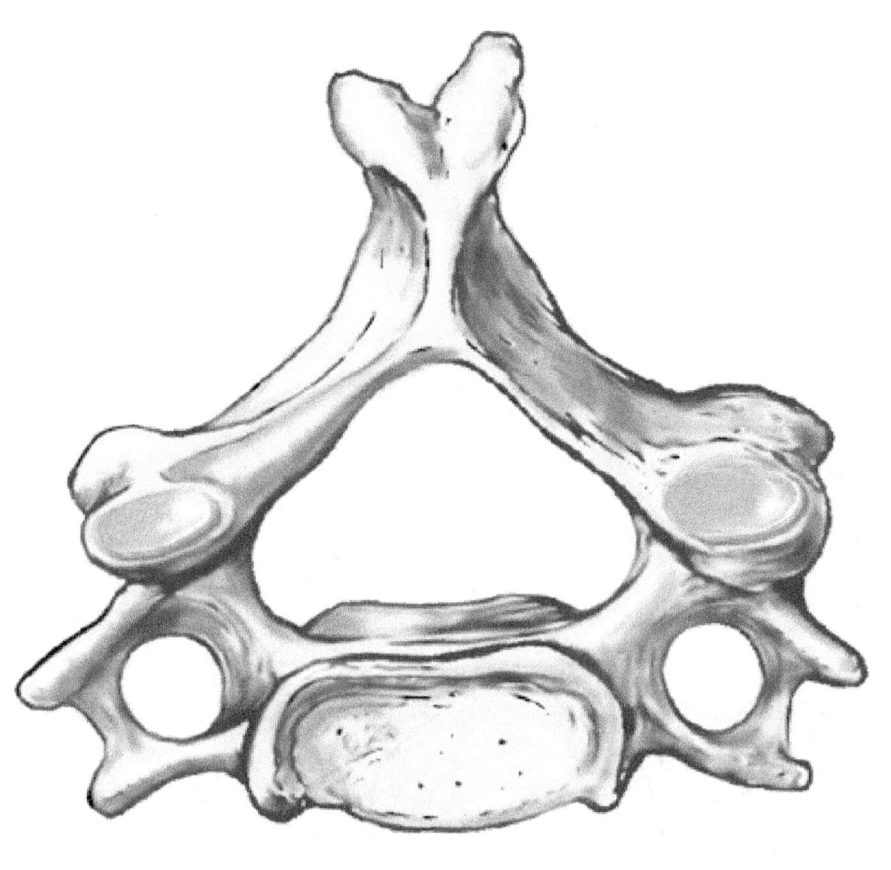

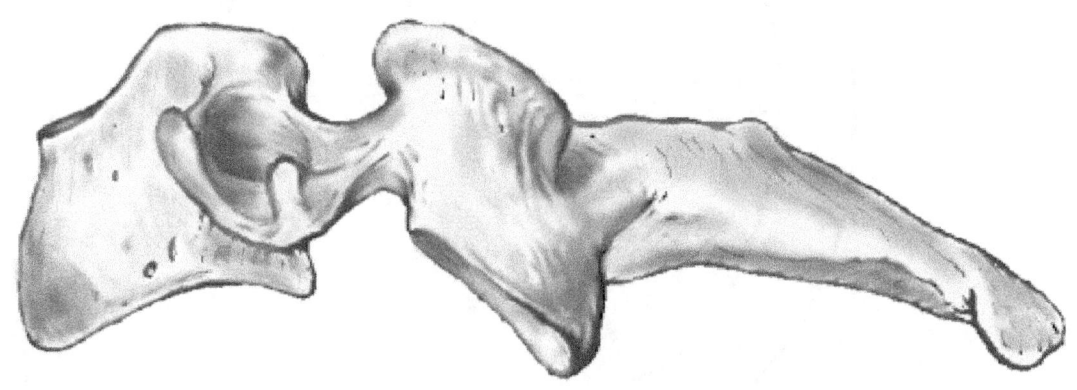

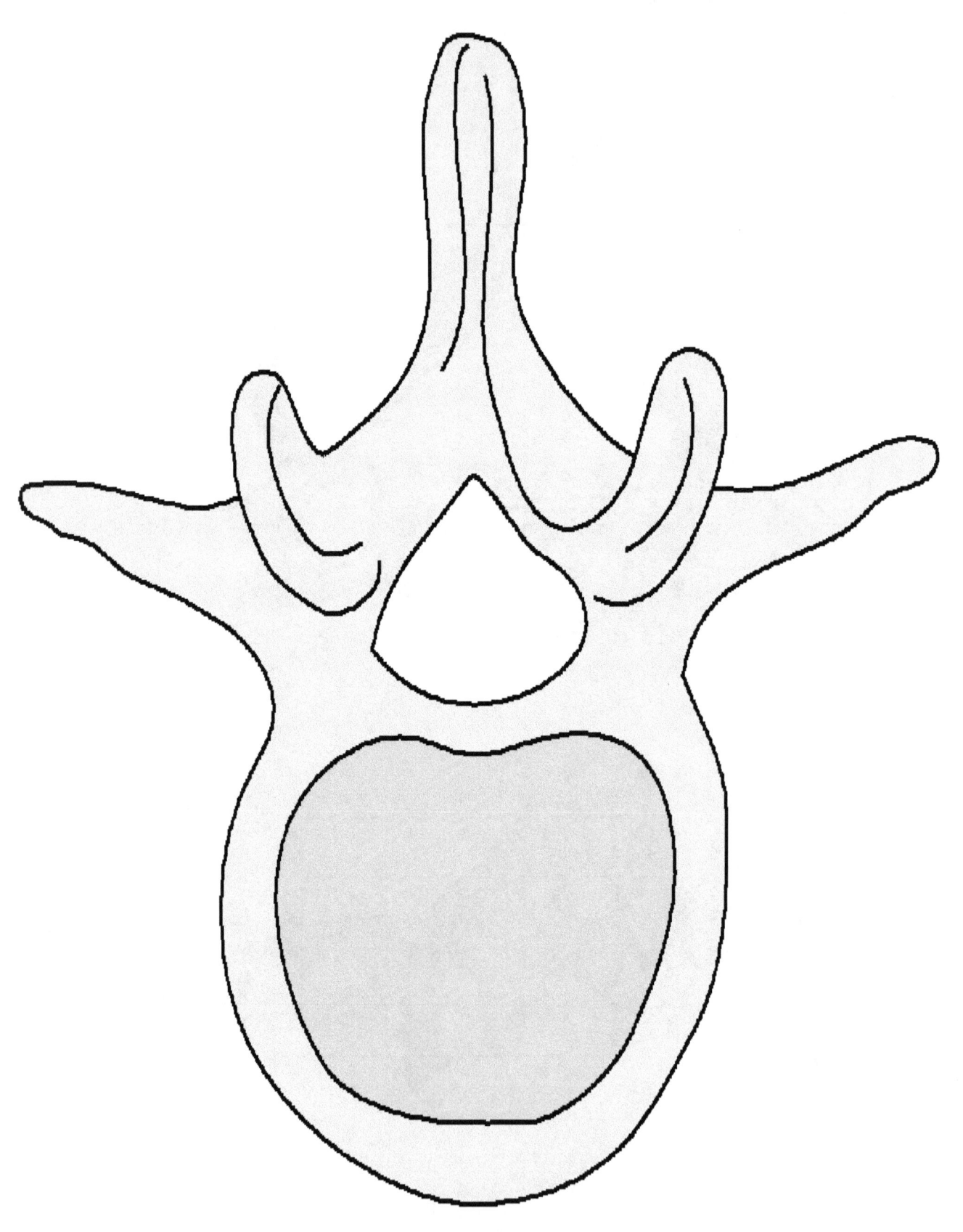

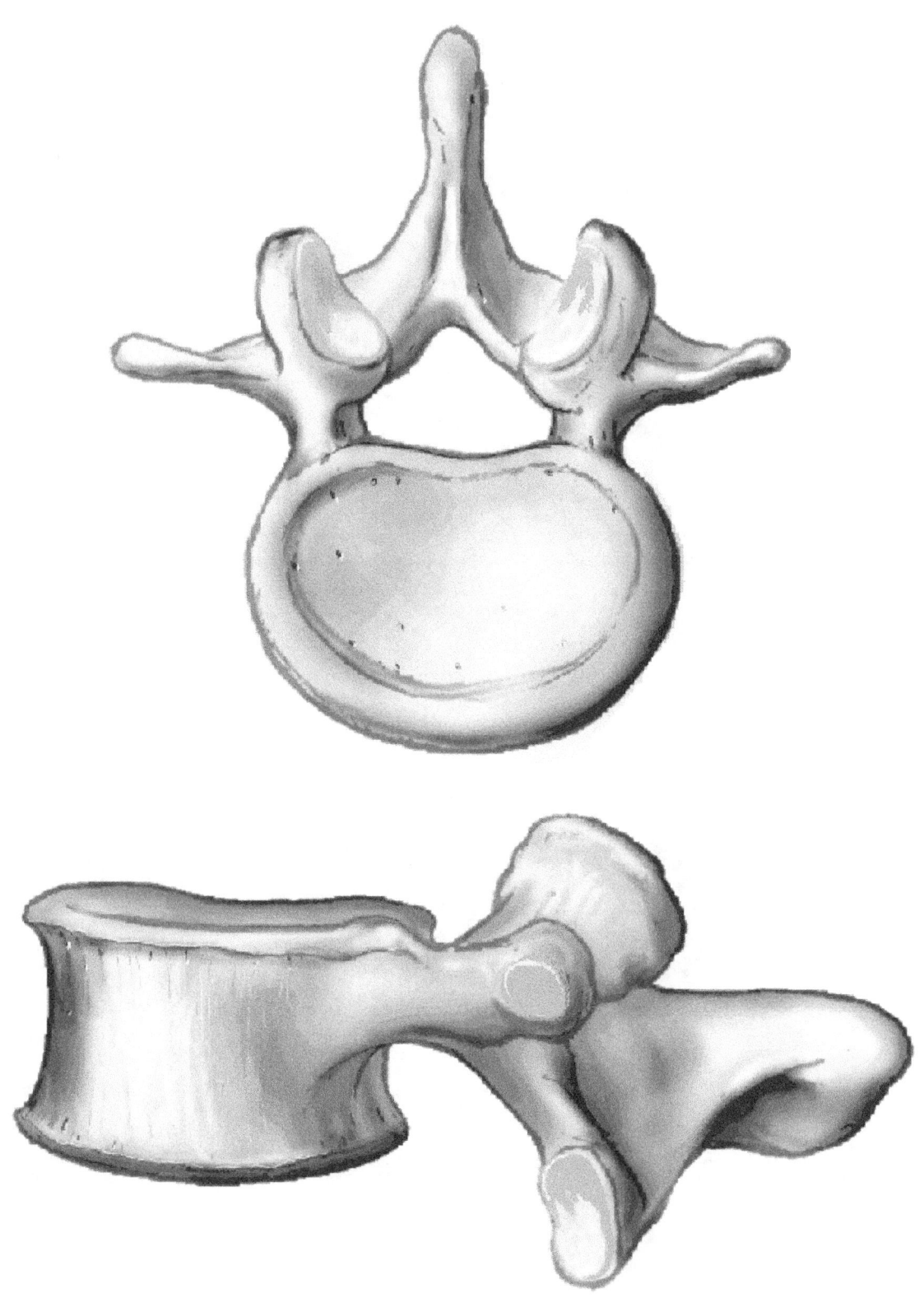

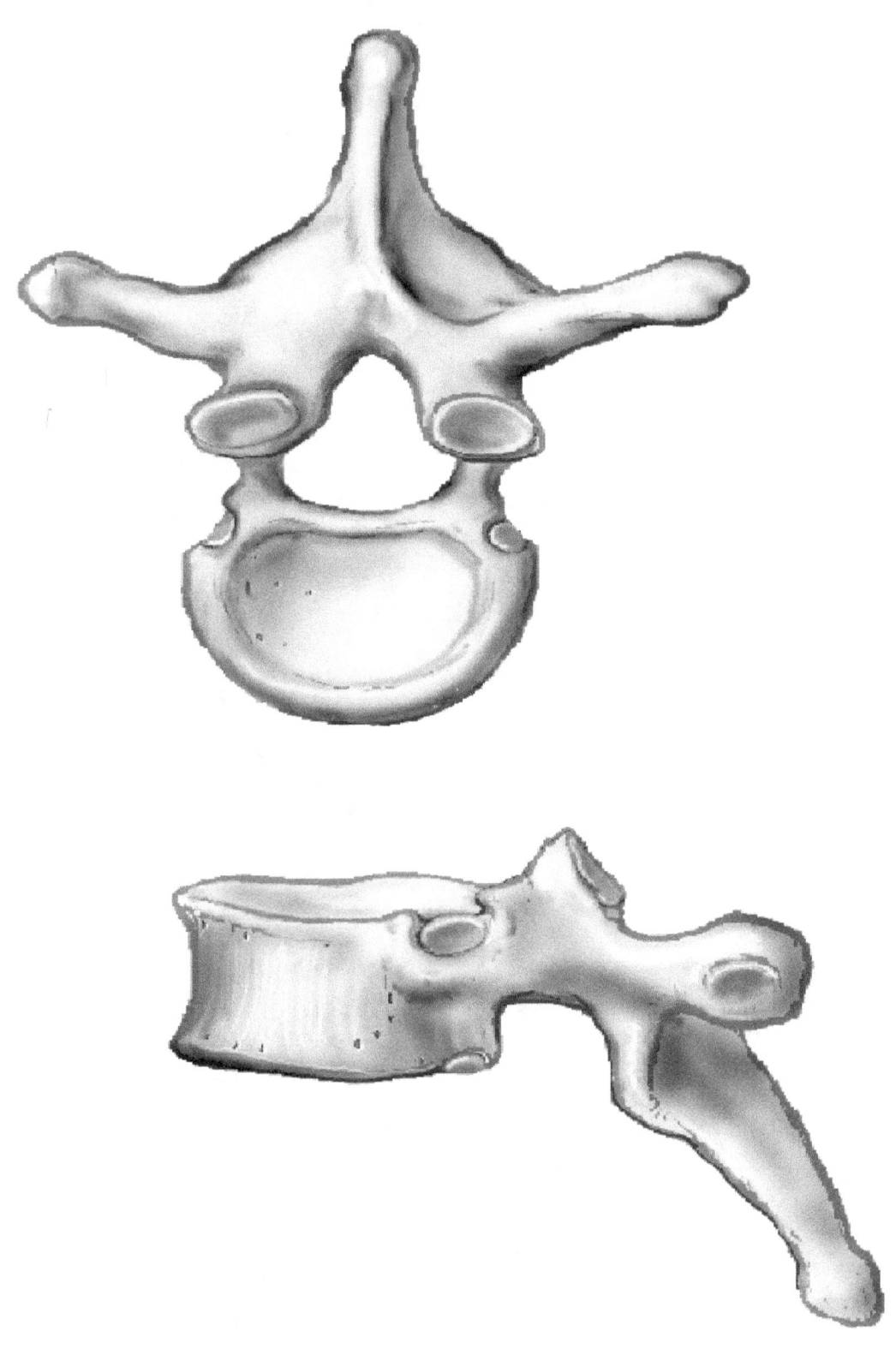

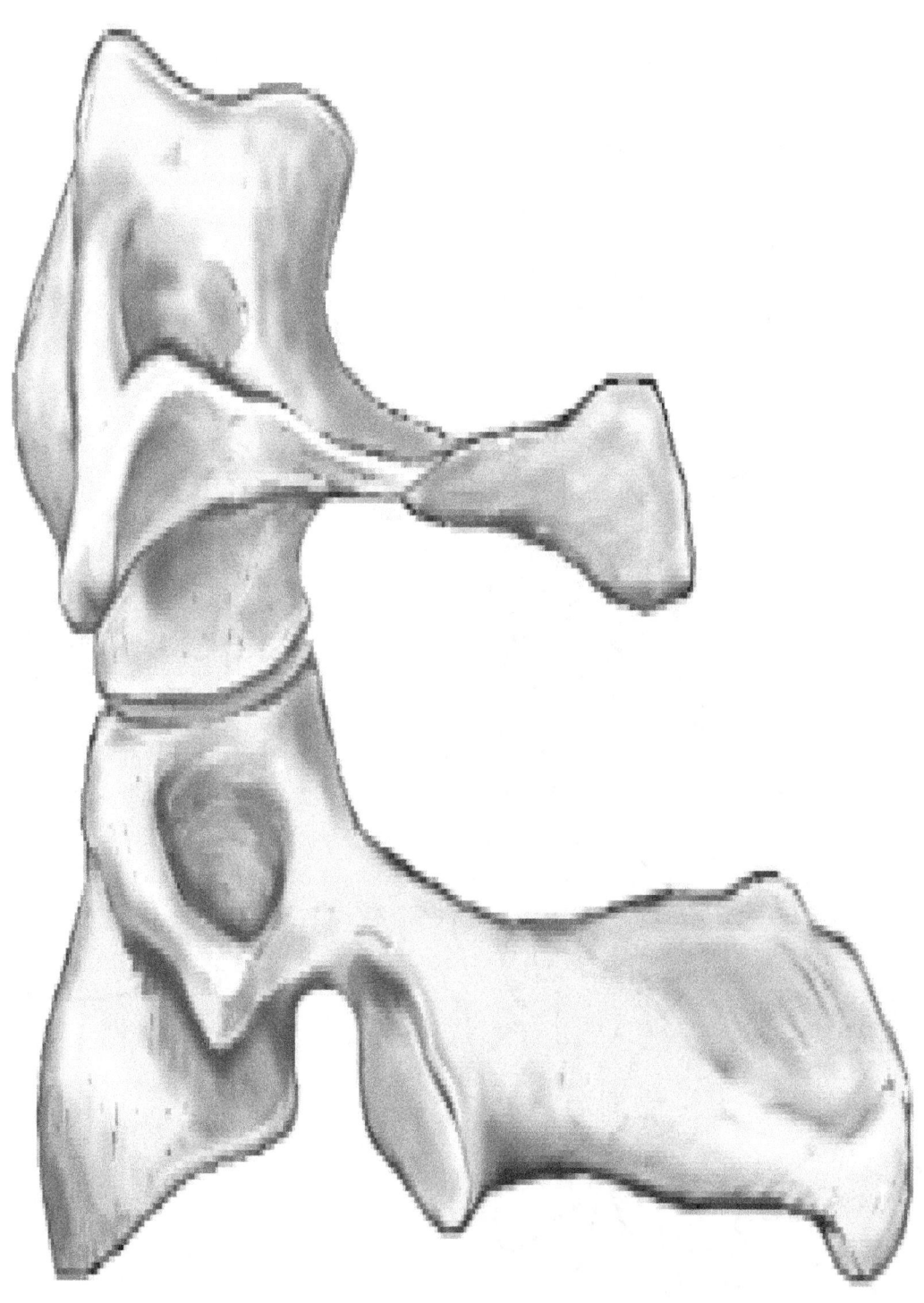

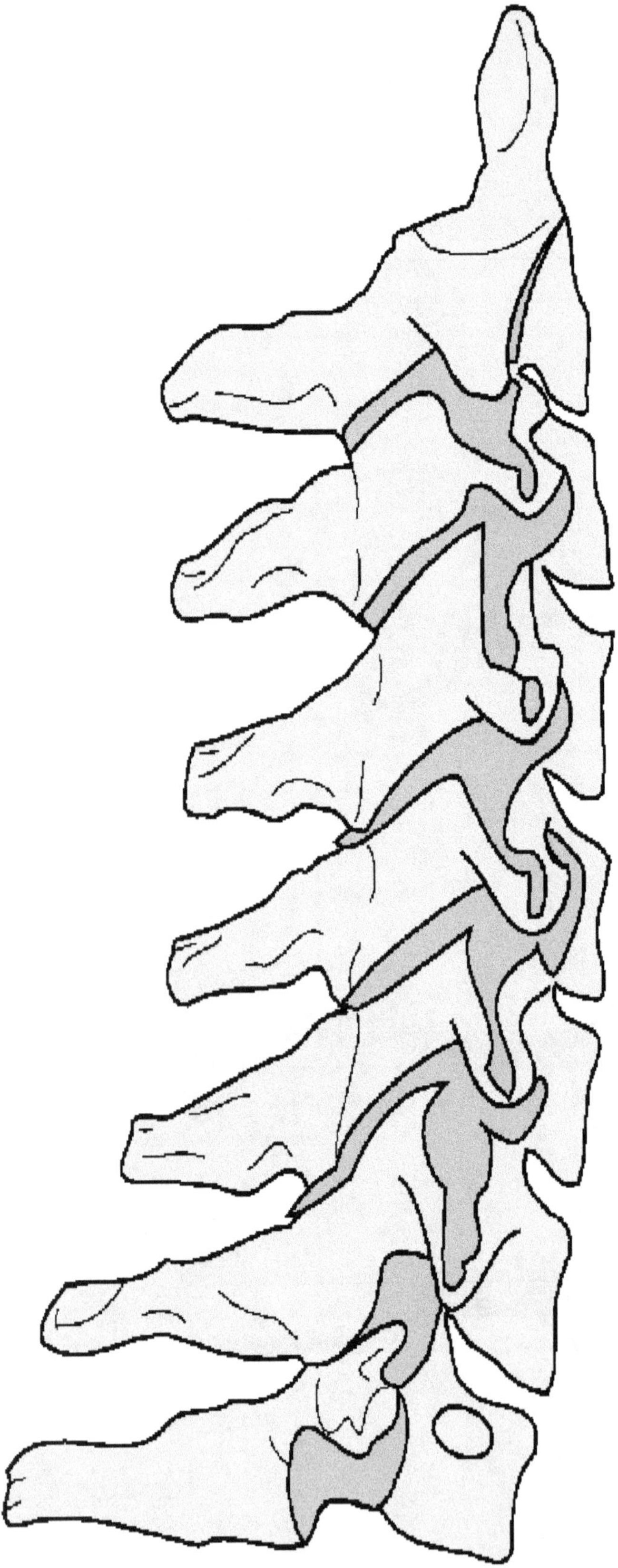

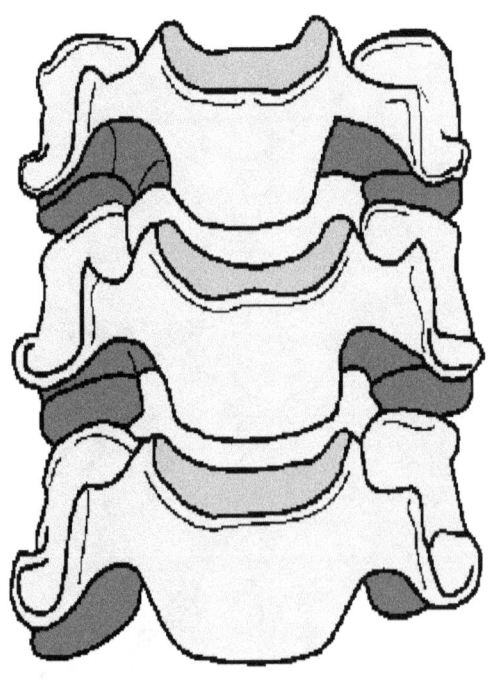

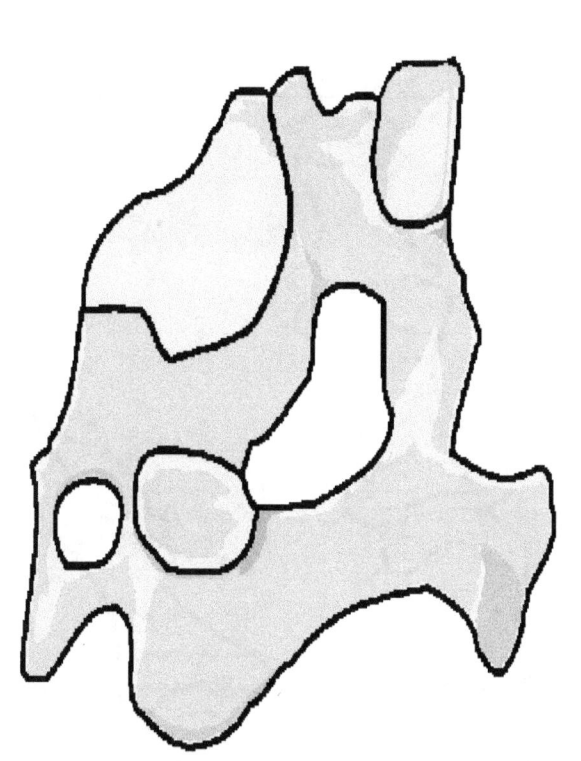

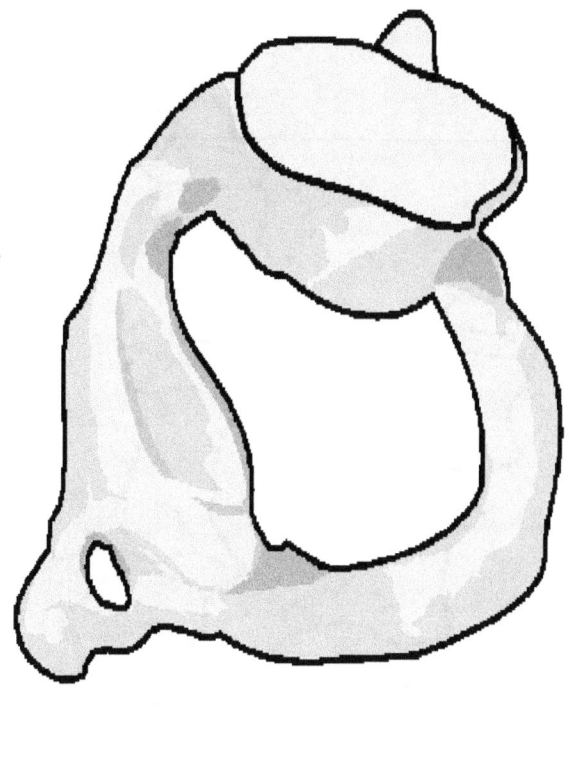

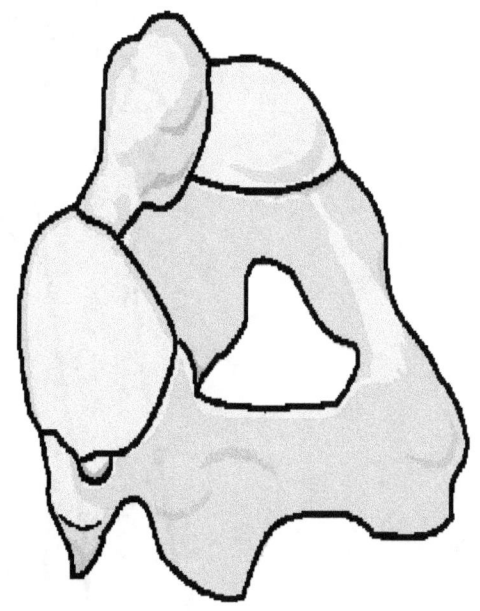

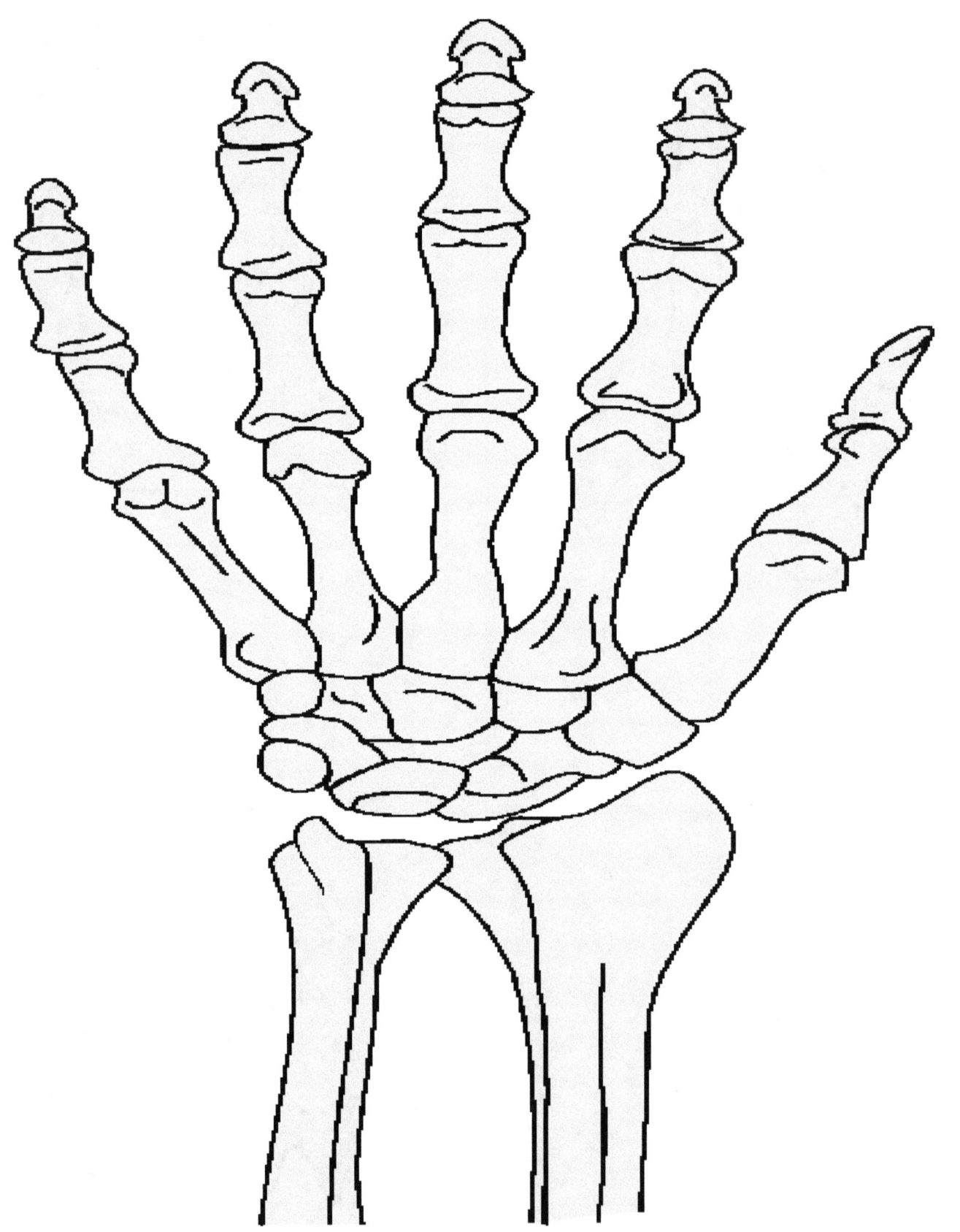

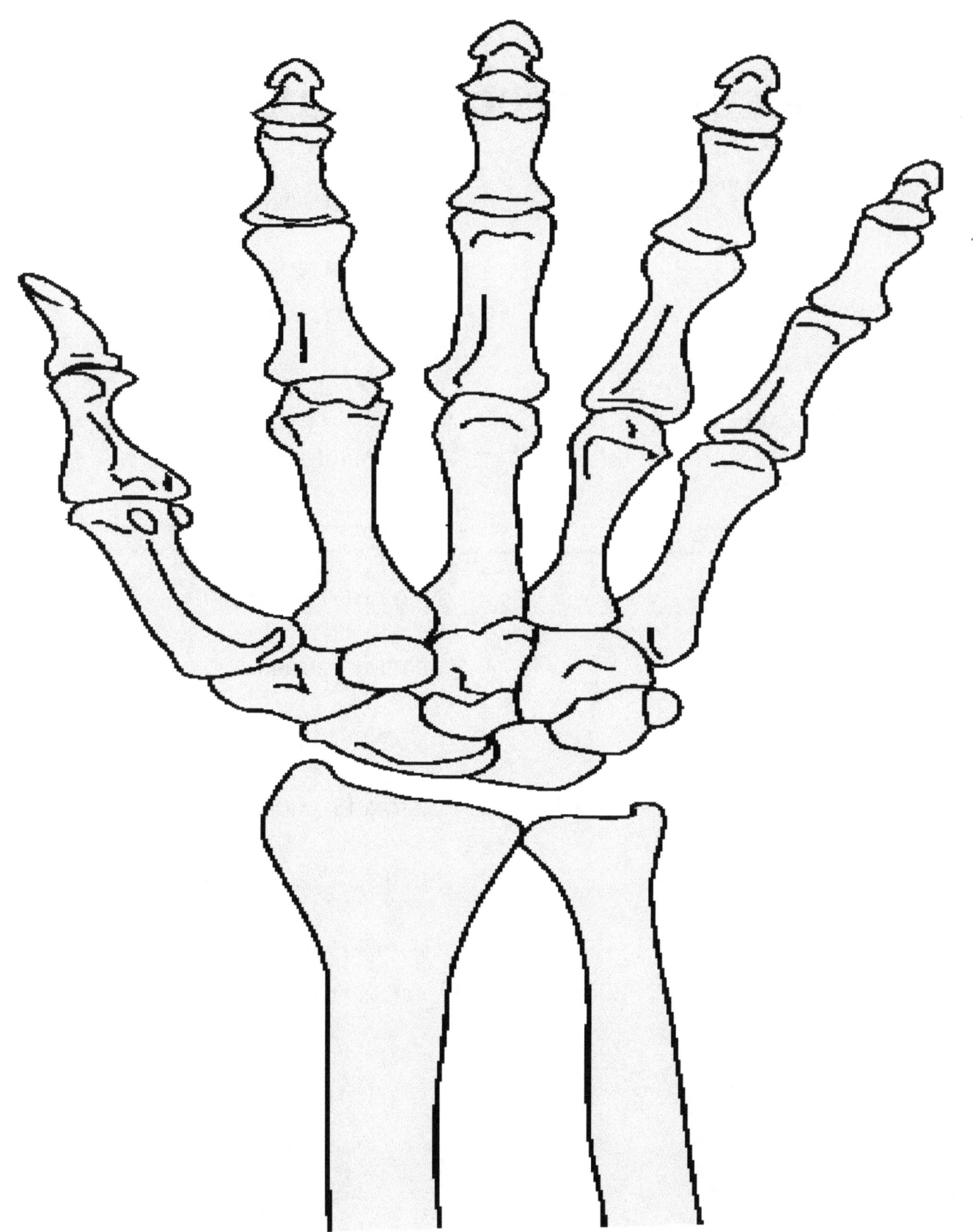

DIGESTIVE & ENDOCRINE SYSTEM 163 - 185

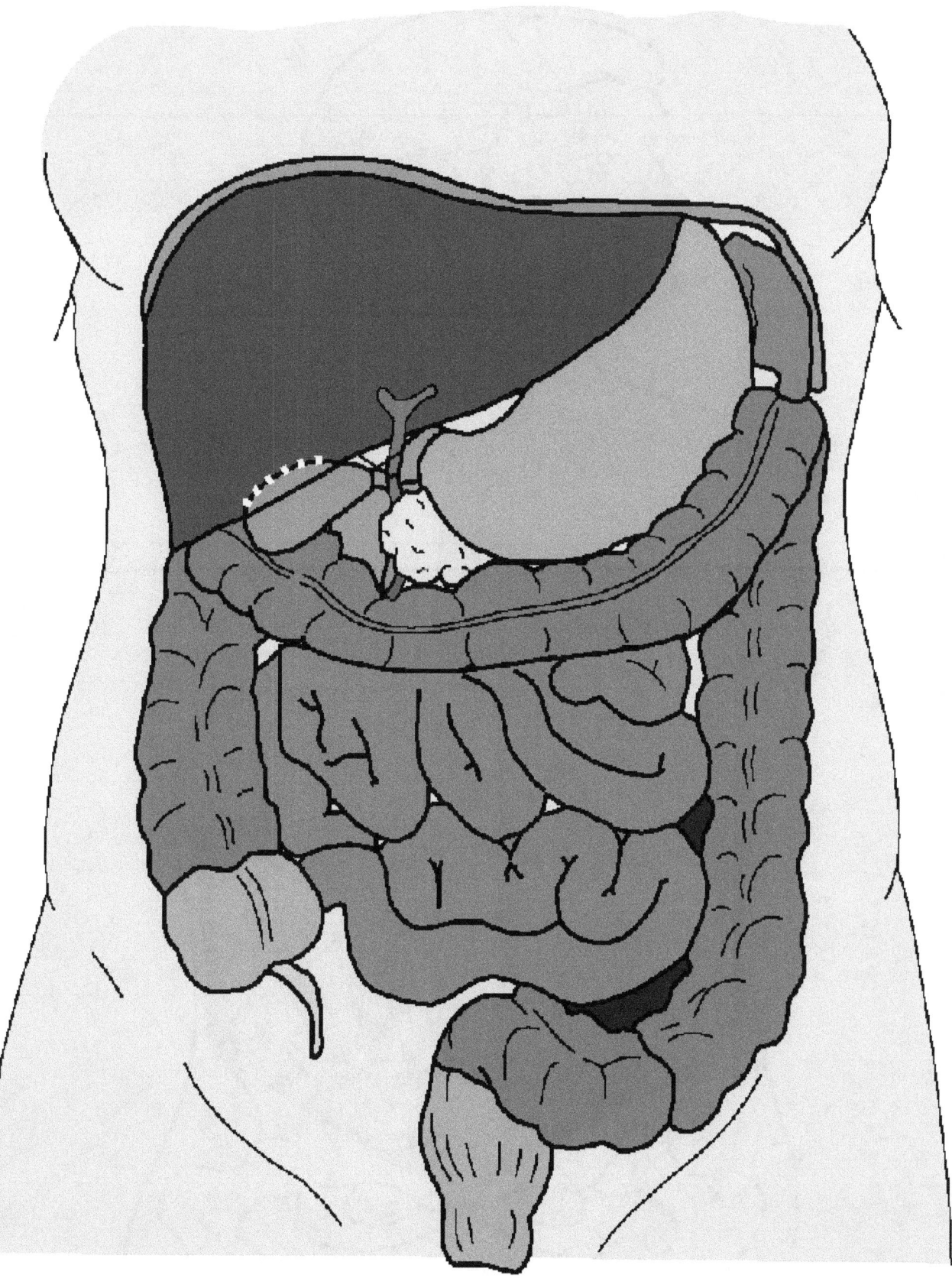

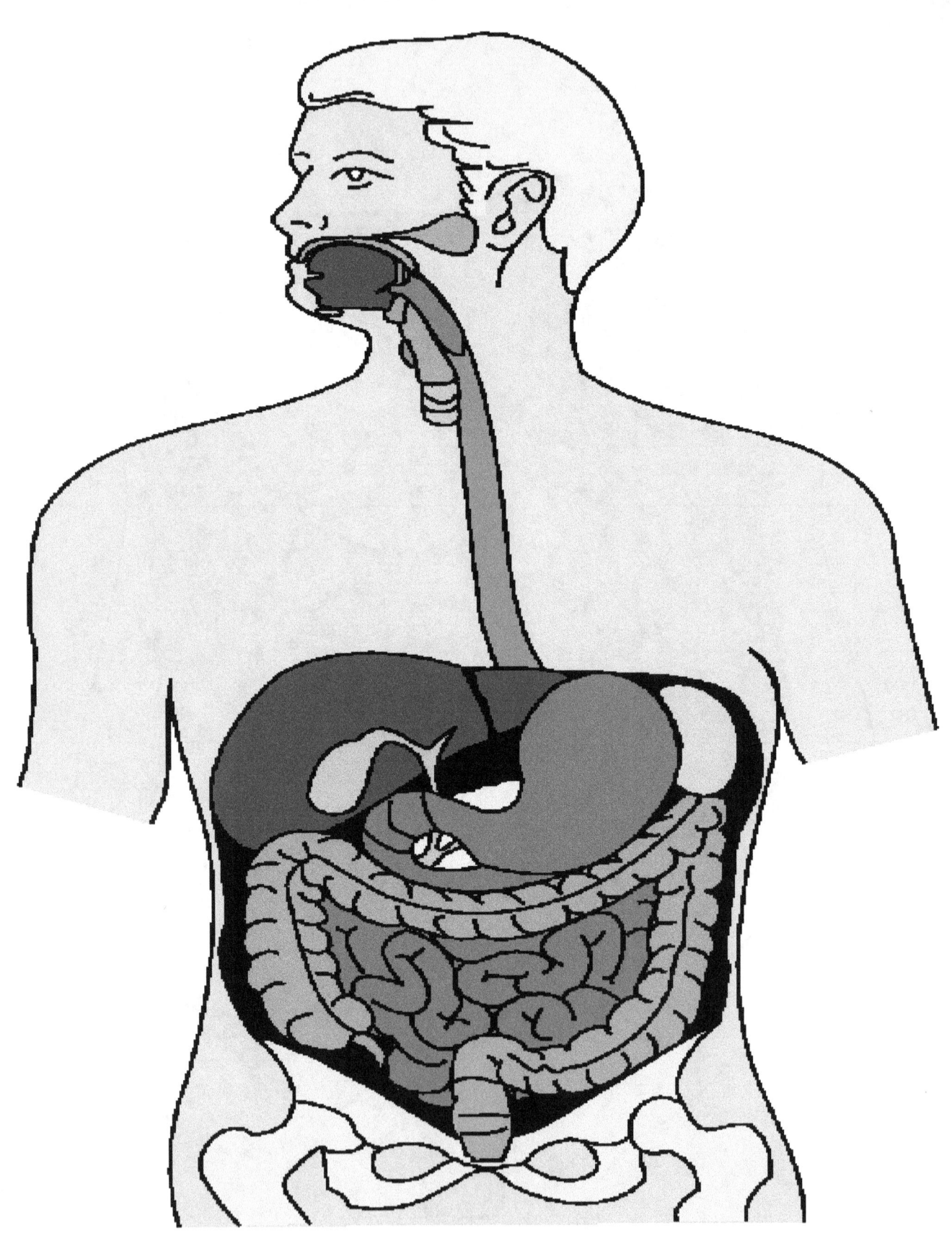

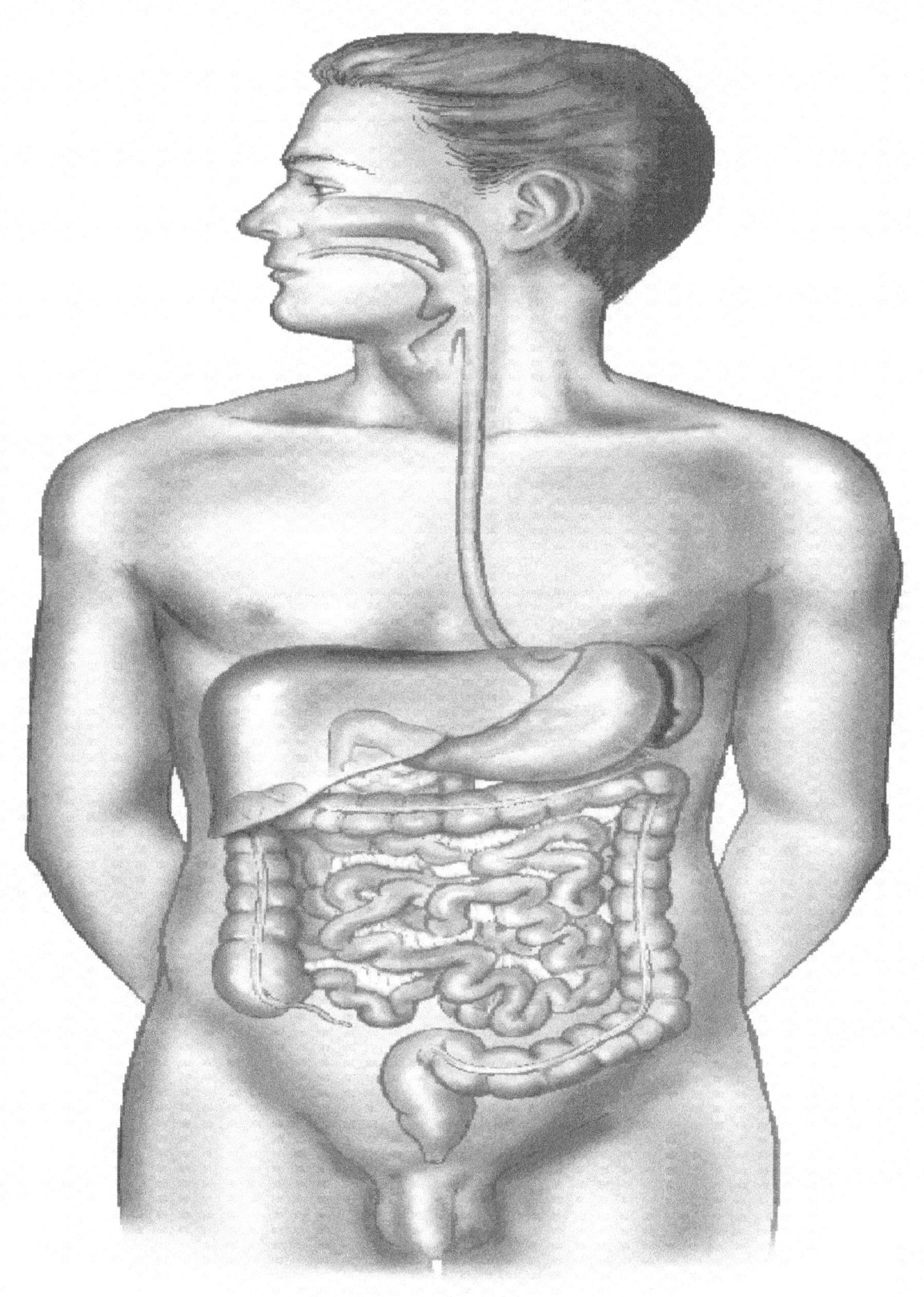

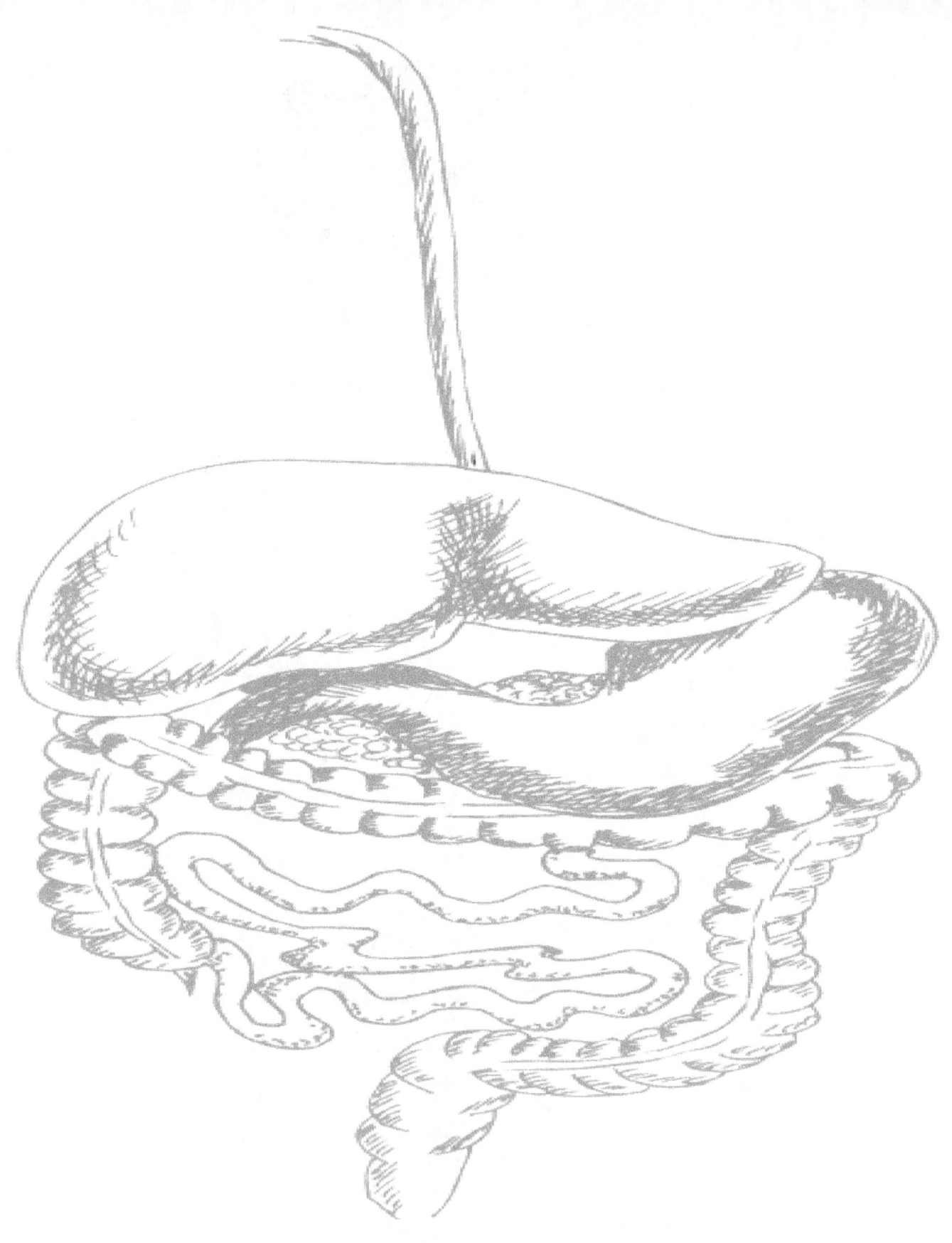

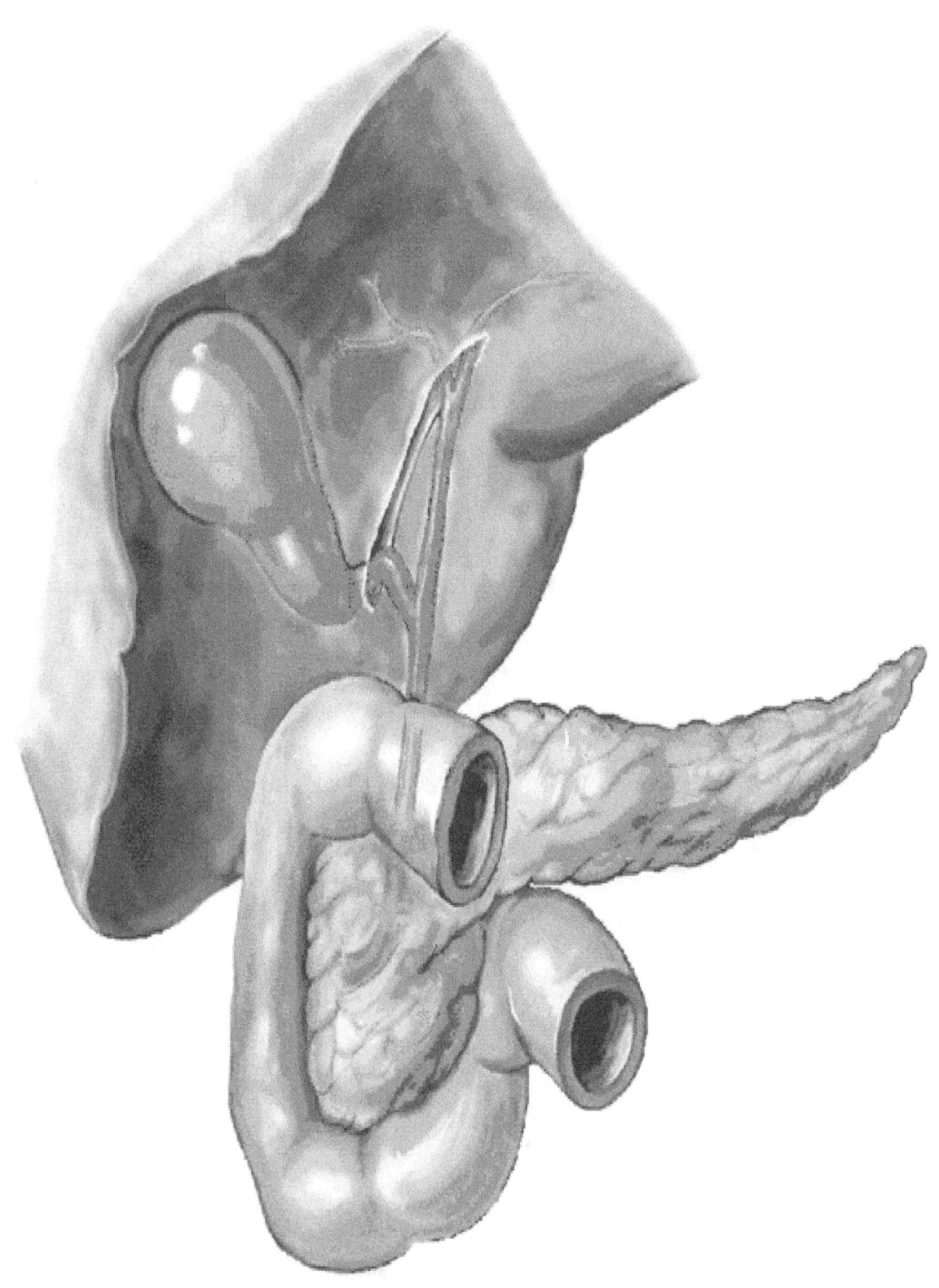

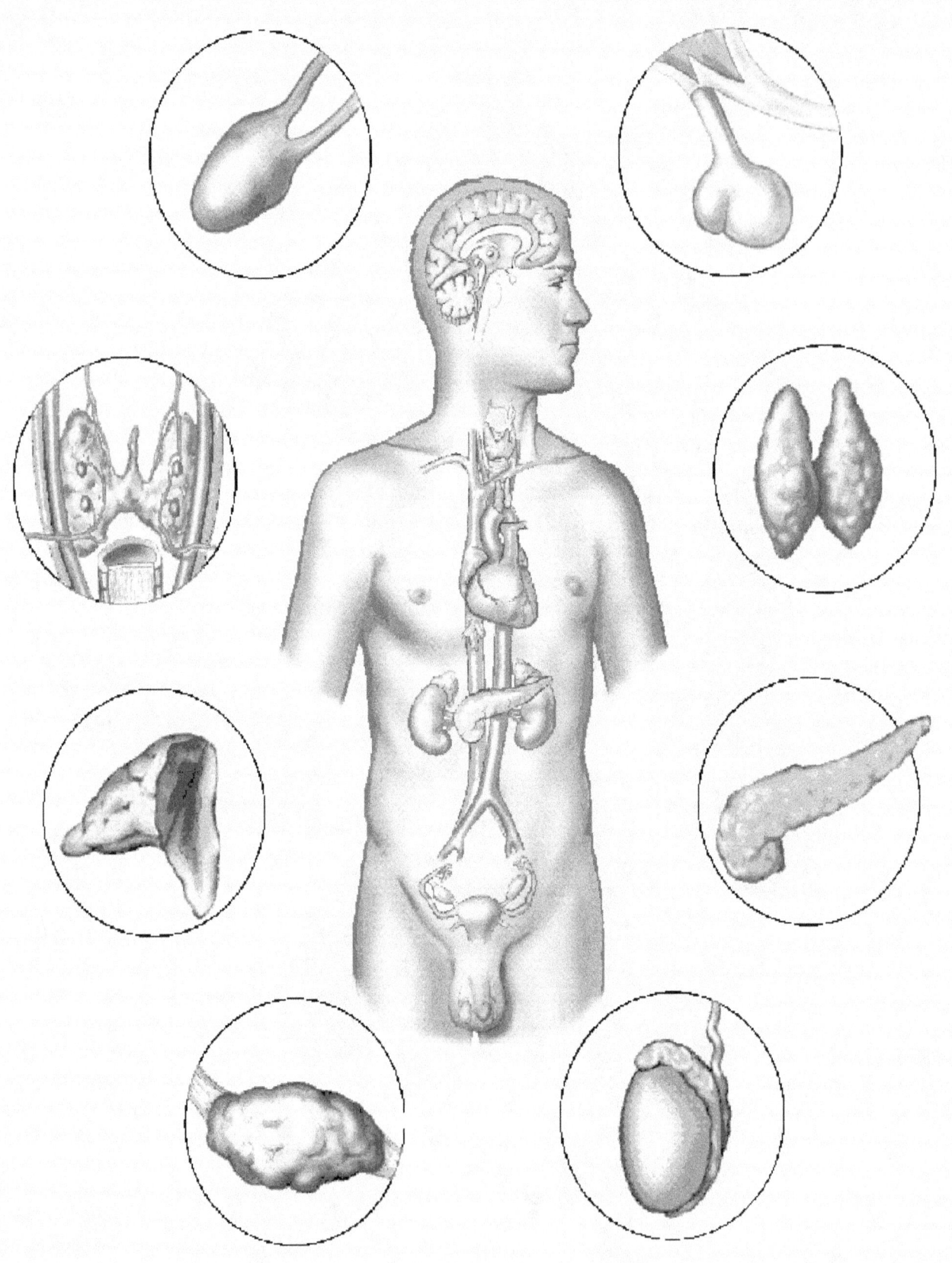

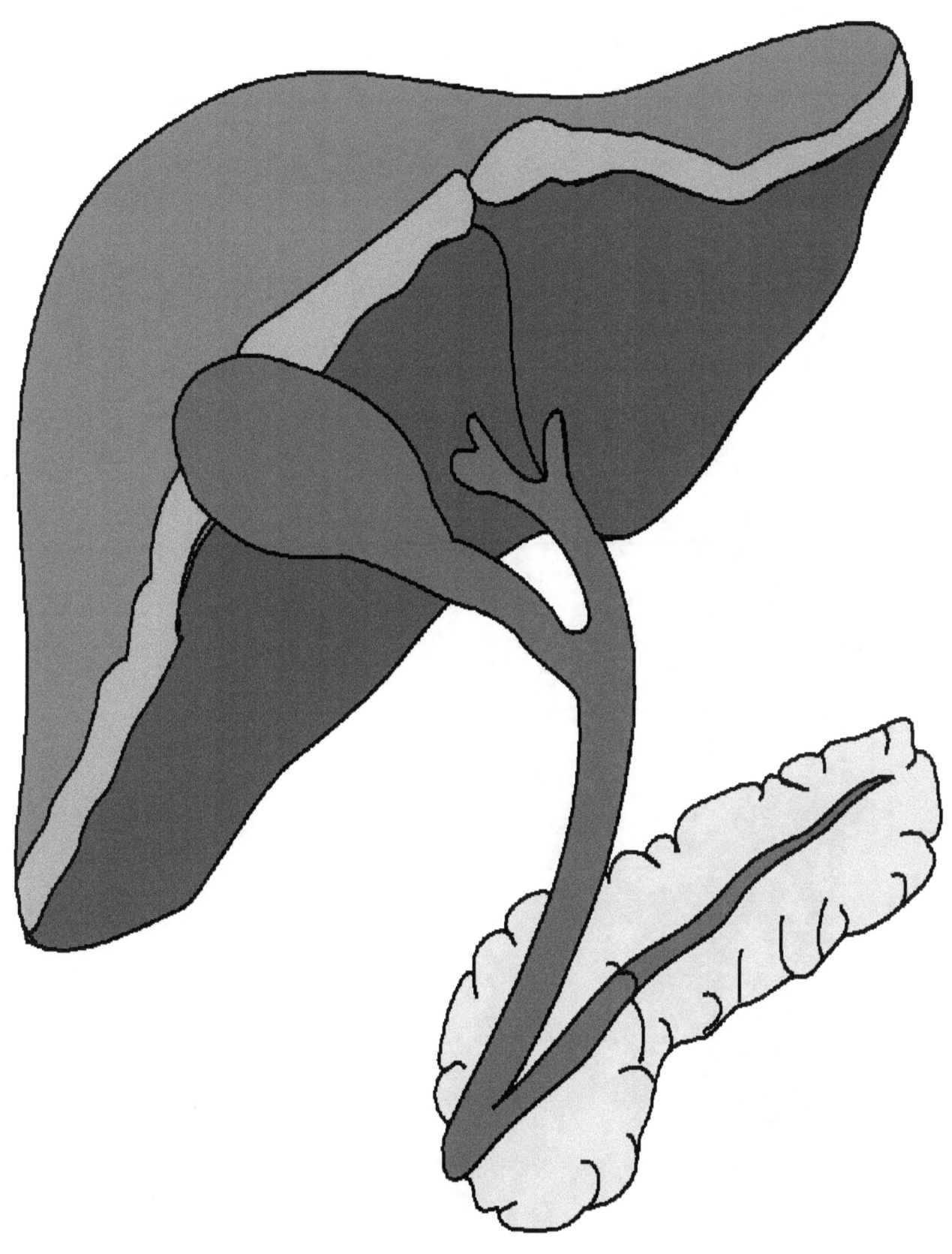

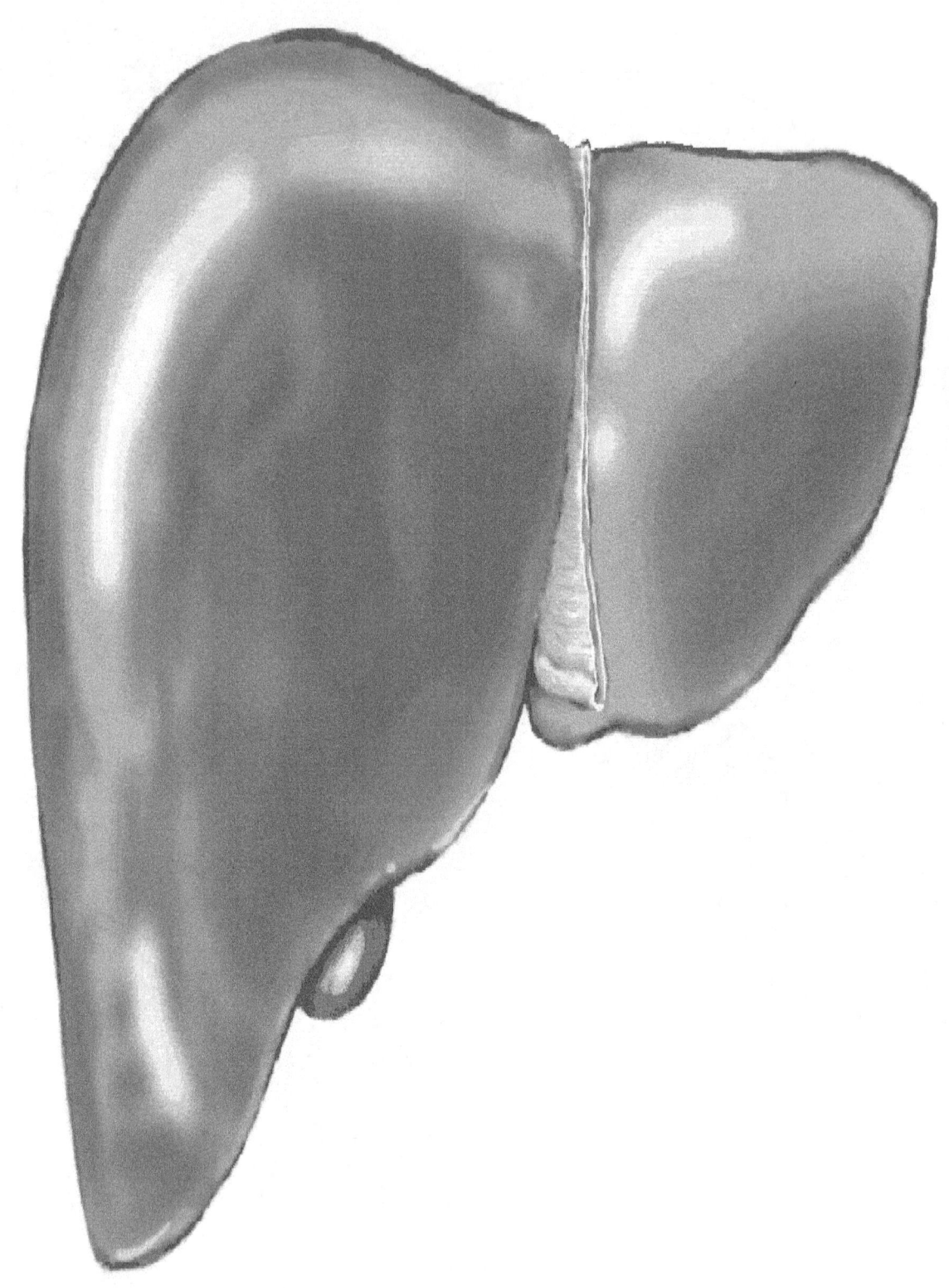

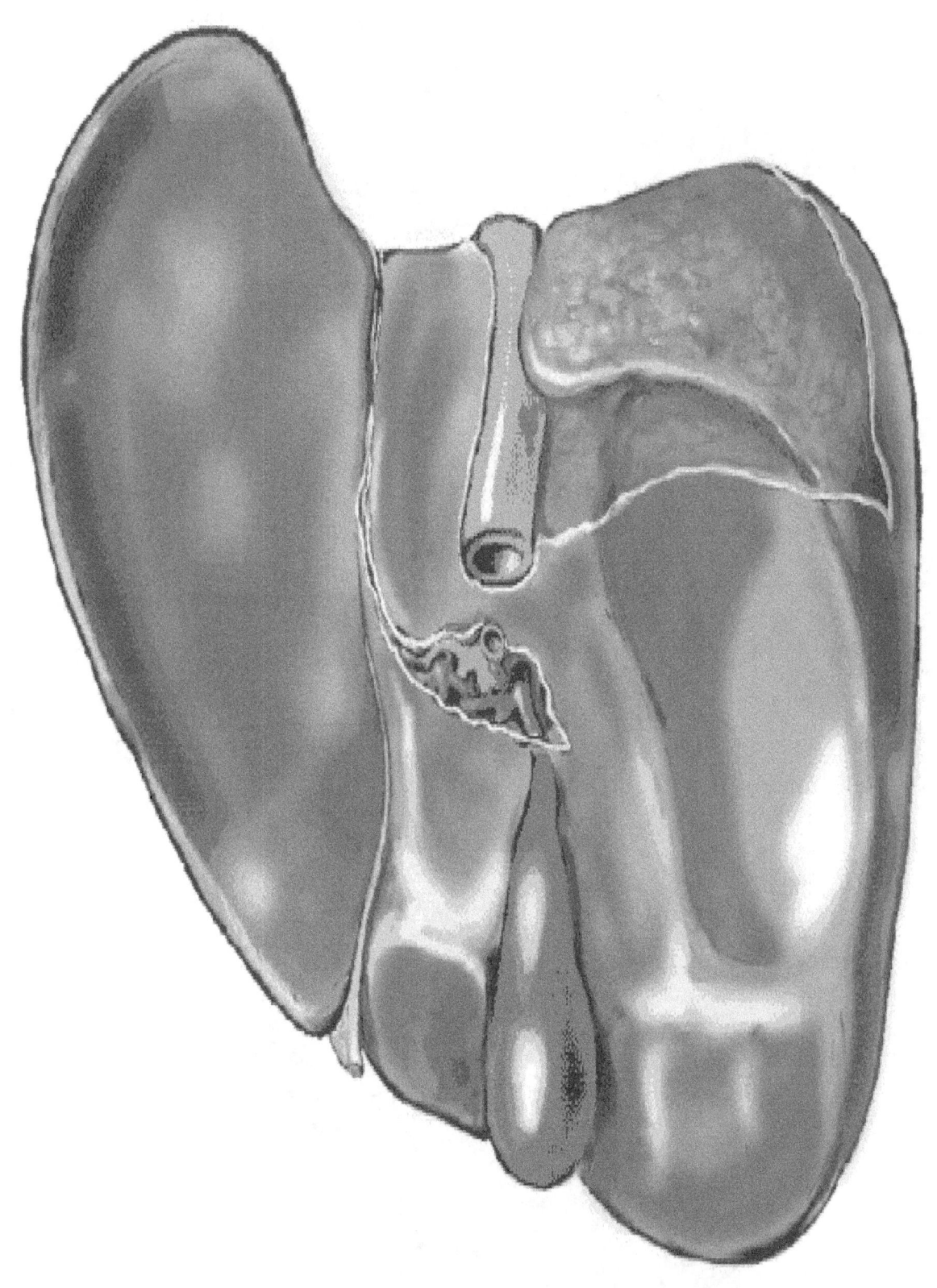

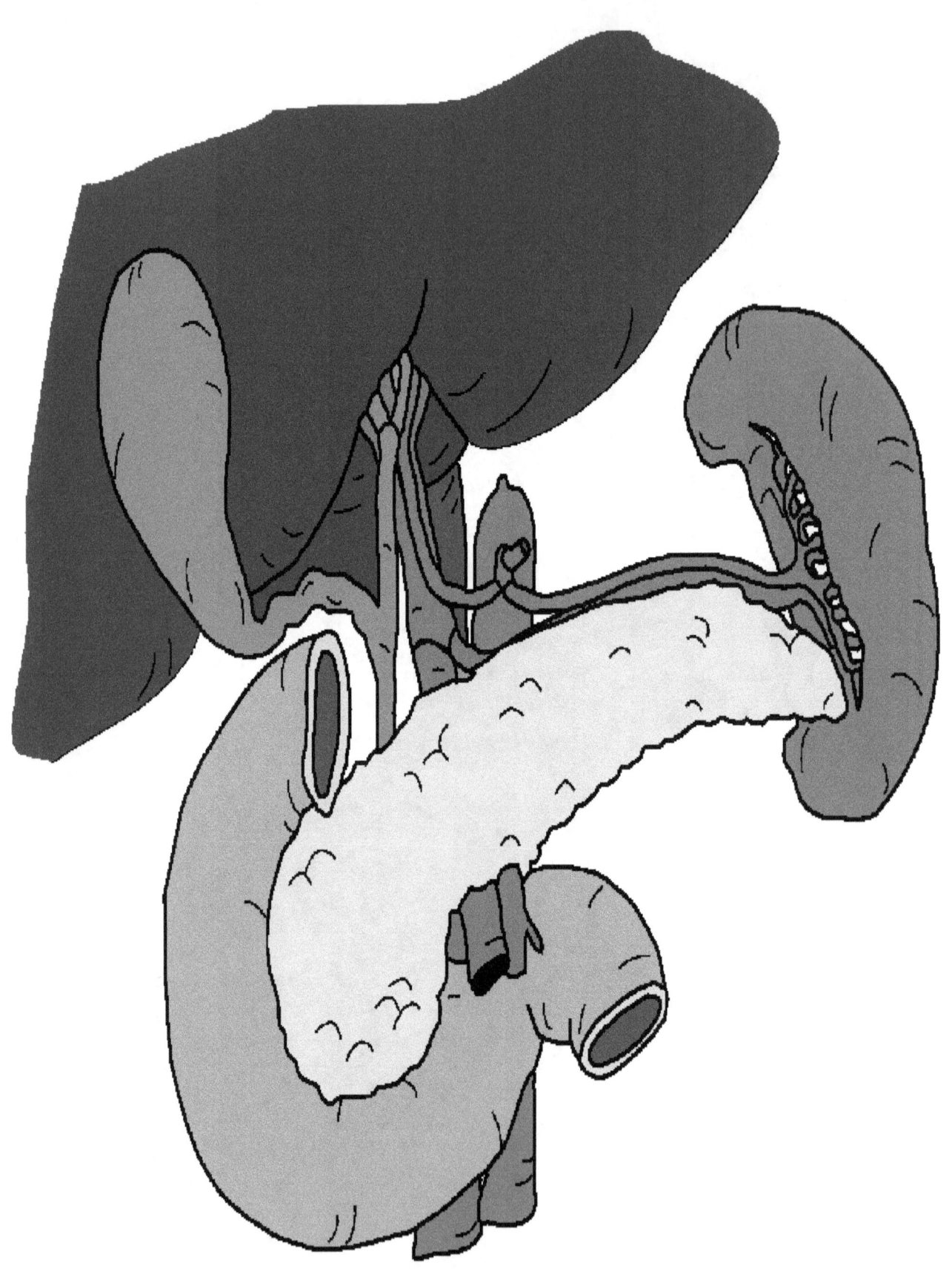

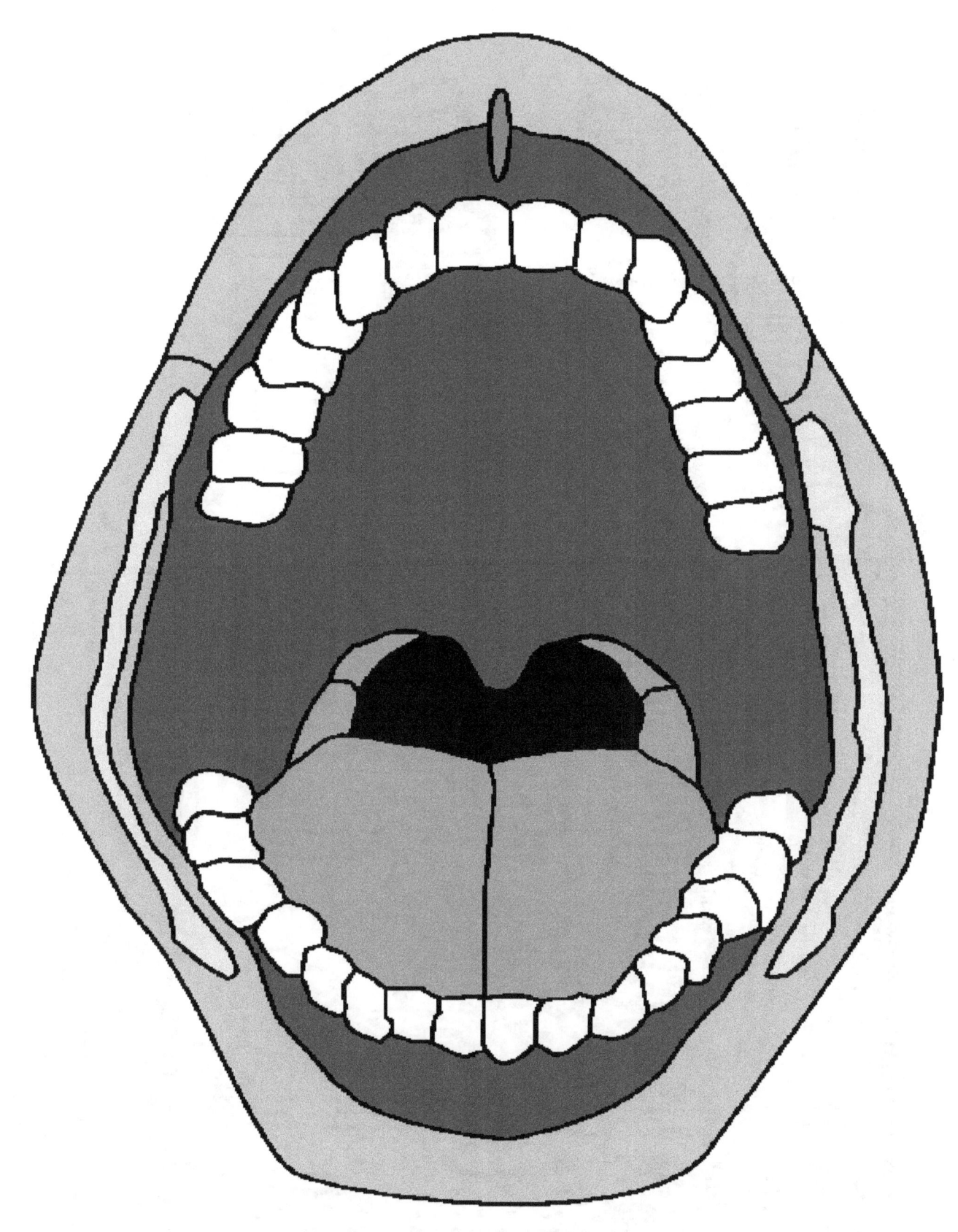

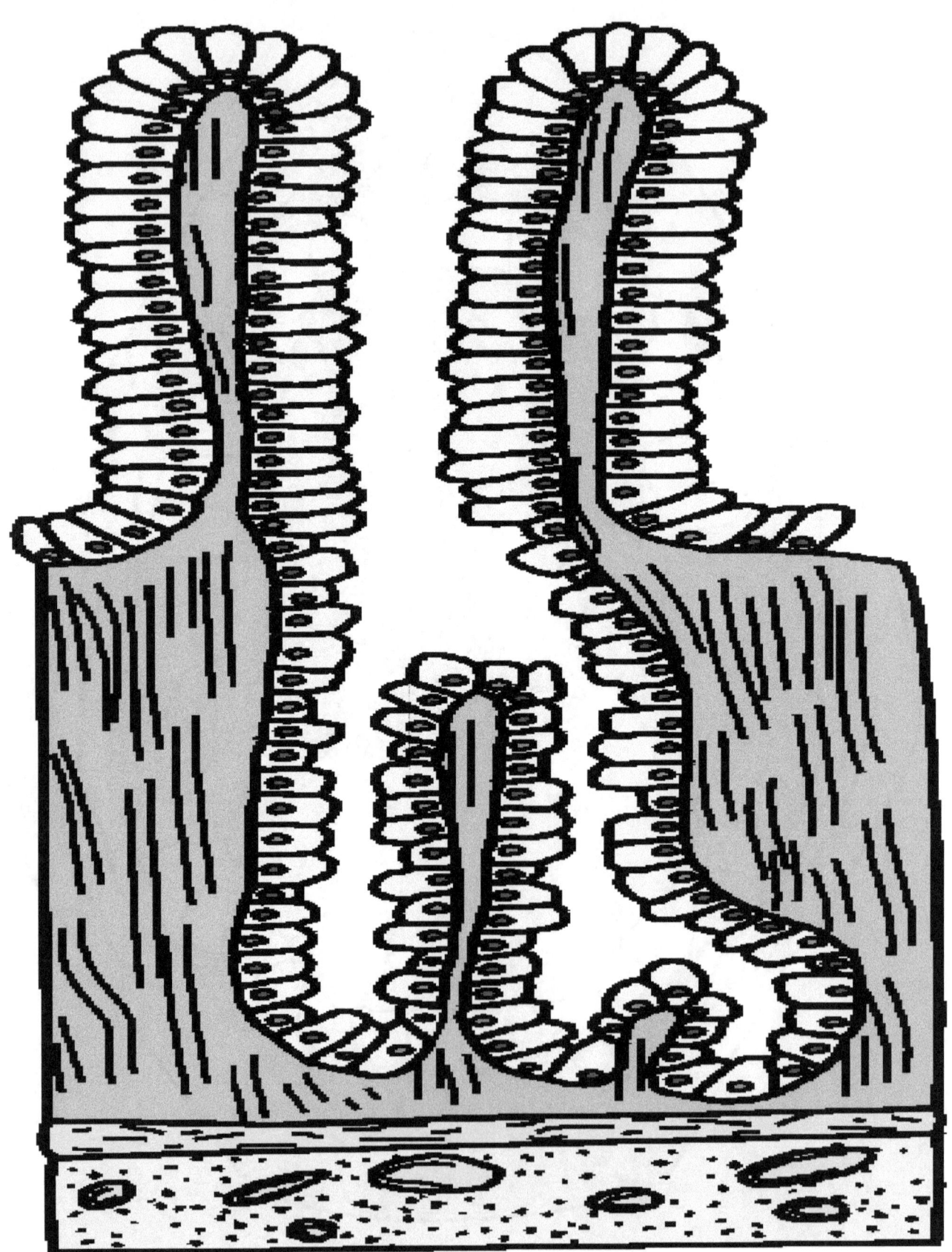

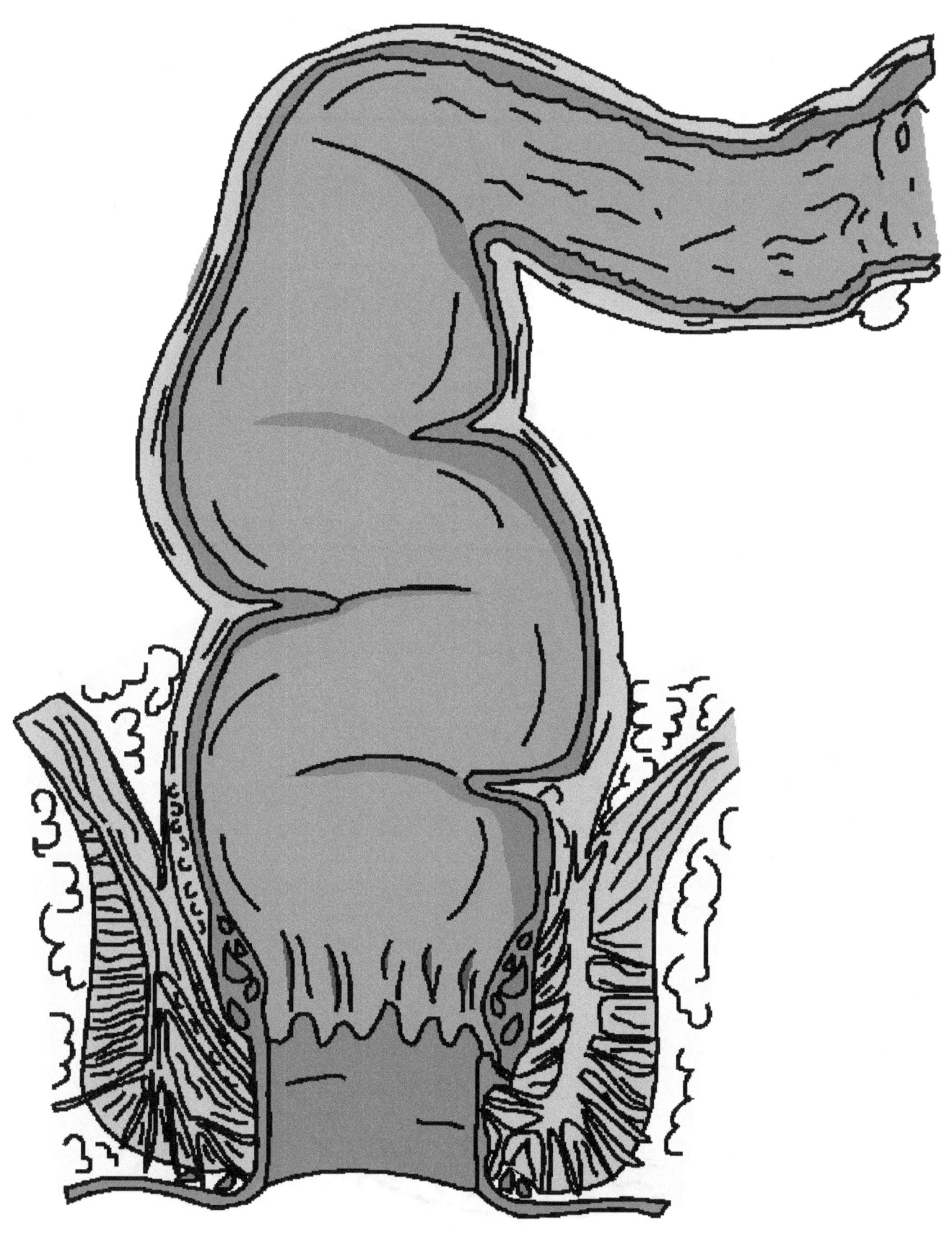

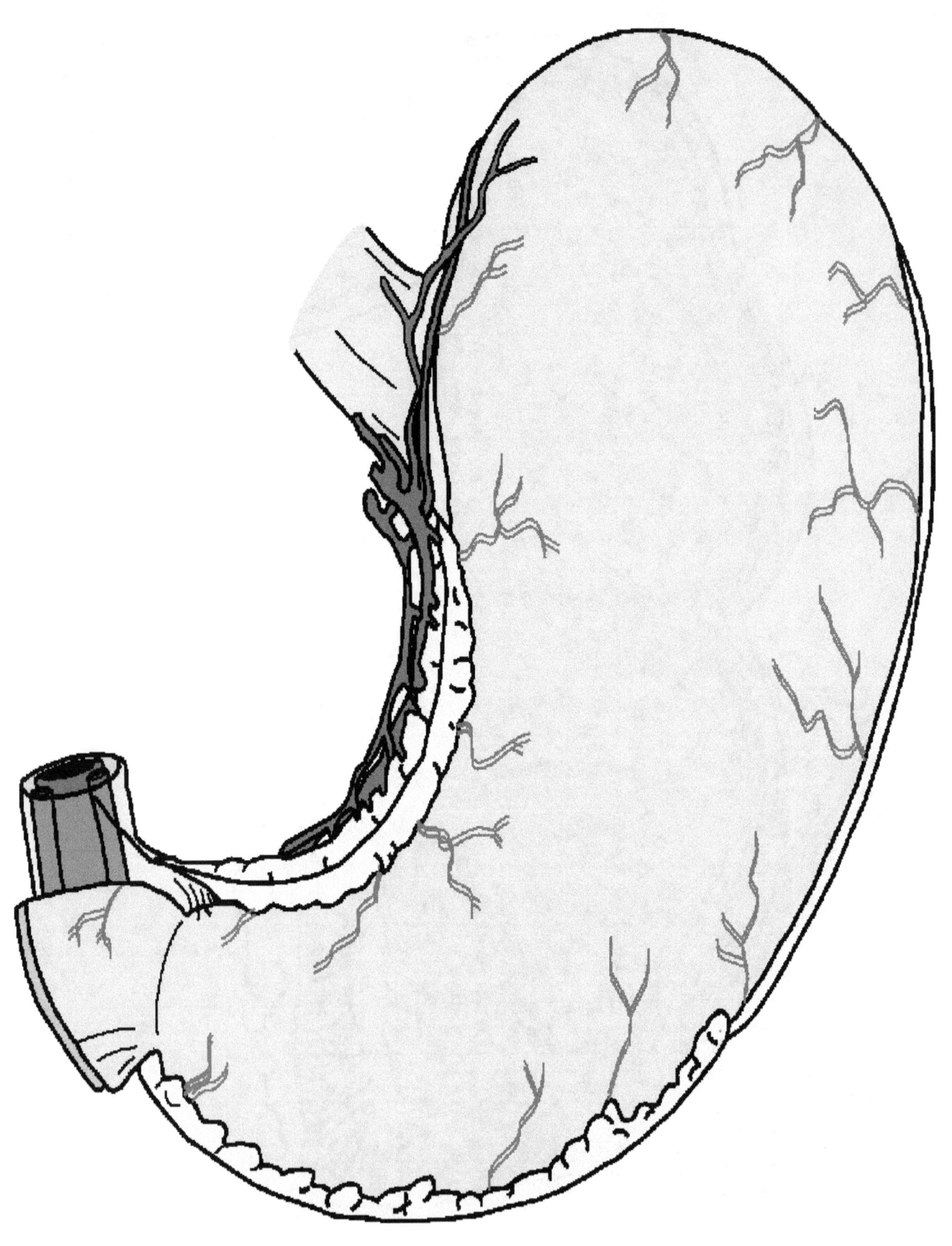

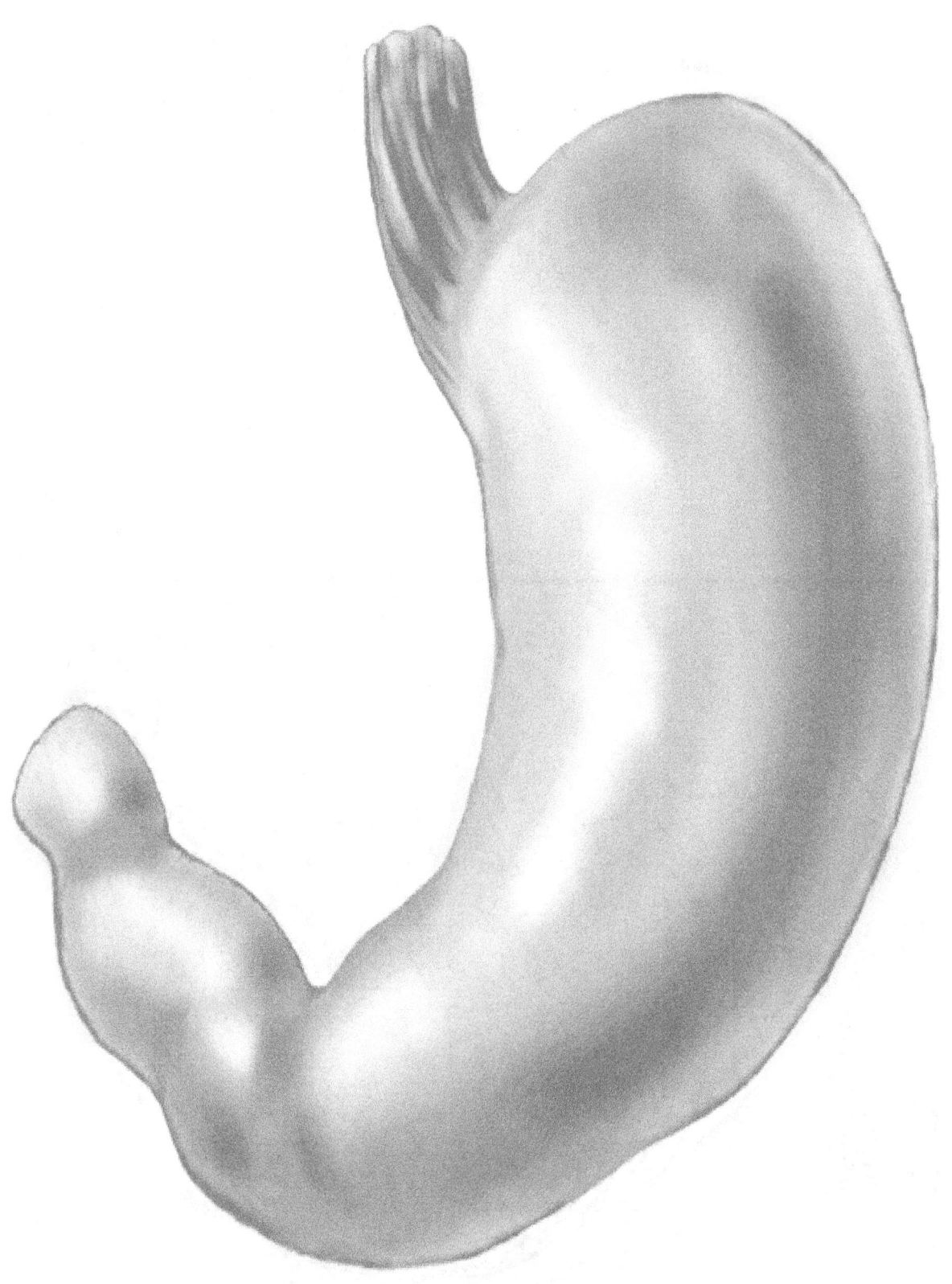

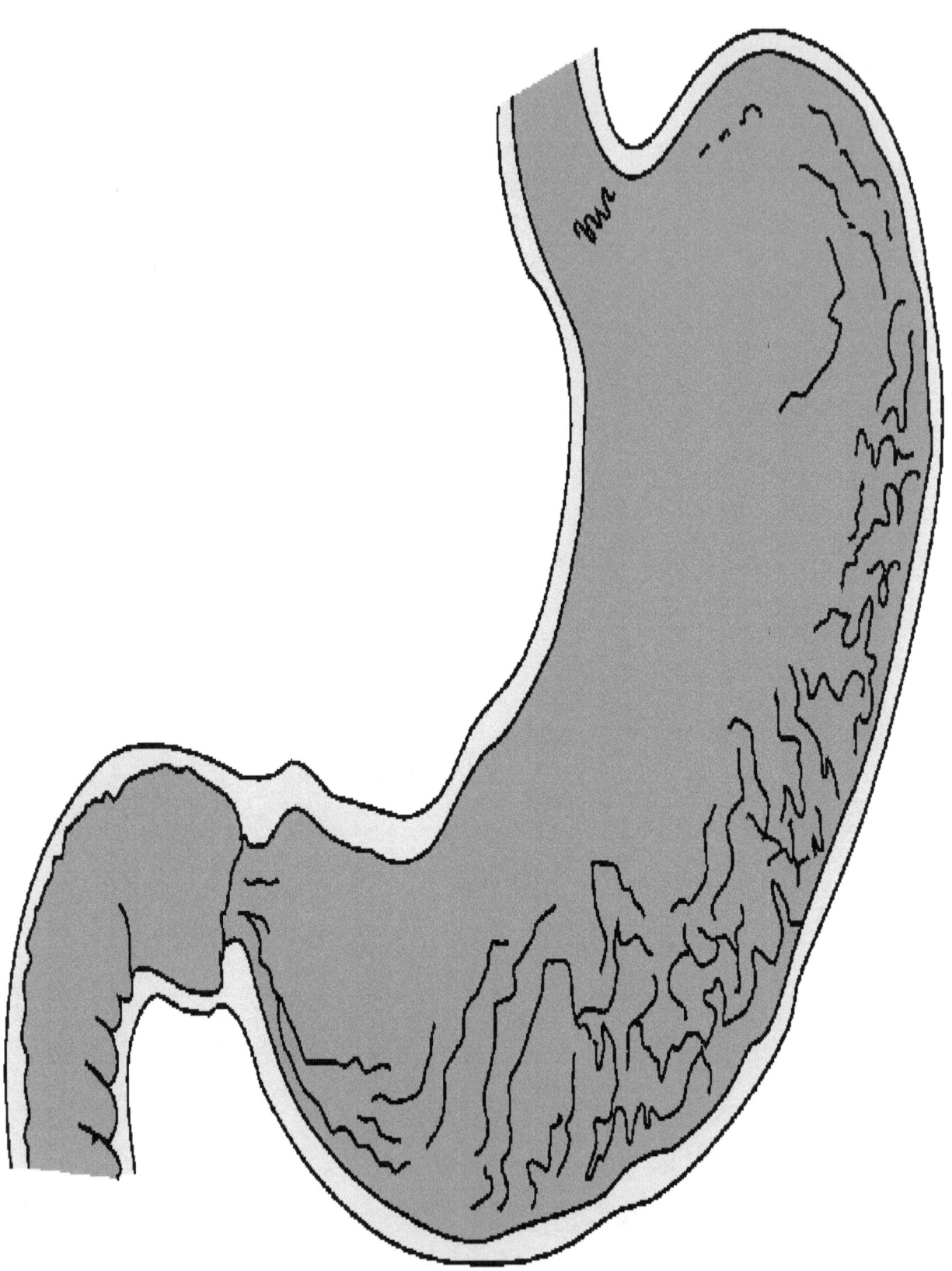

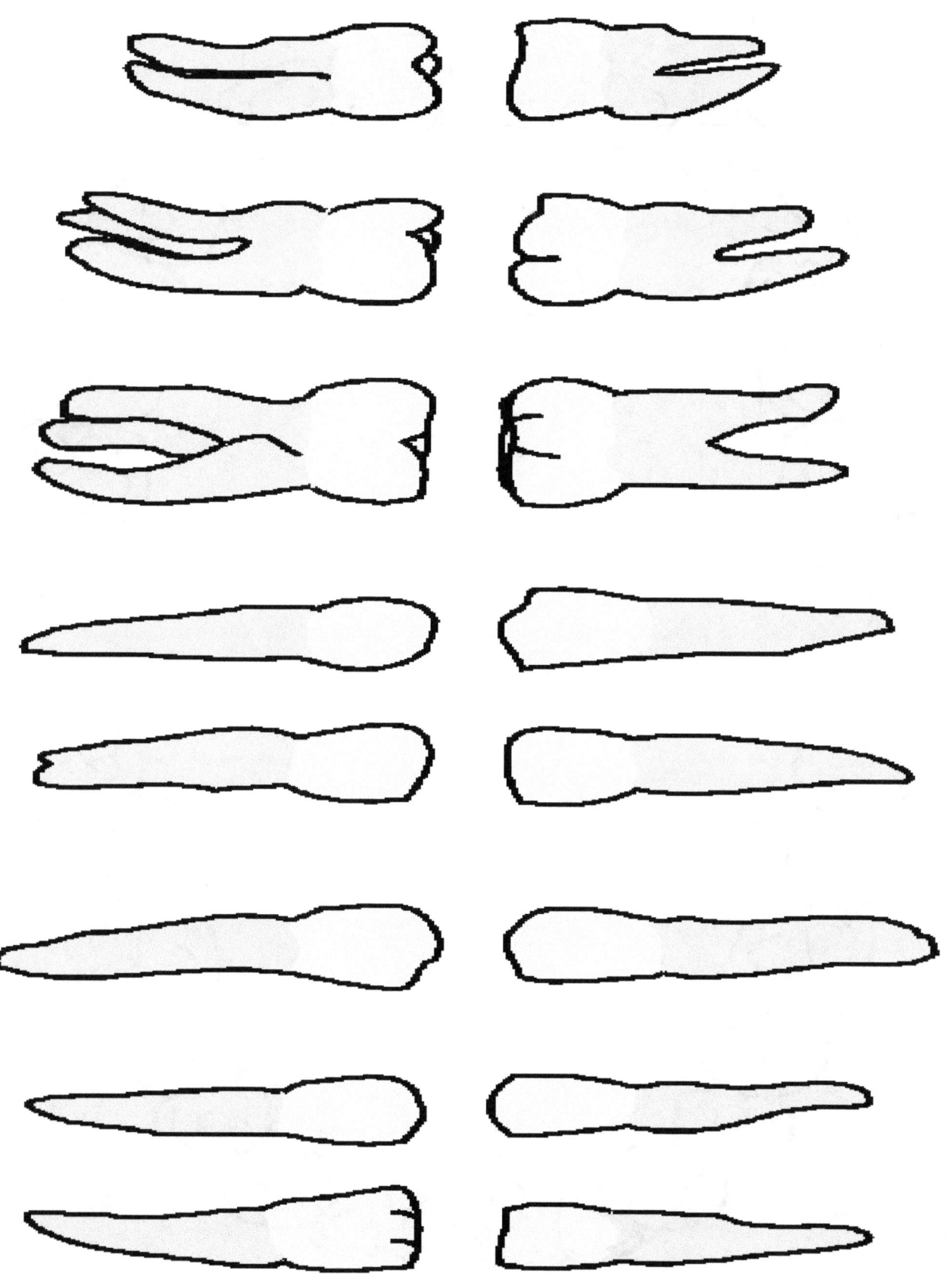

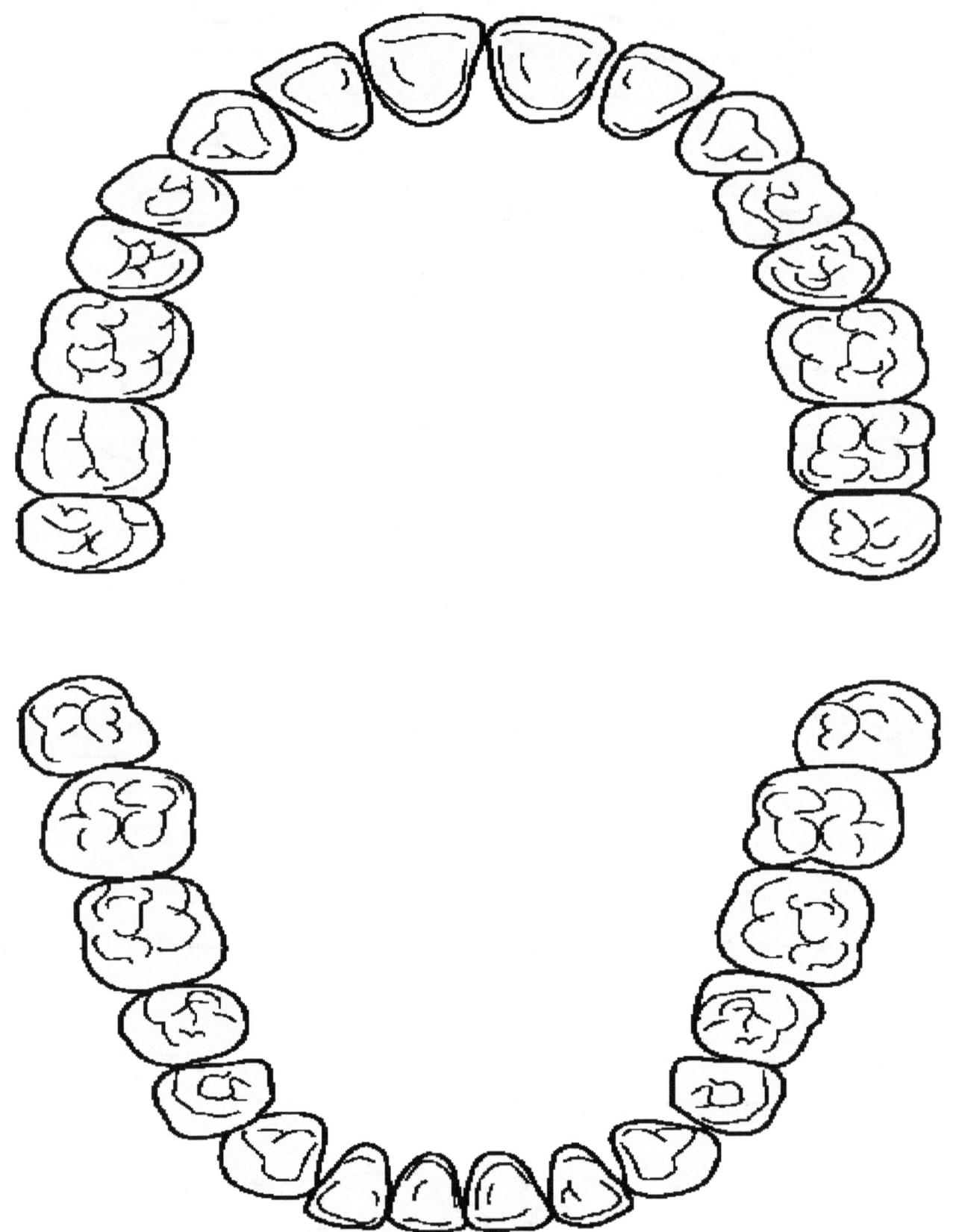

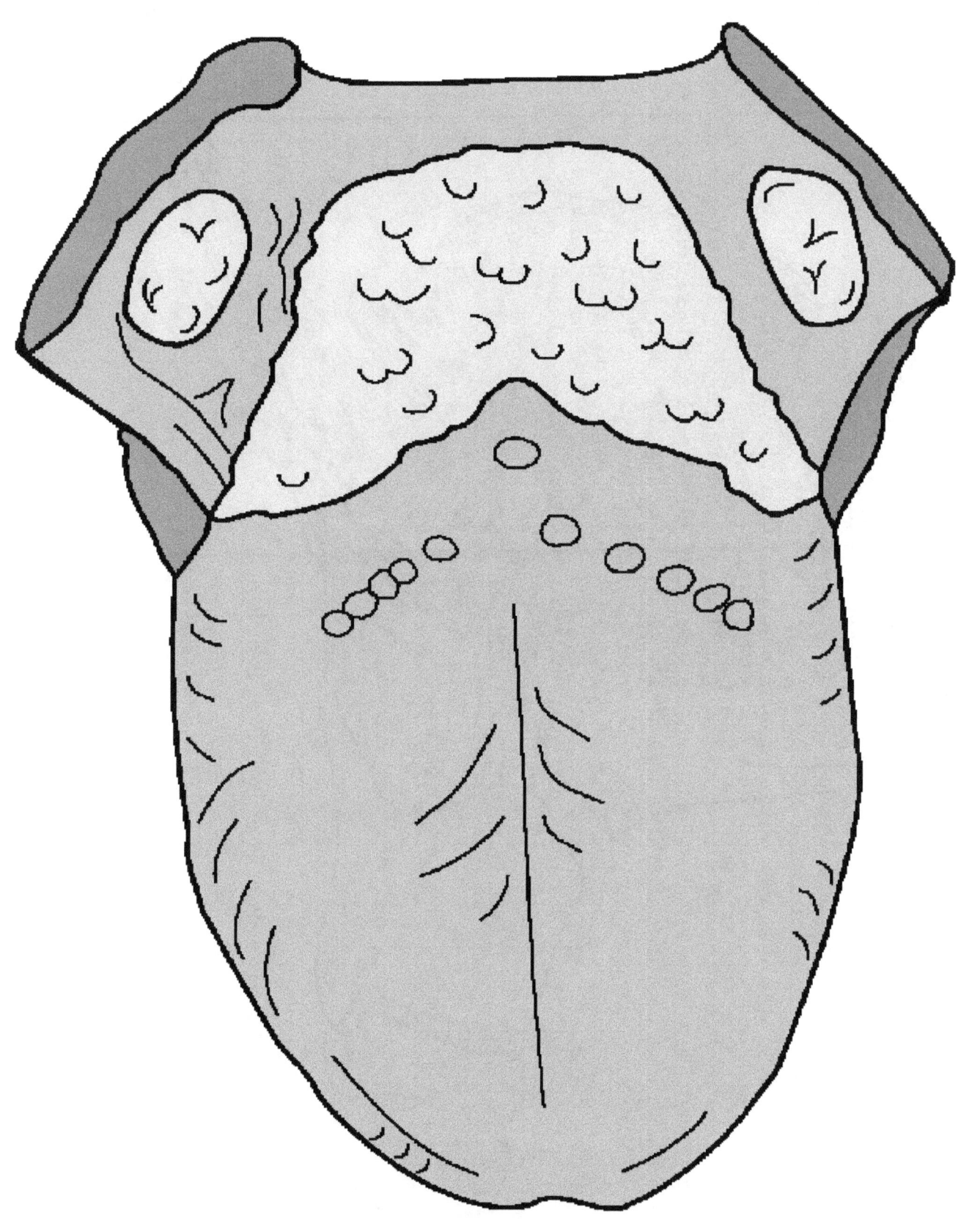

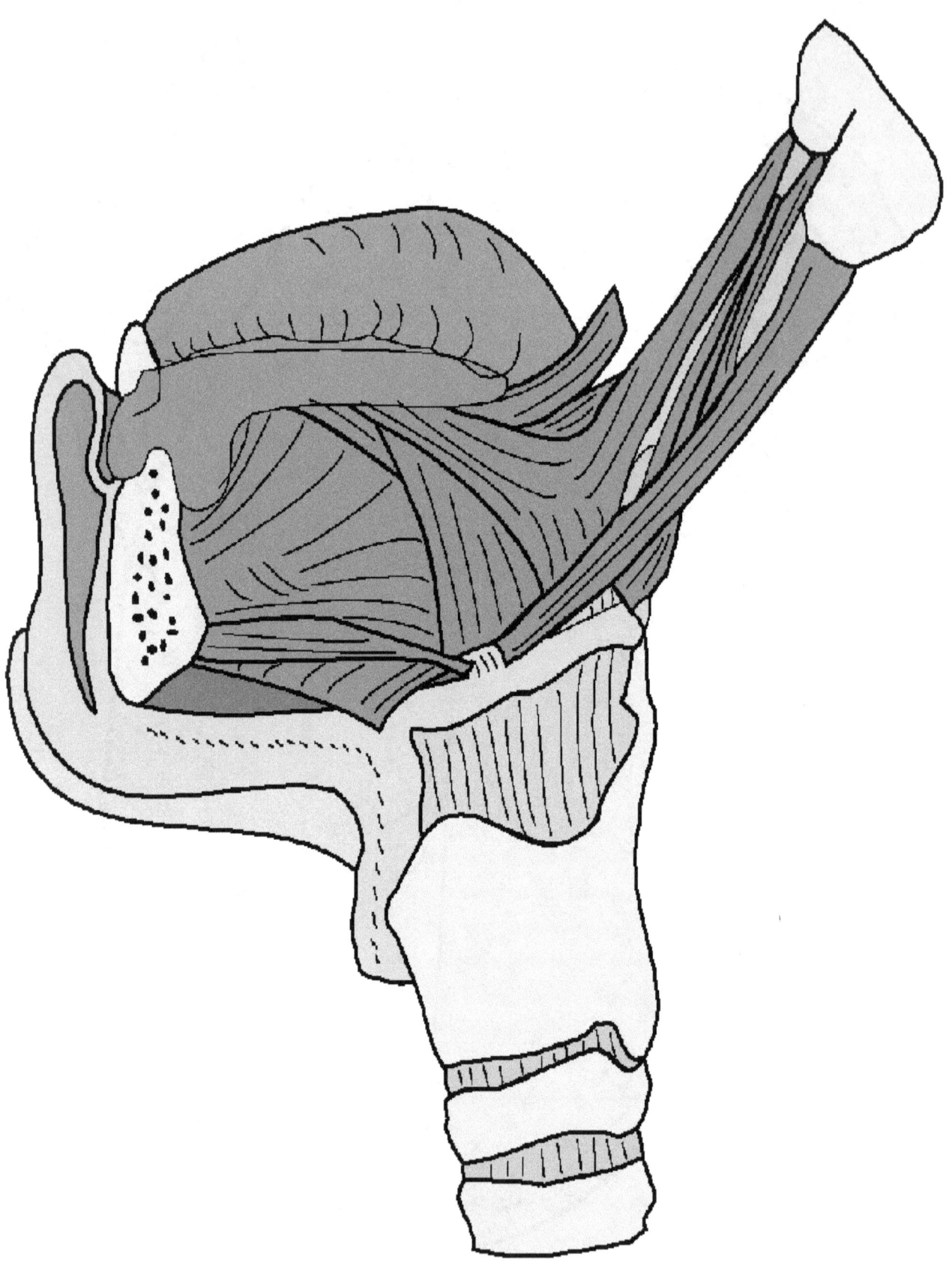

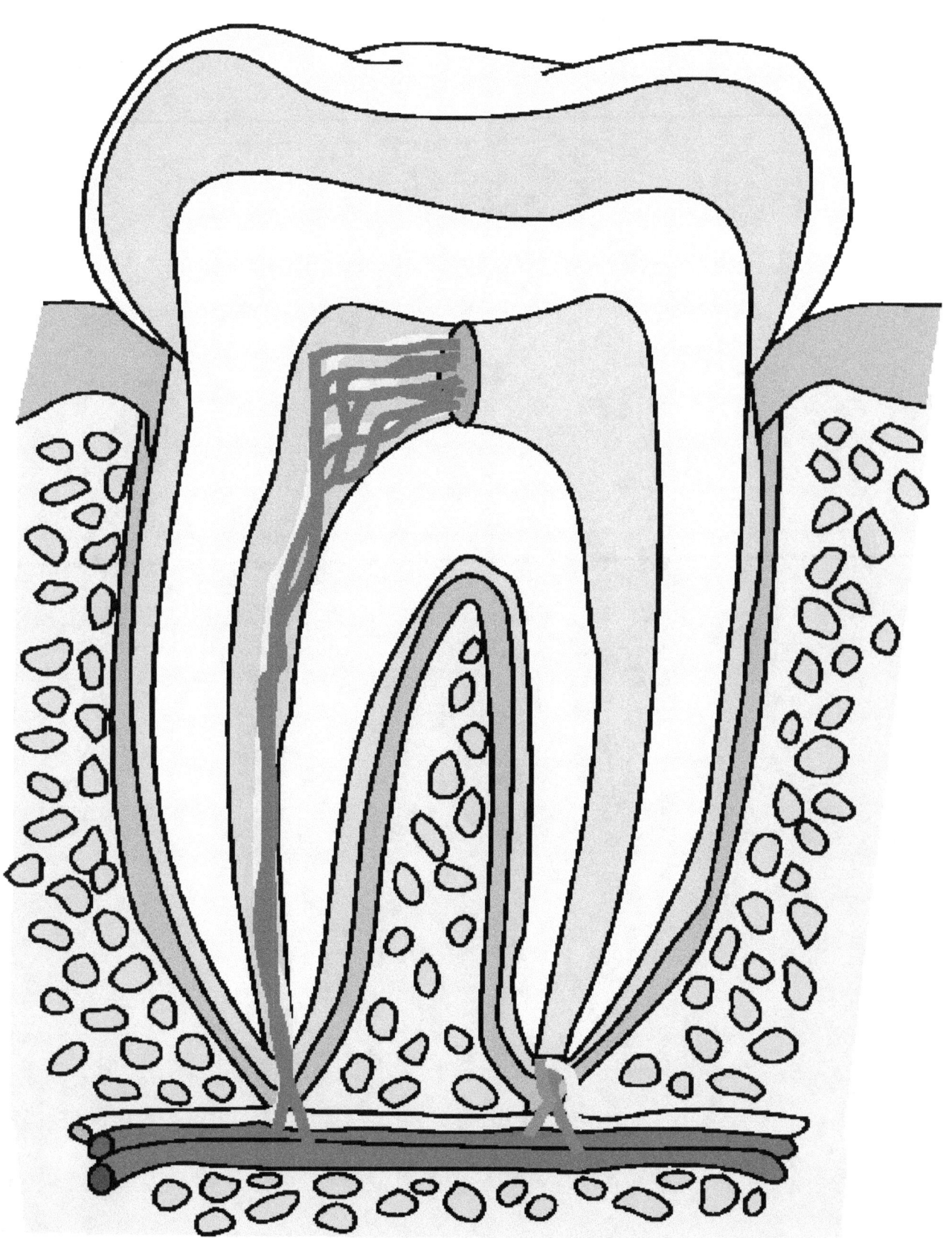

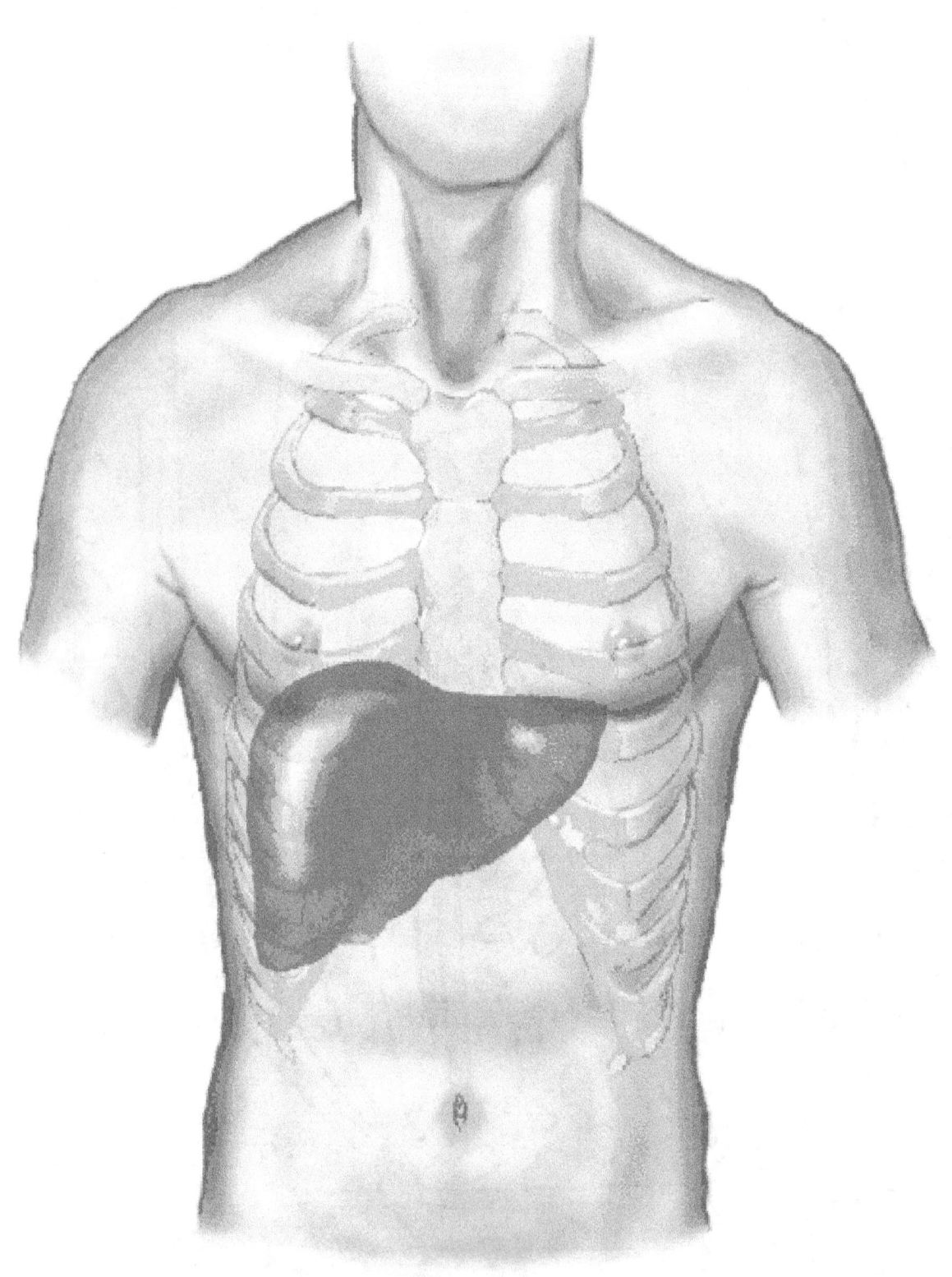

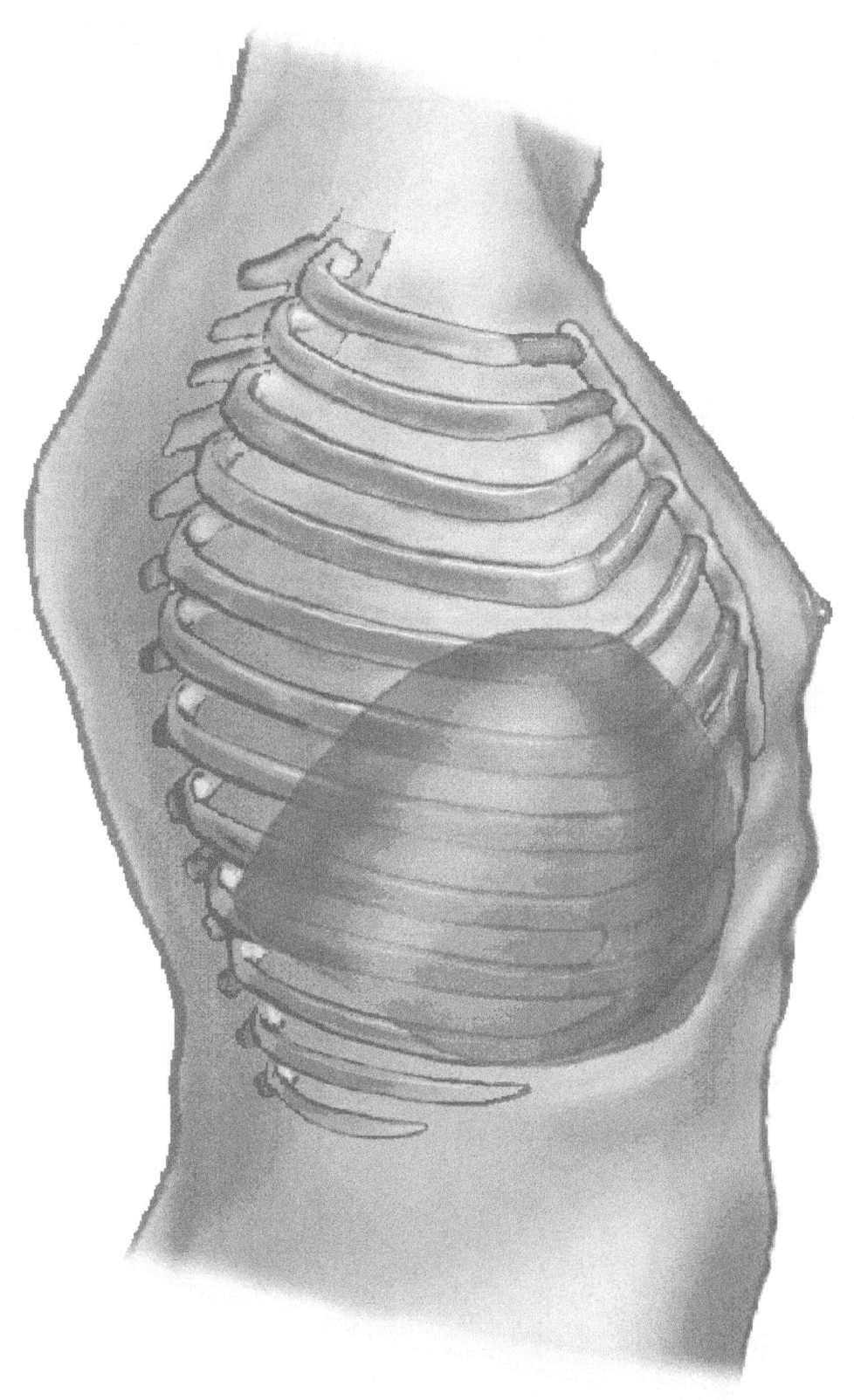

Nervous System 187 - 222

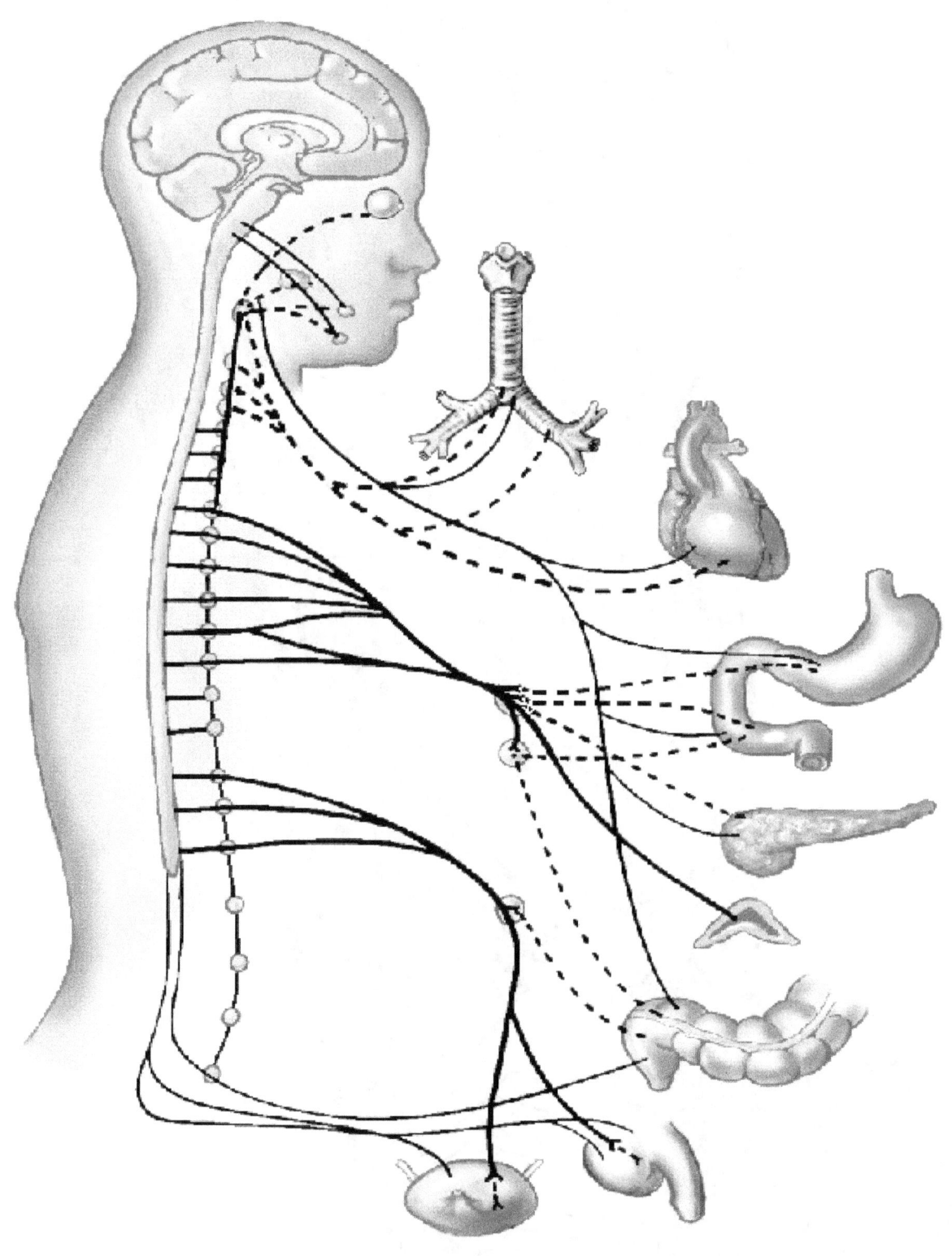

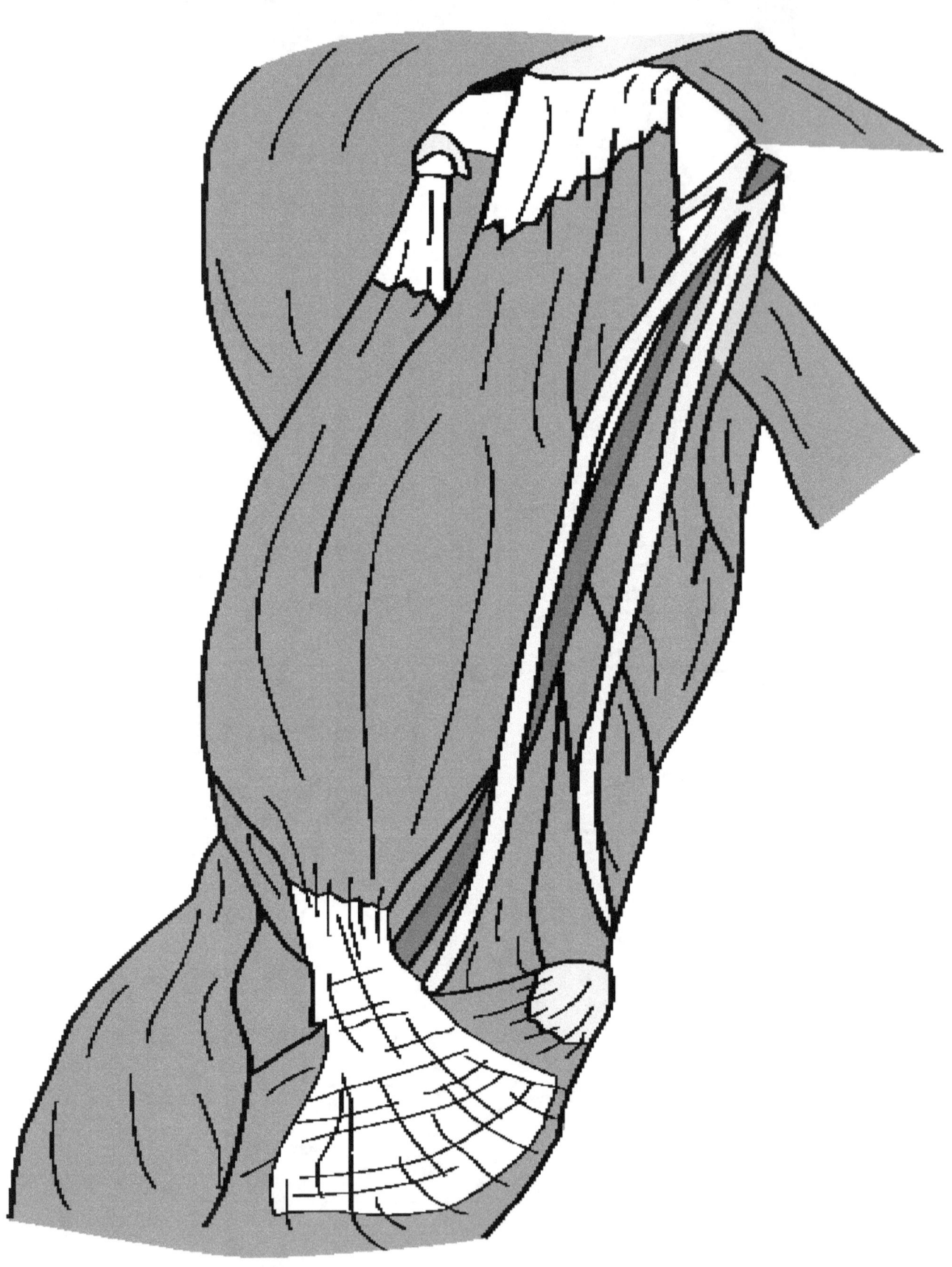

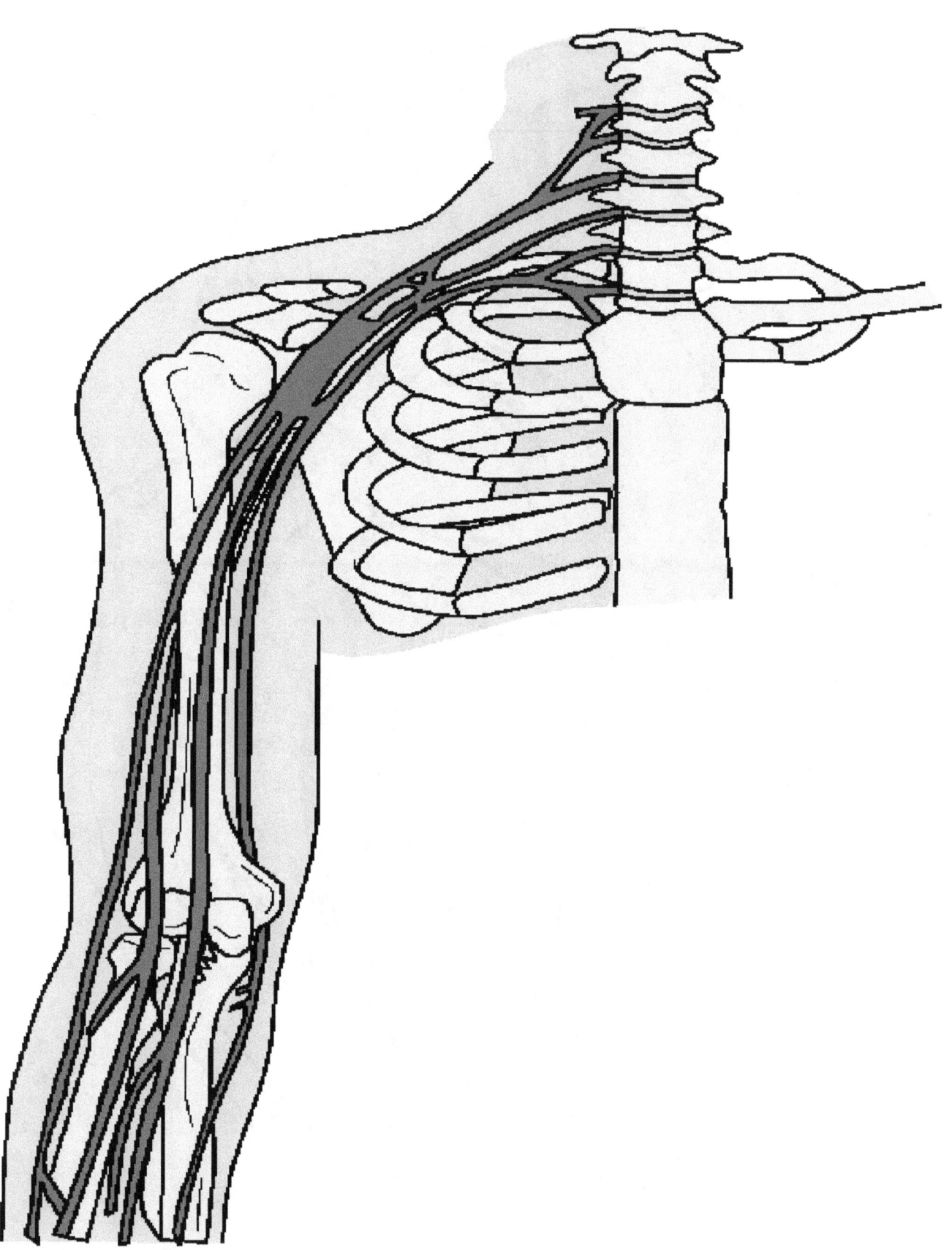

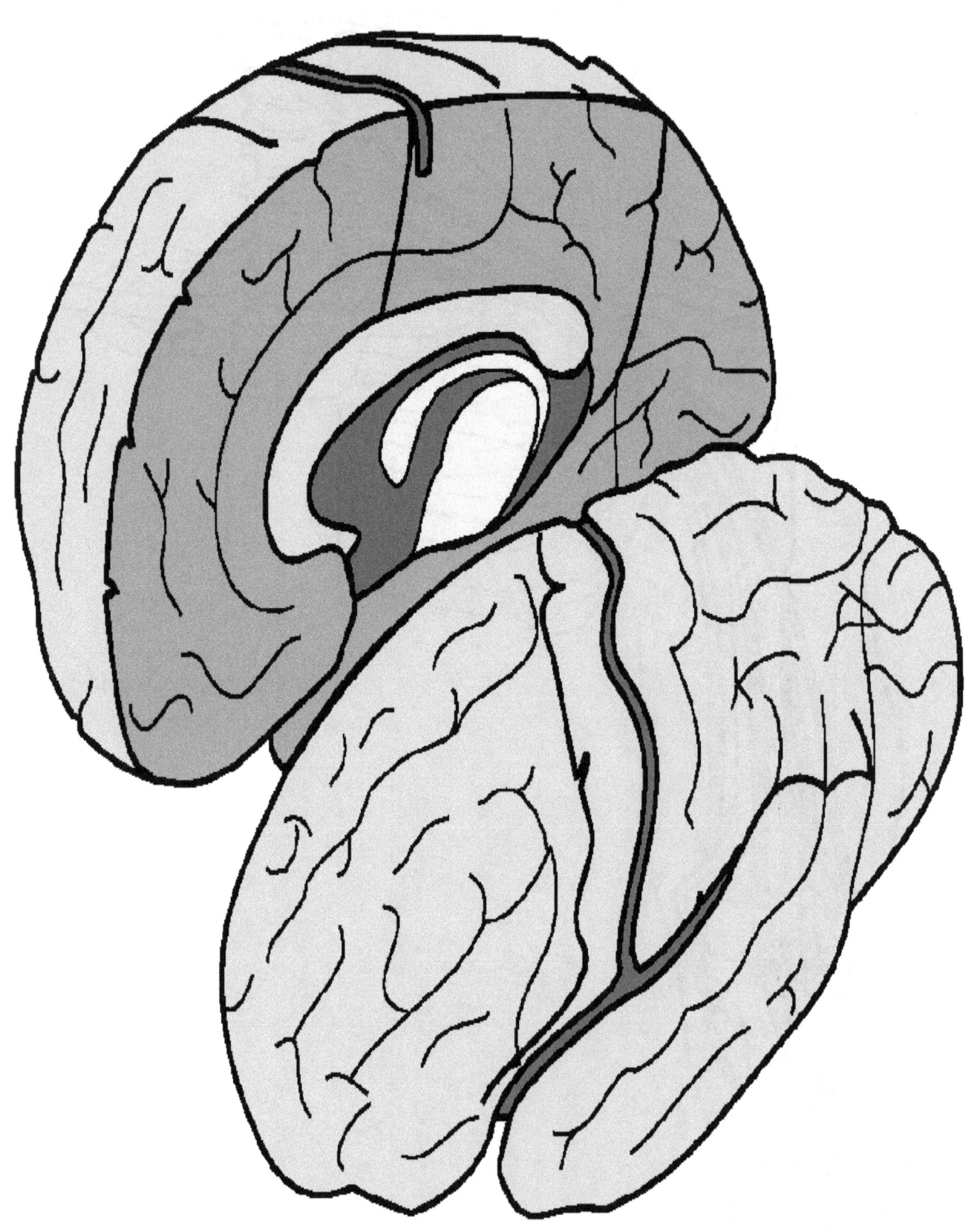

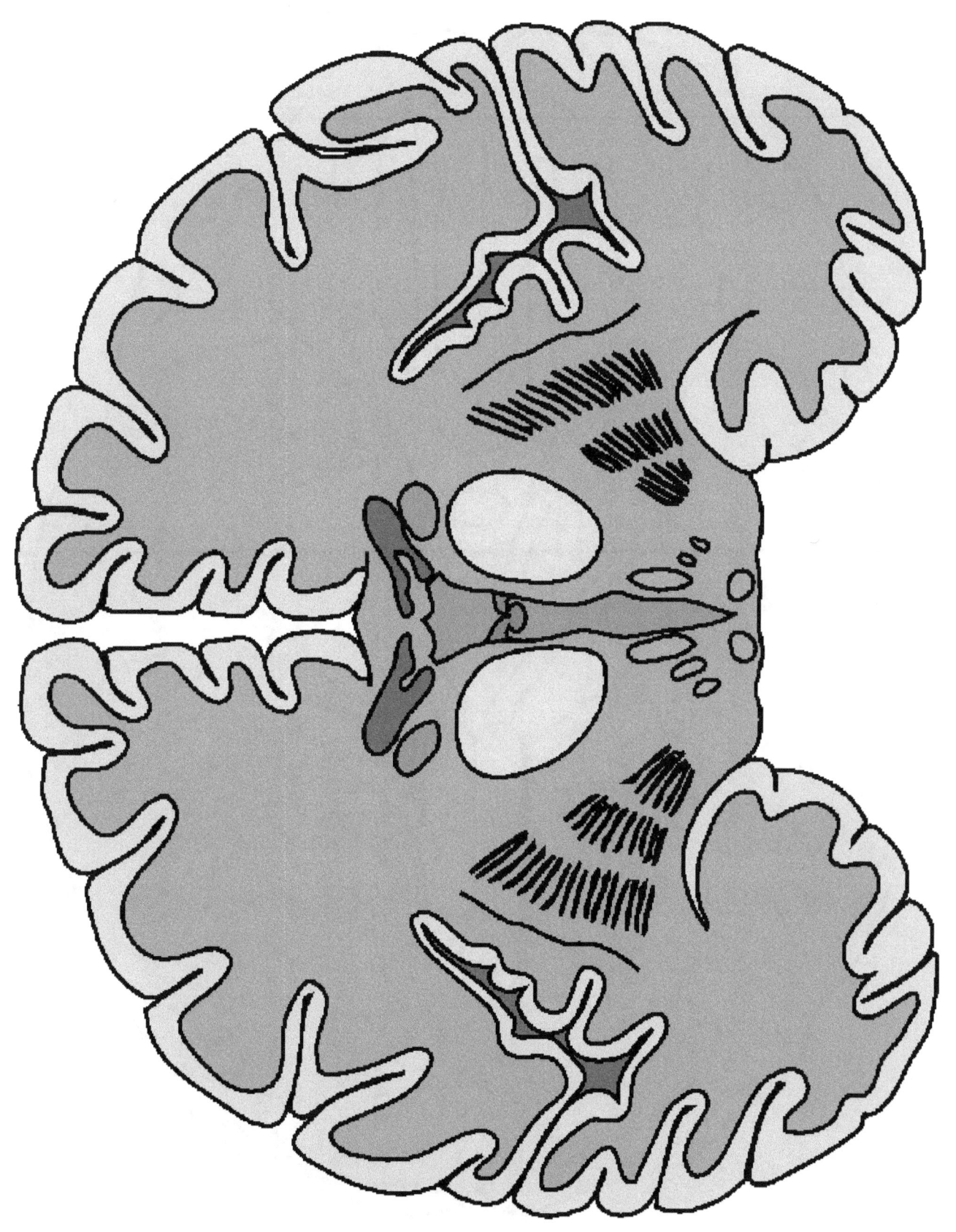

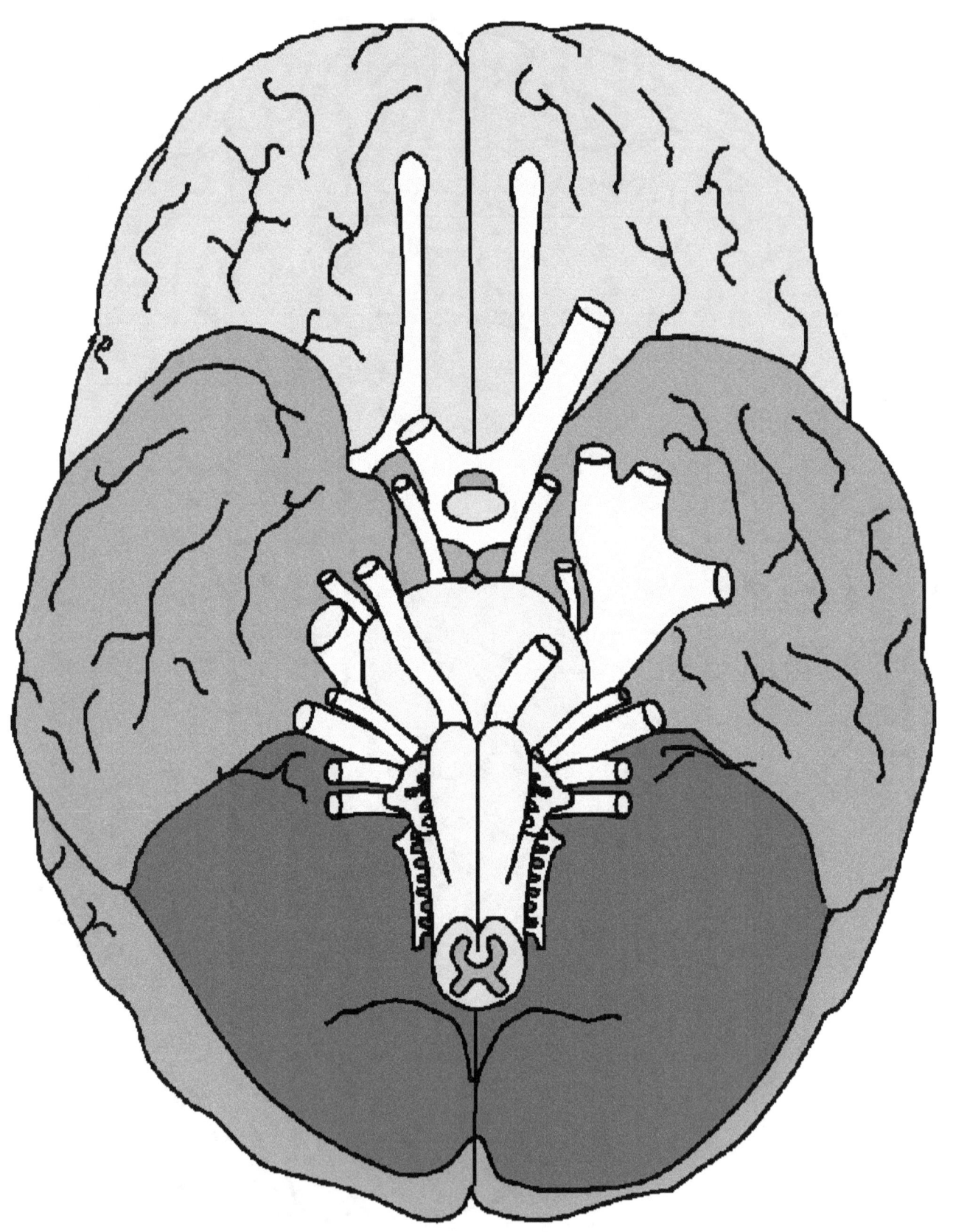

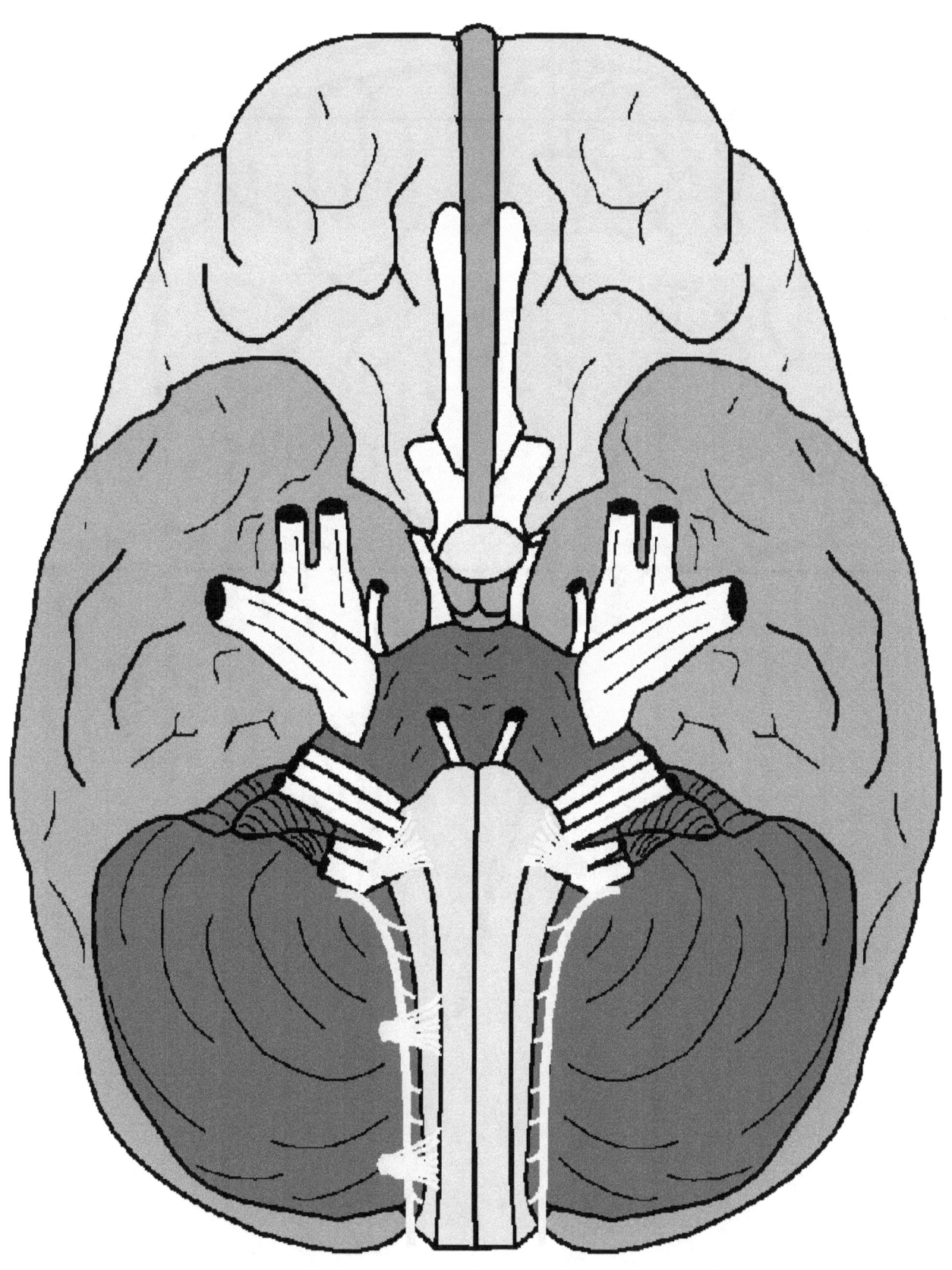

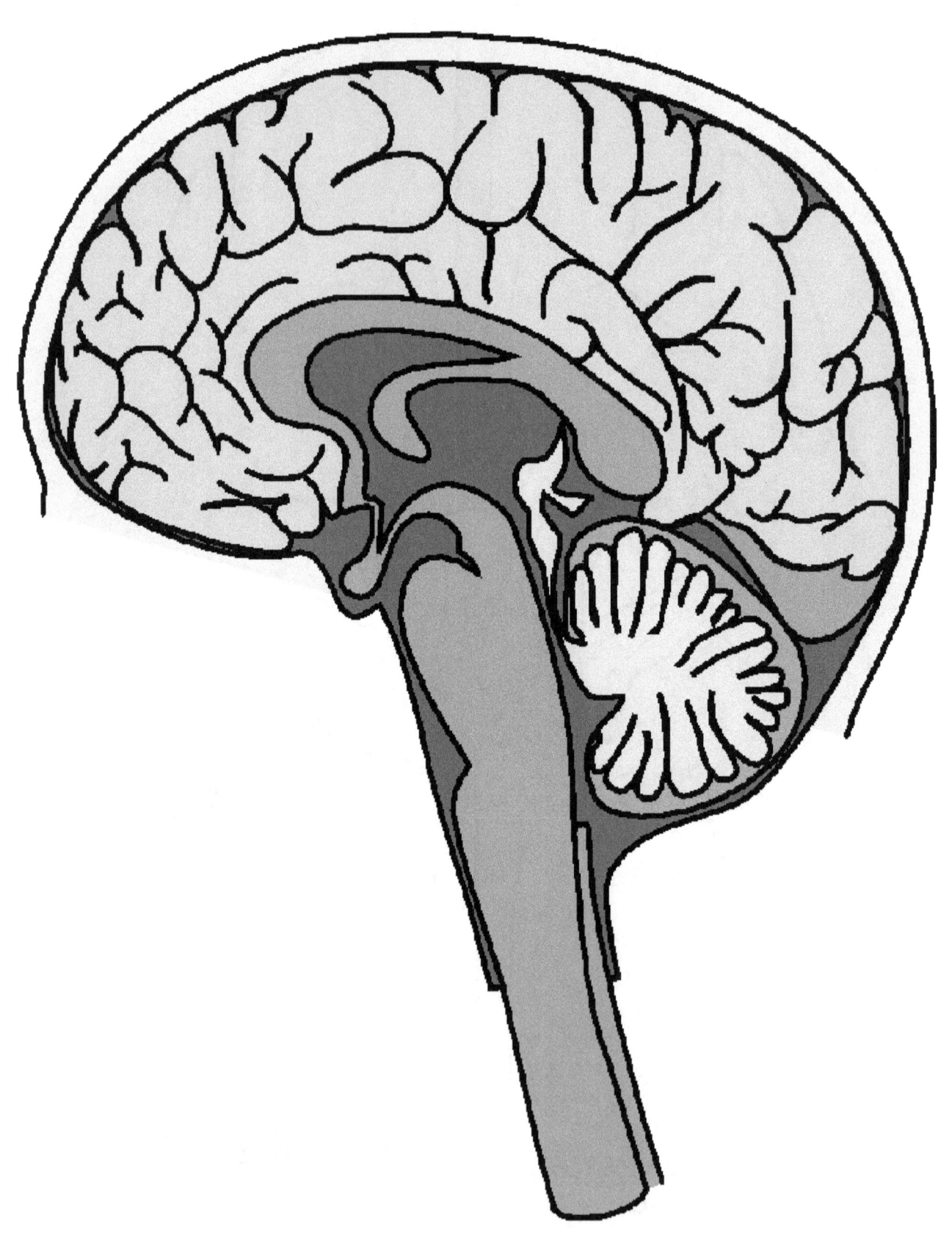

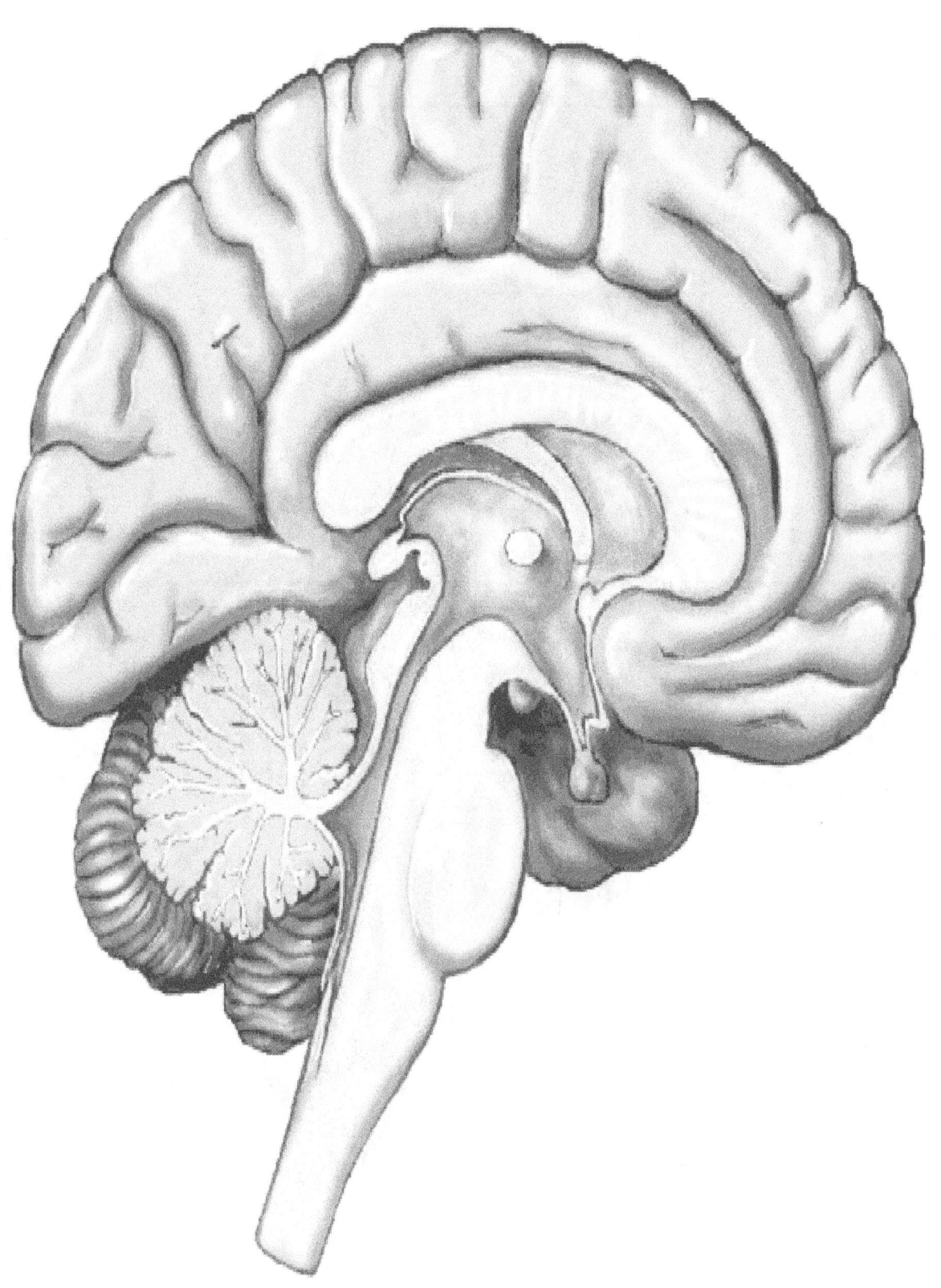

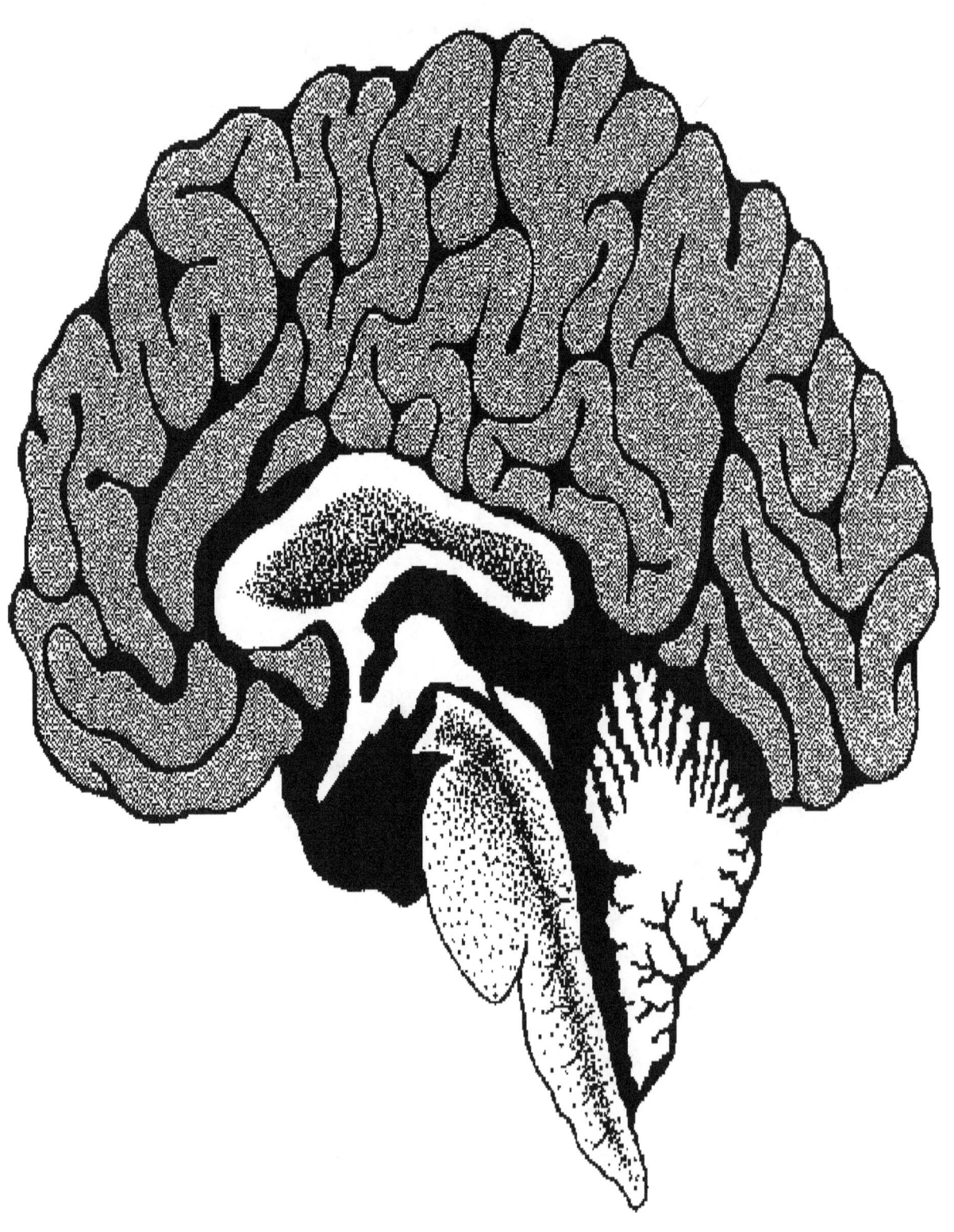

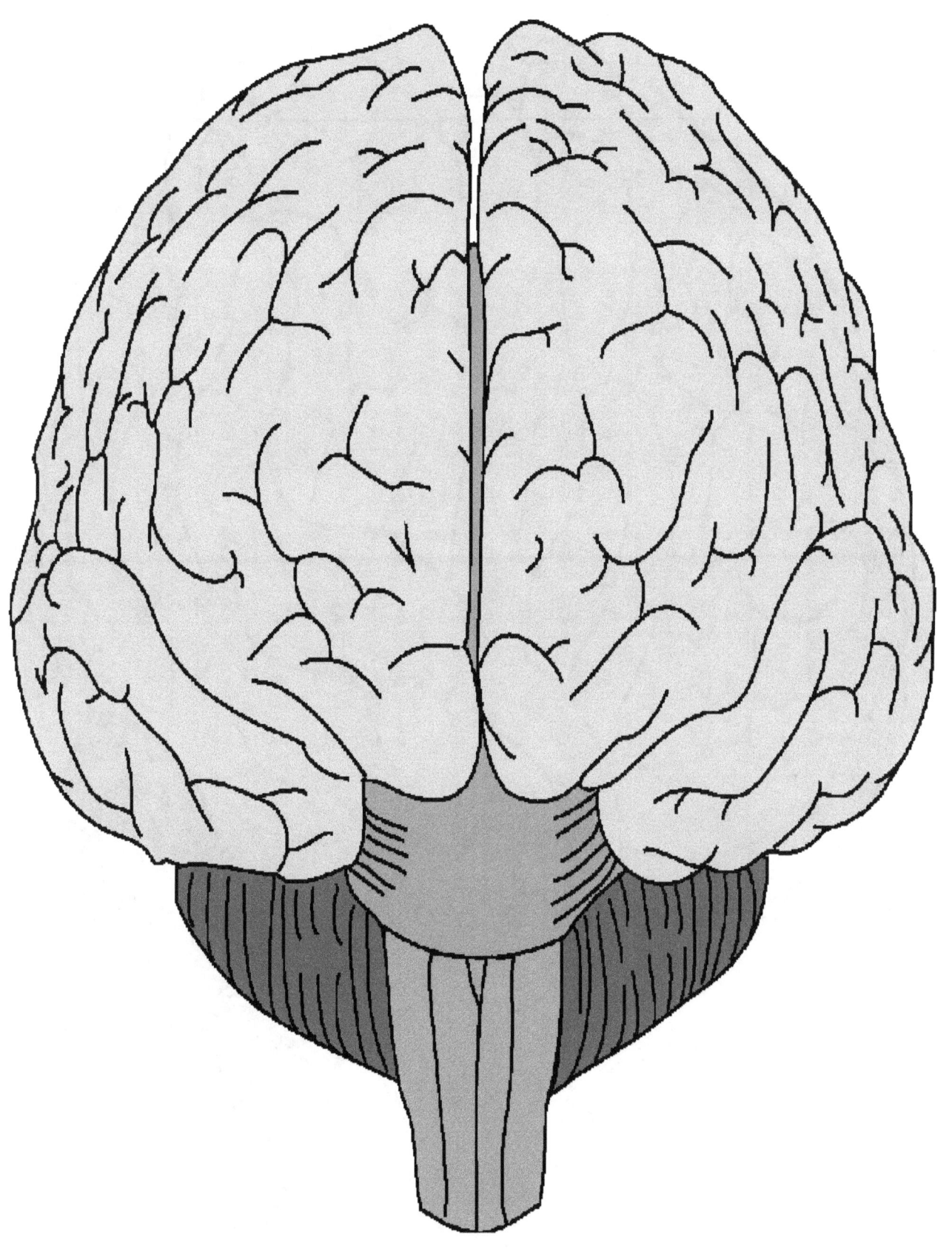

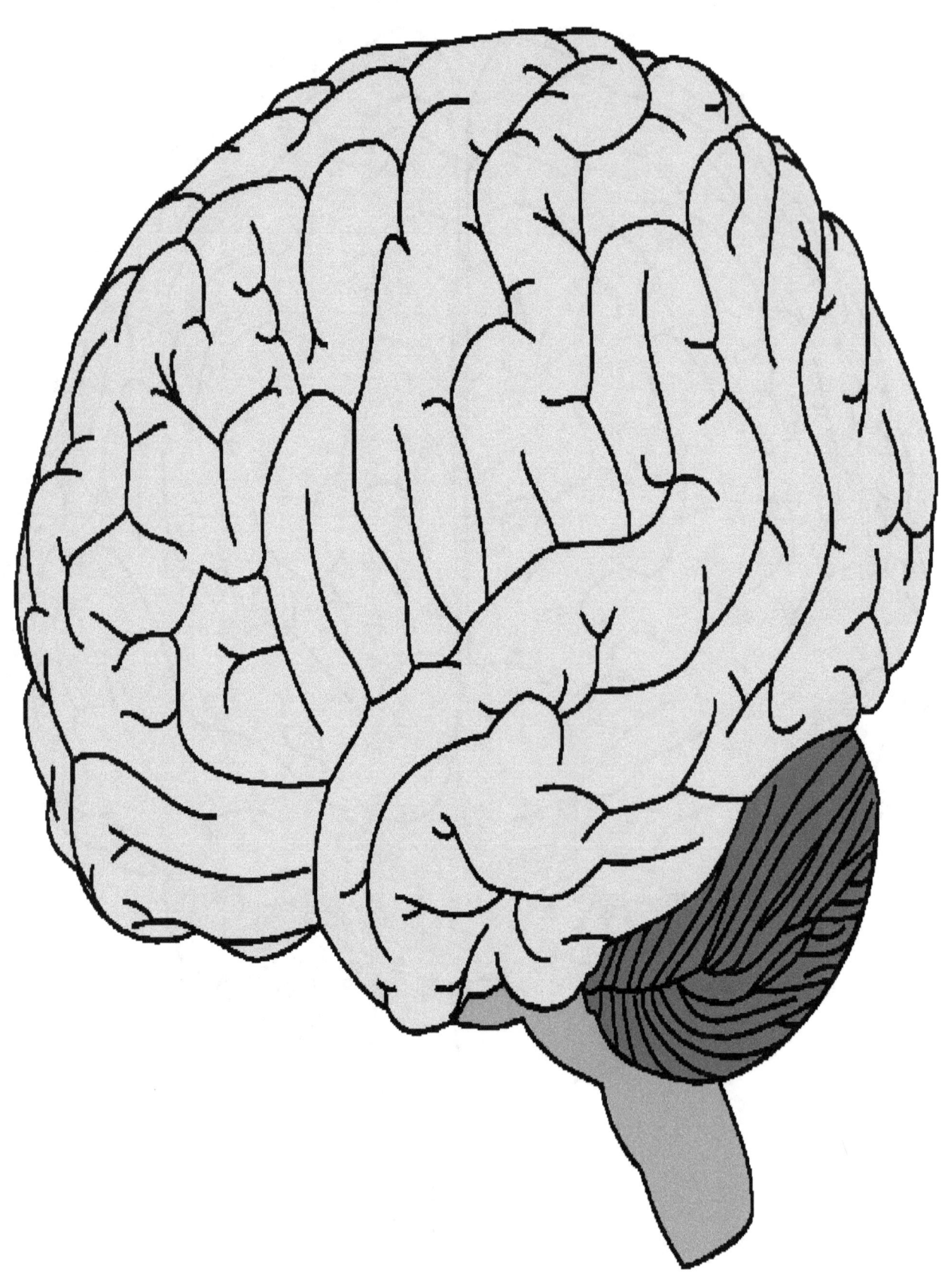

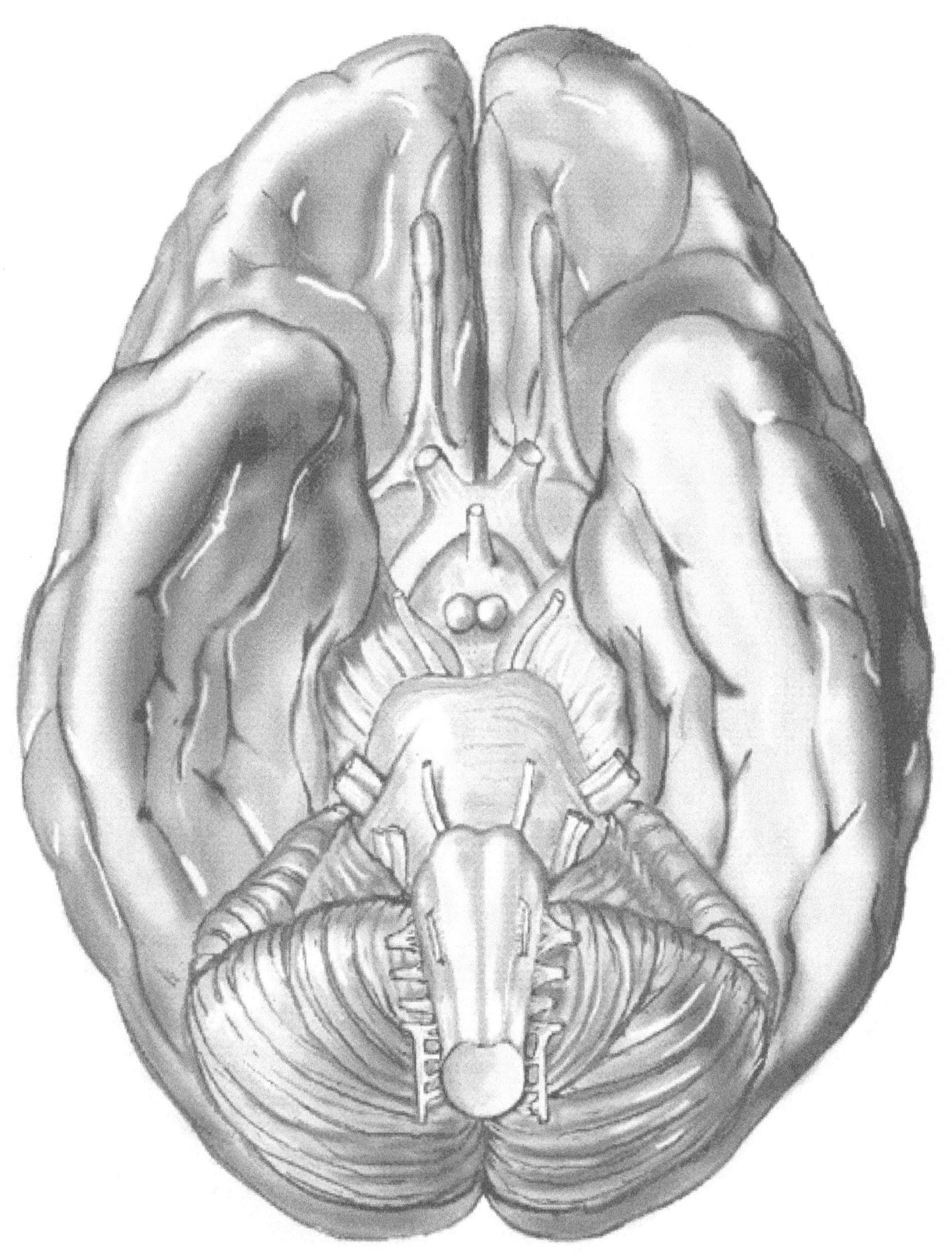

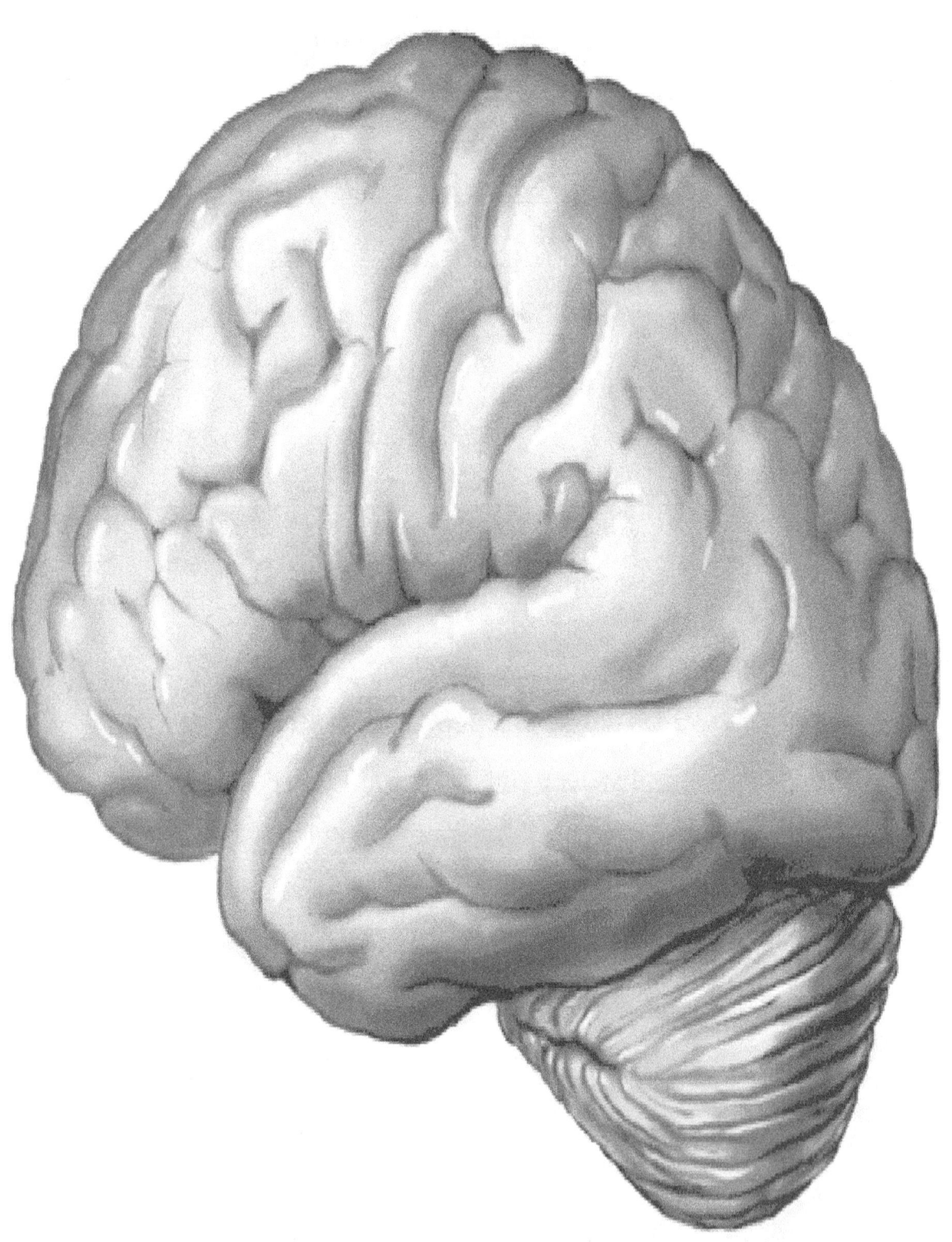

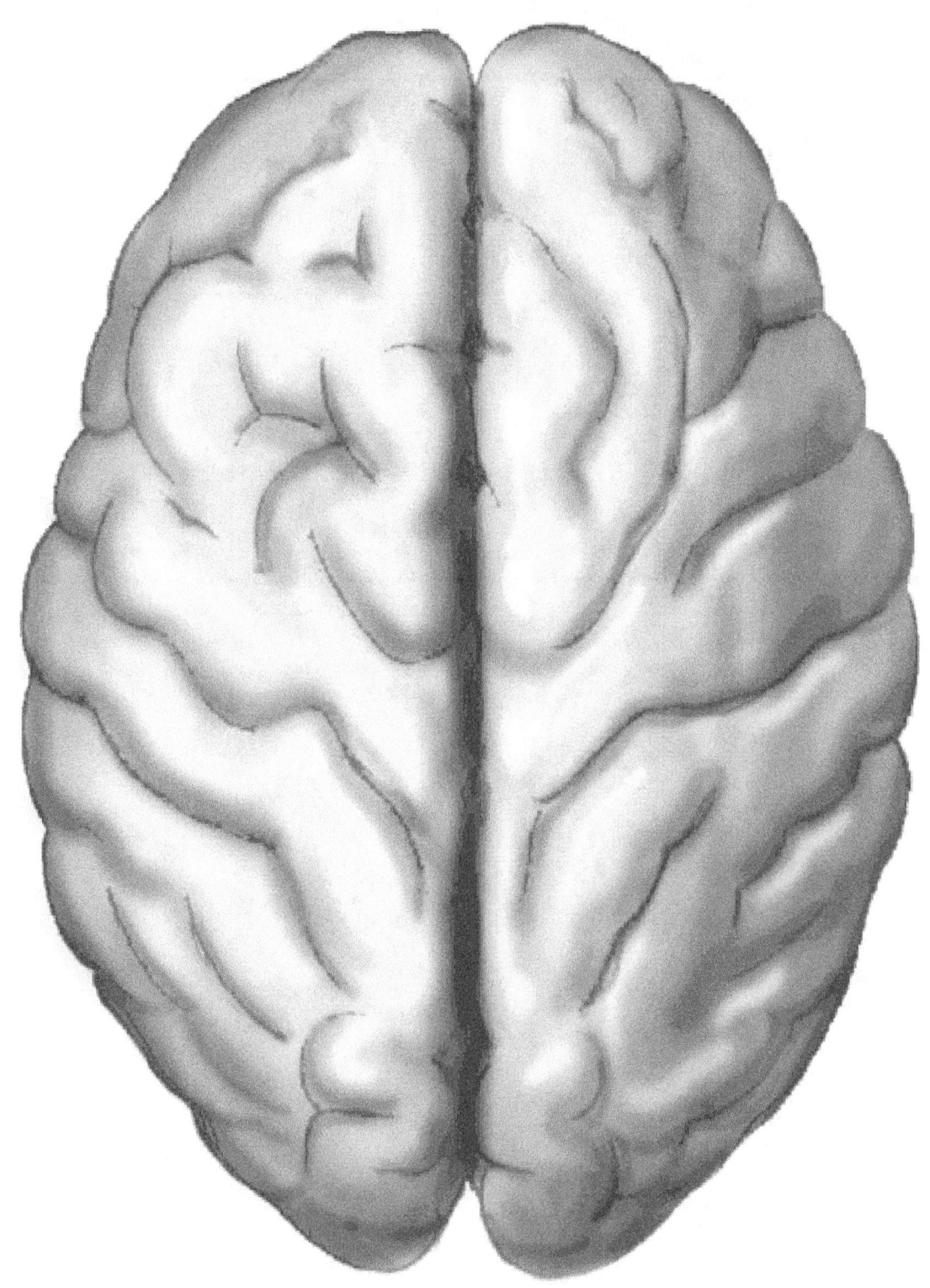

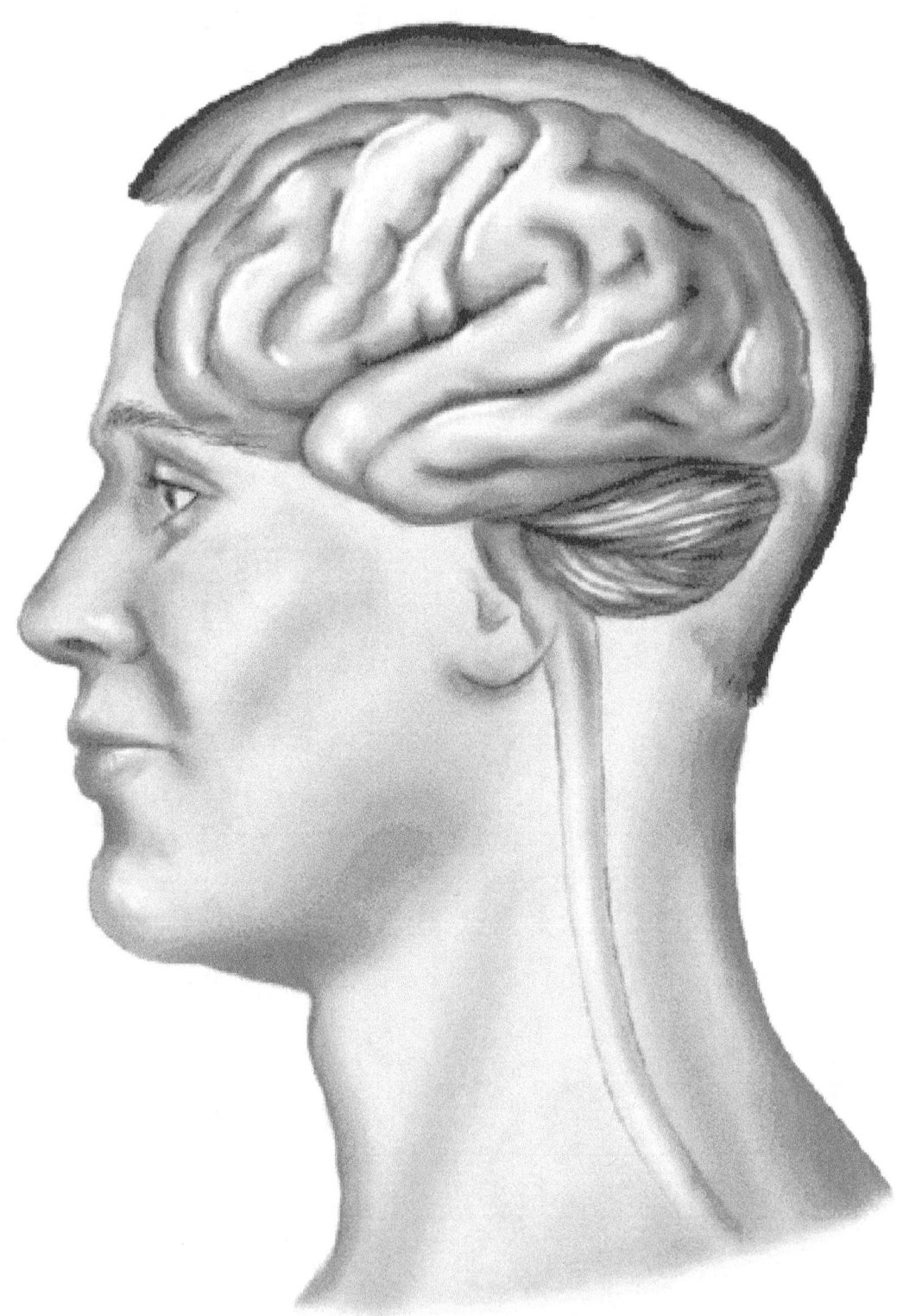

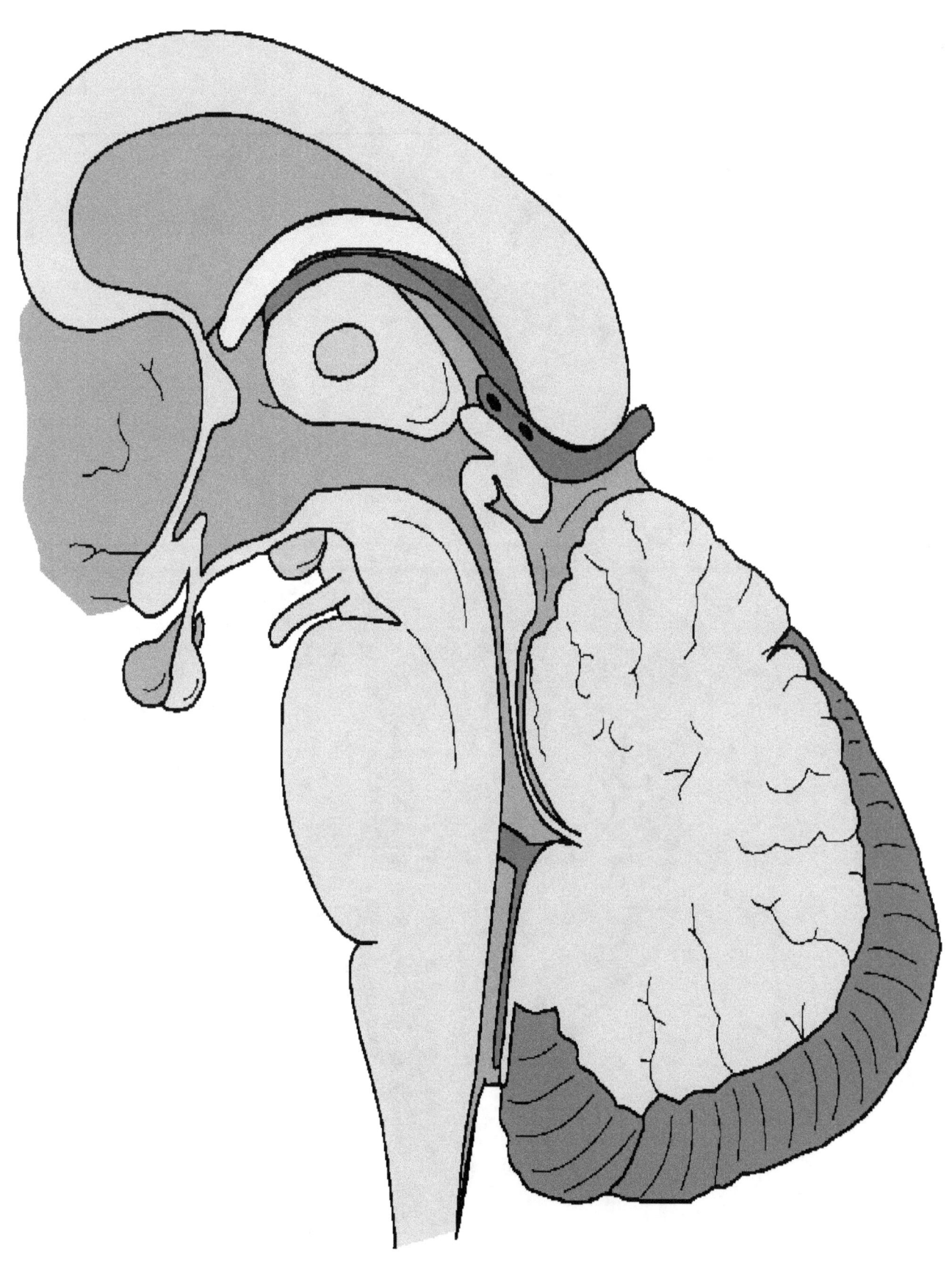

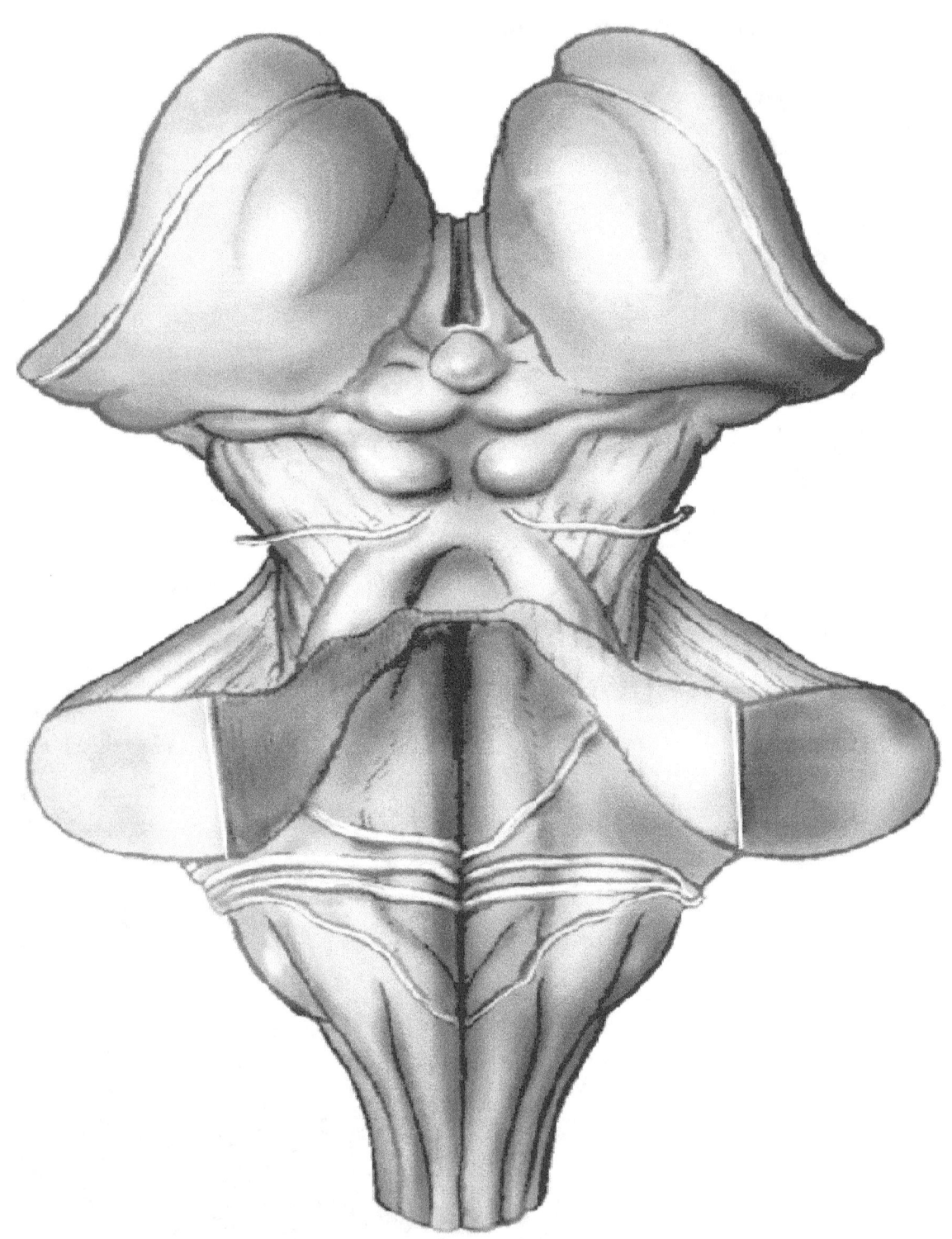

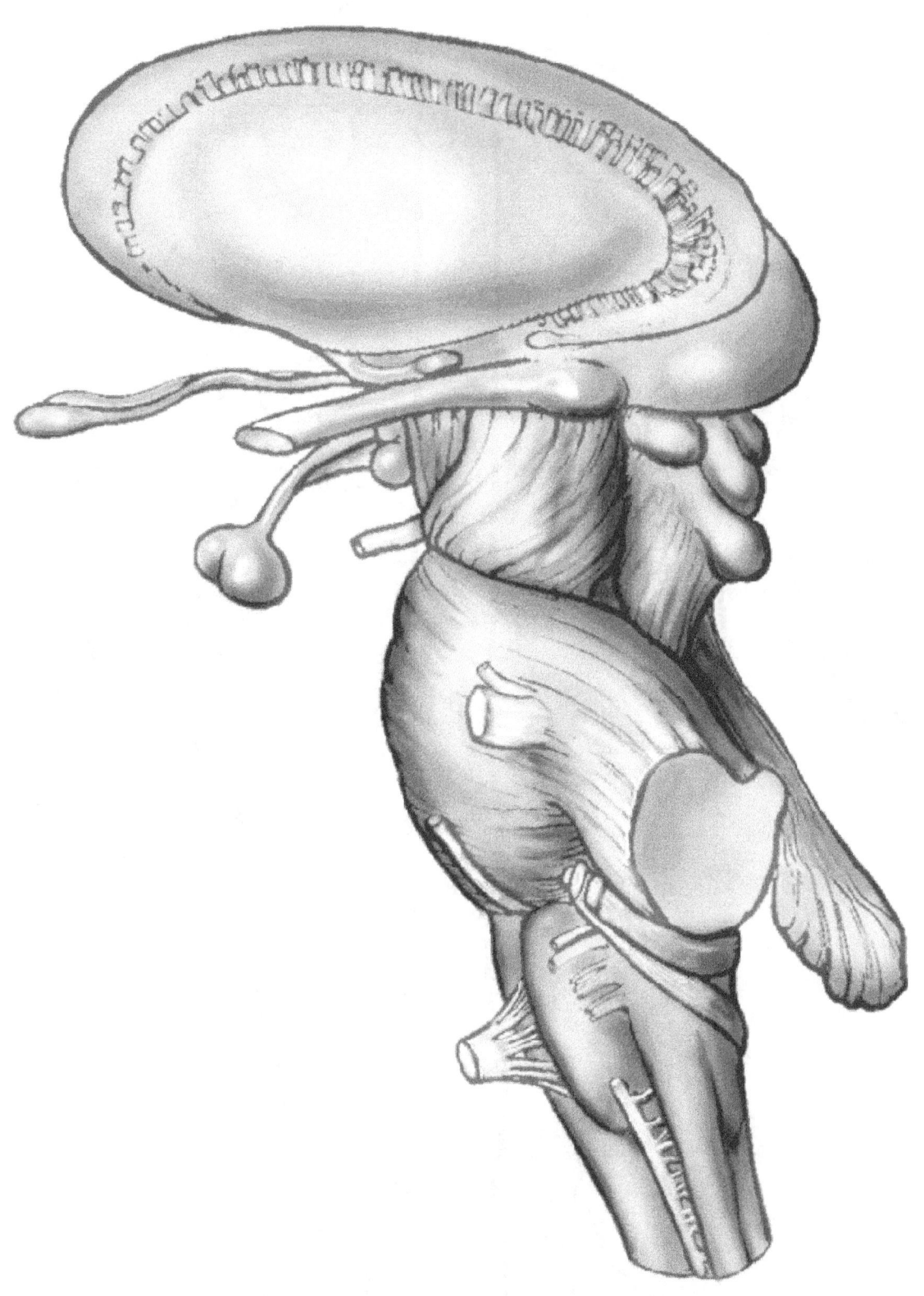

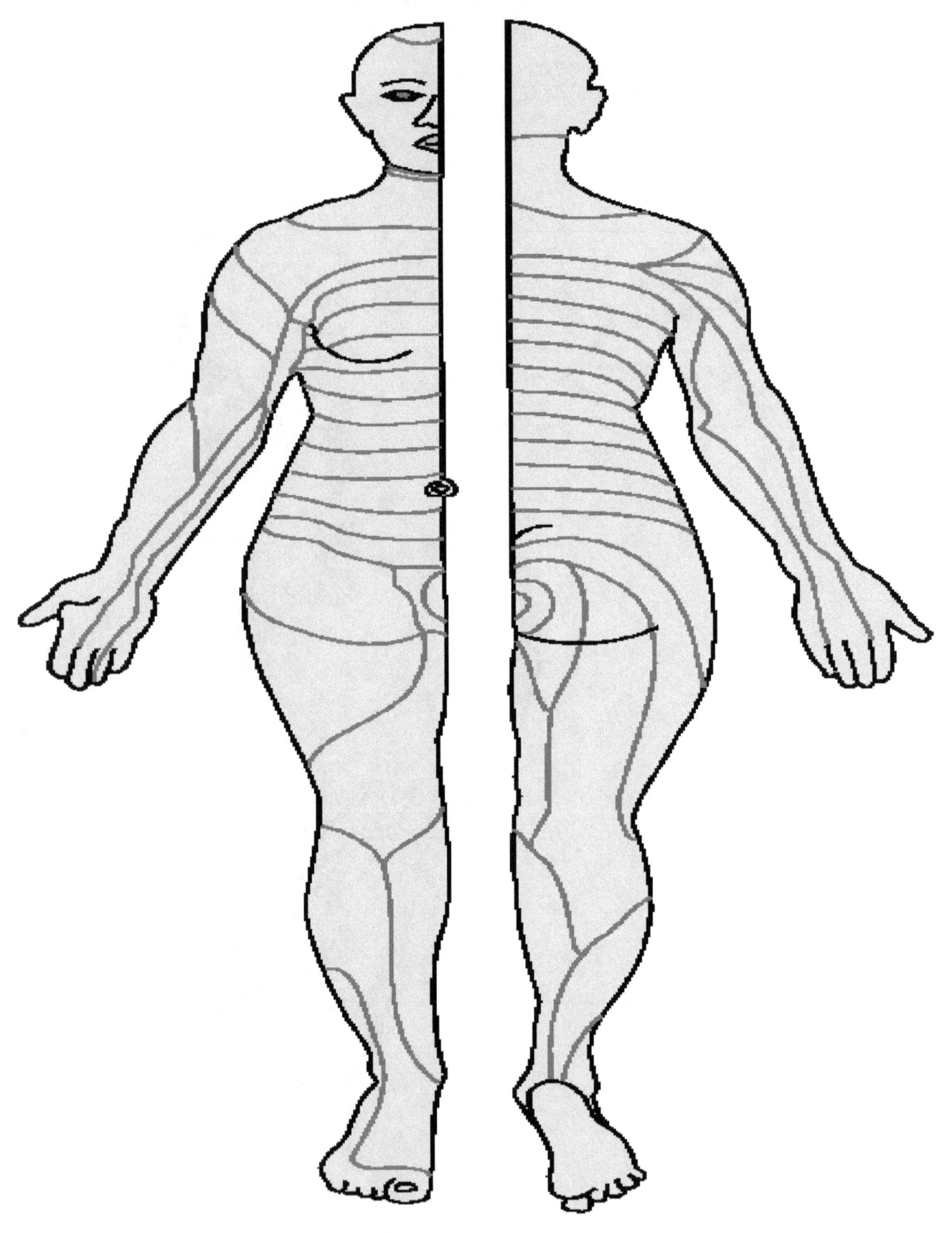

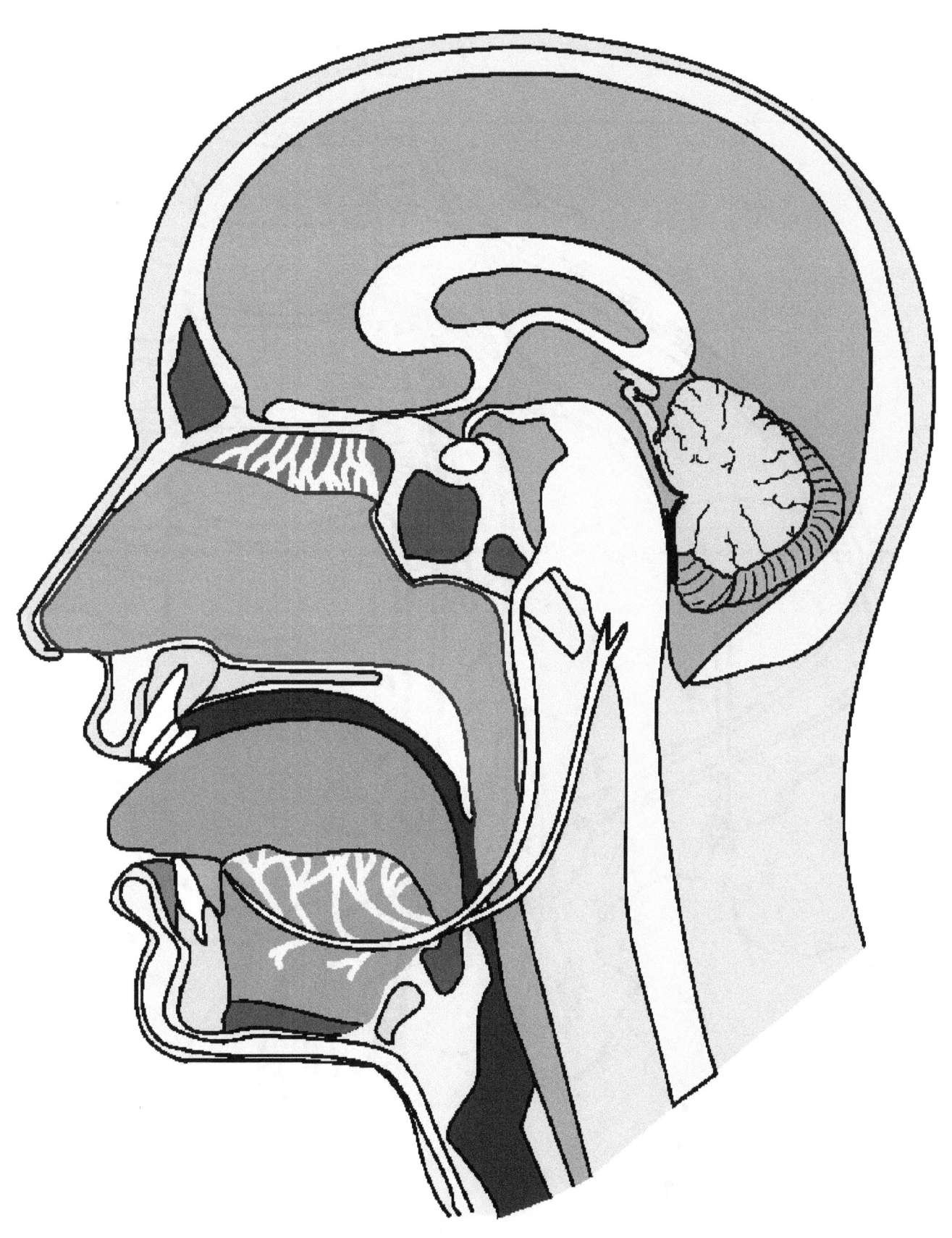

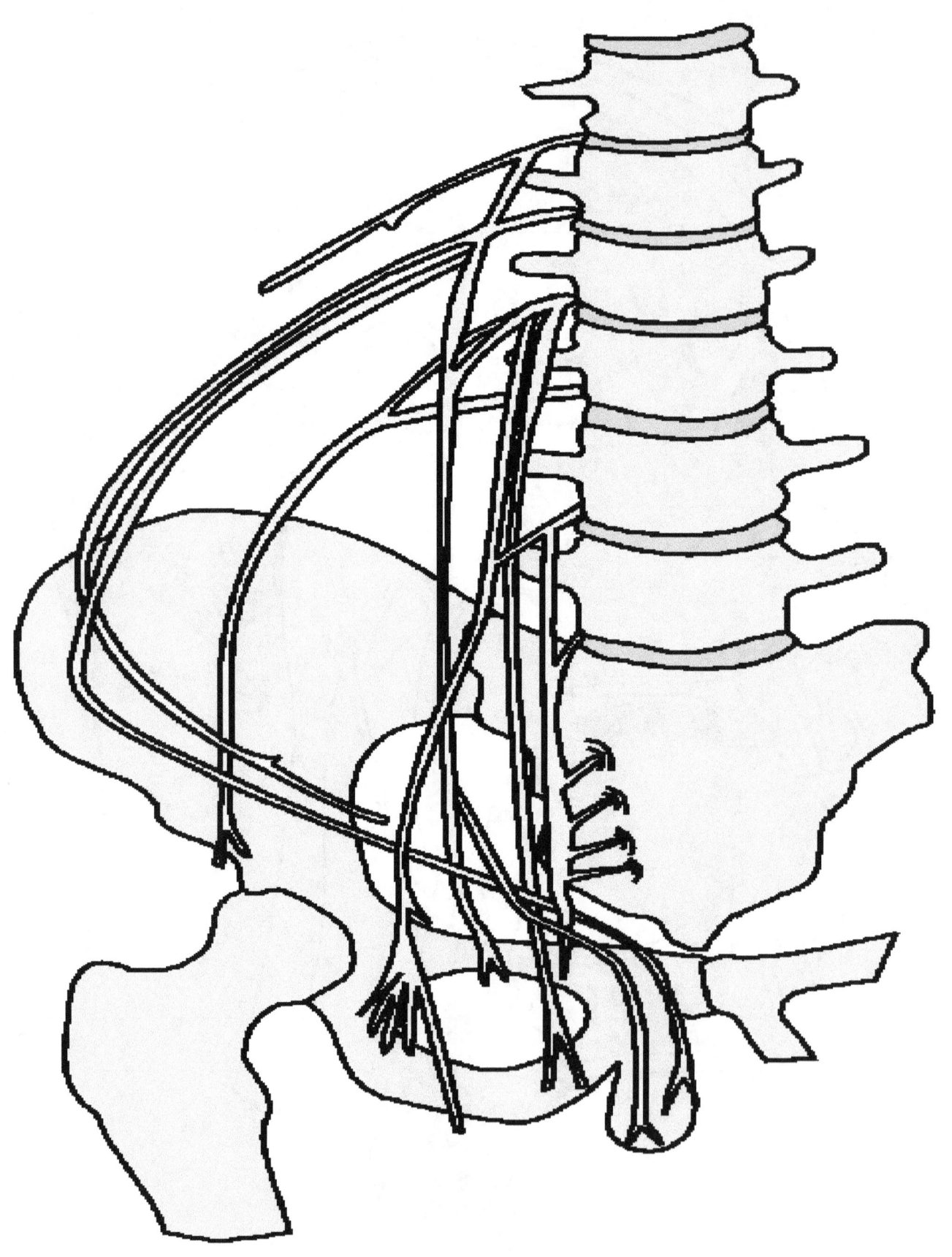

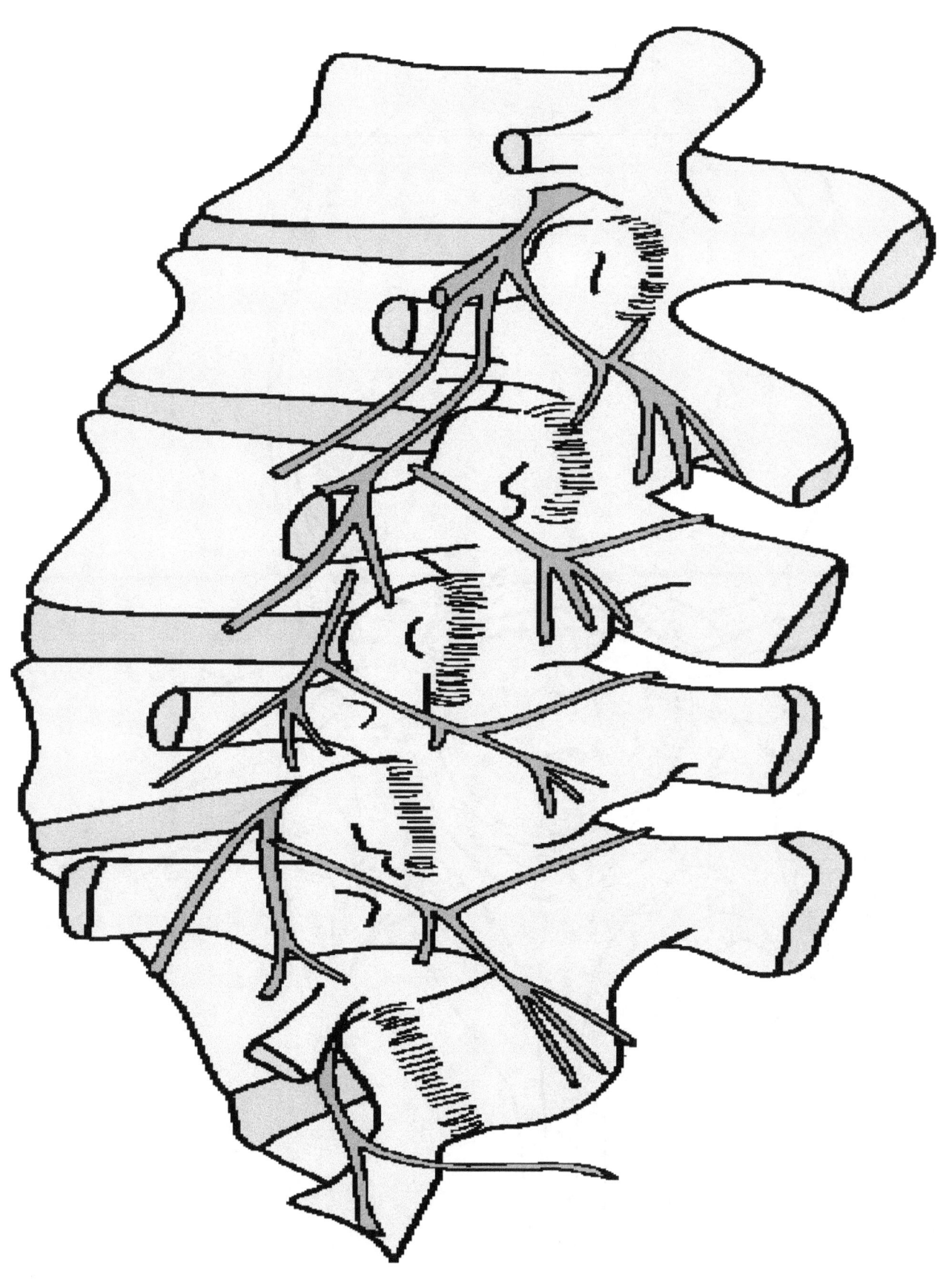

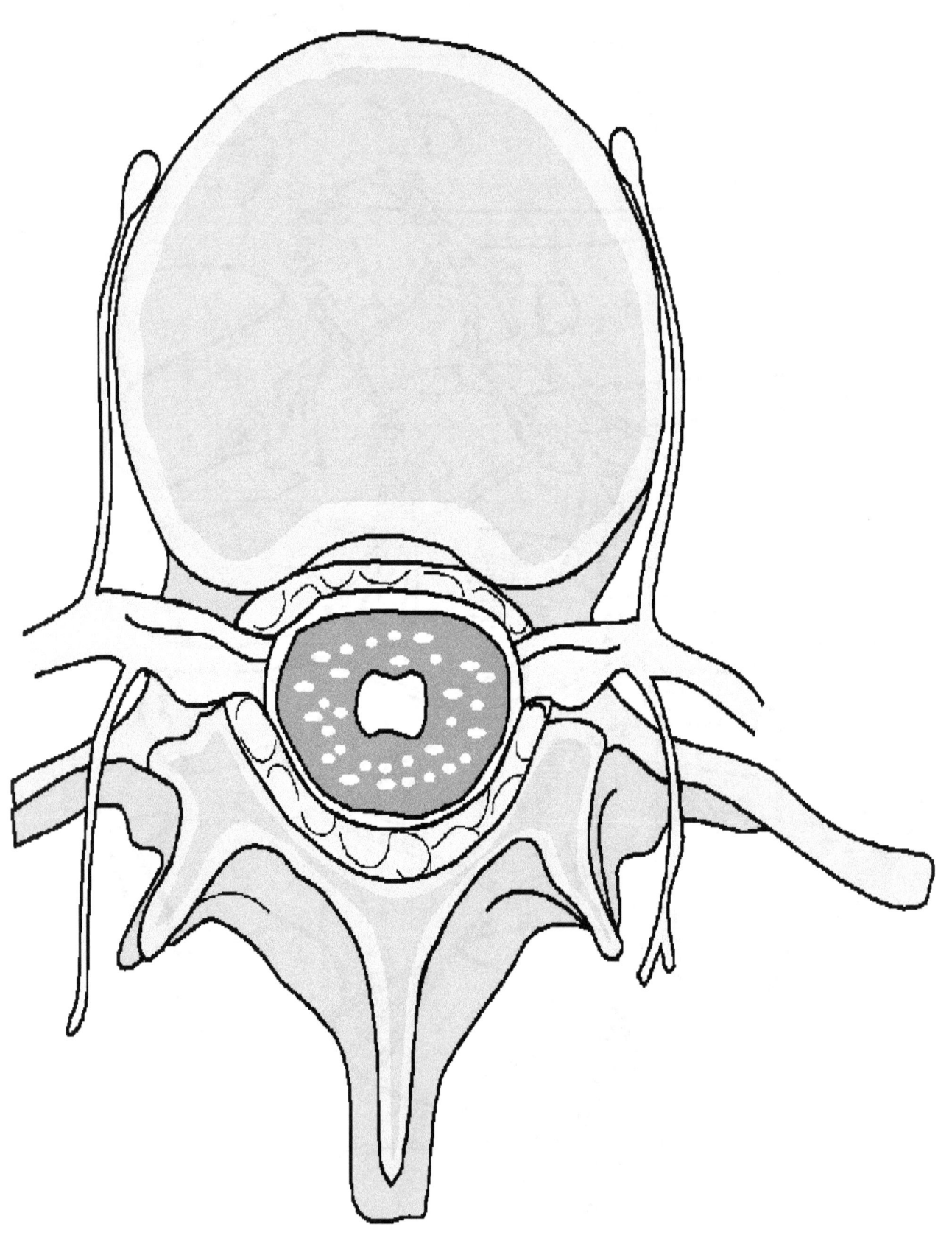

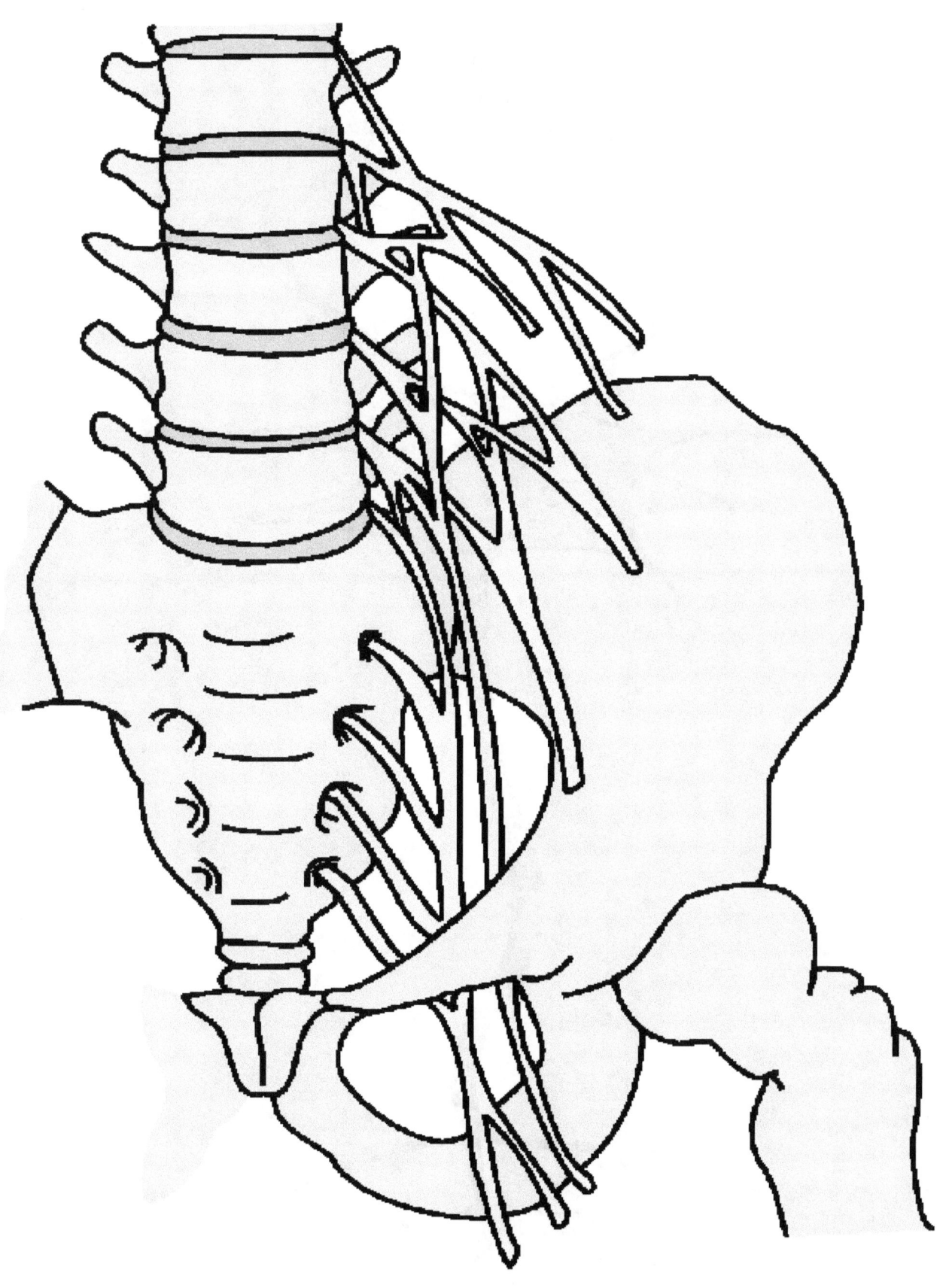

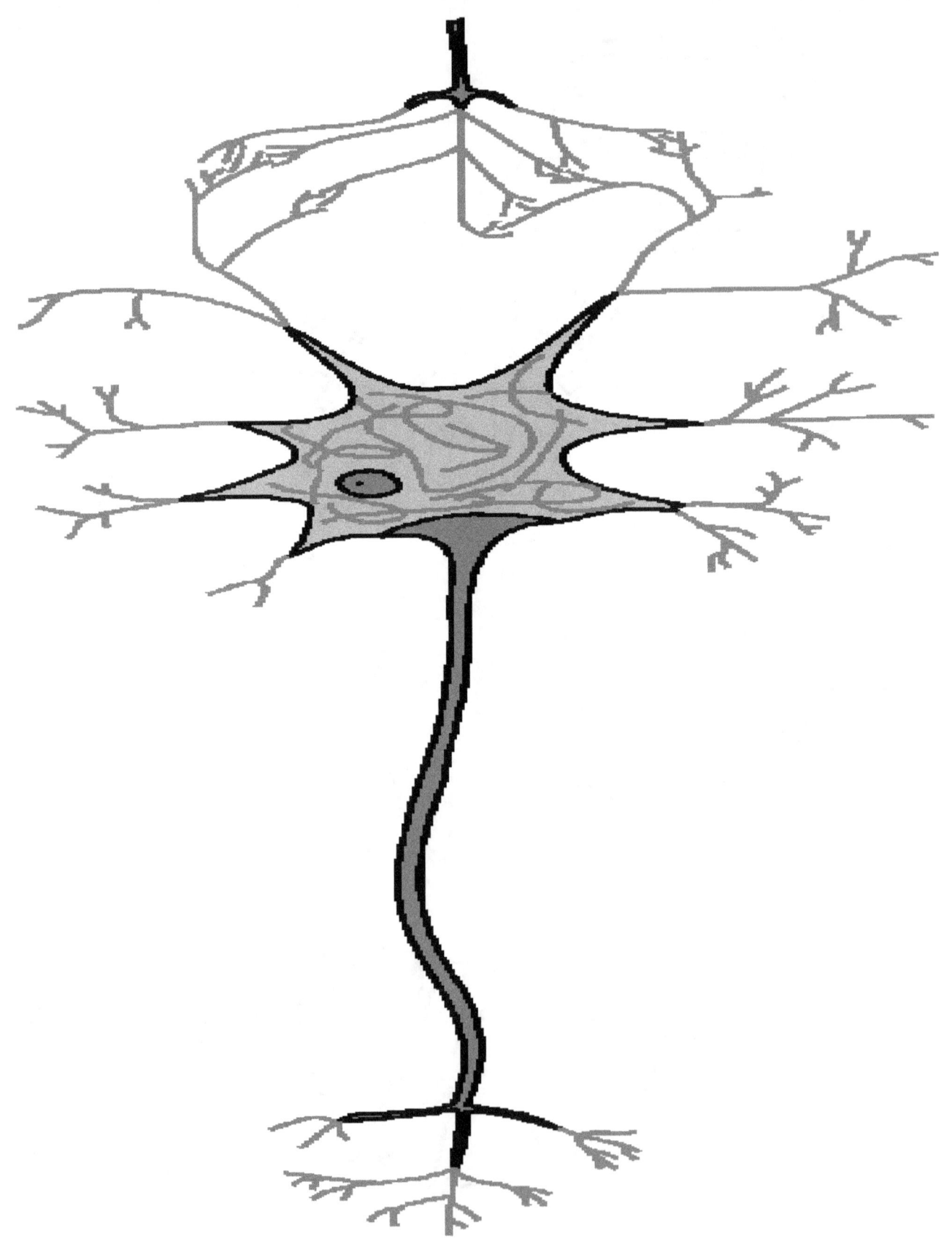

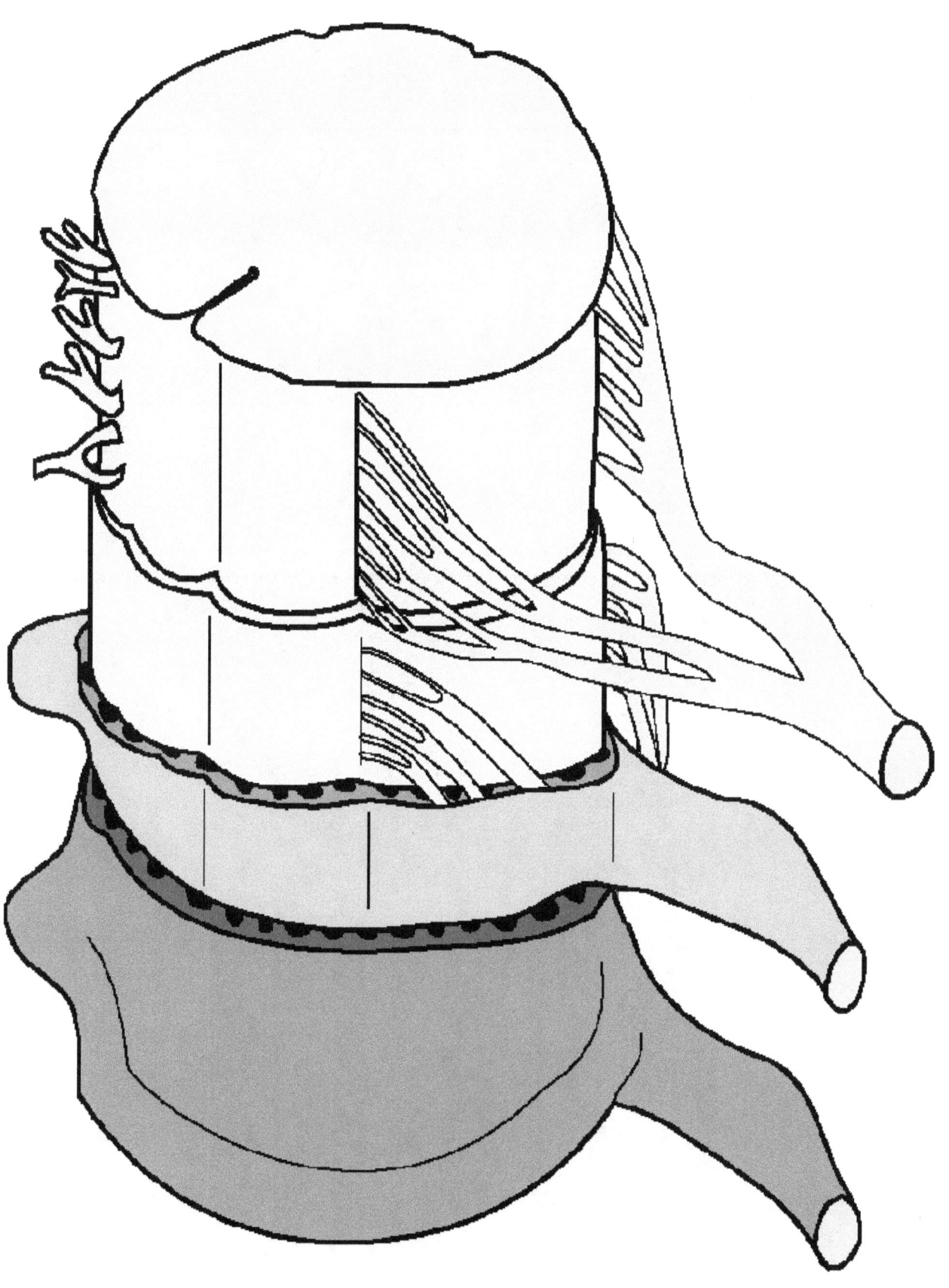

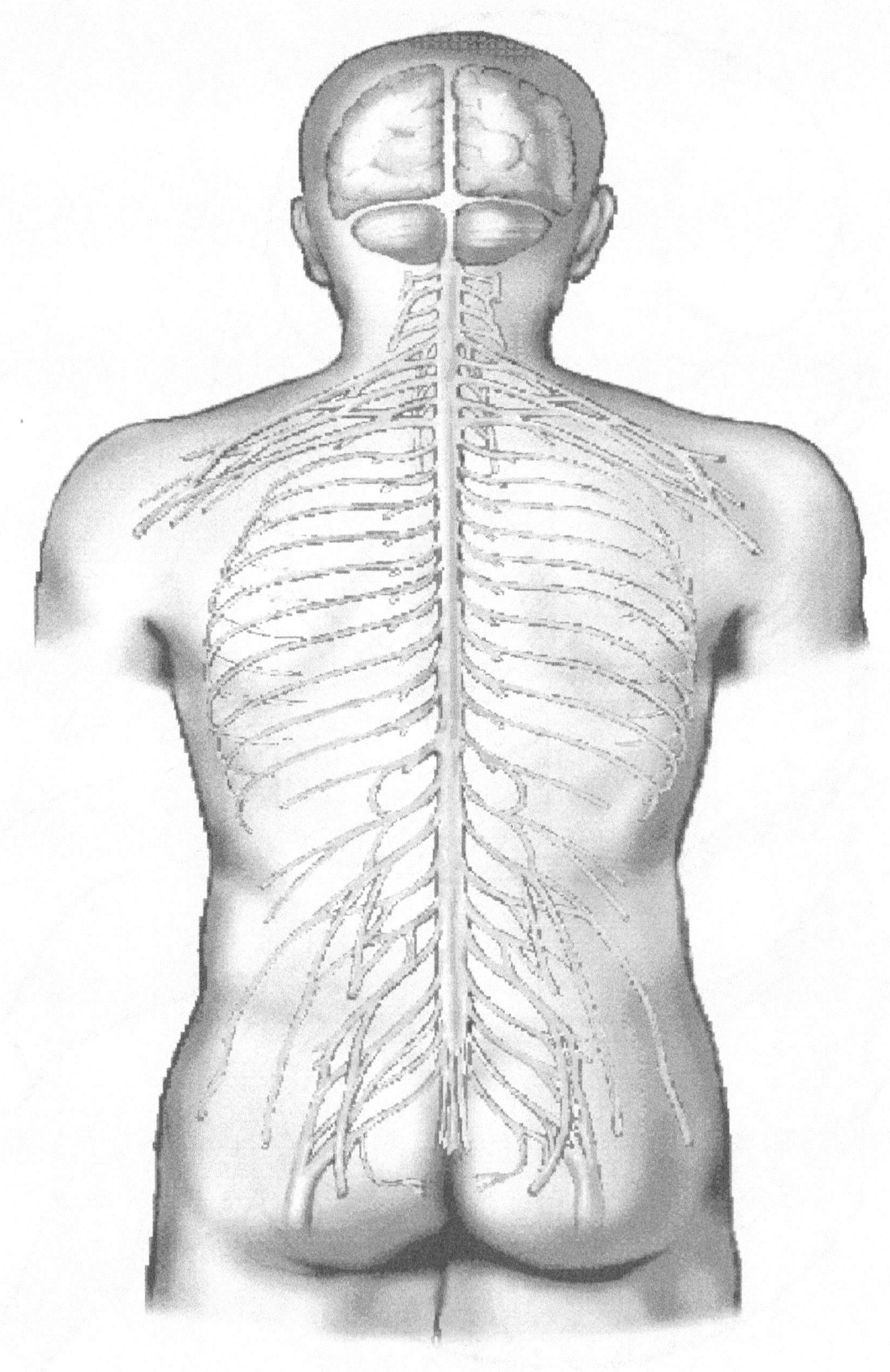

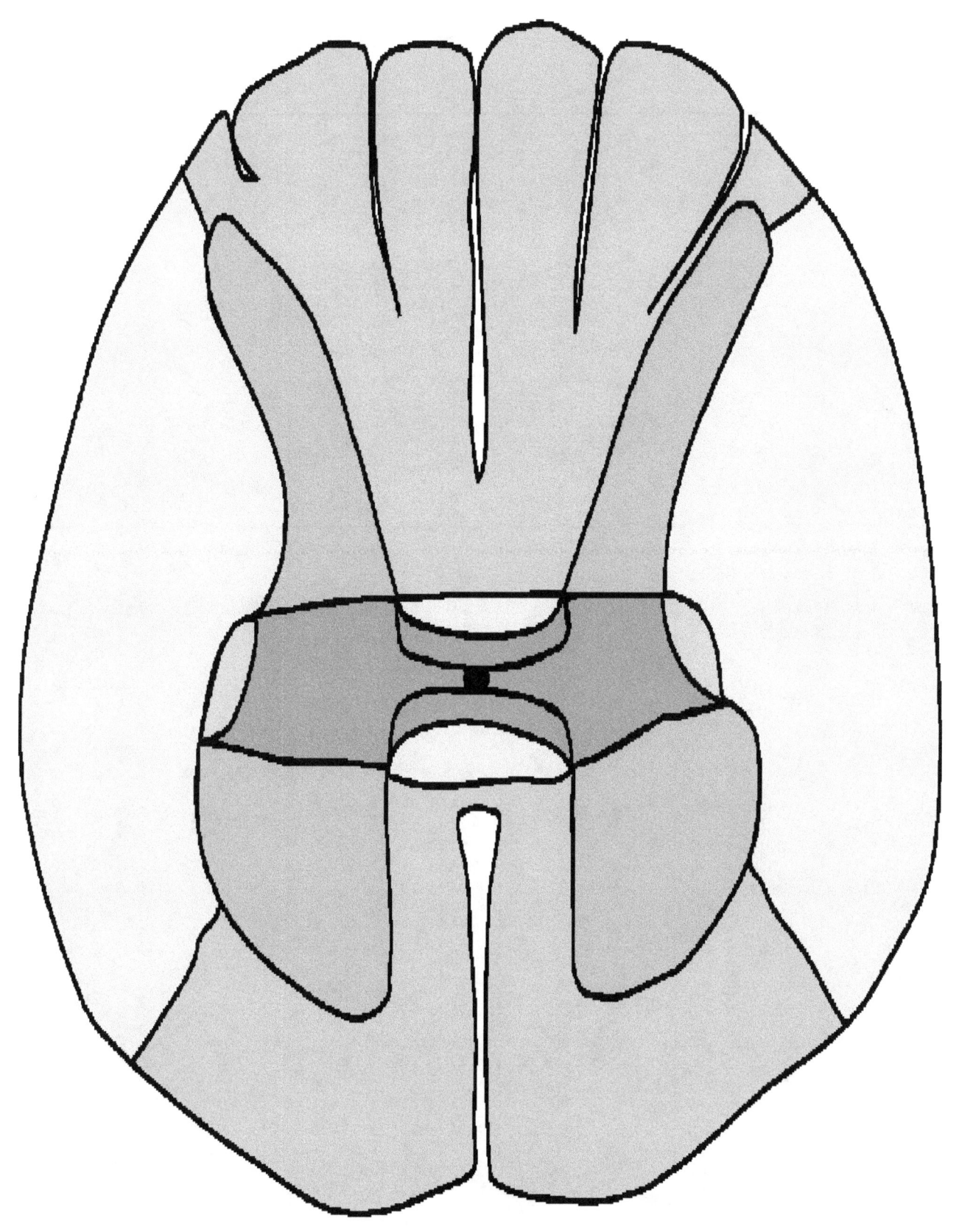

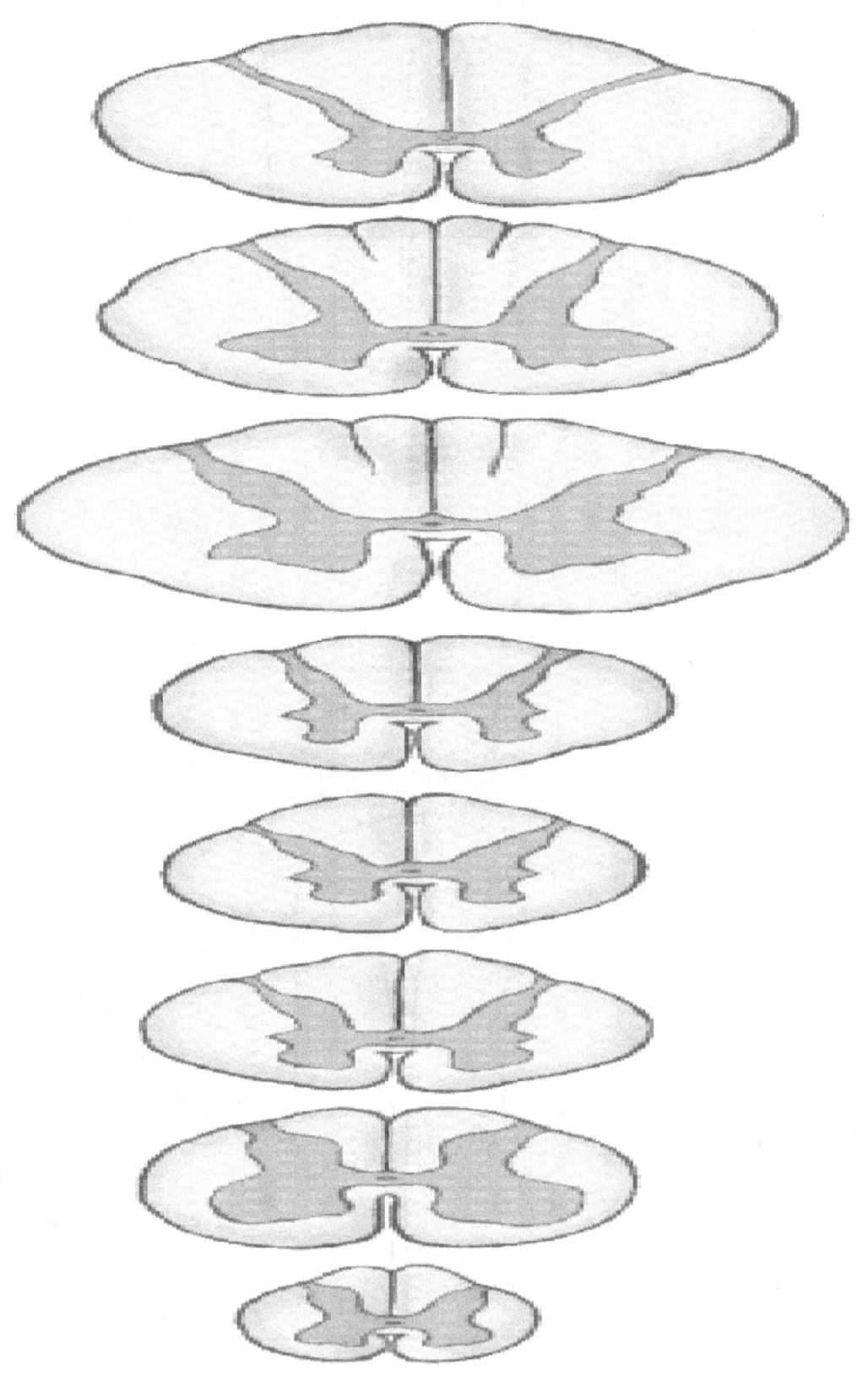

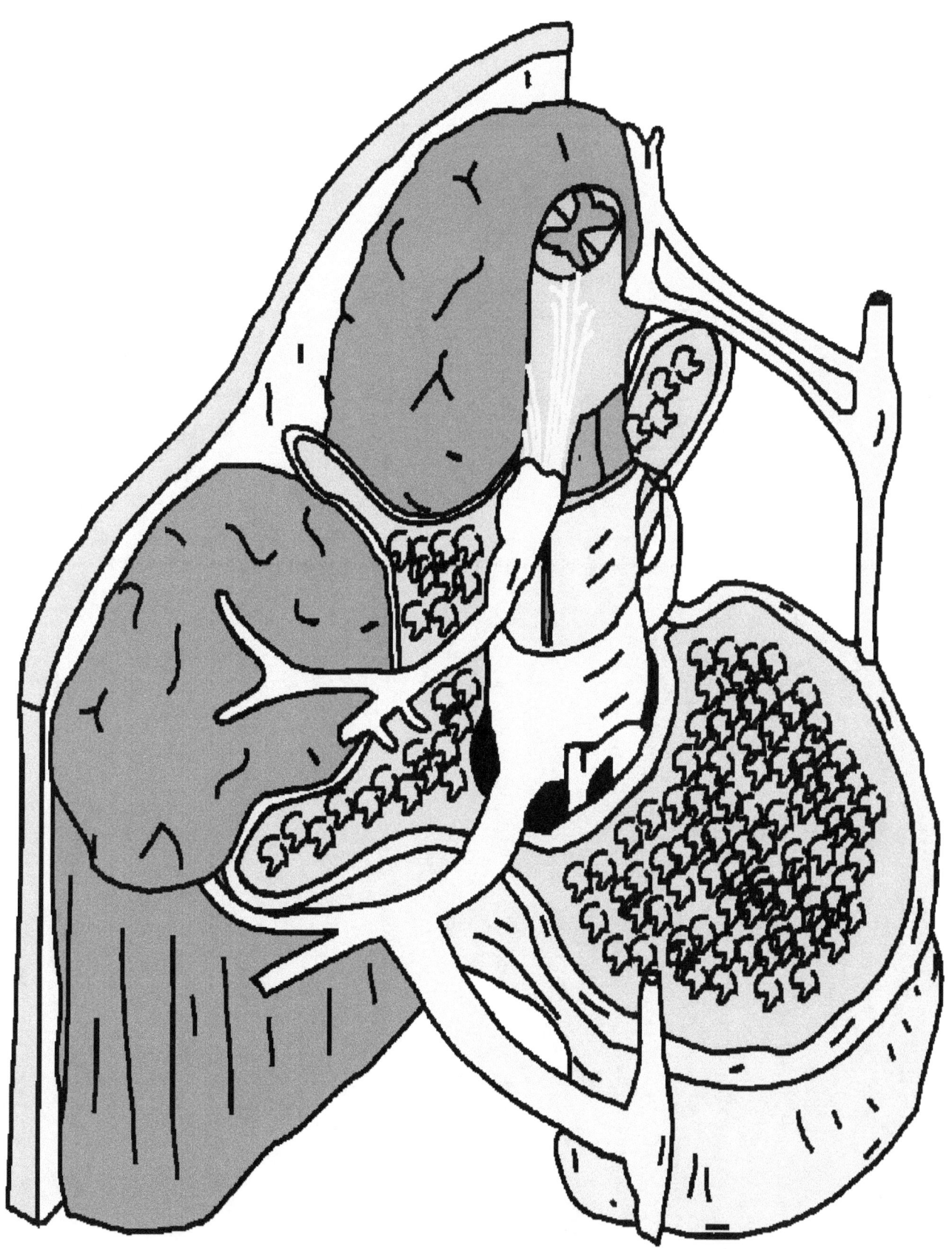

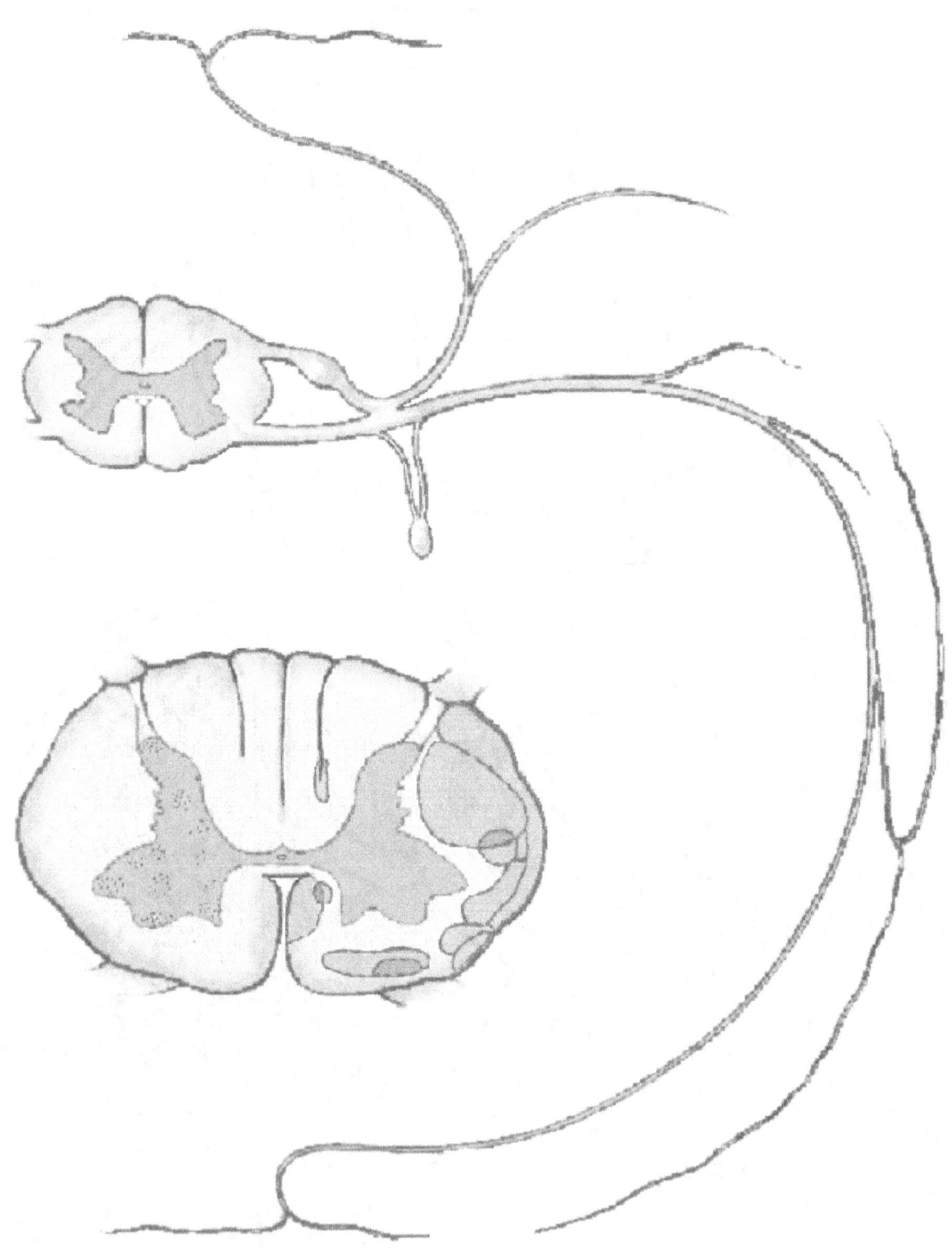

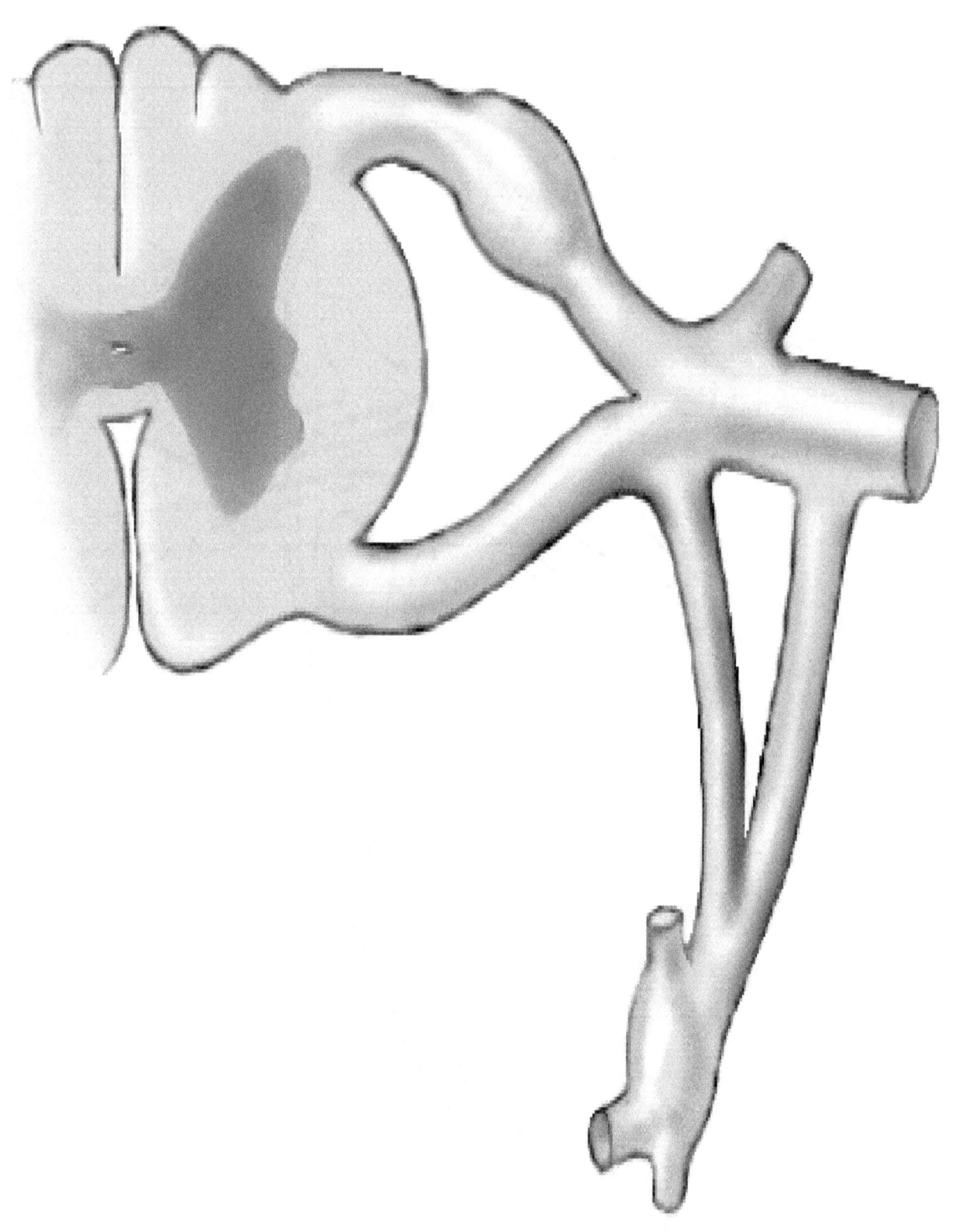

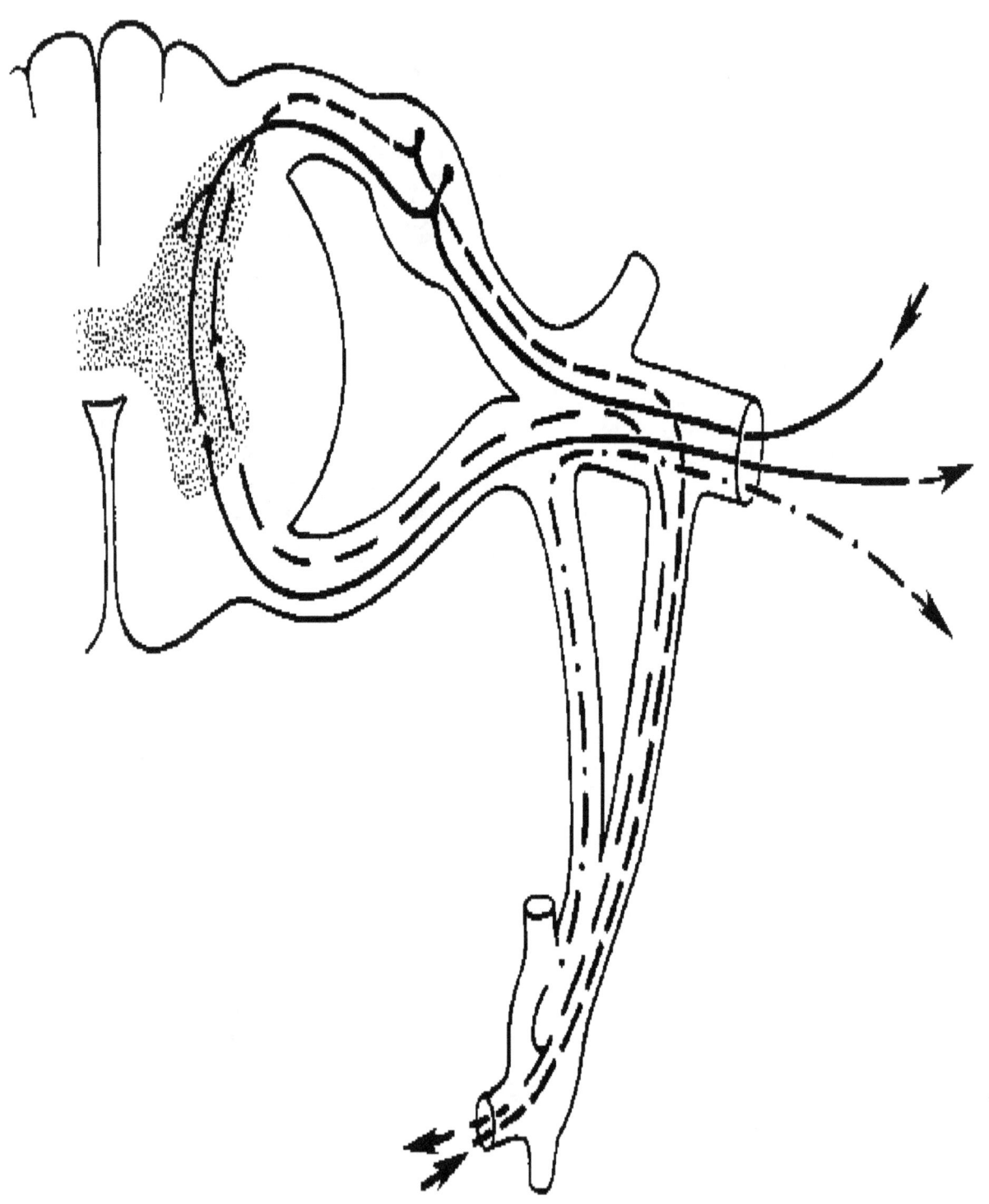

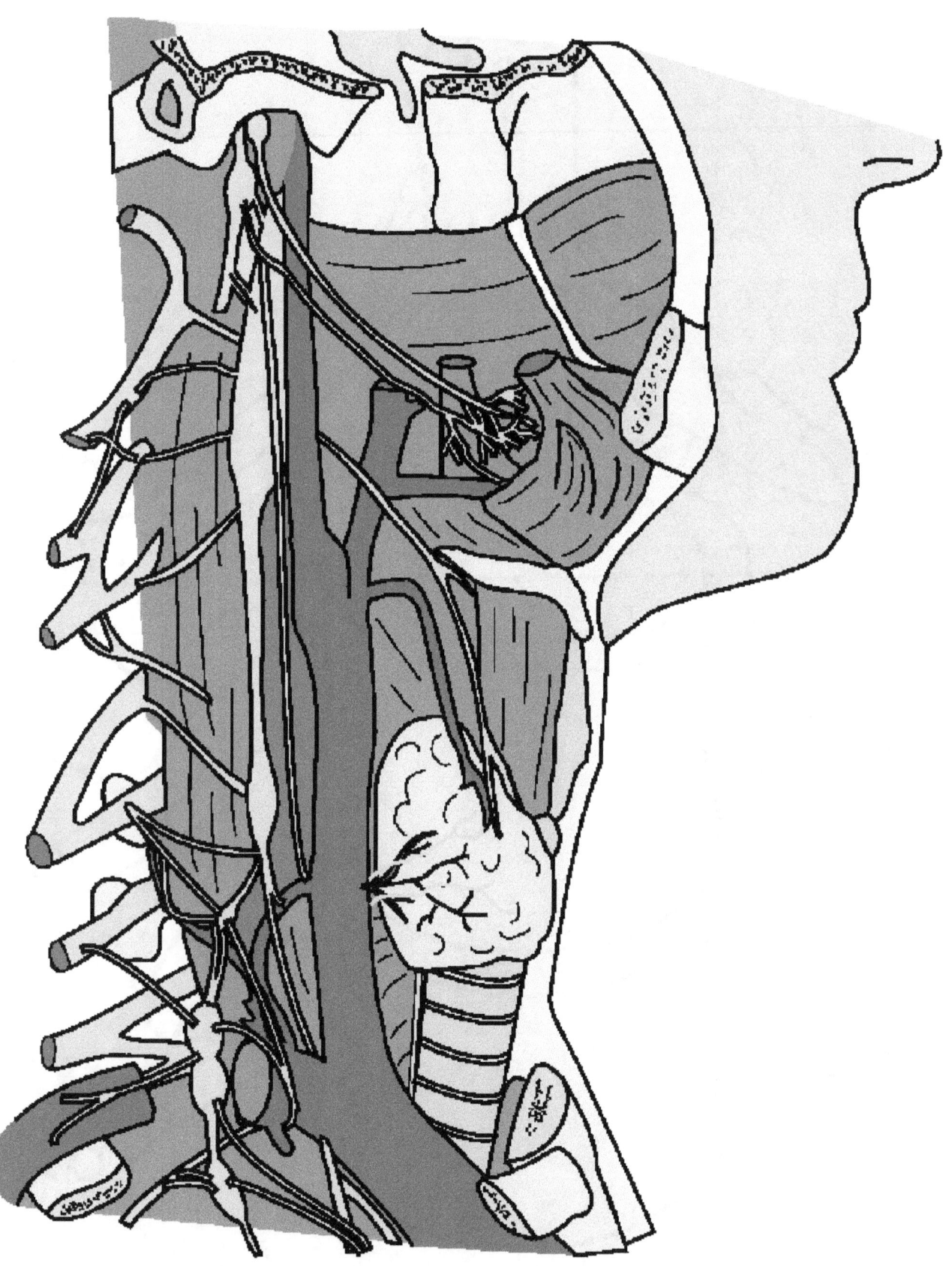

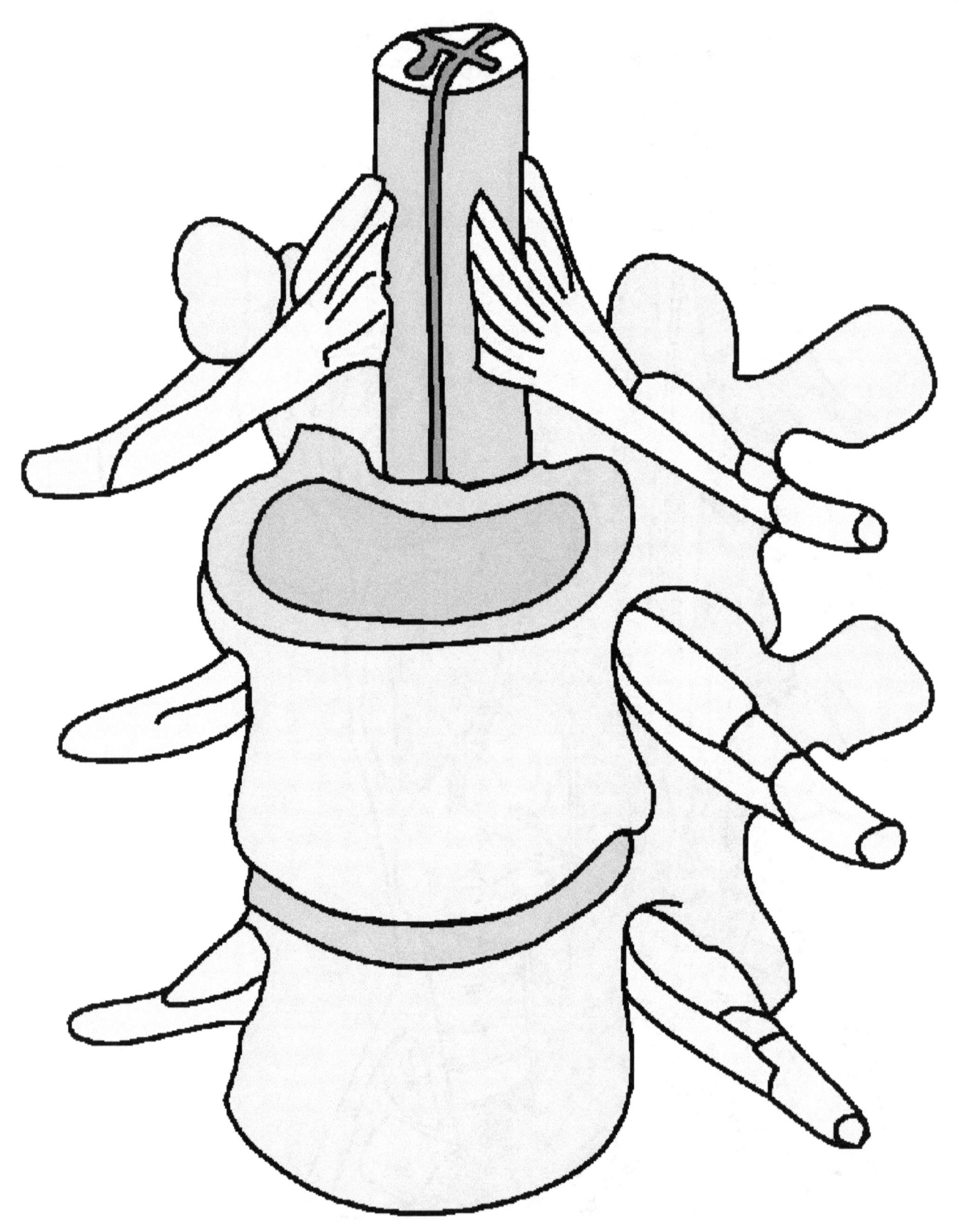

Respiratory System 224-237

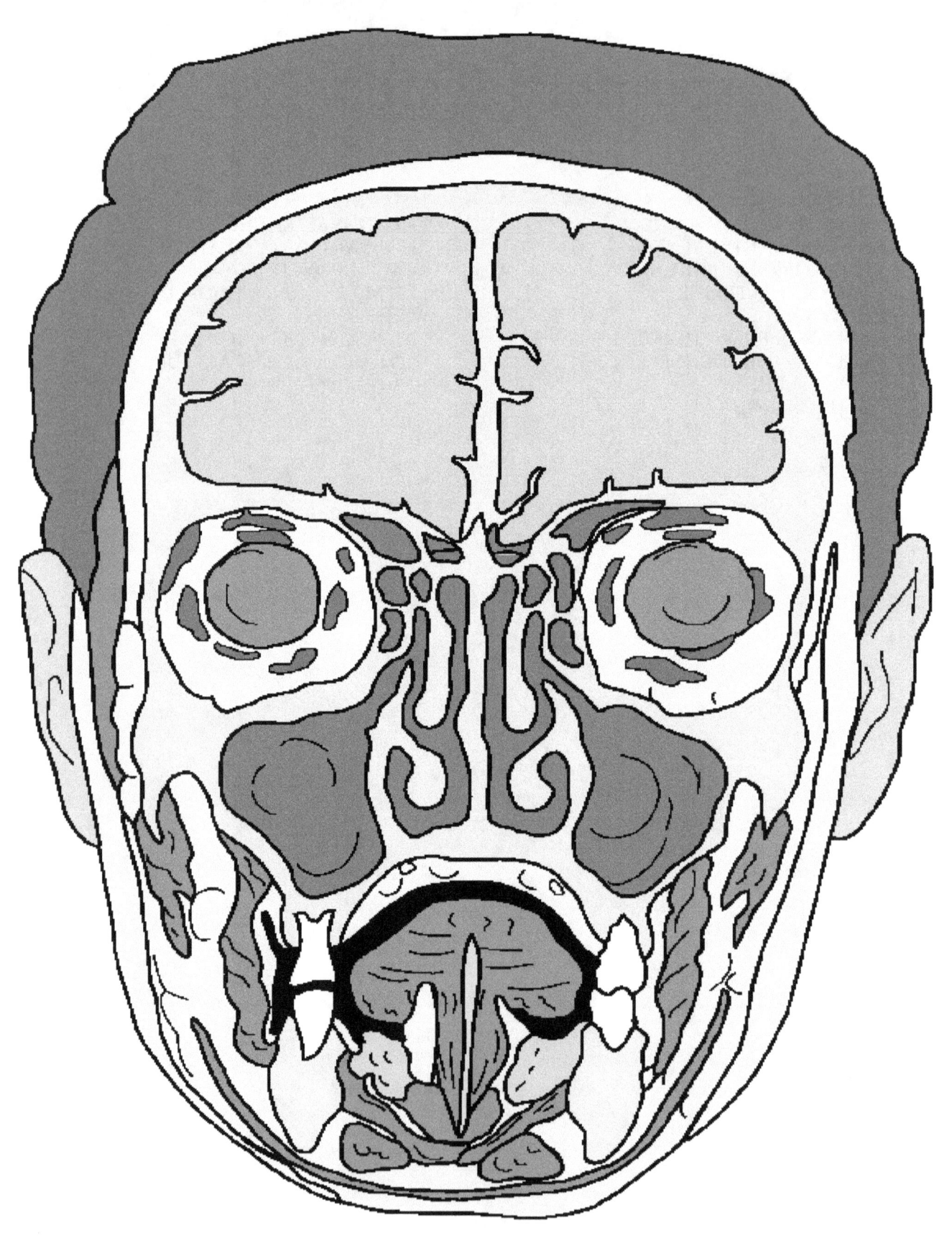

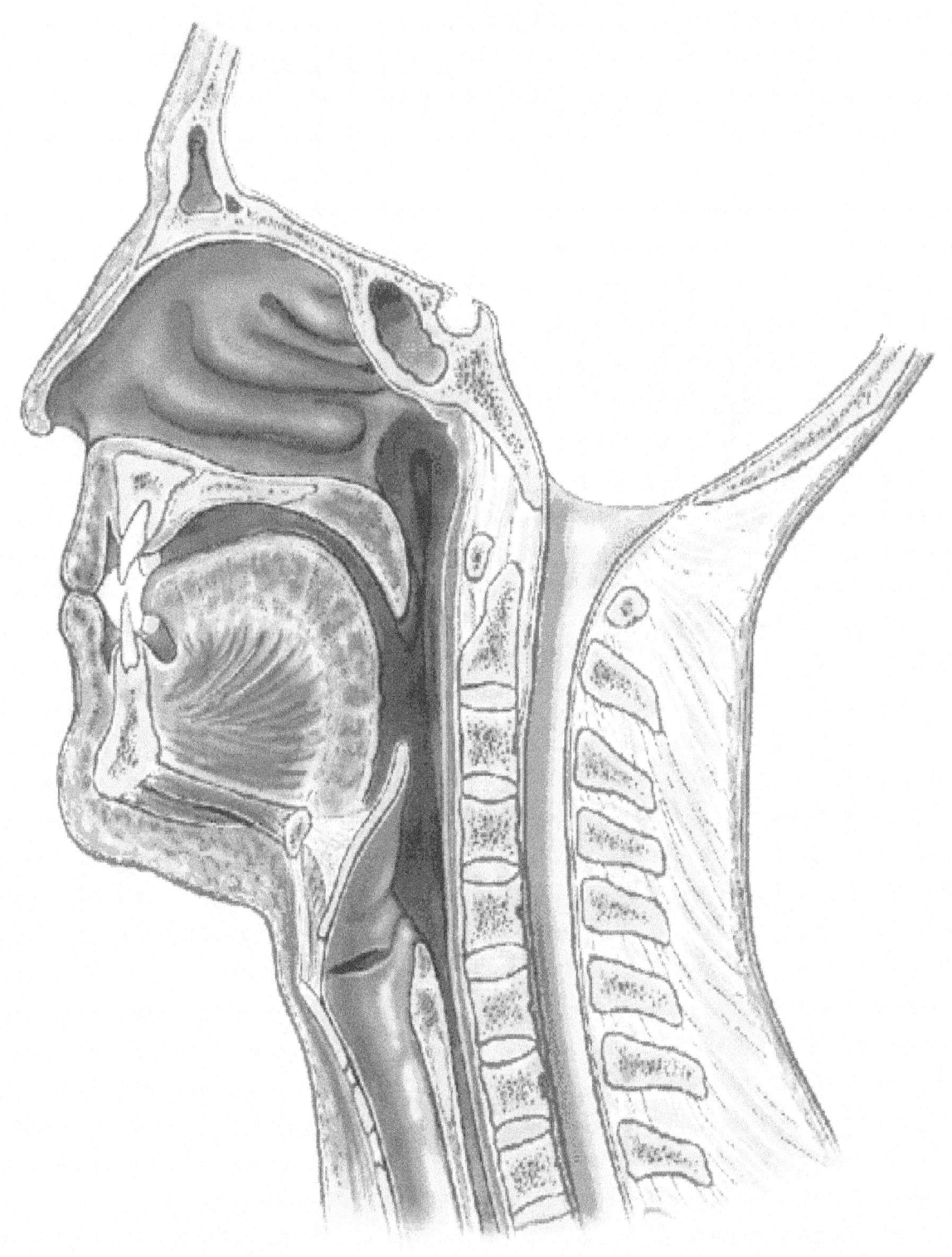

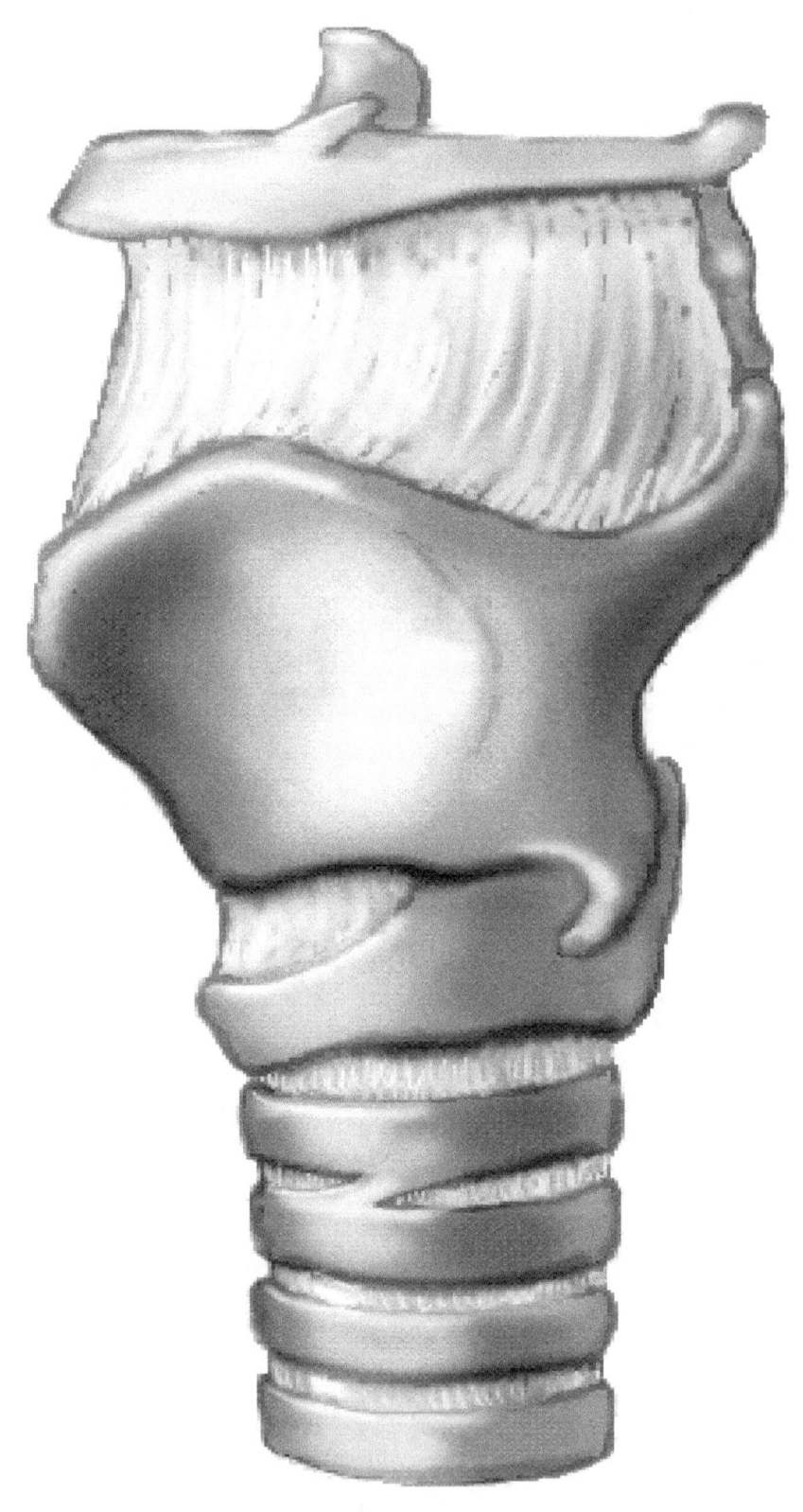

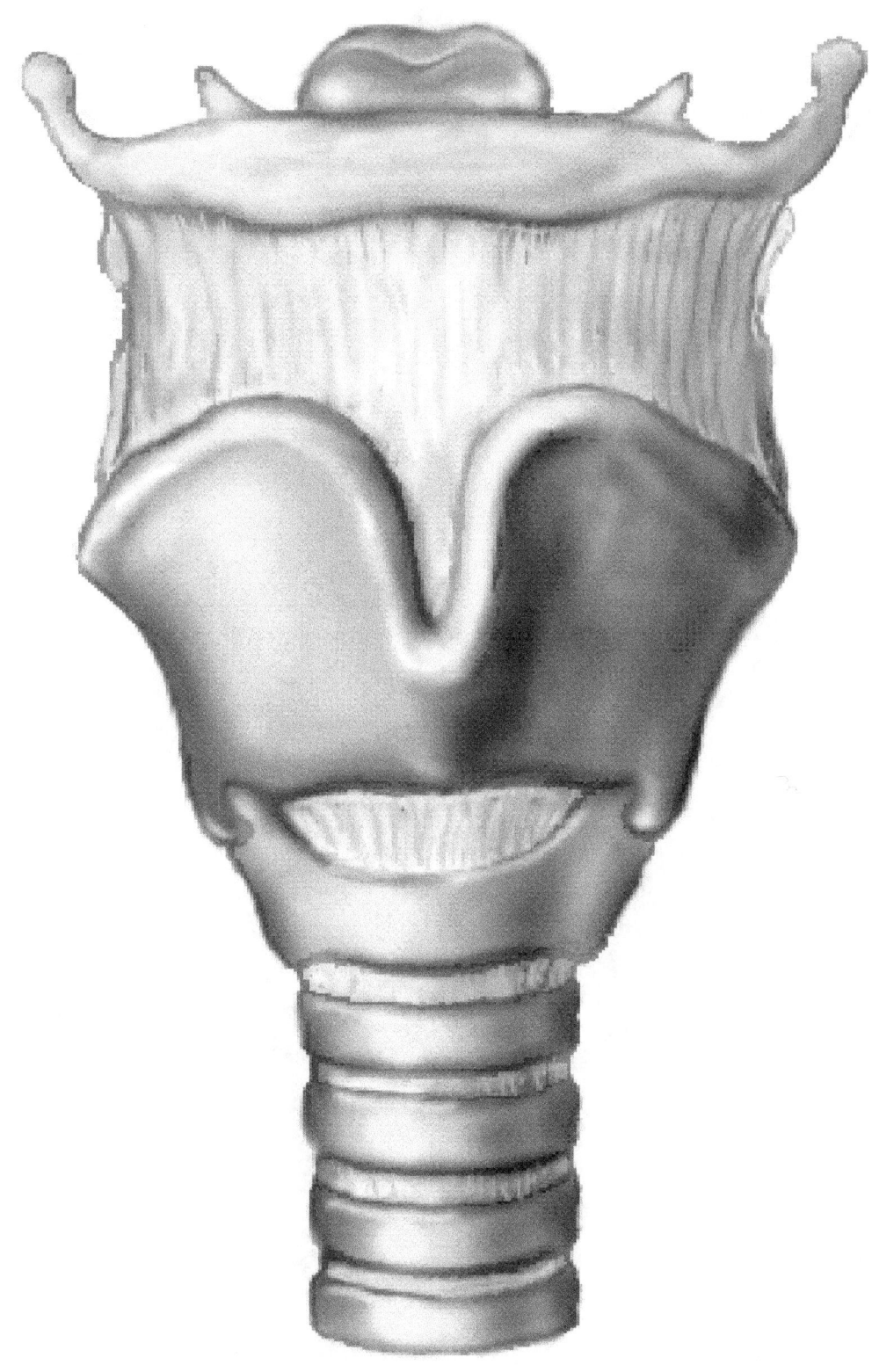

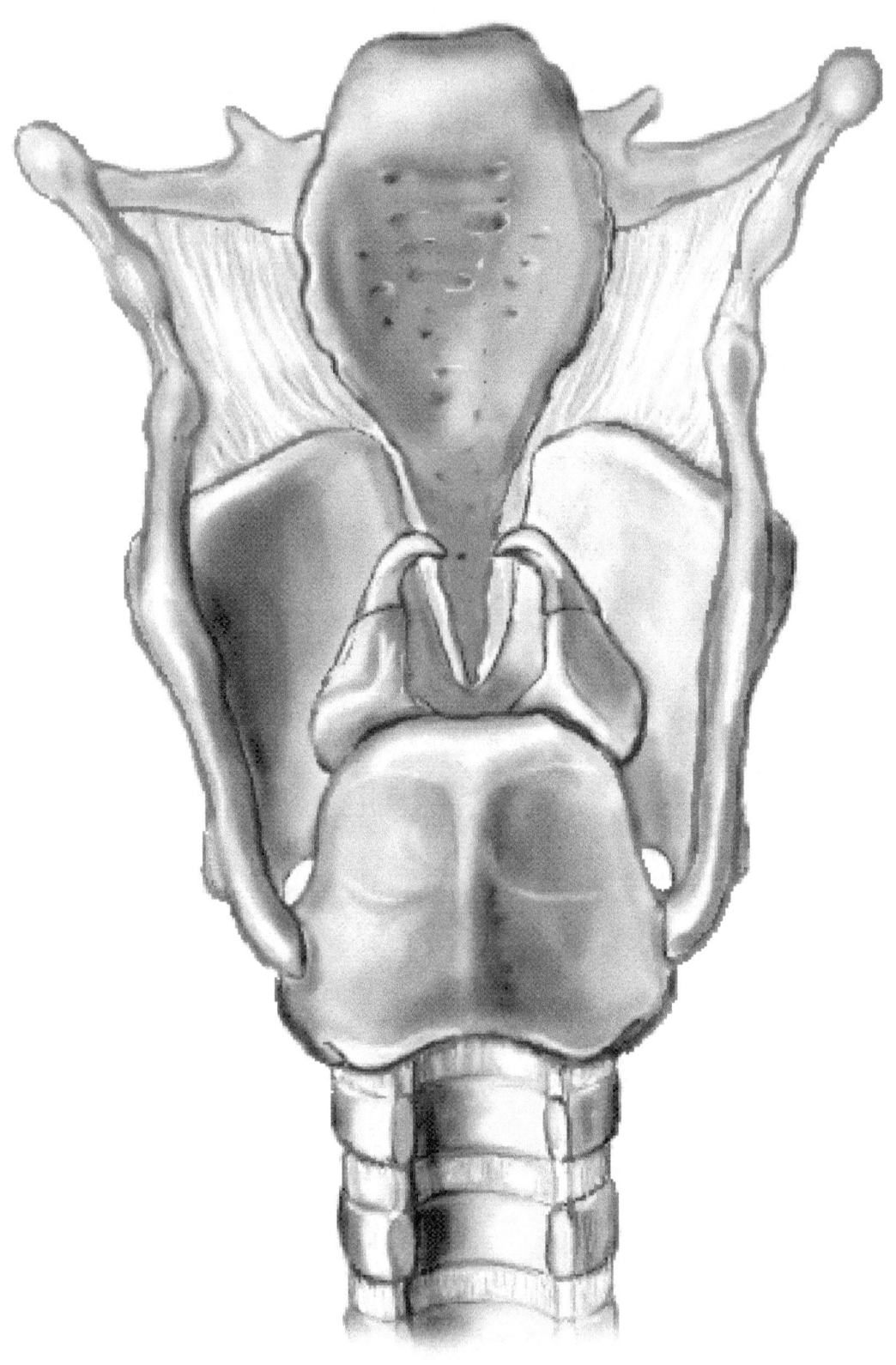

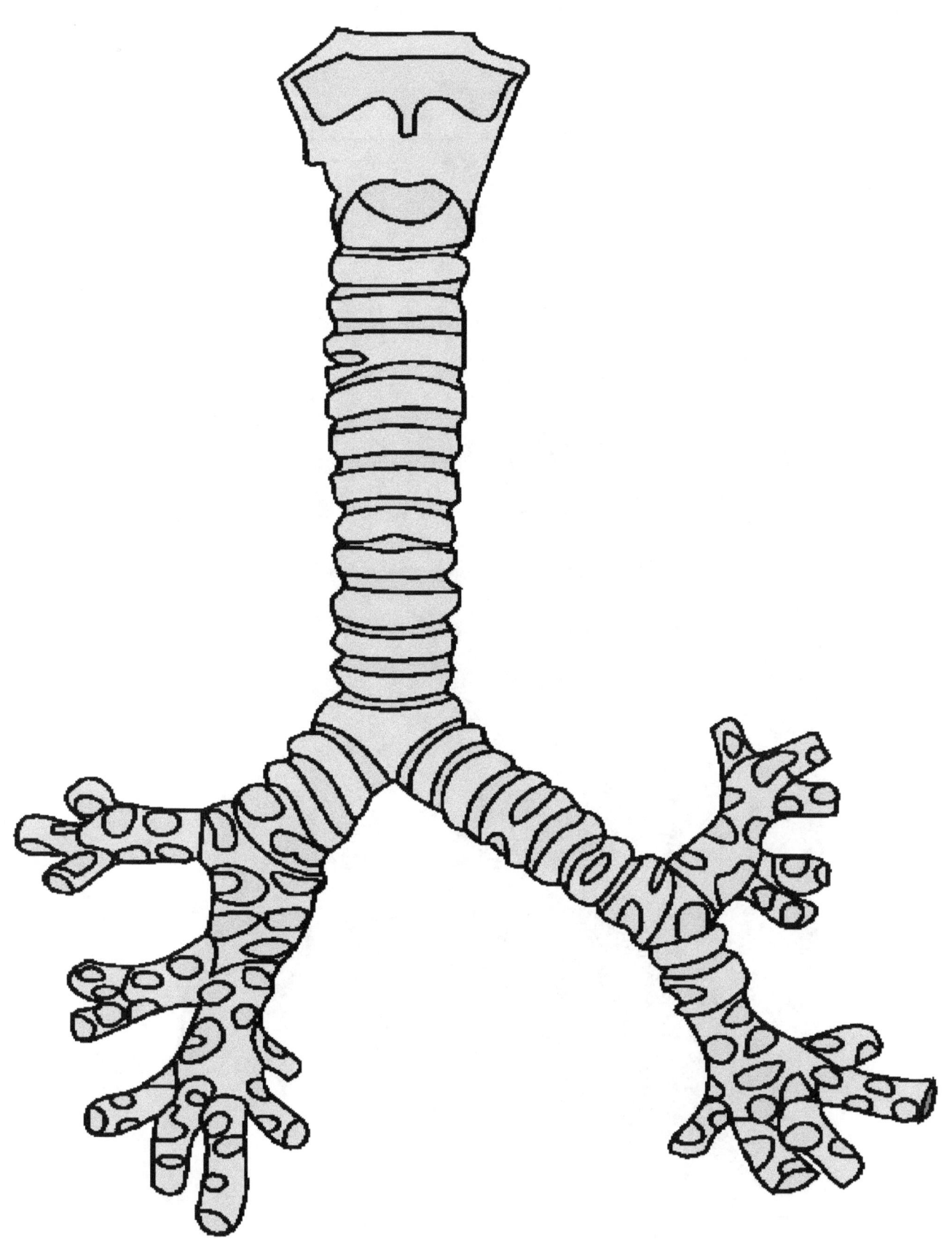

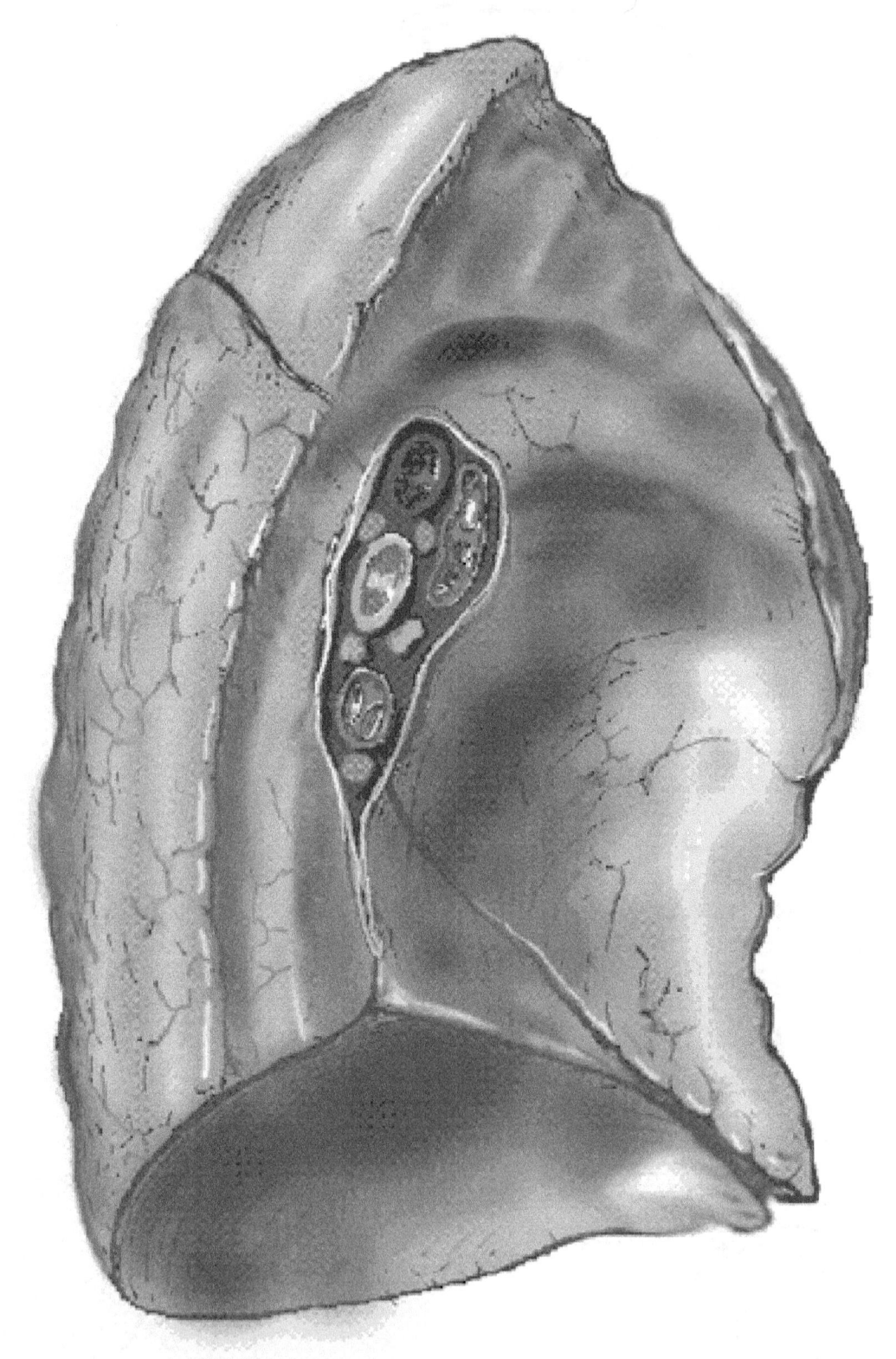

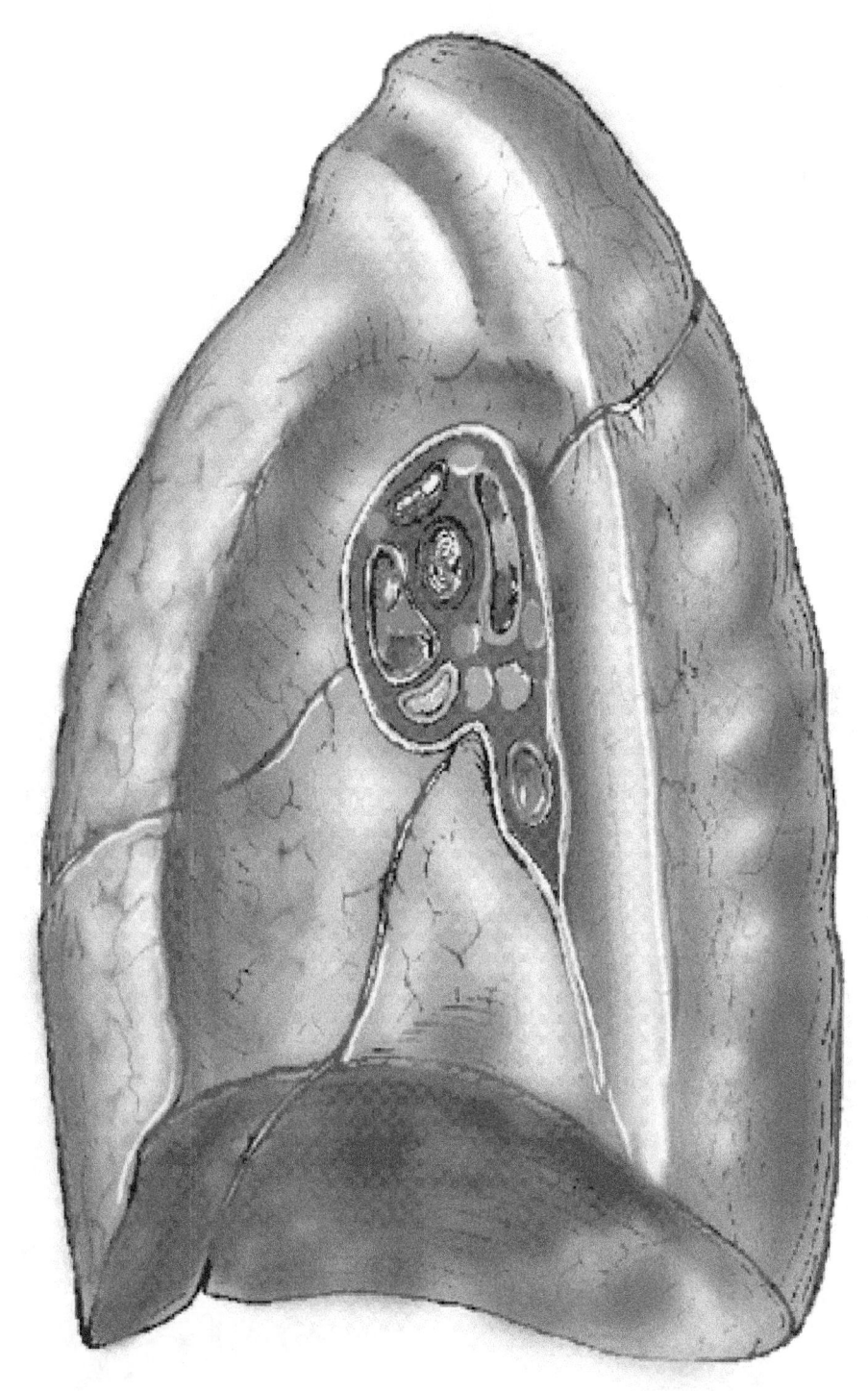

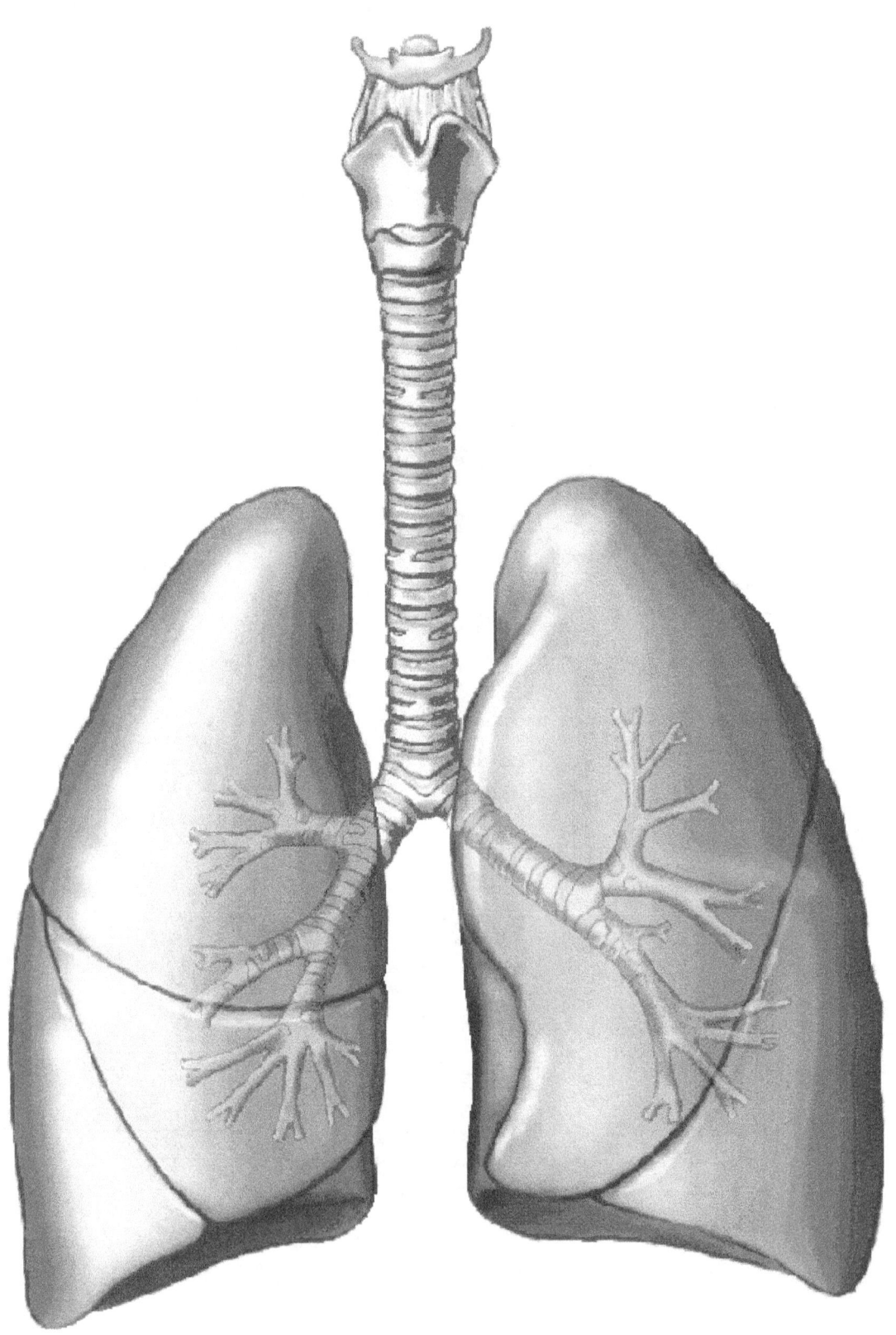

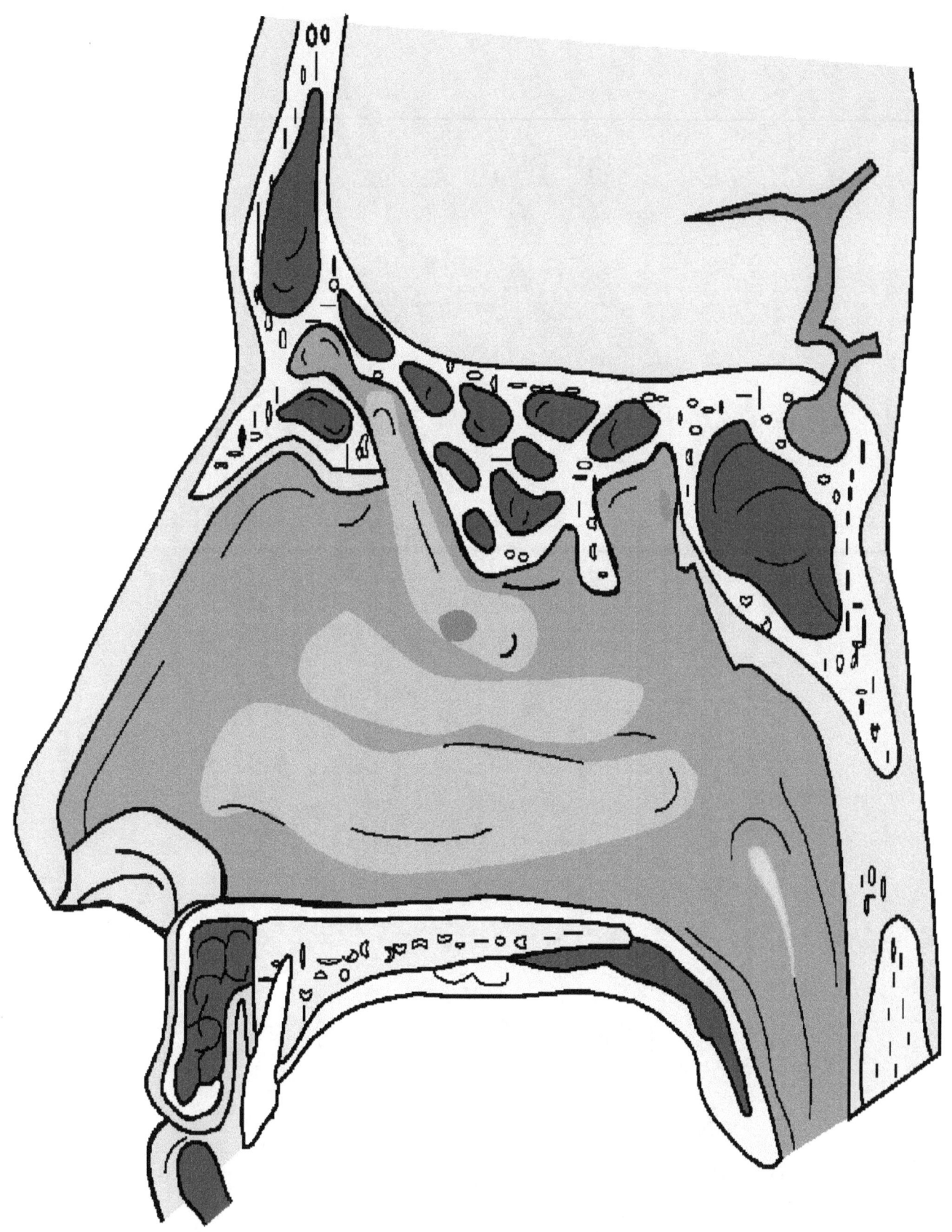

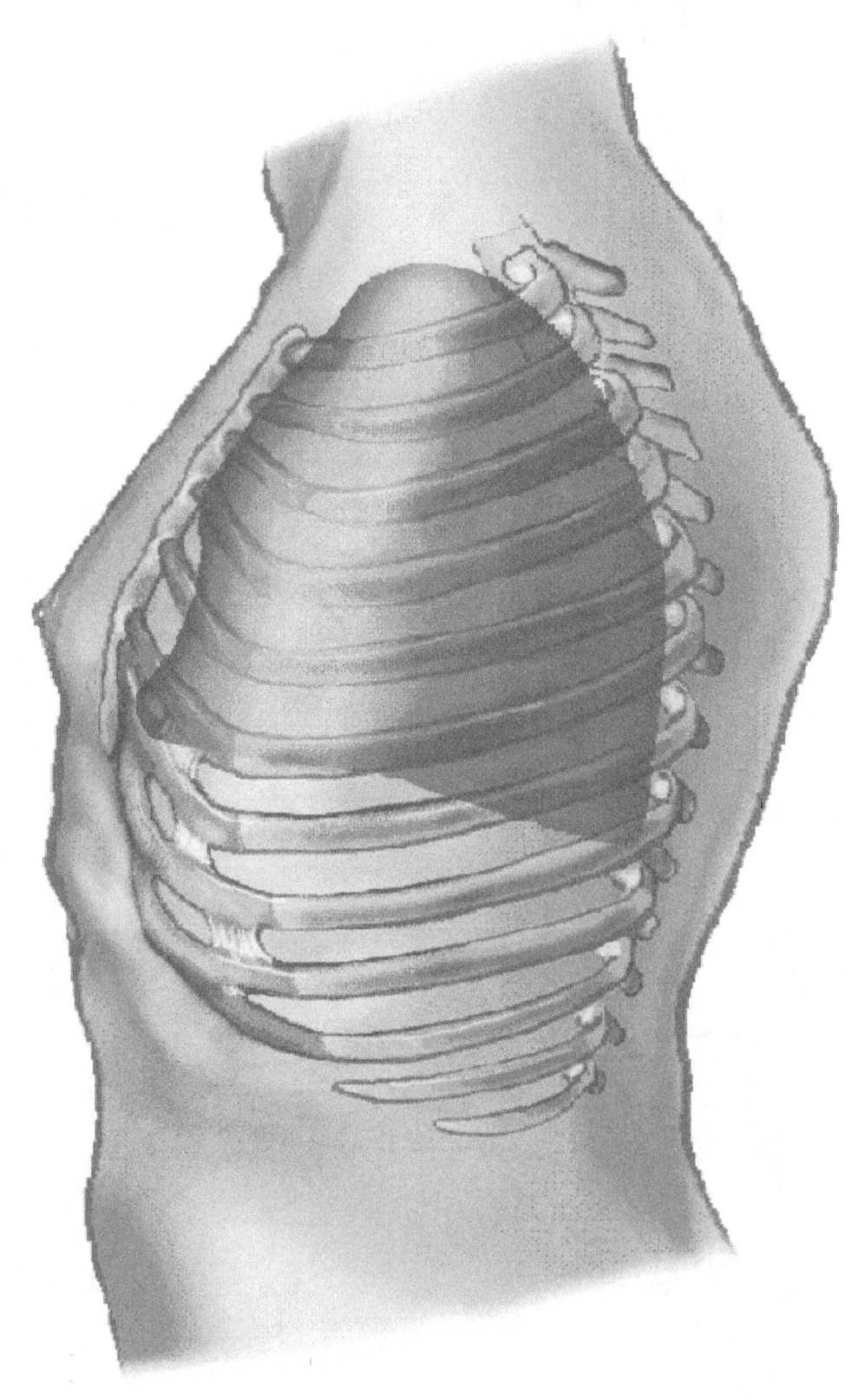

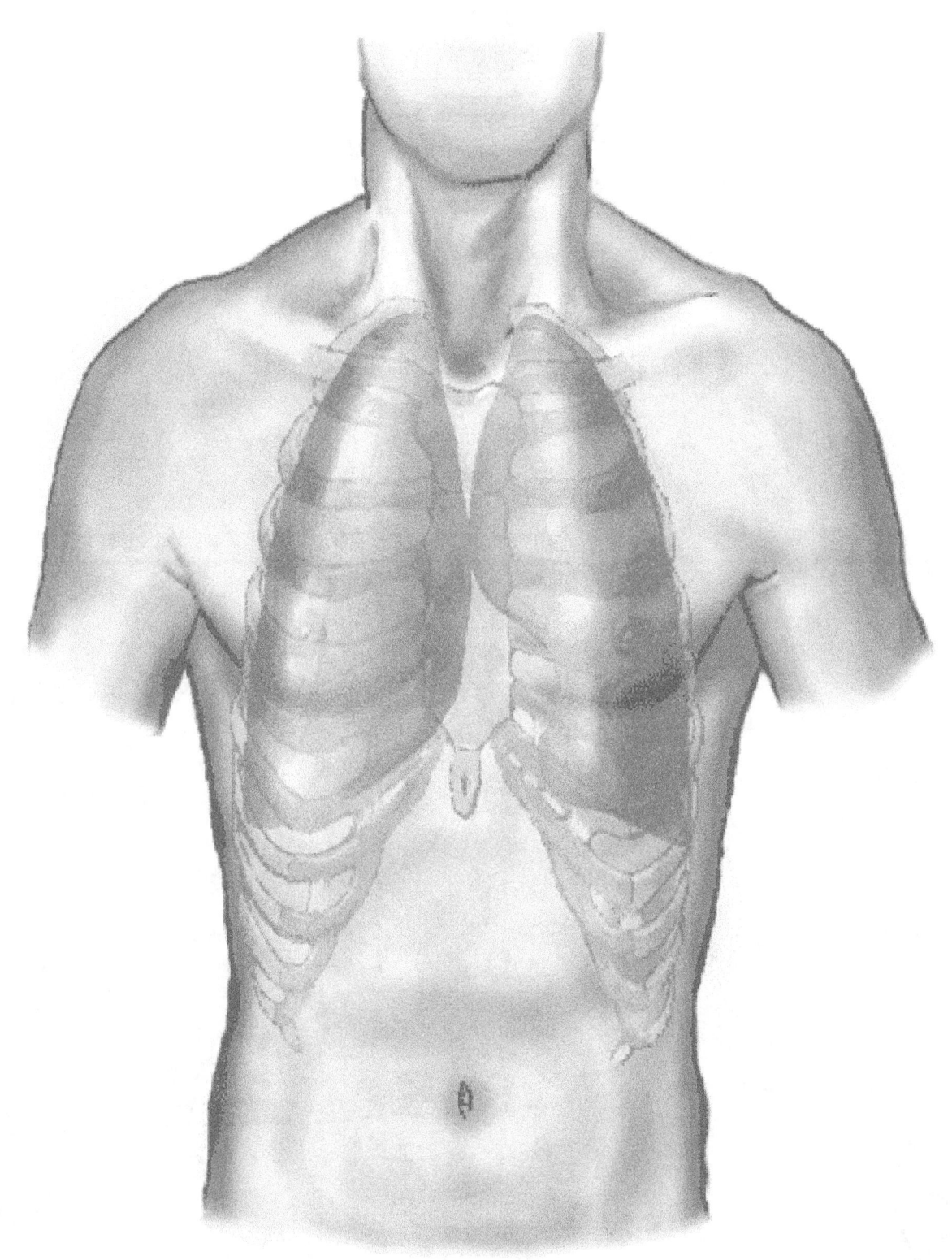

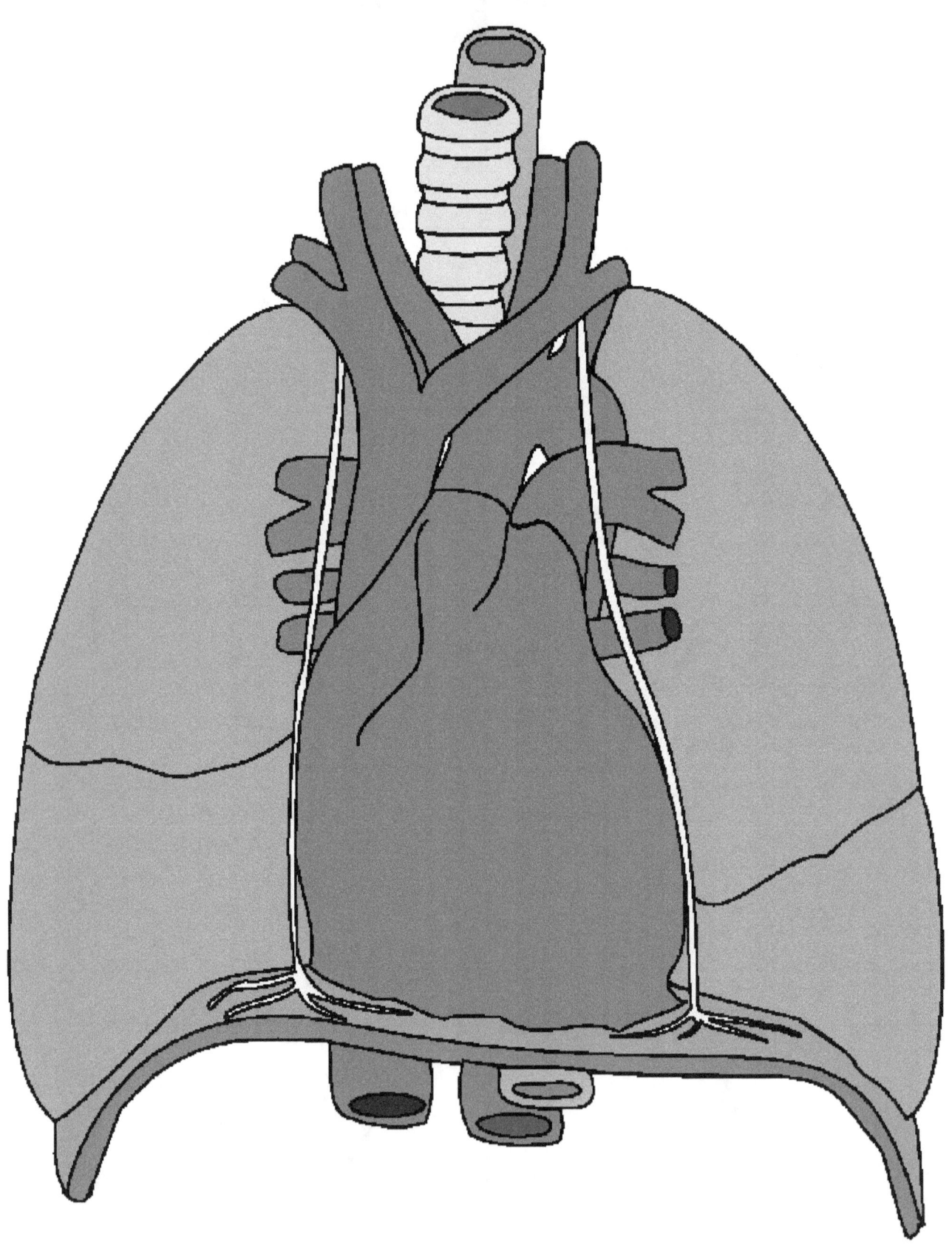

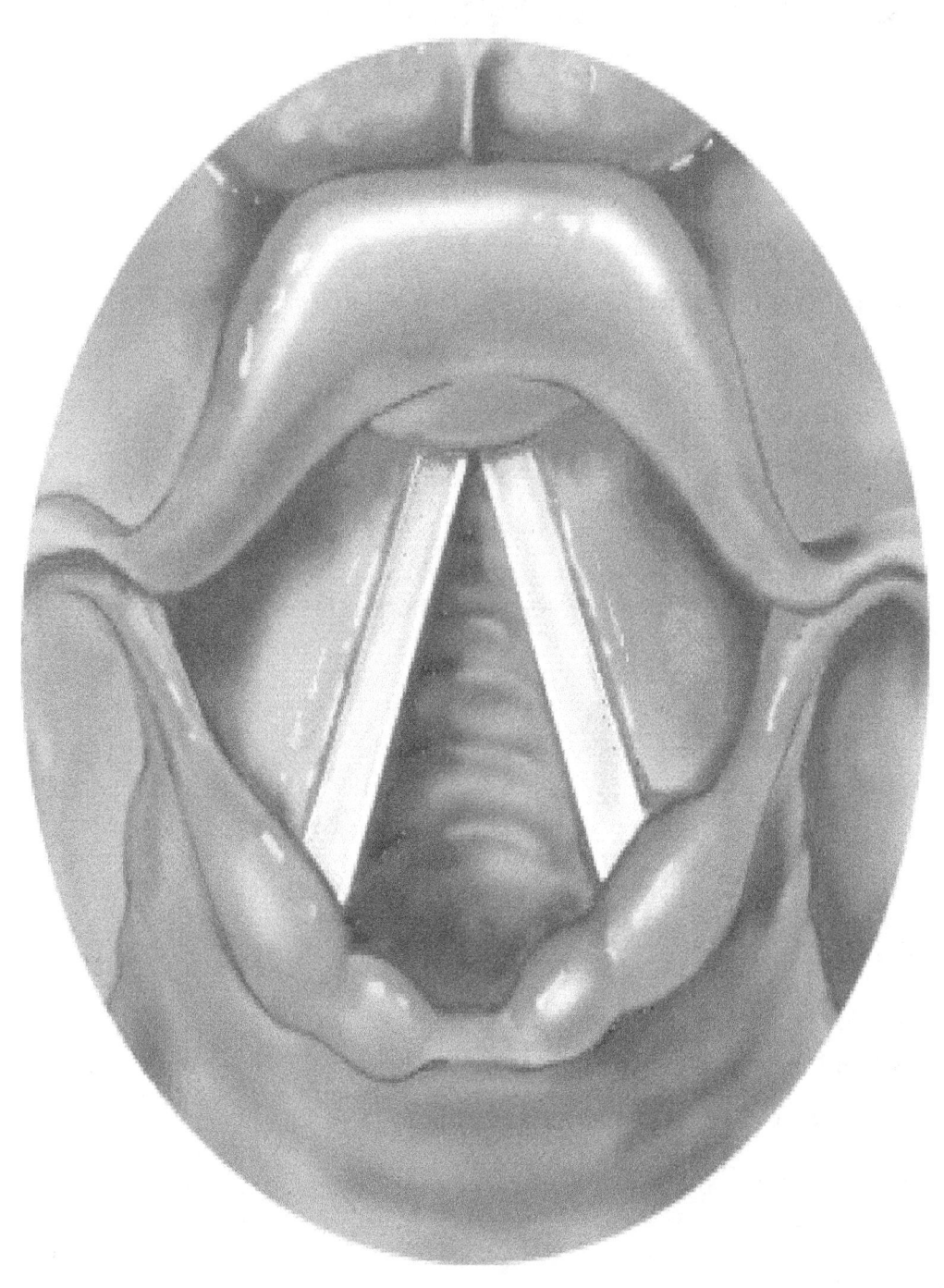

Urogenital System 239- 263

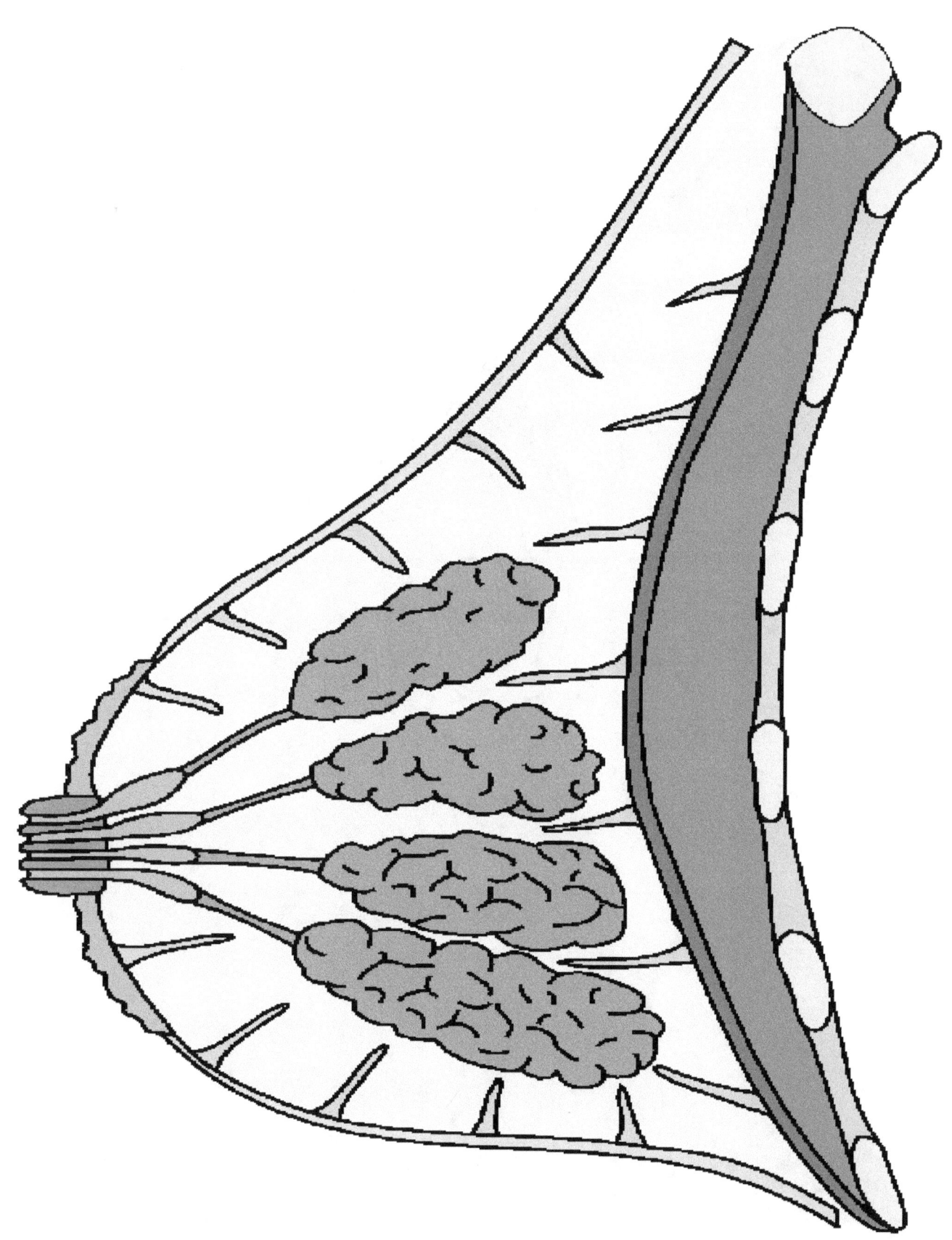

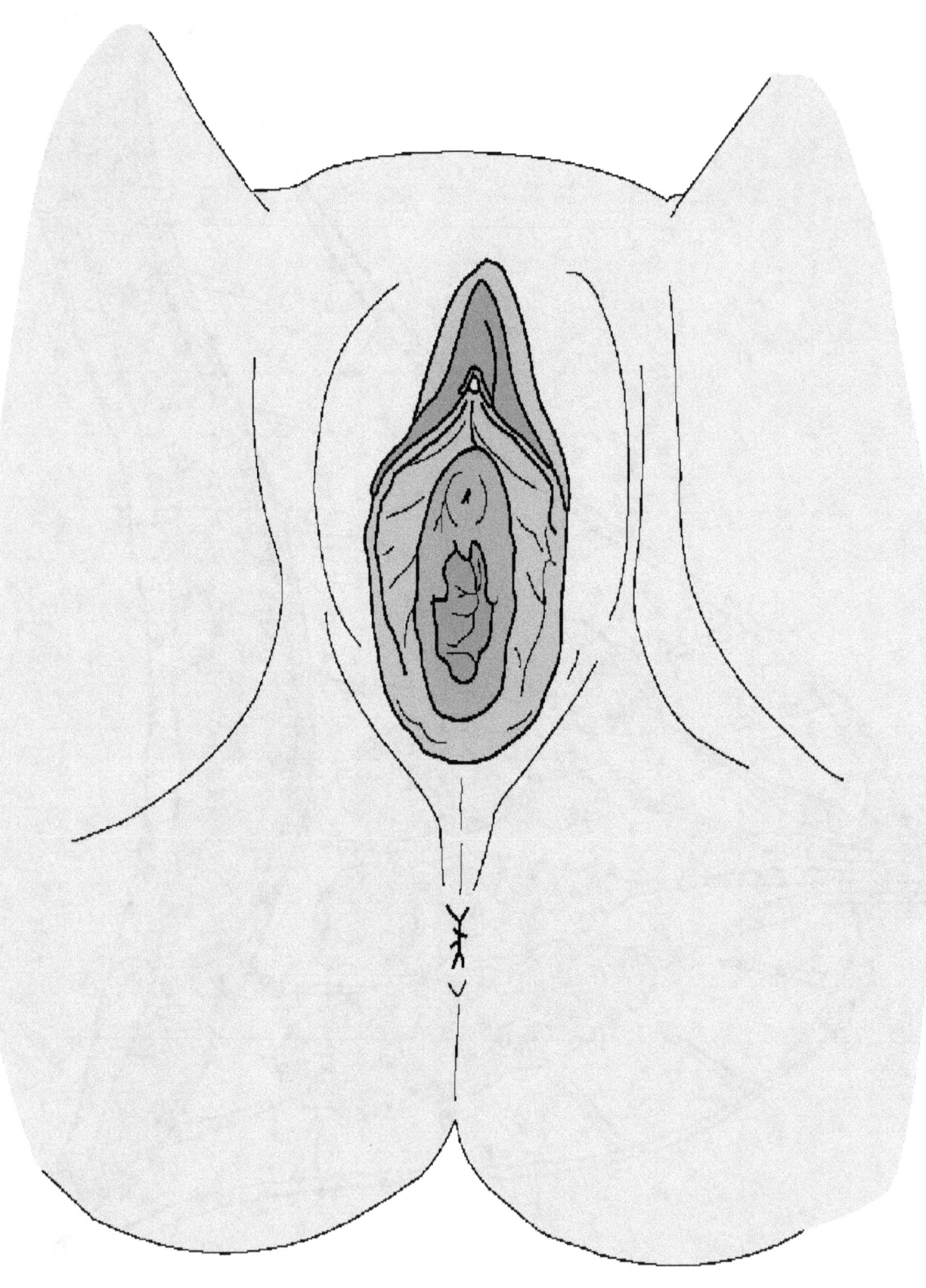

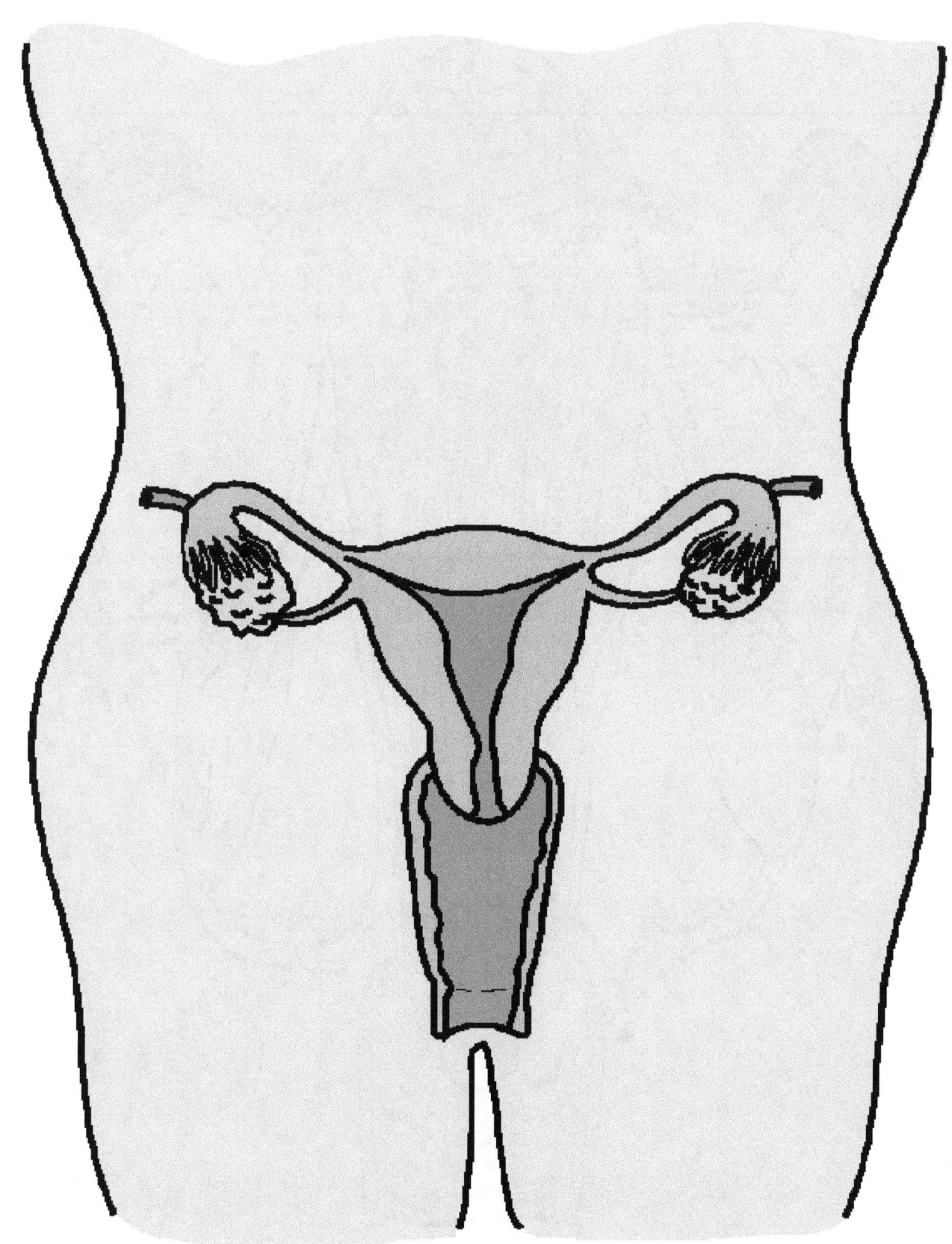

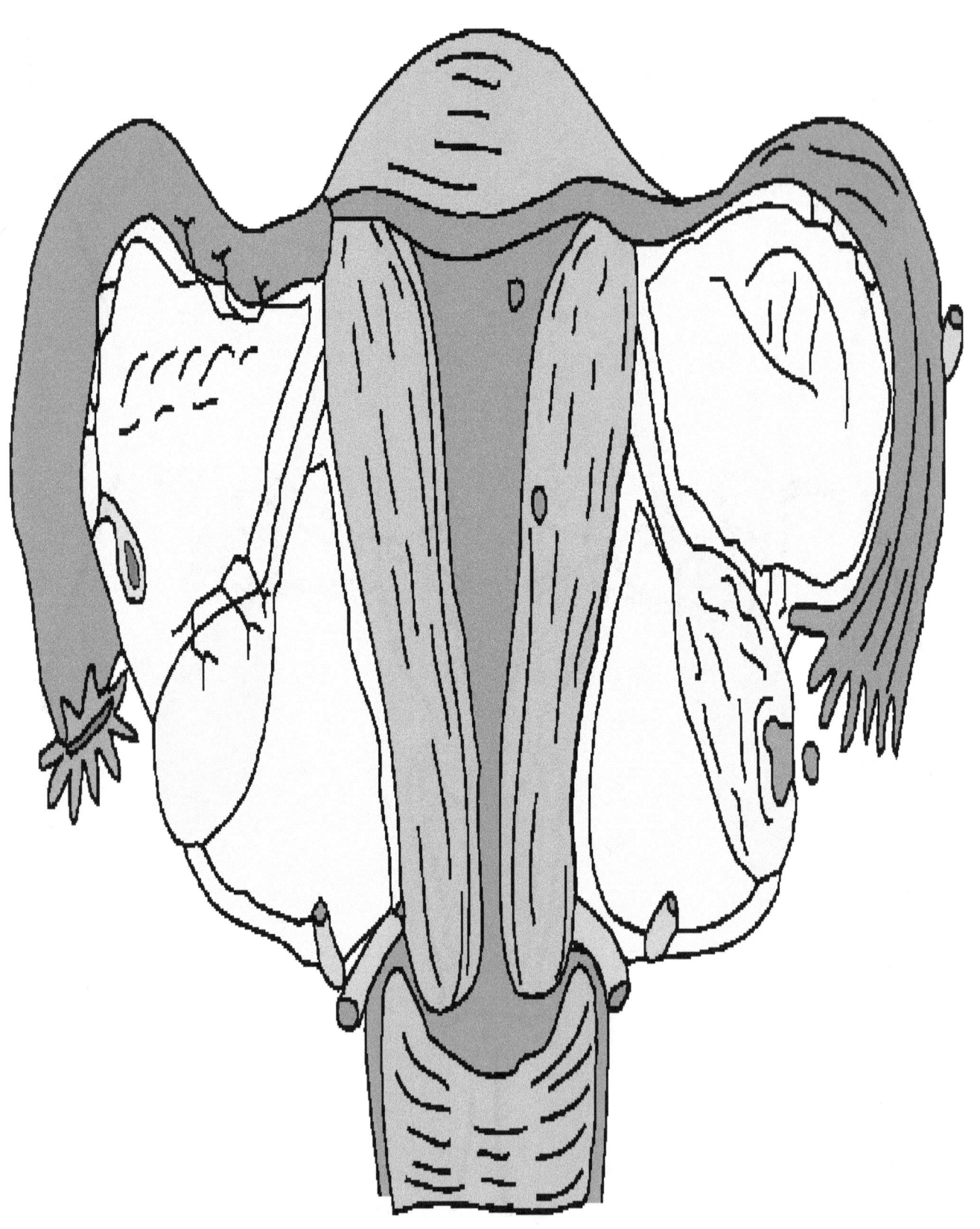

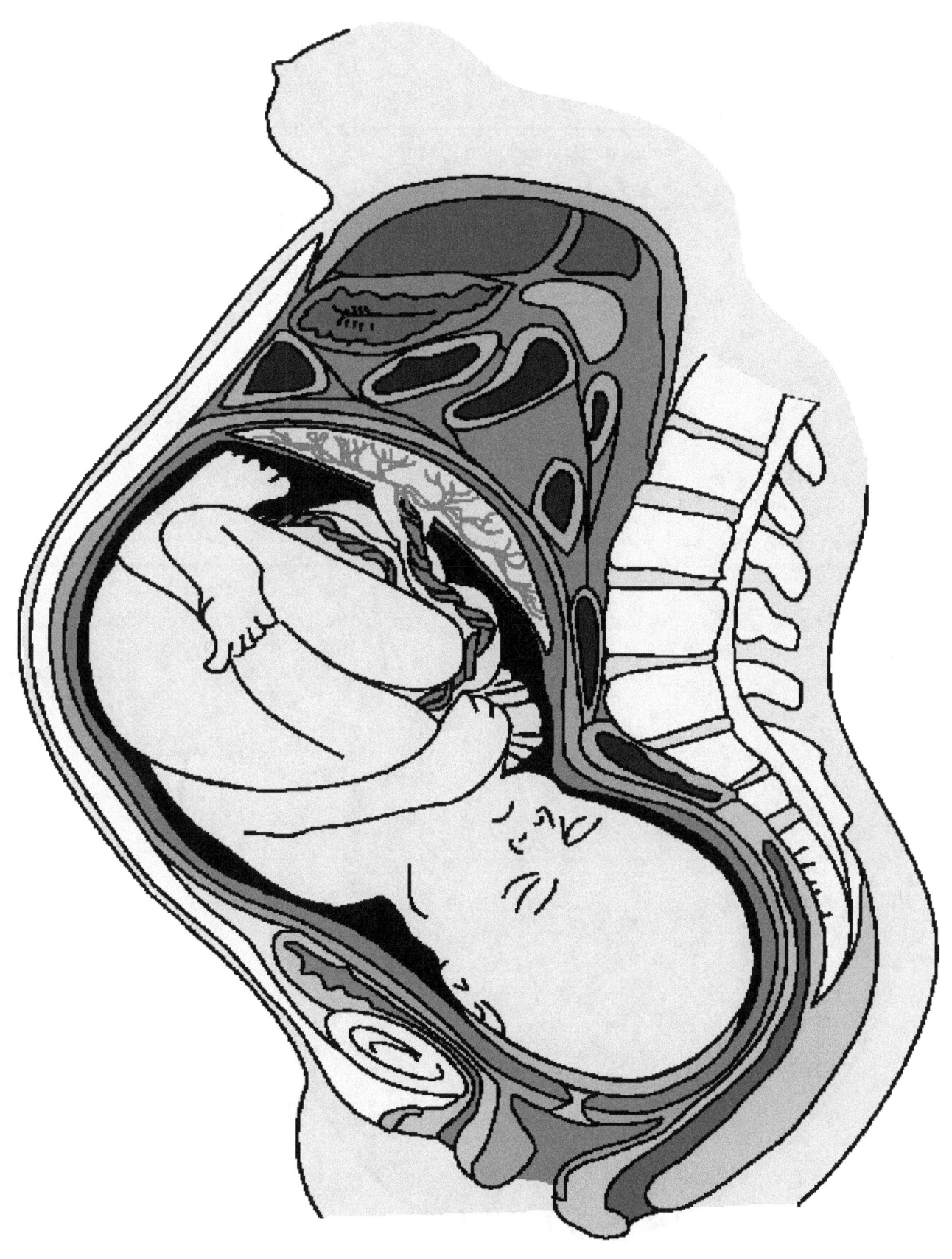

243

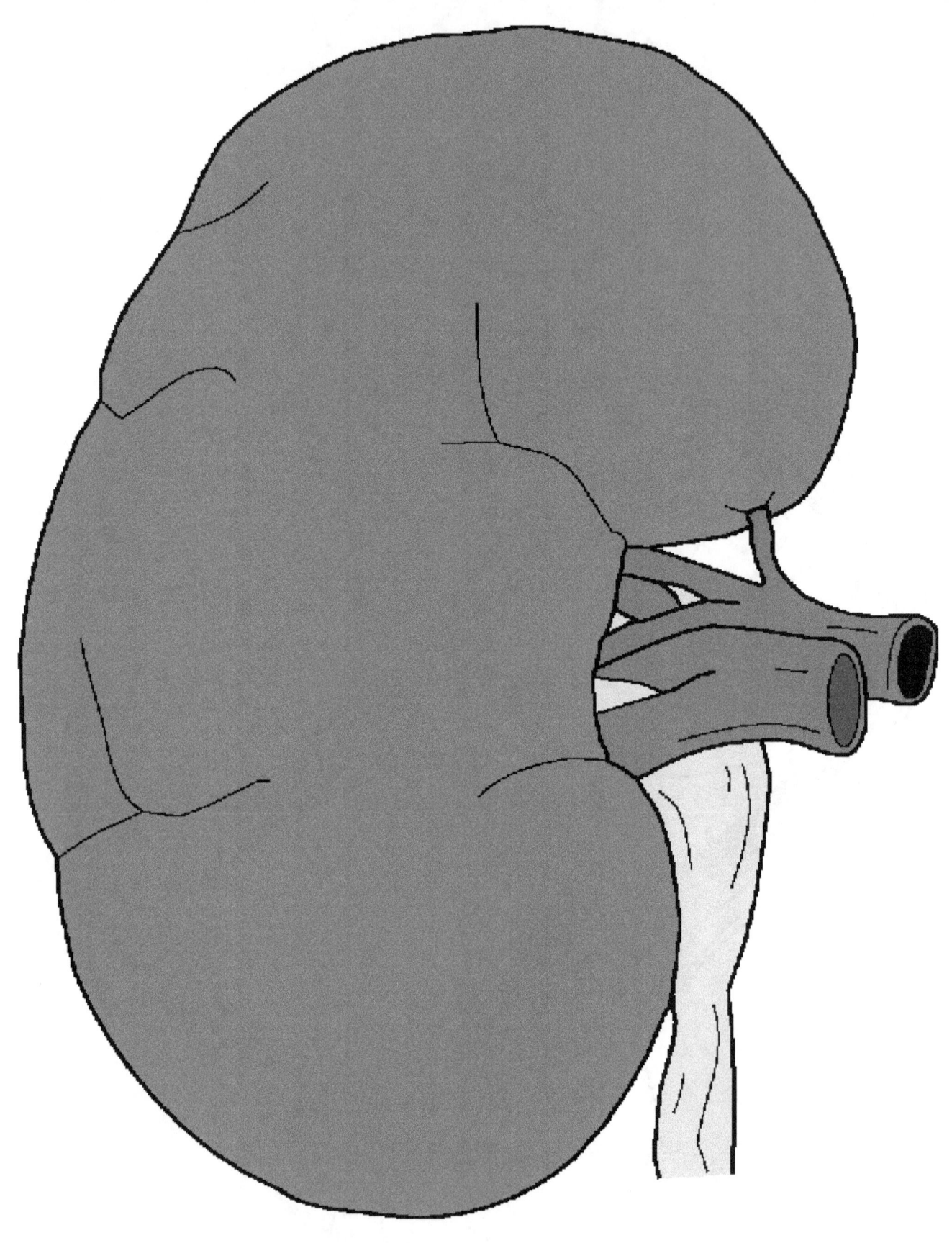

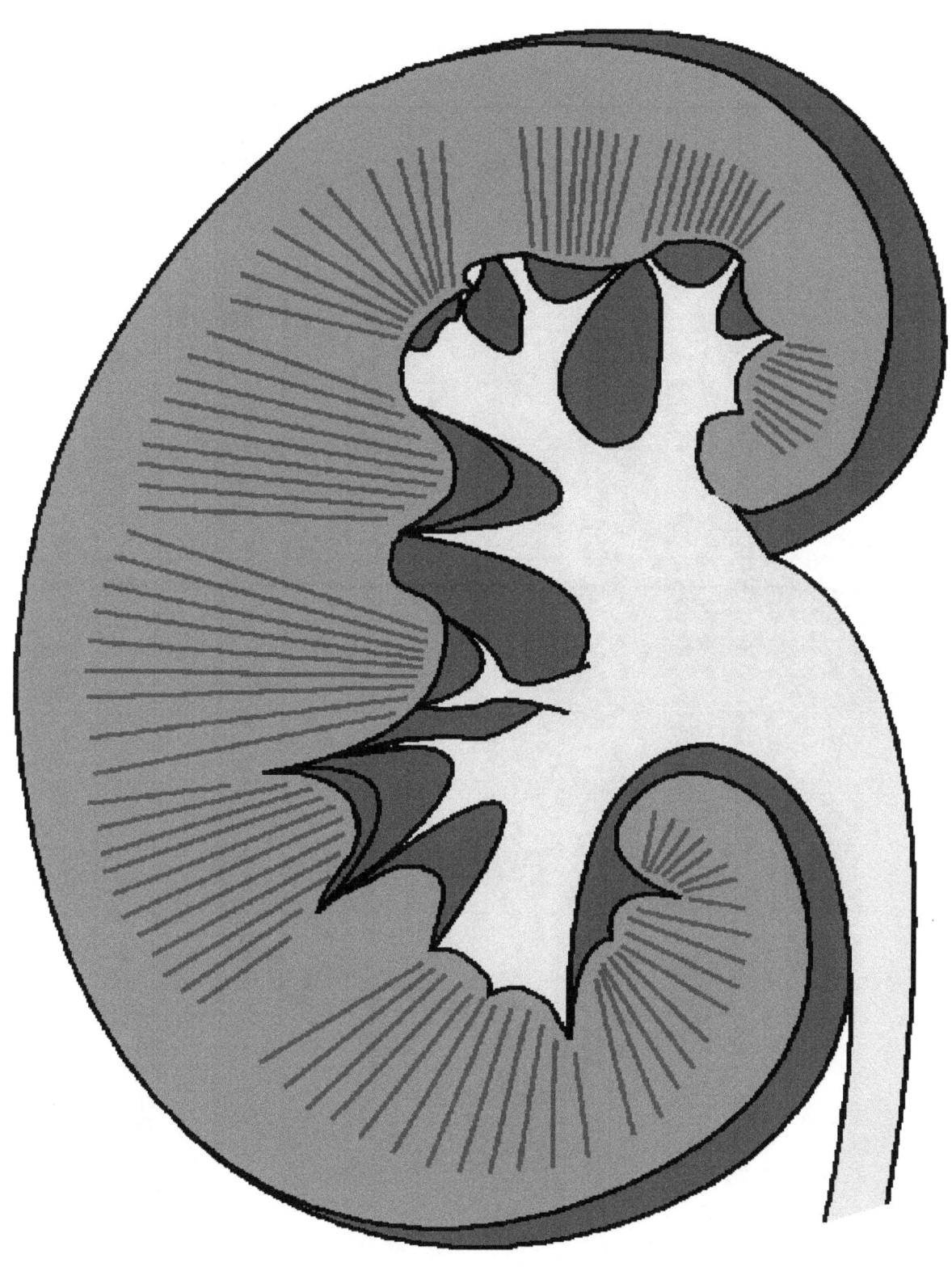

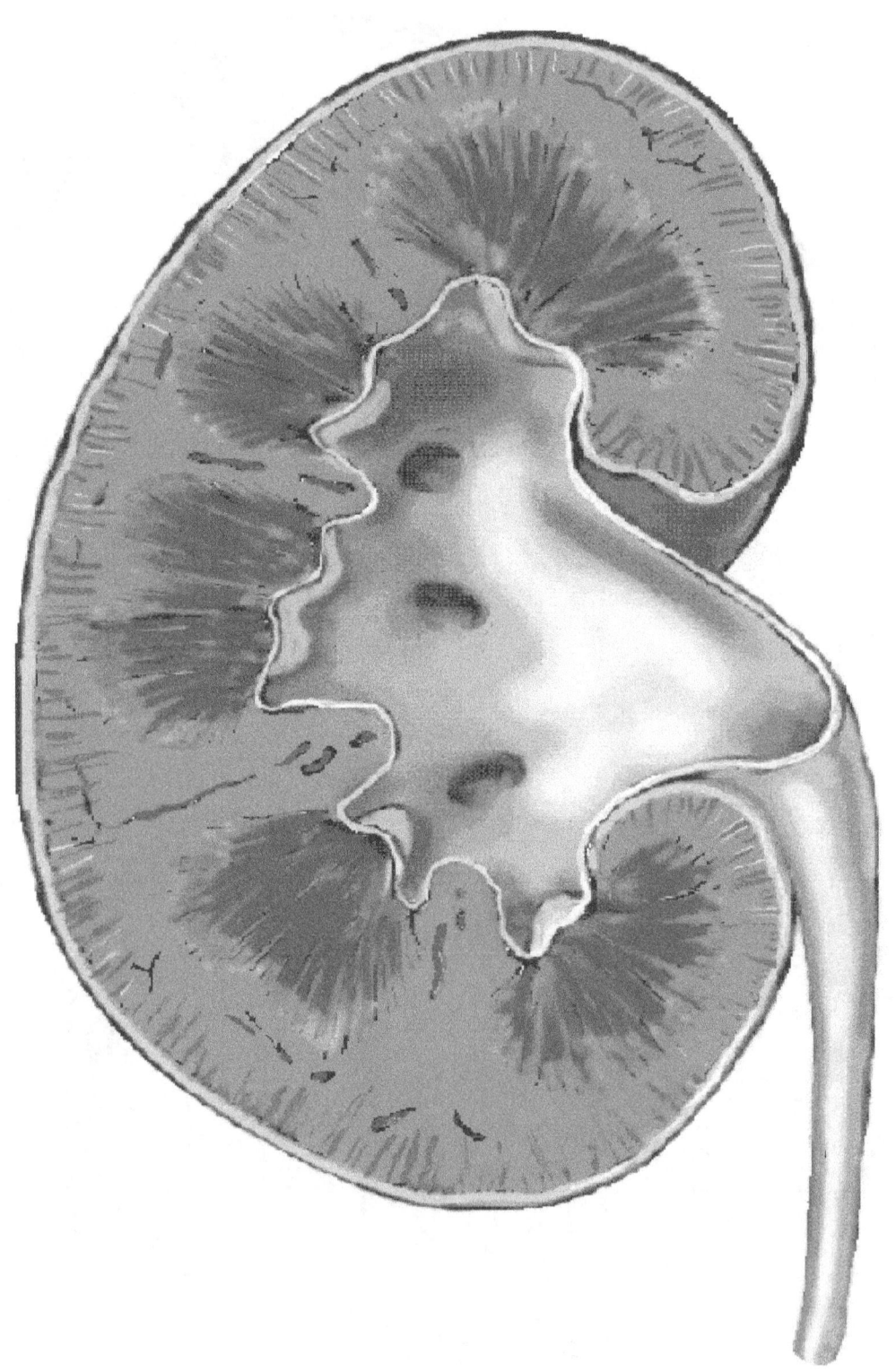

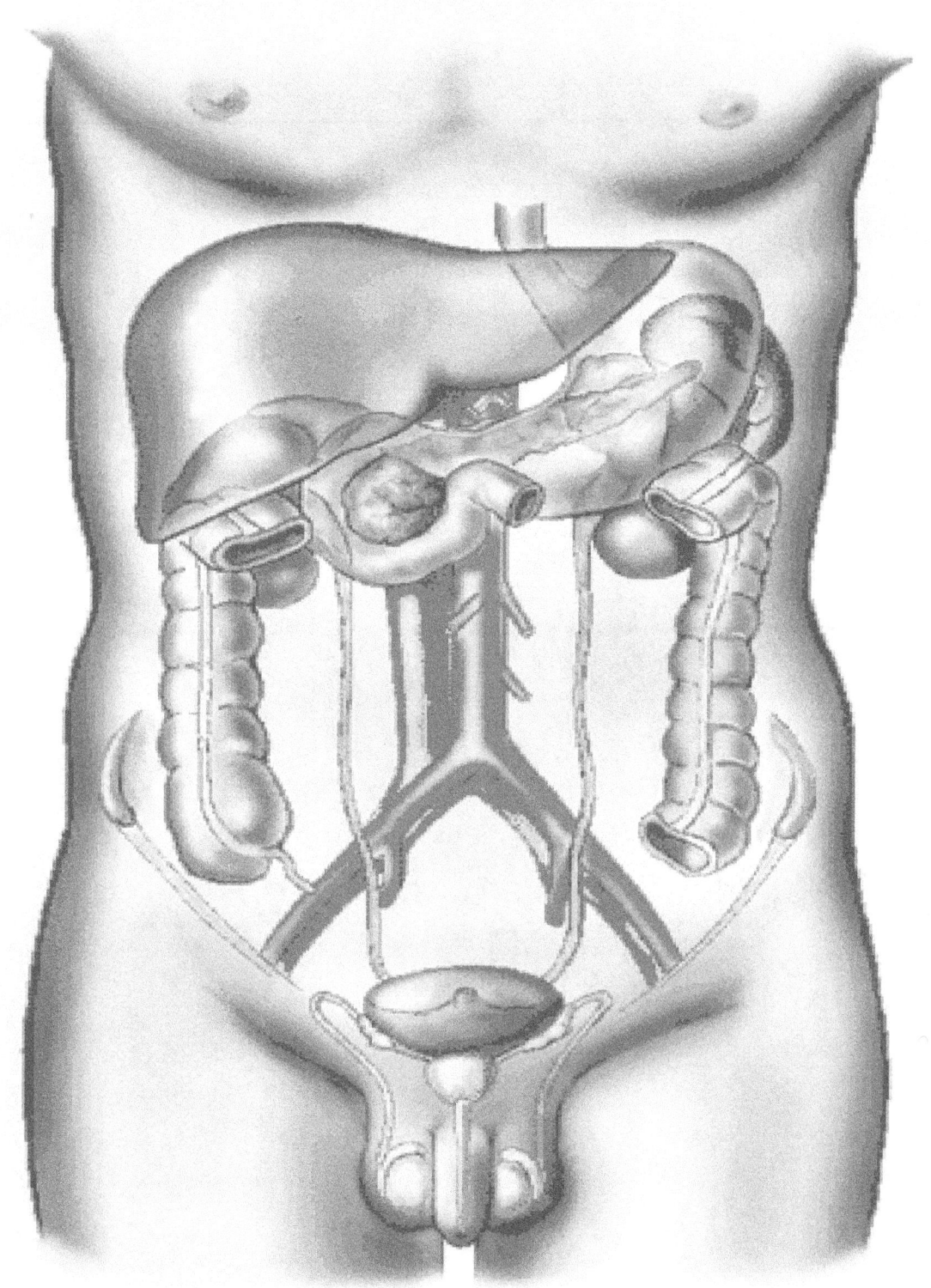

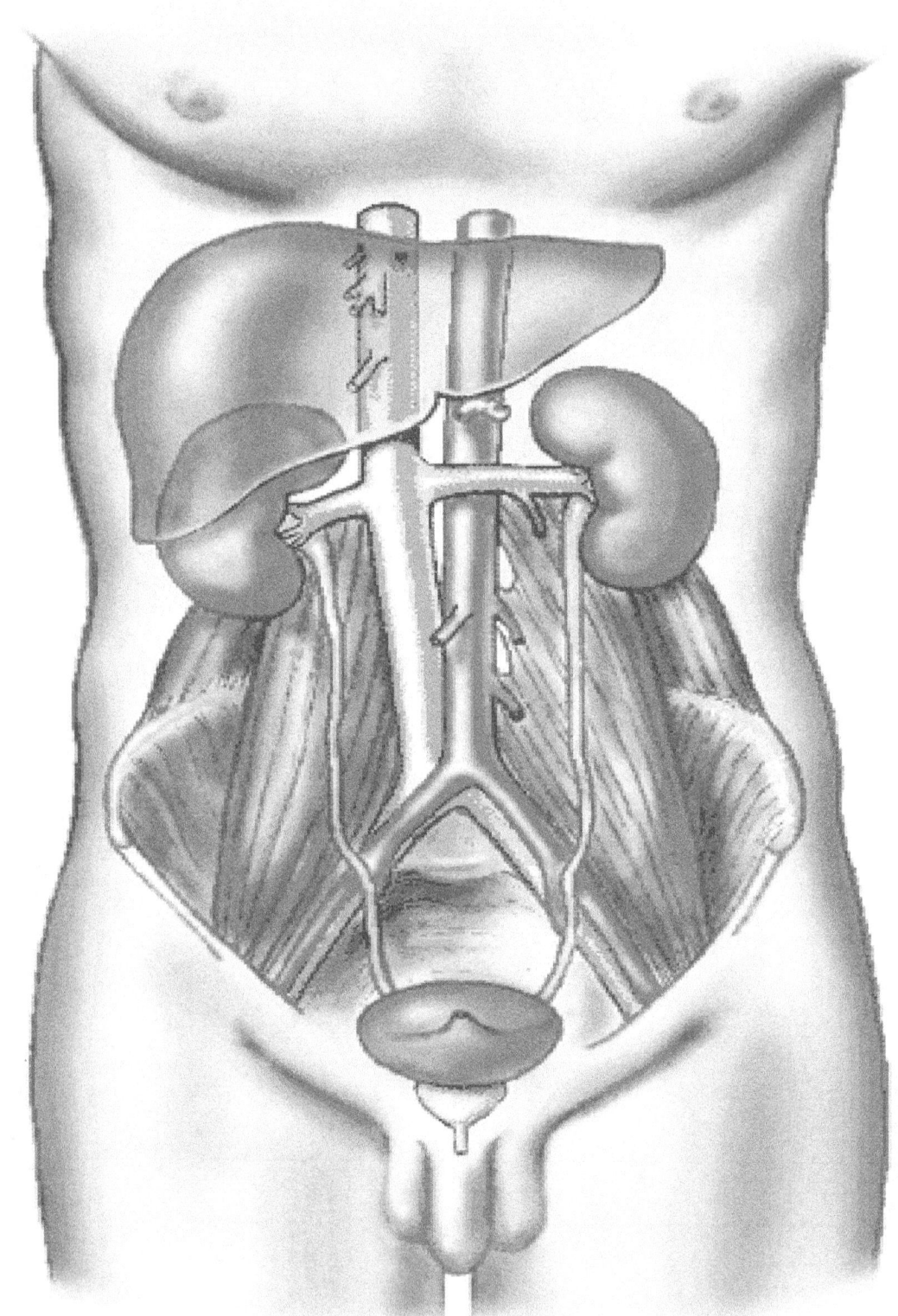

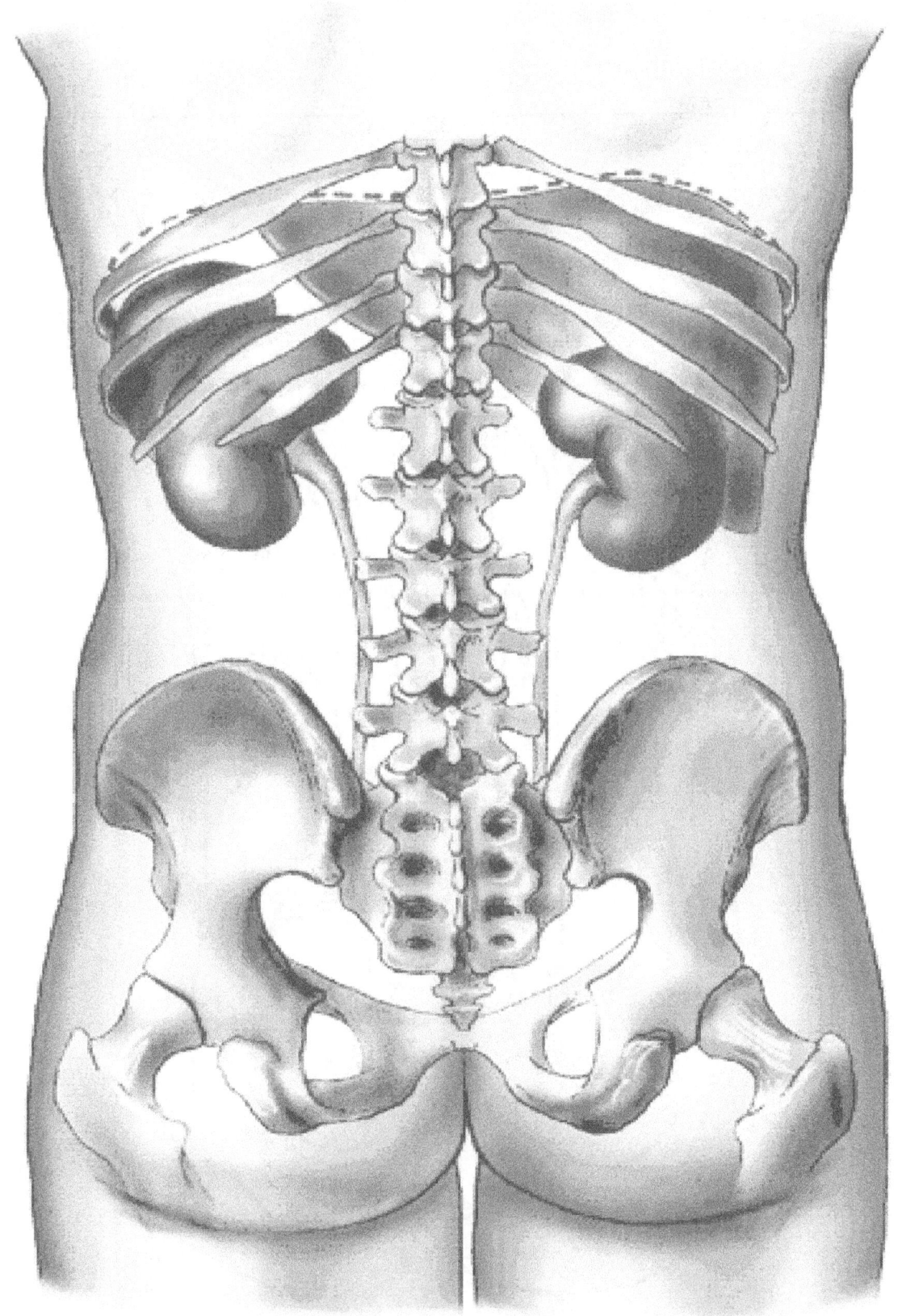

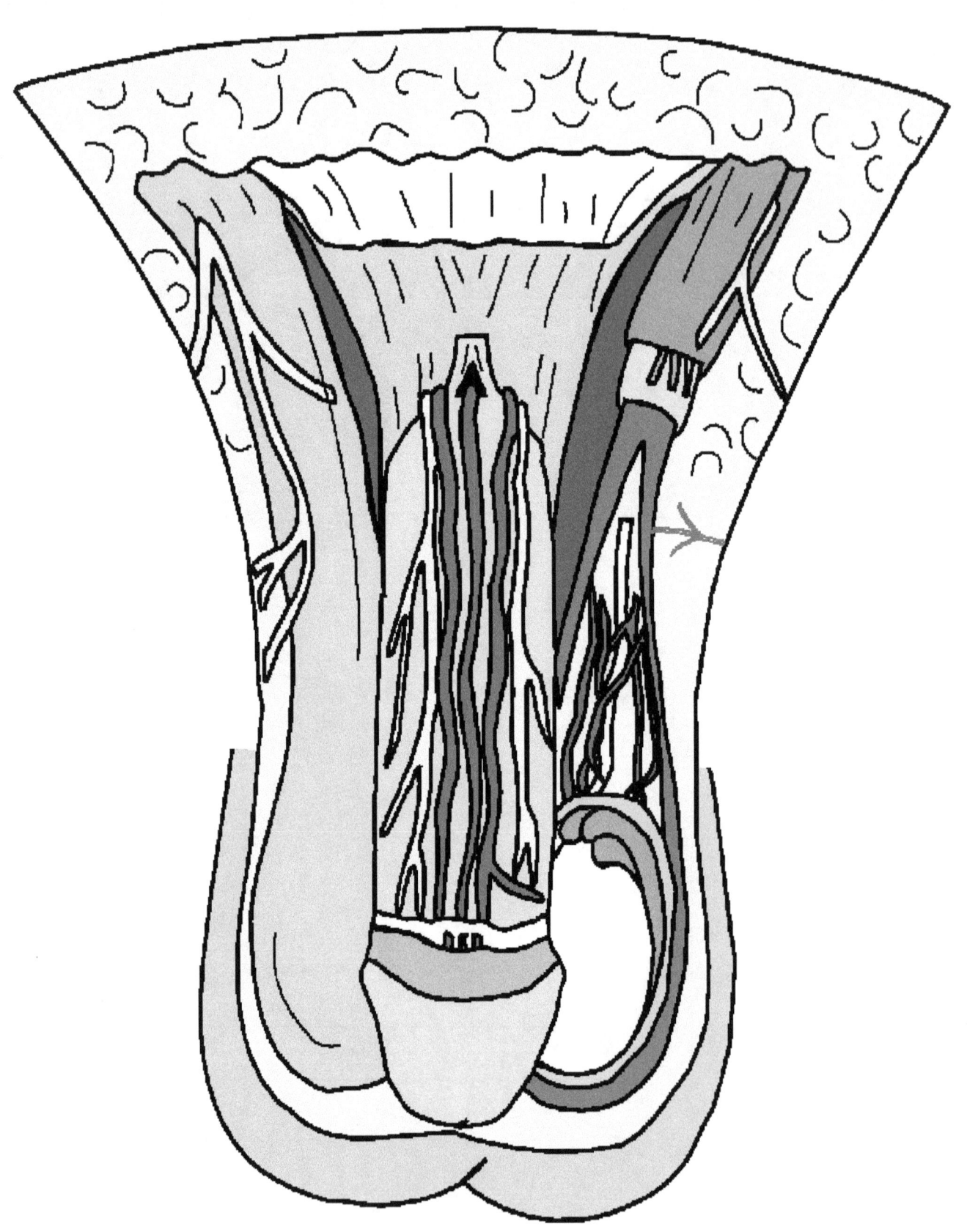

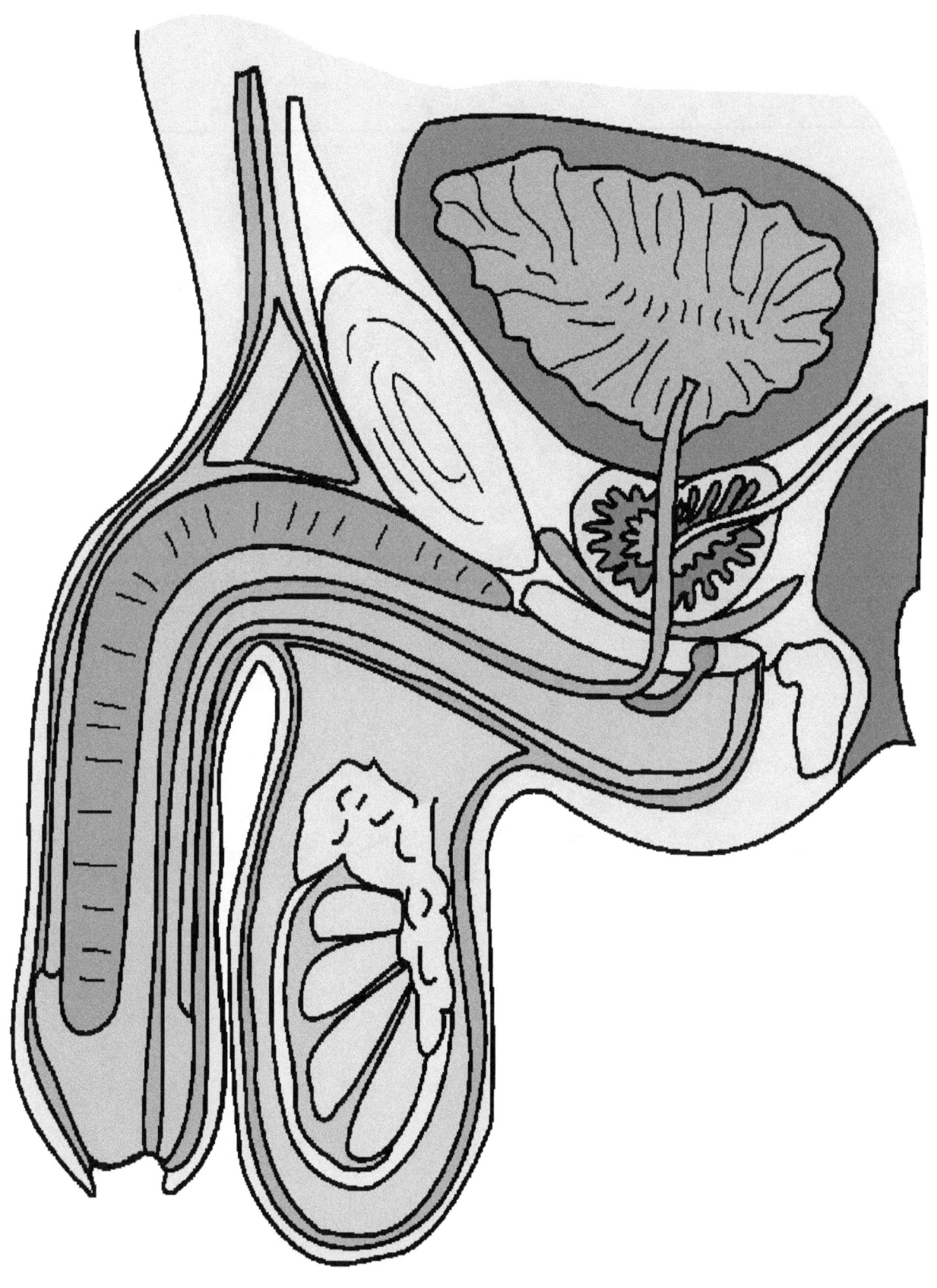

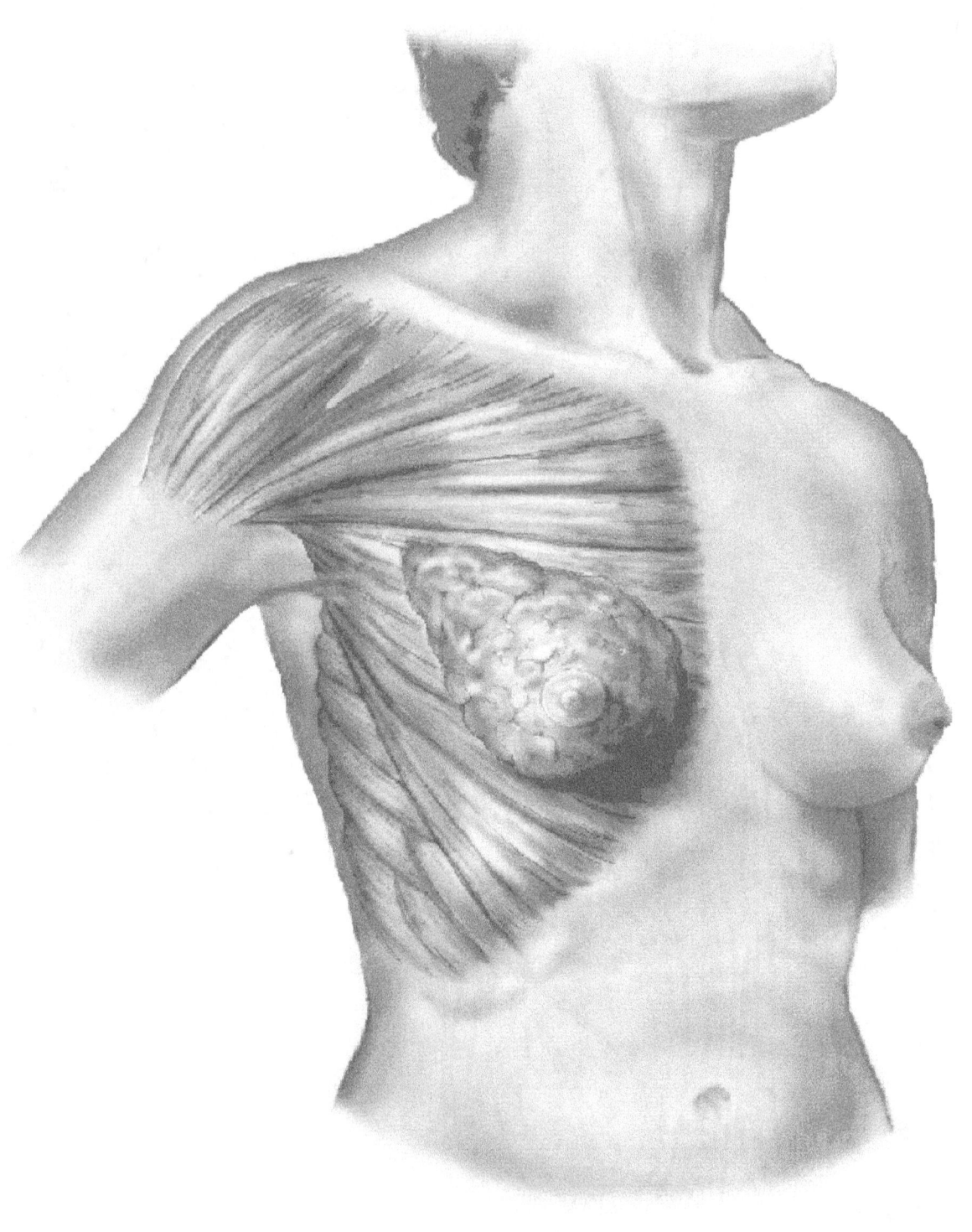

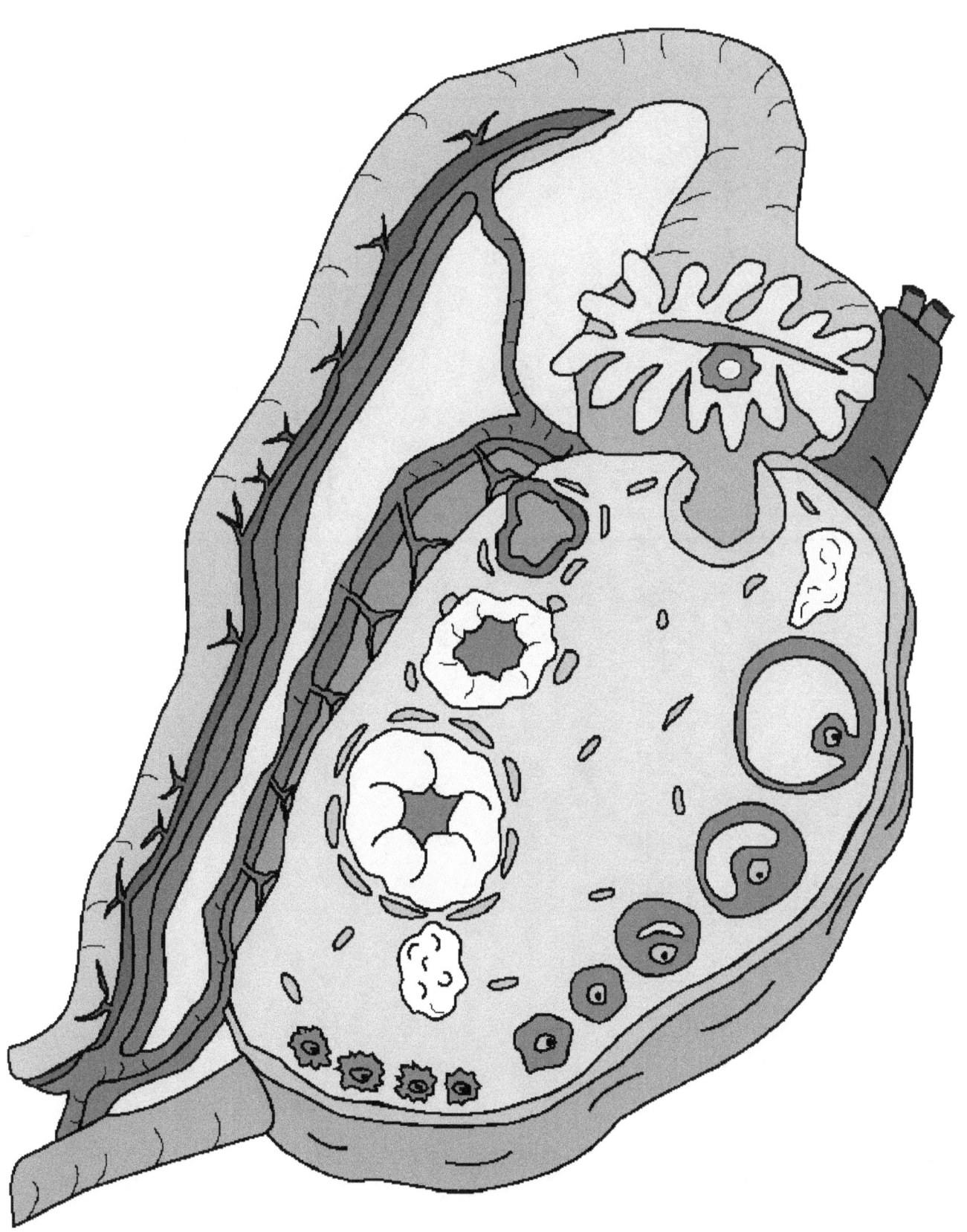

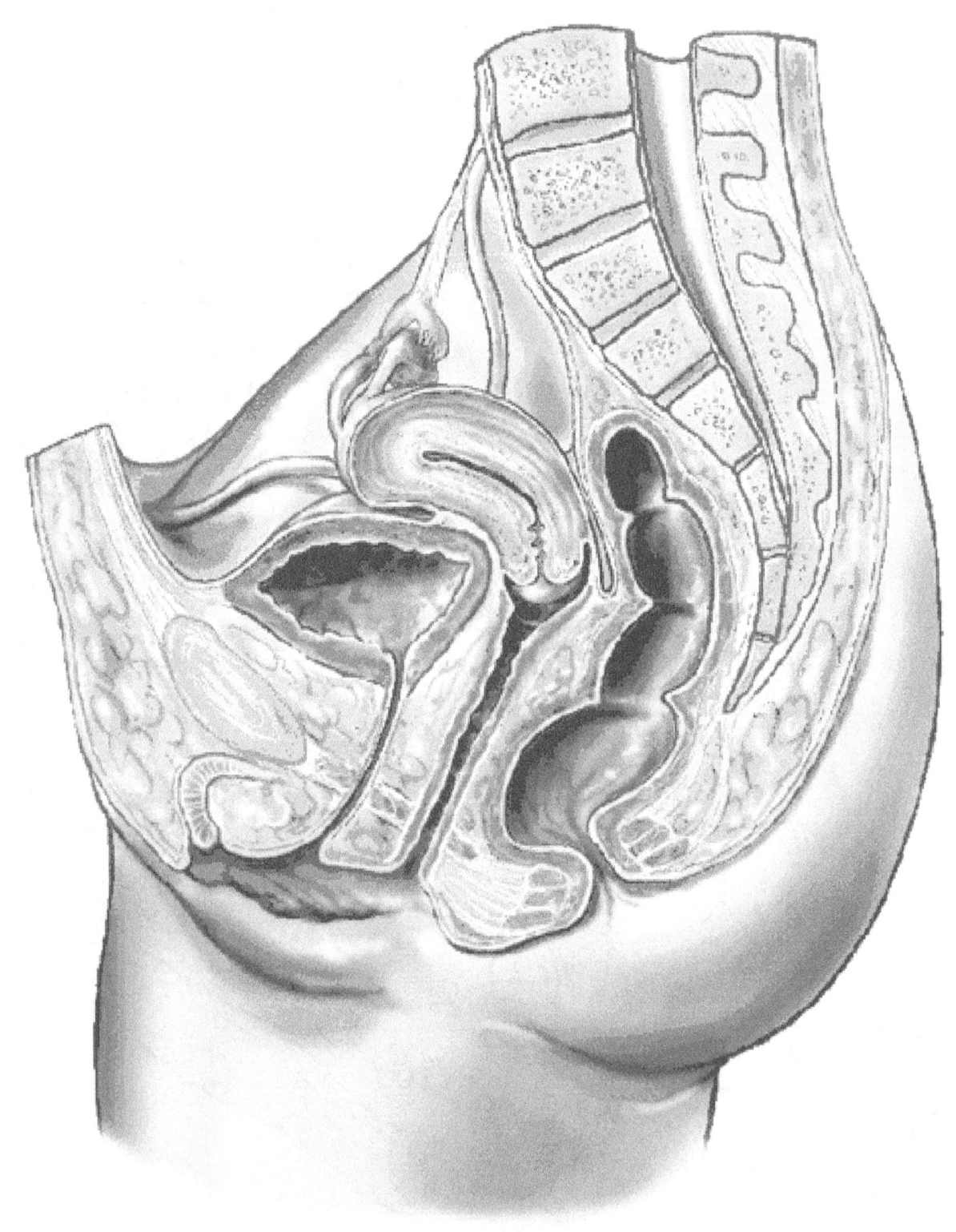

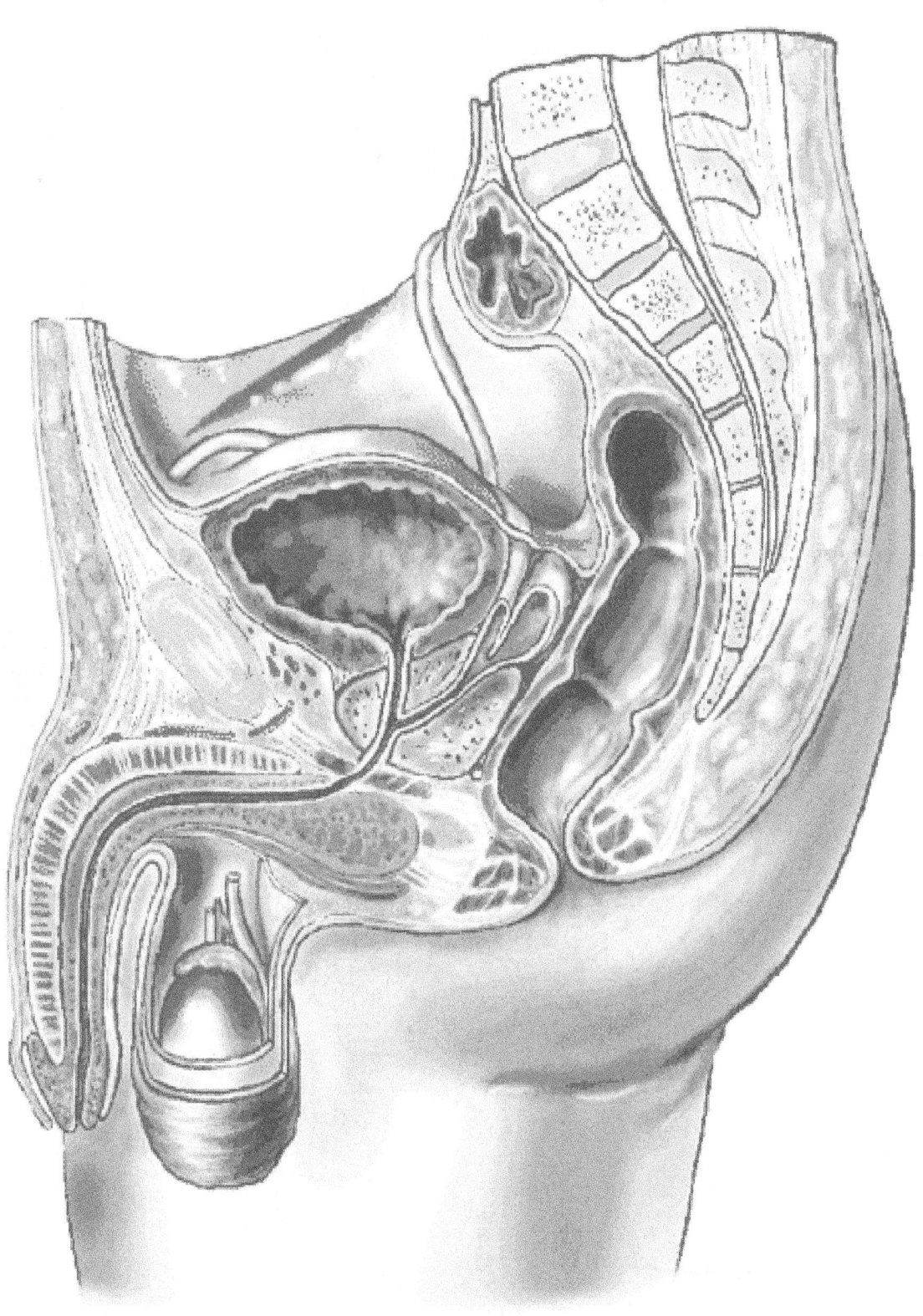

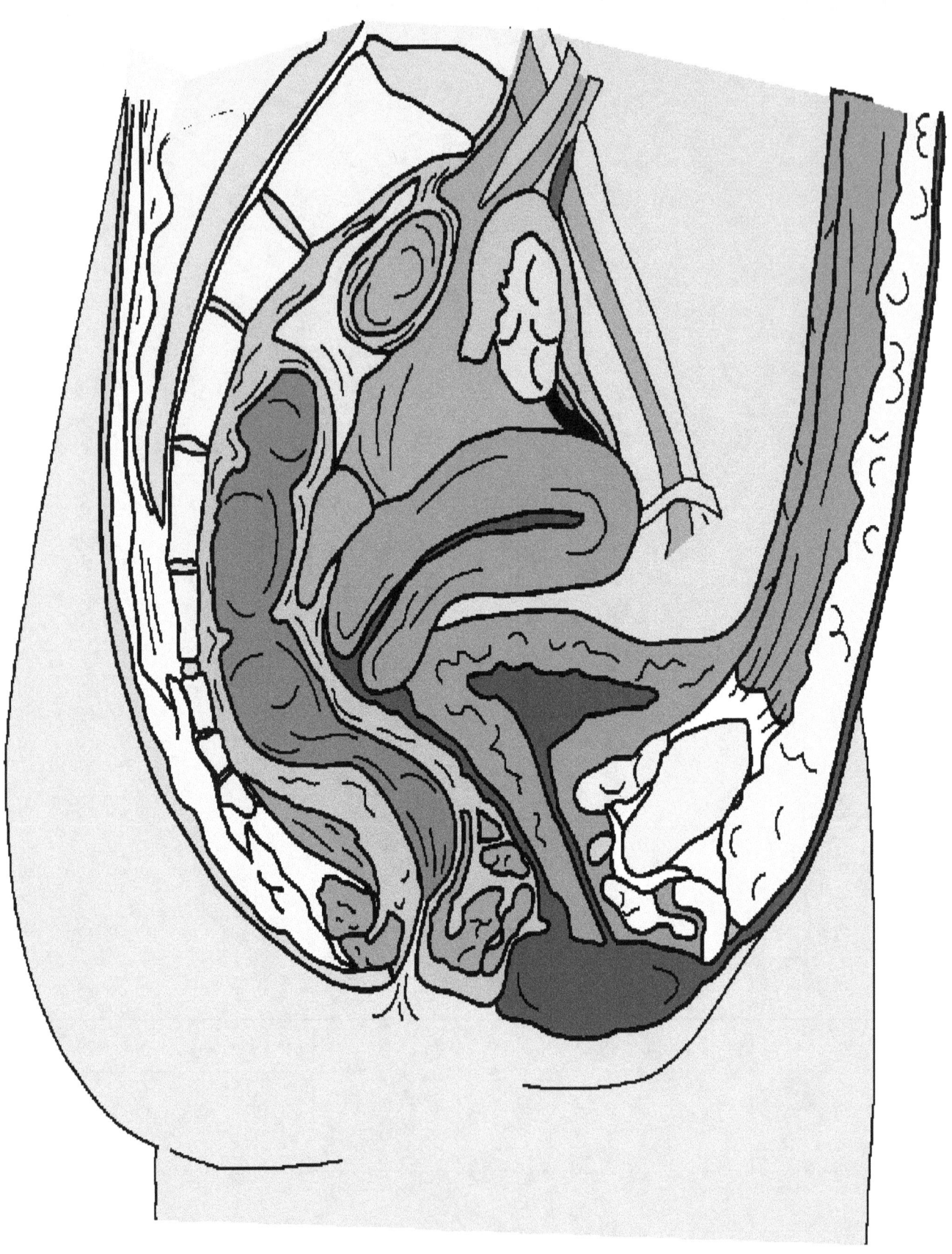

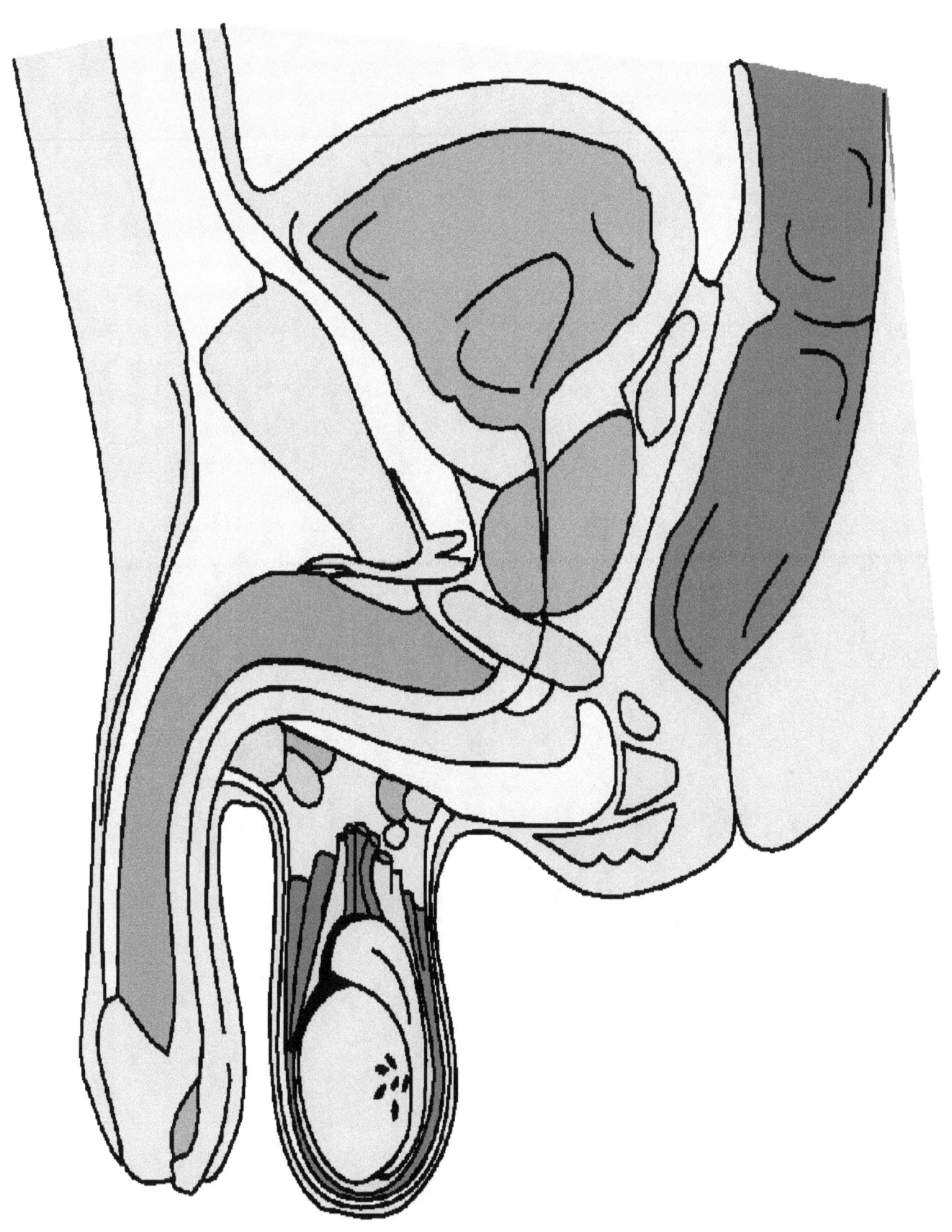

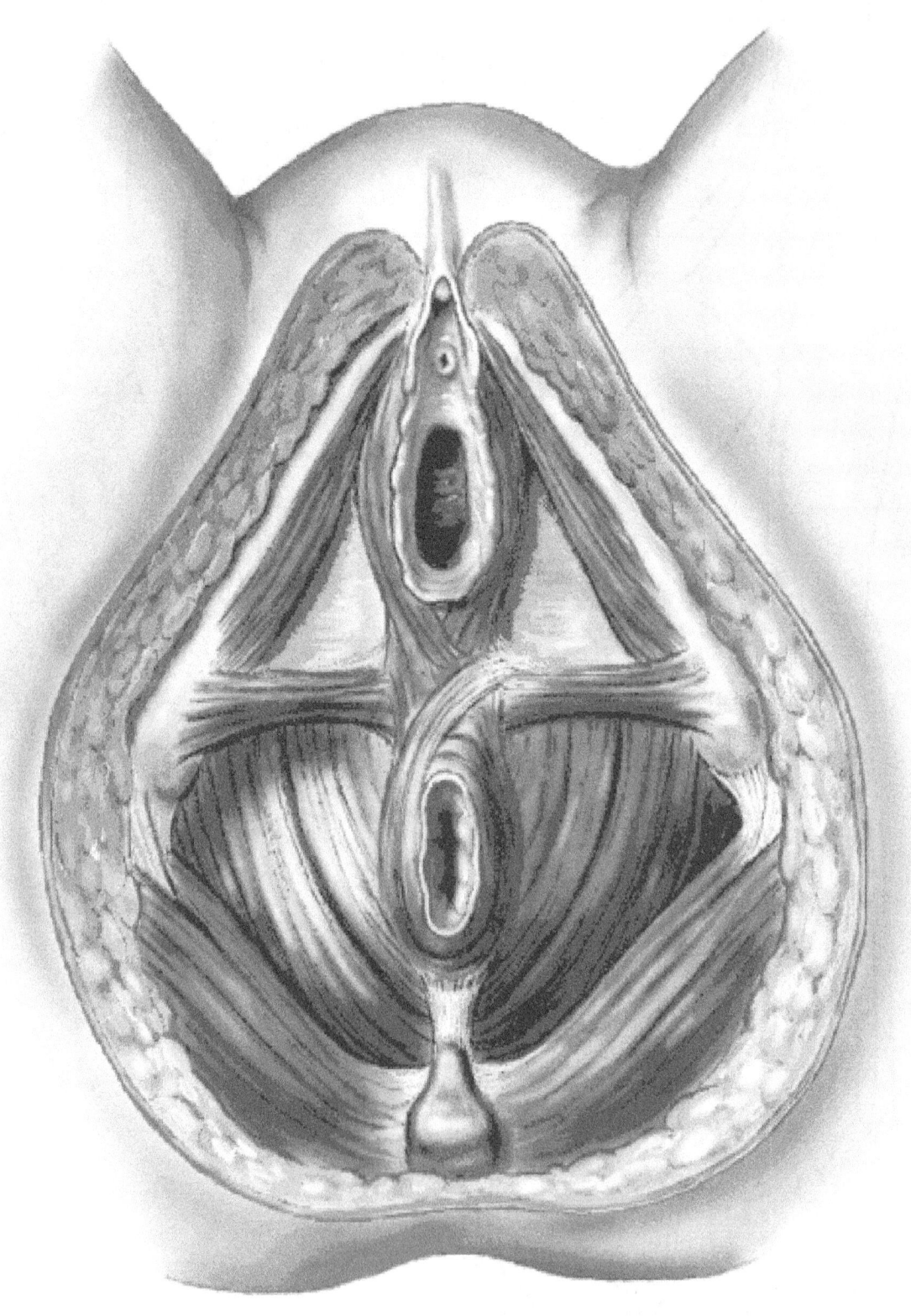

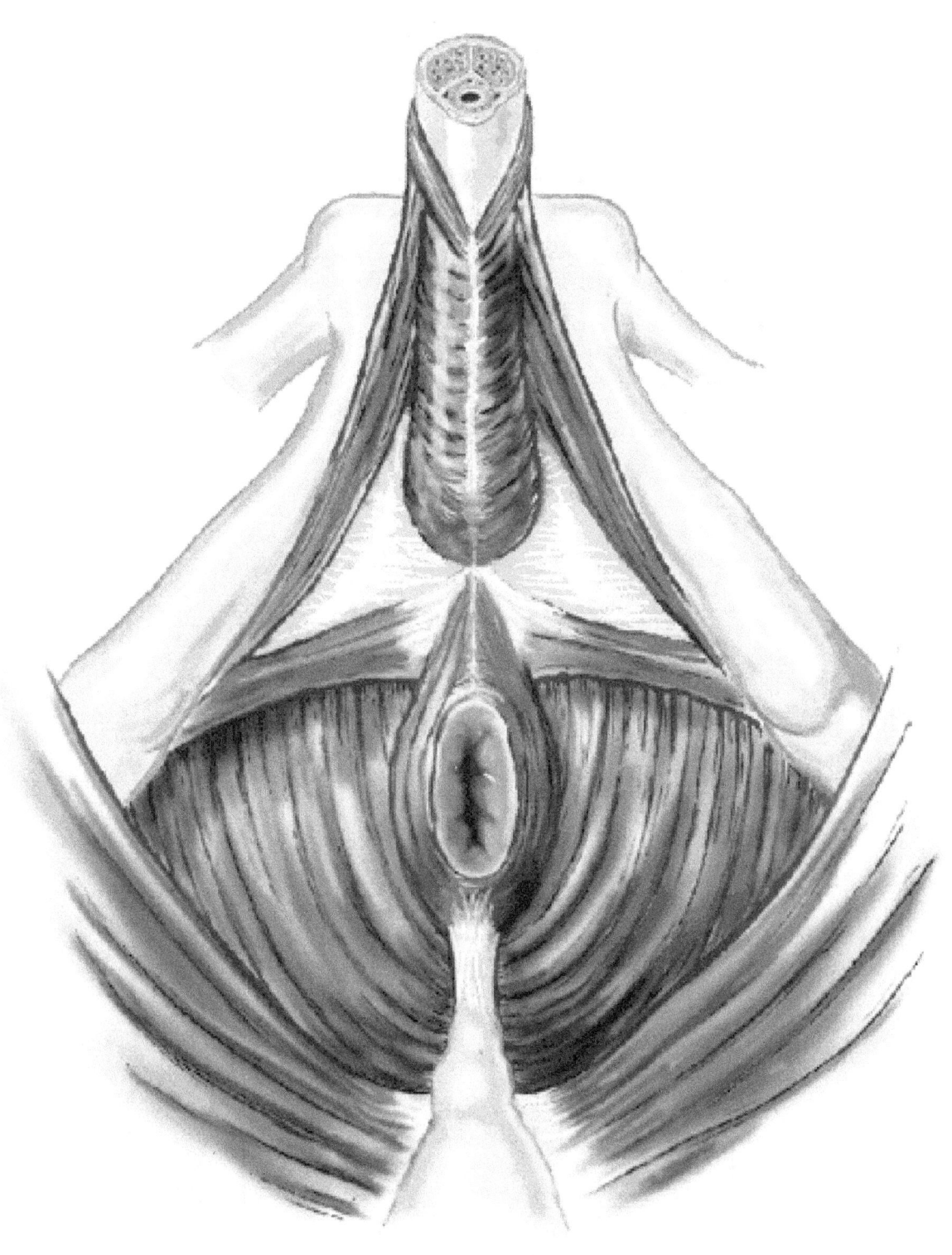

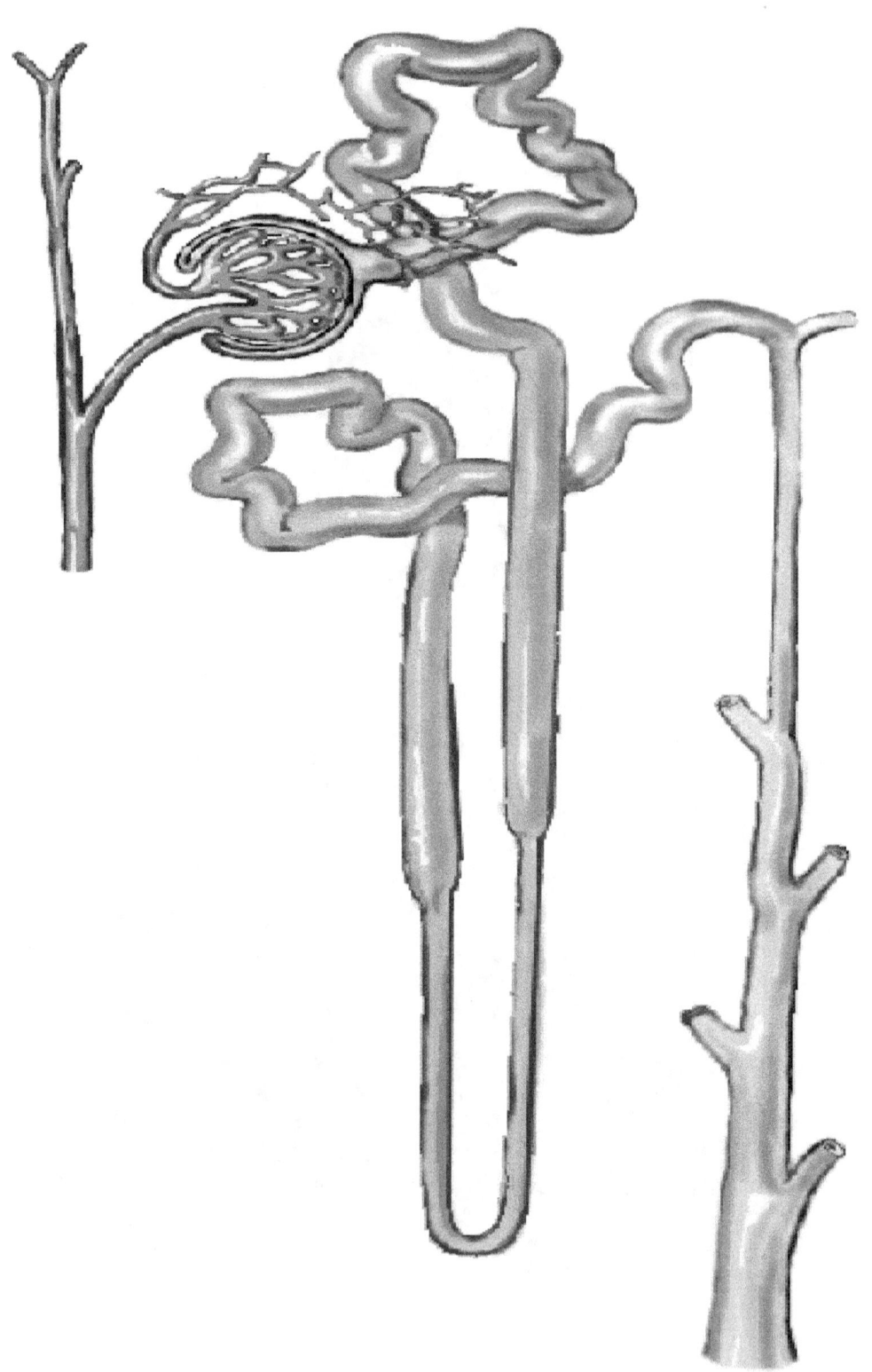

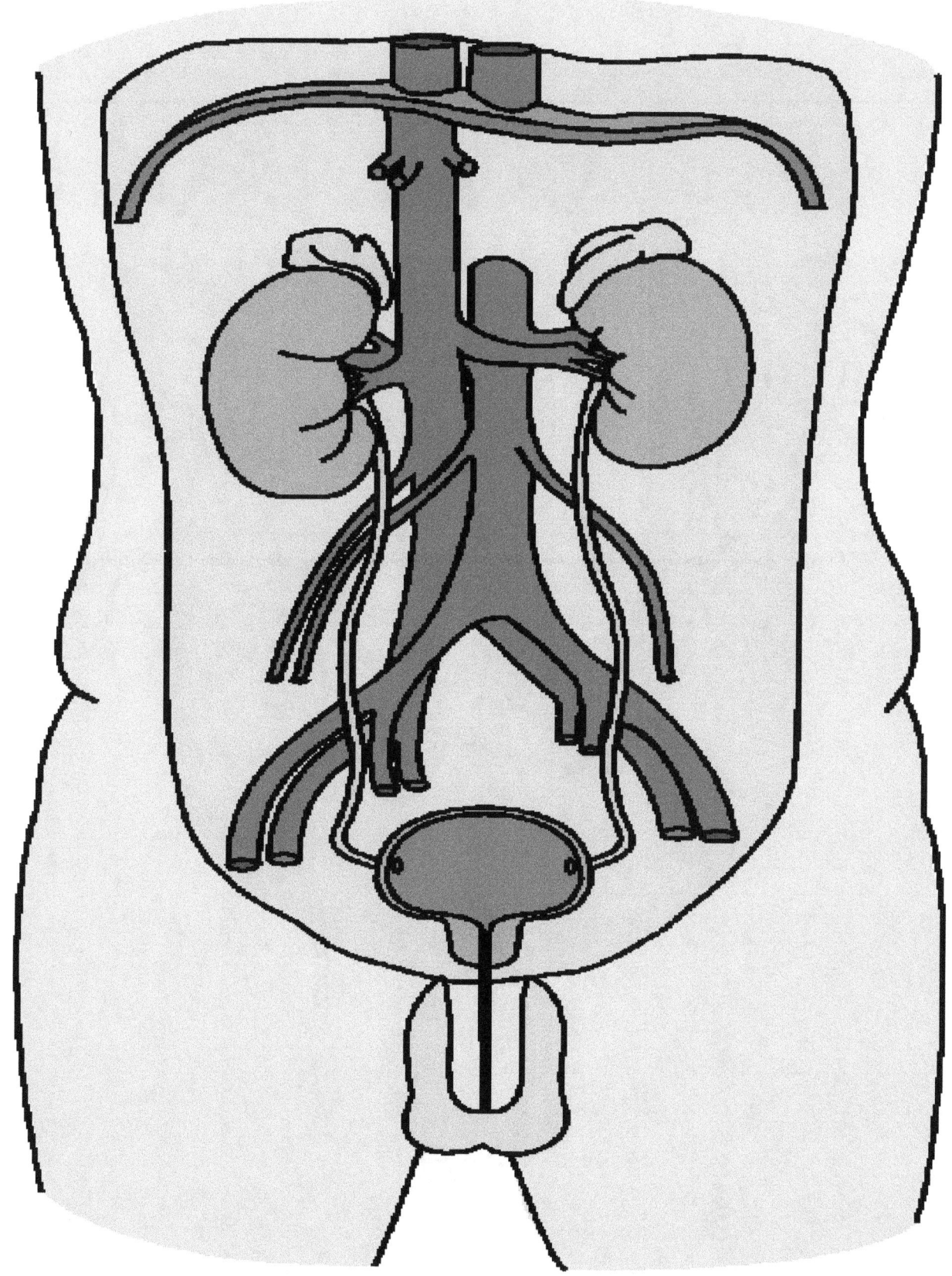

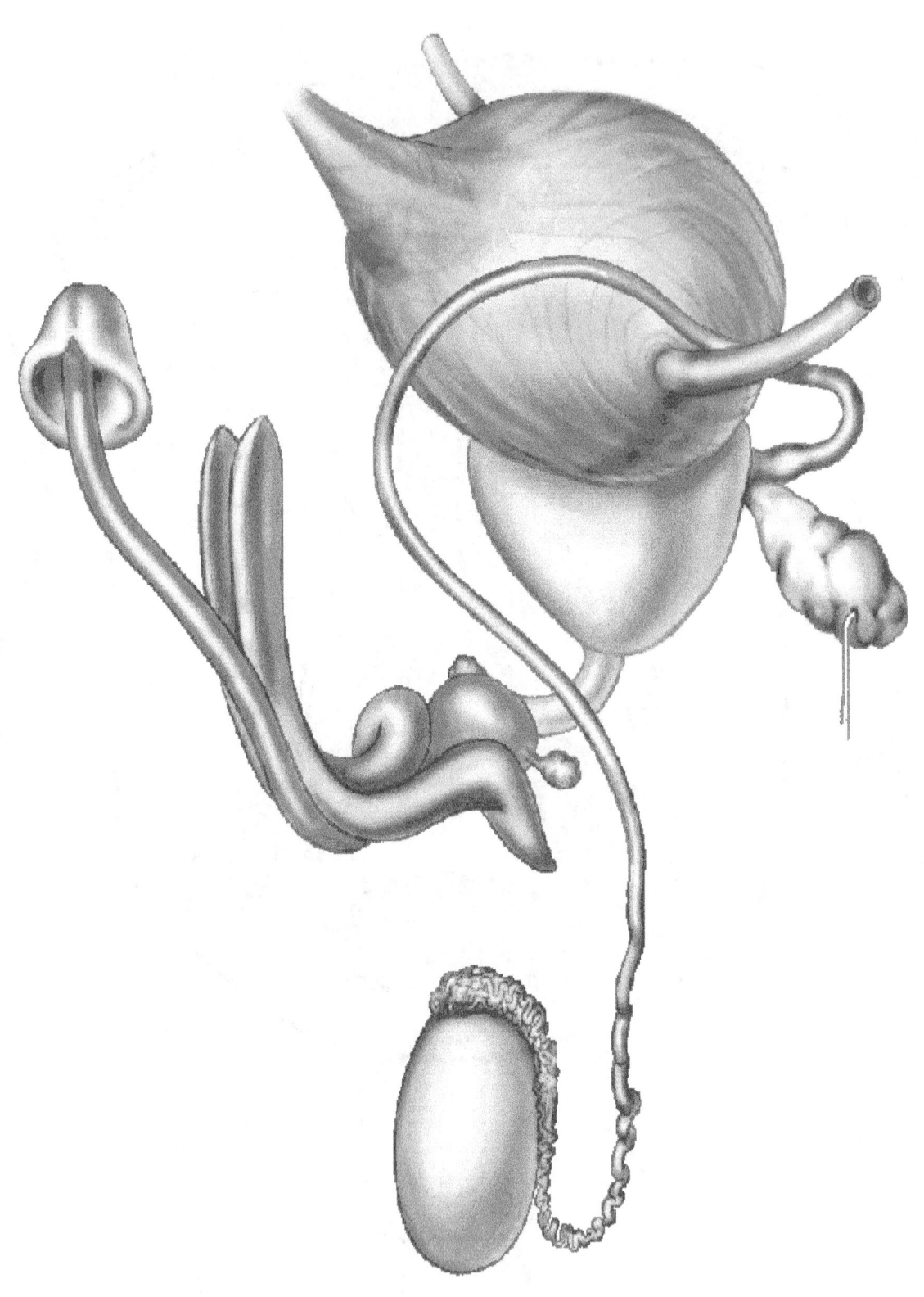

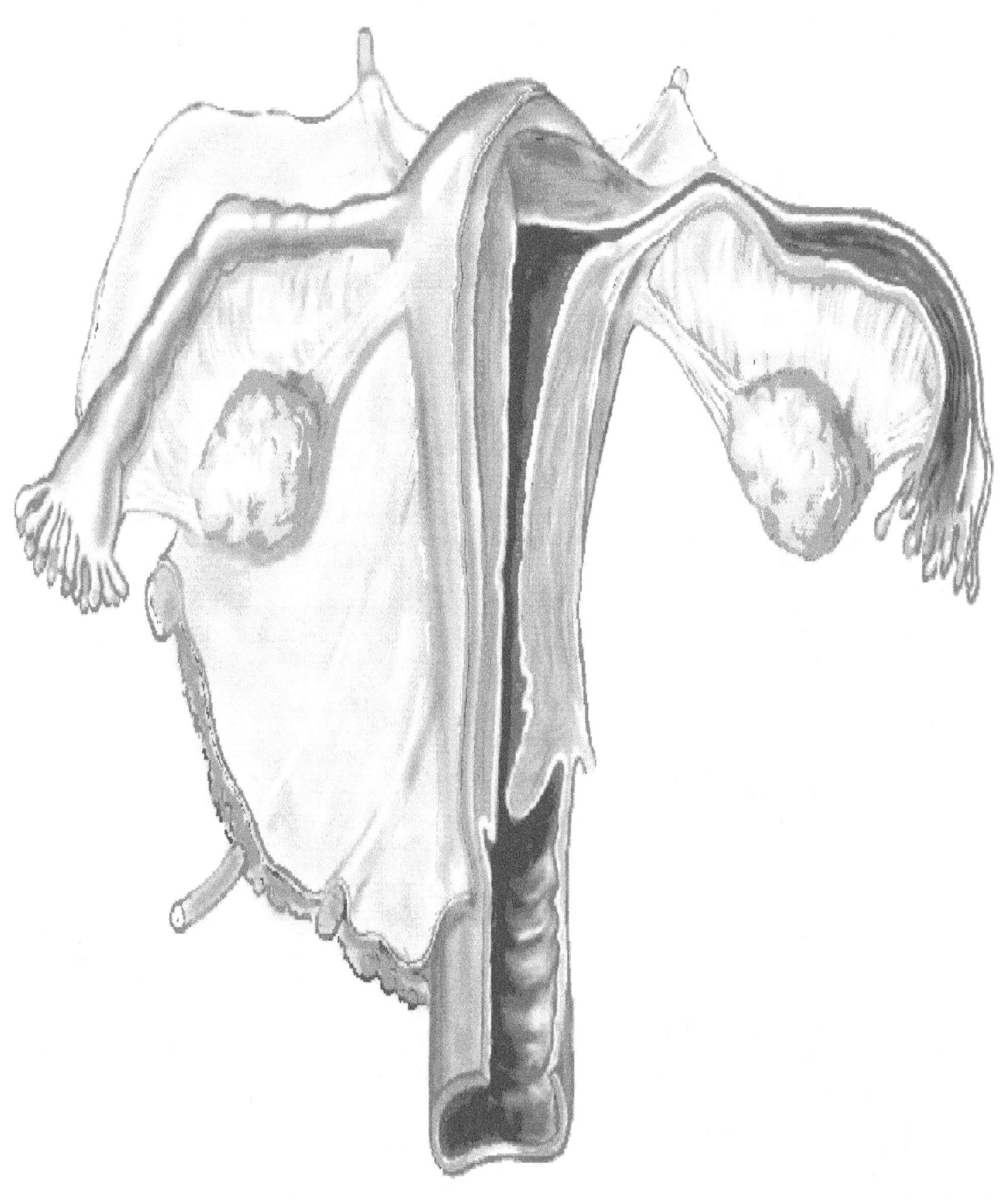

CardioVascular System 265-329

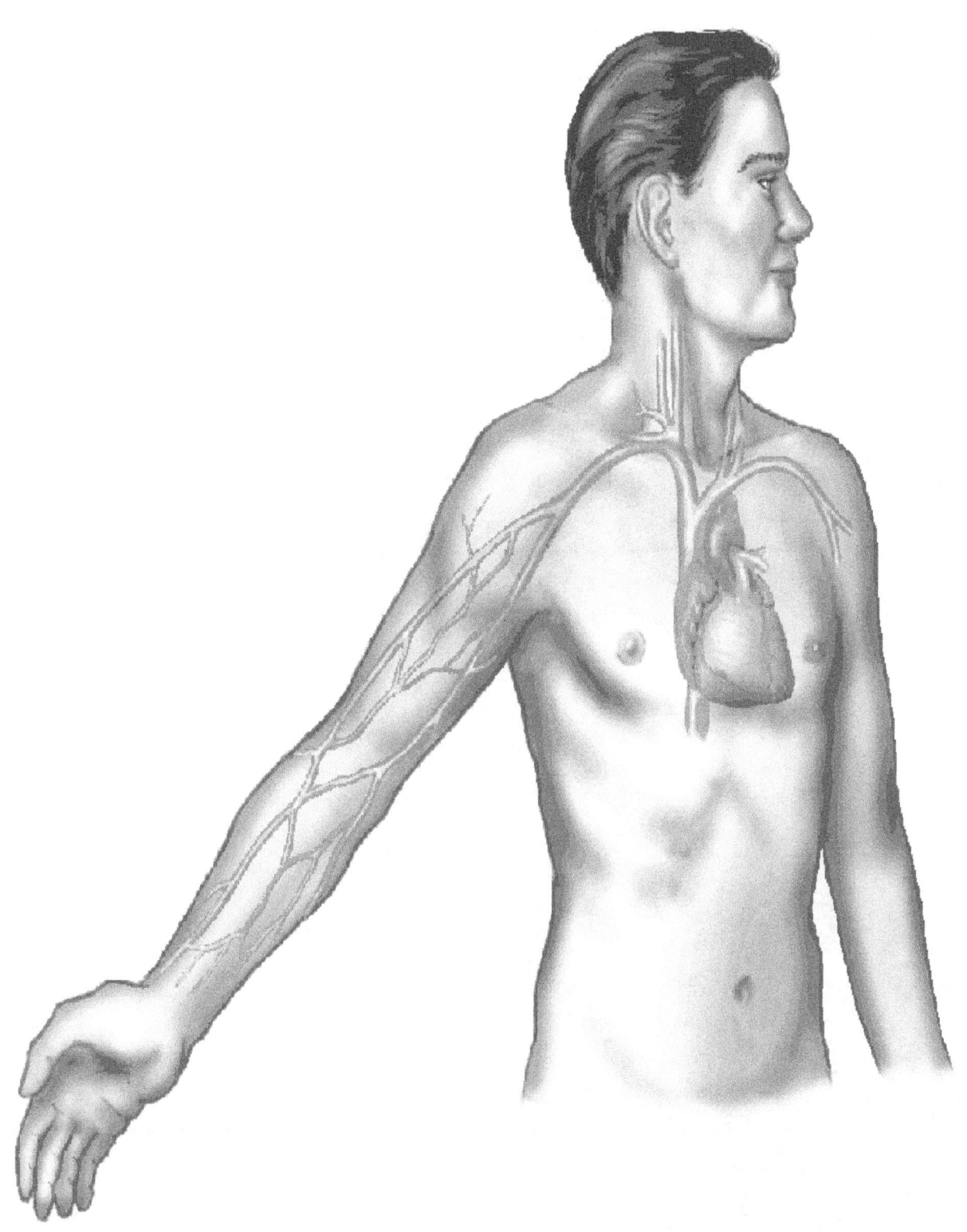

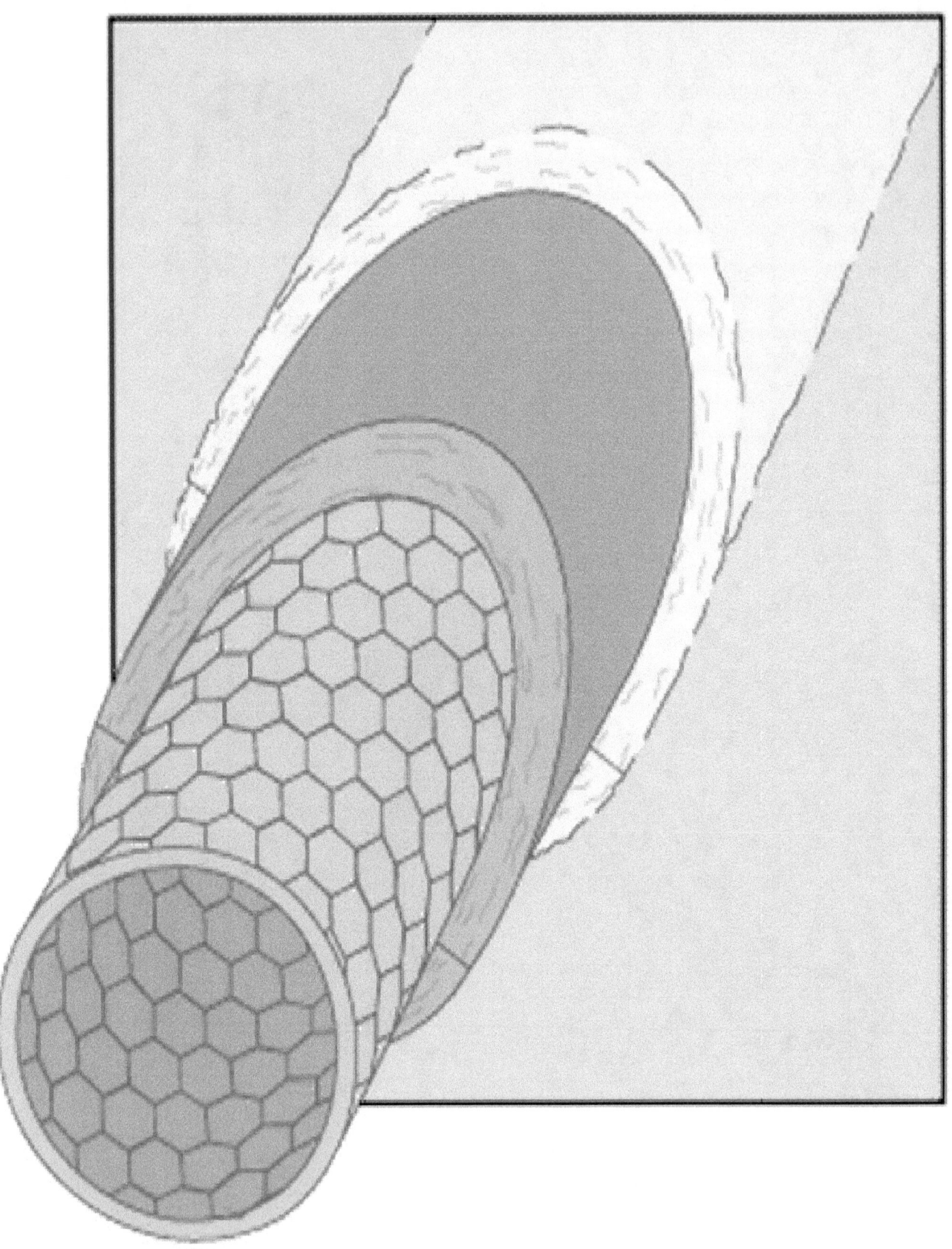

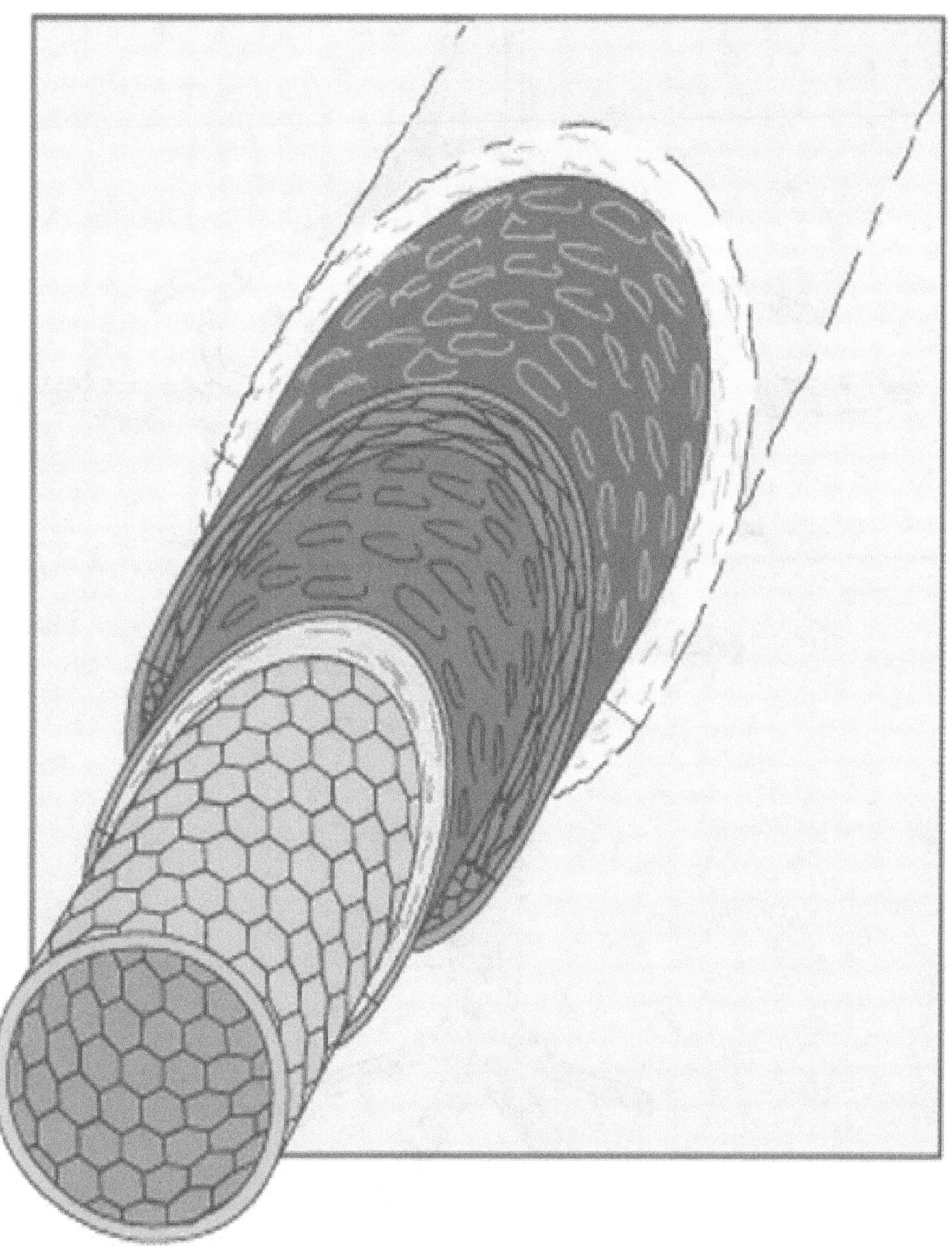

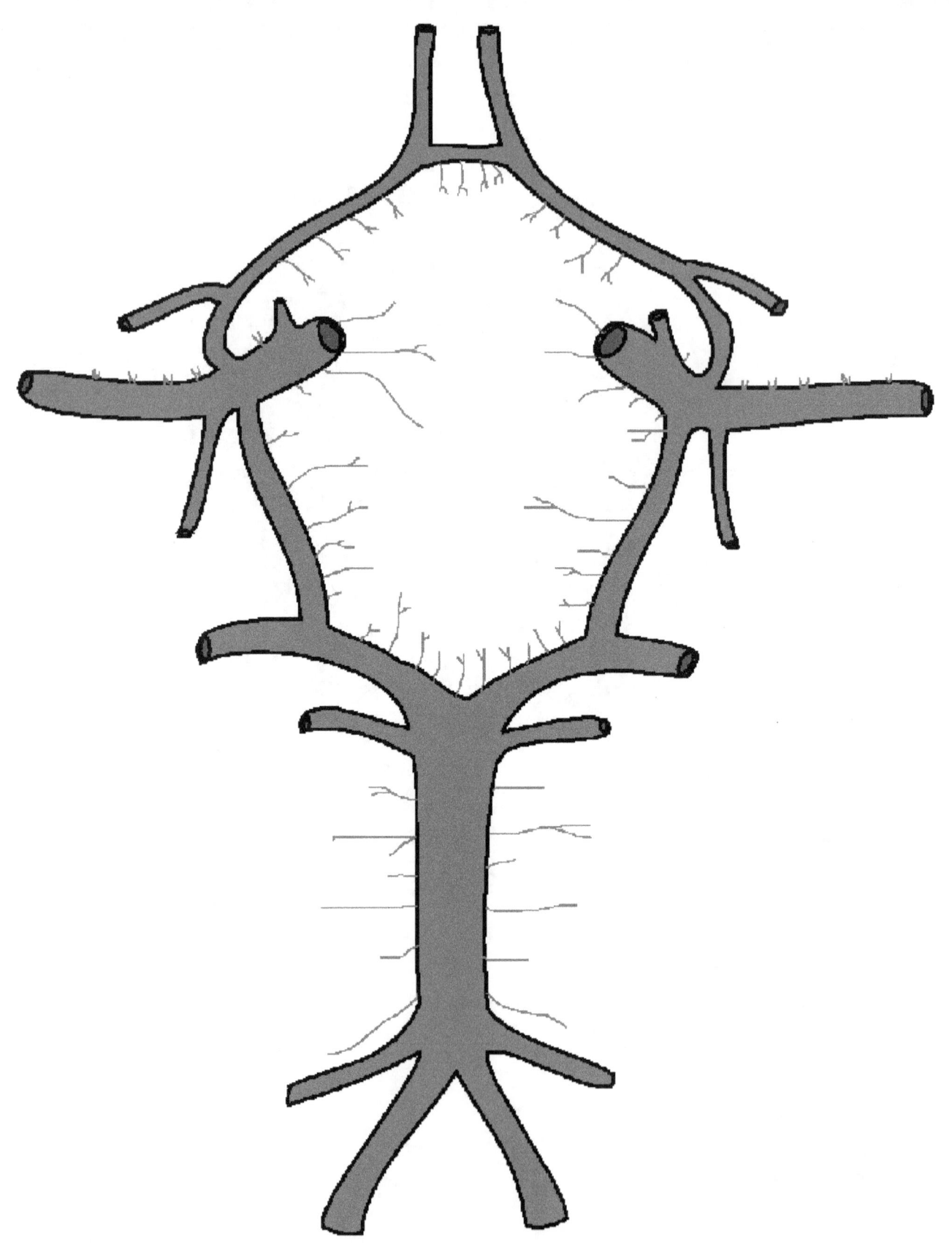

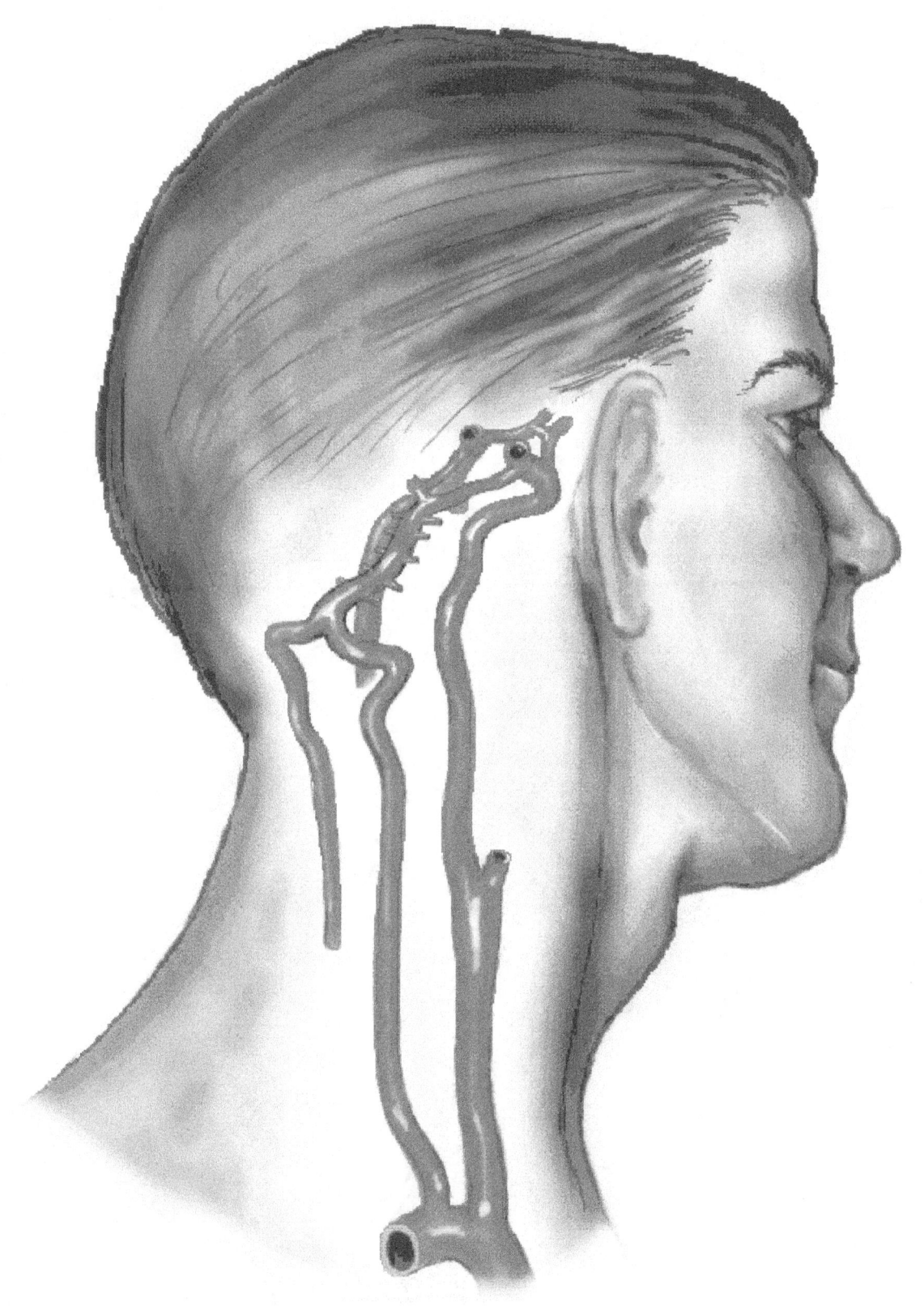

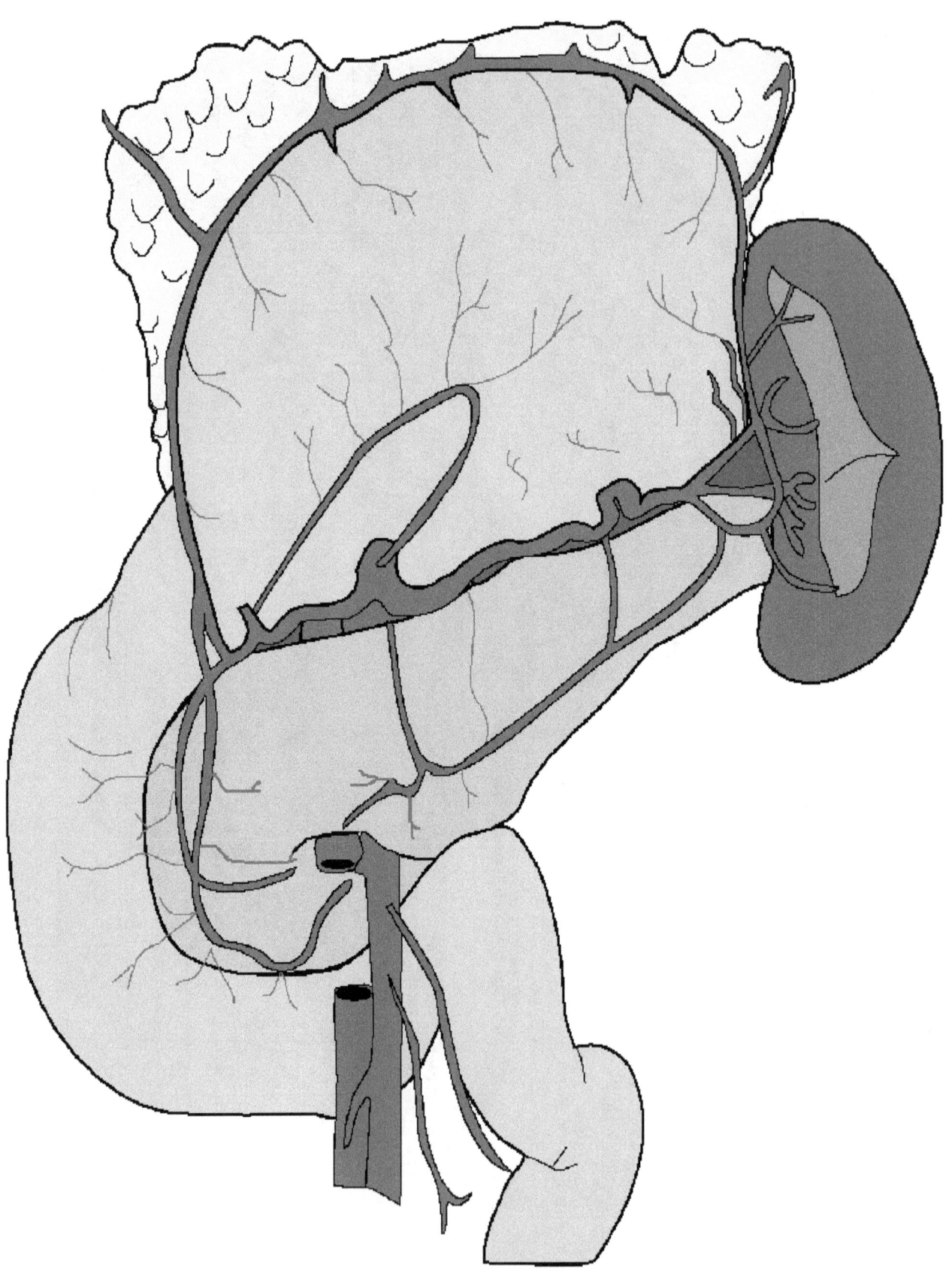

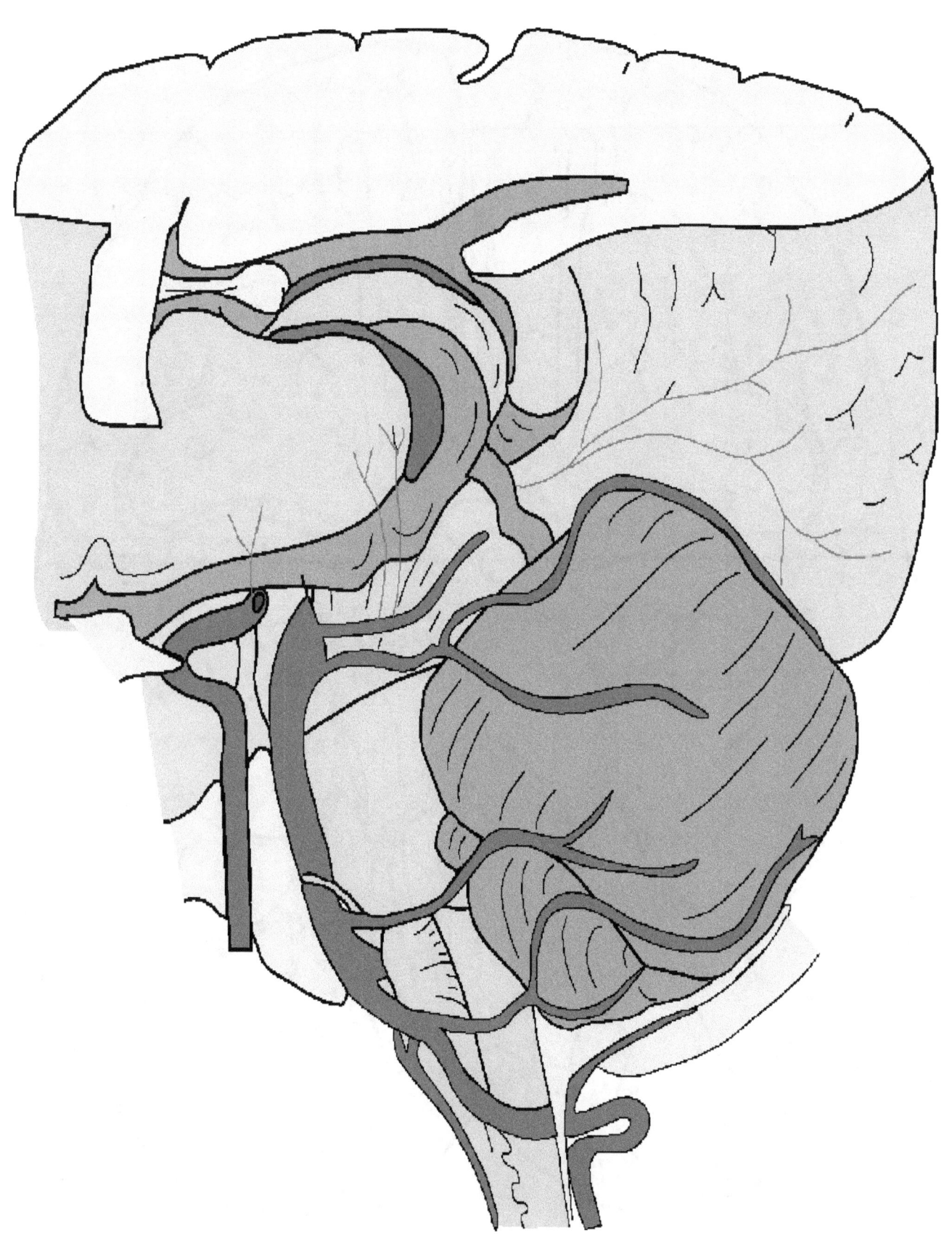

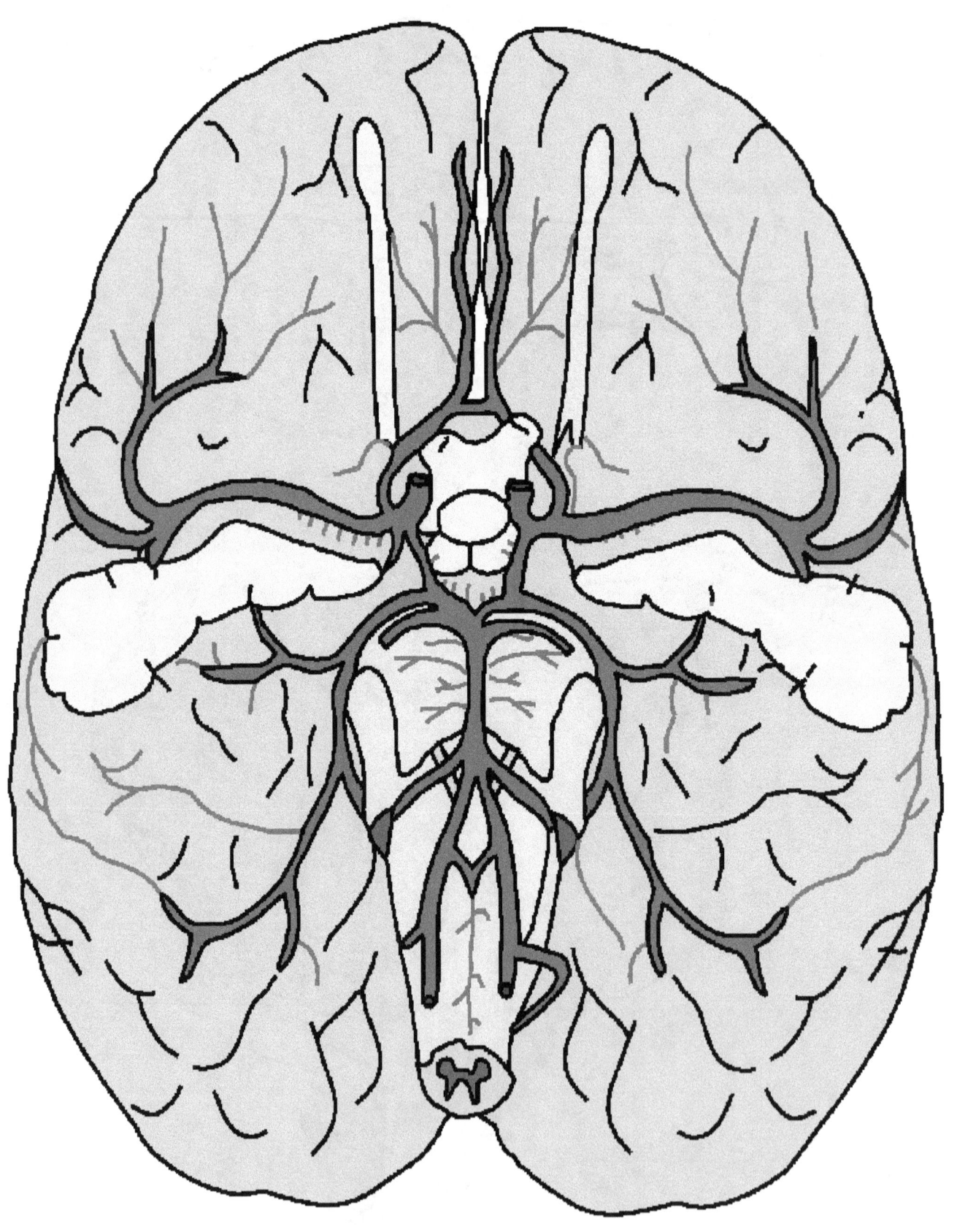

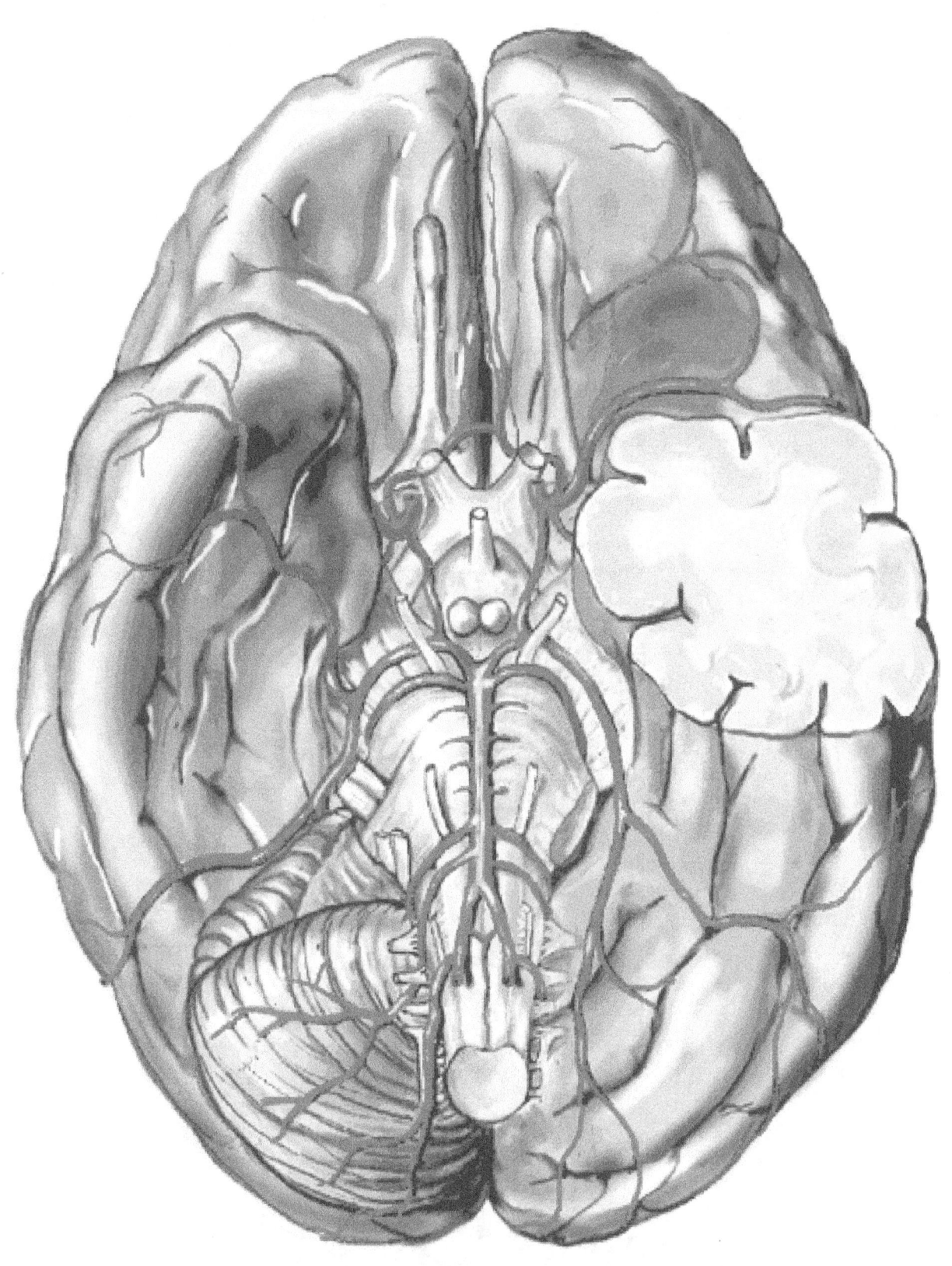

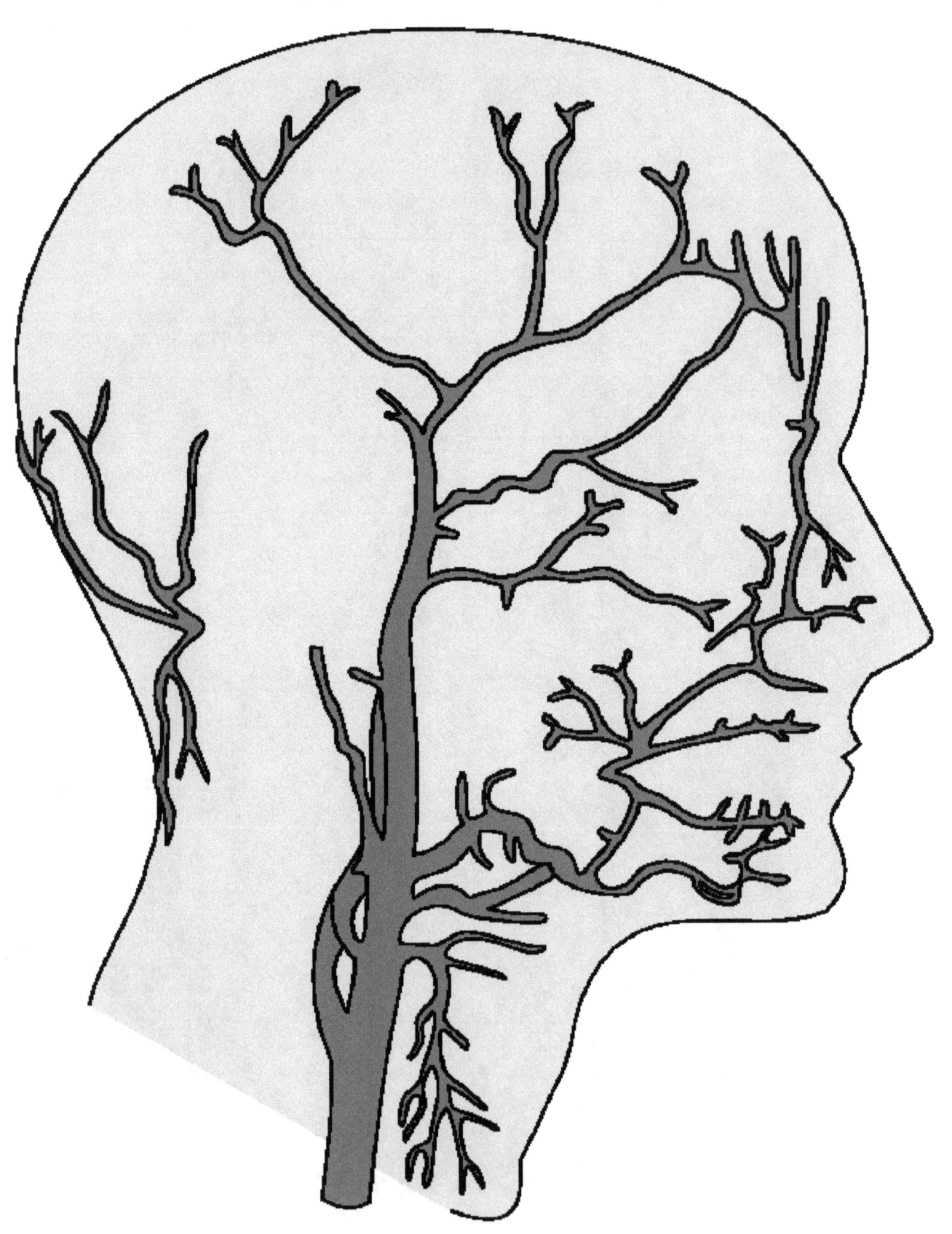

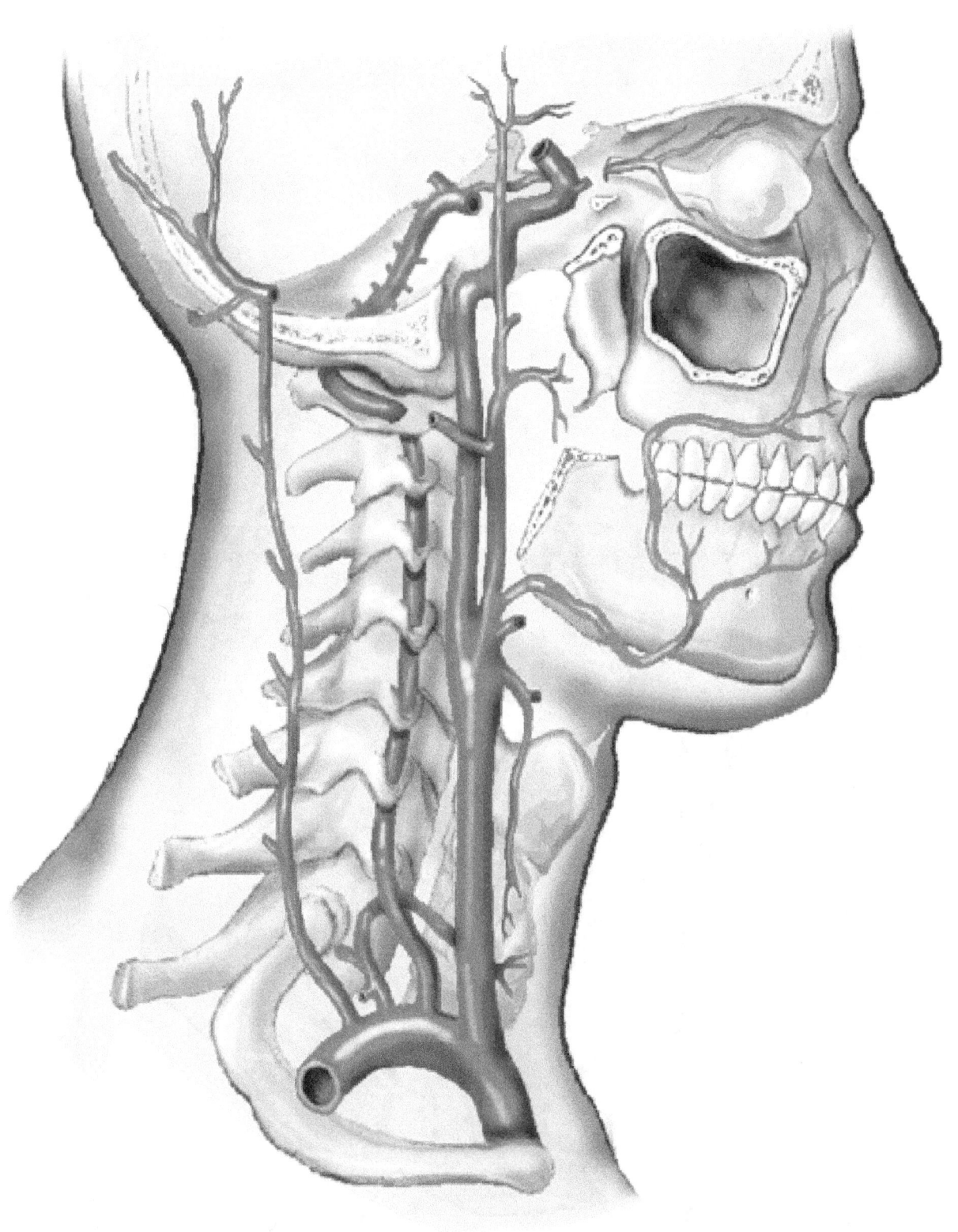

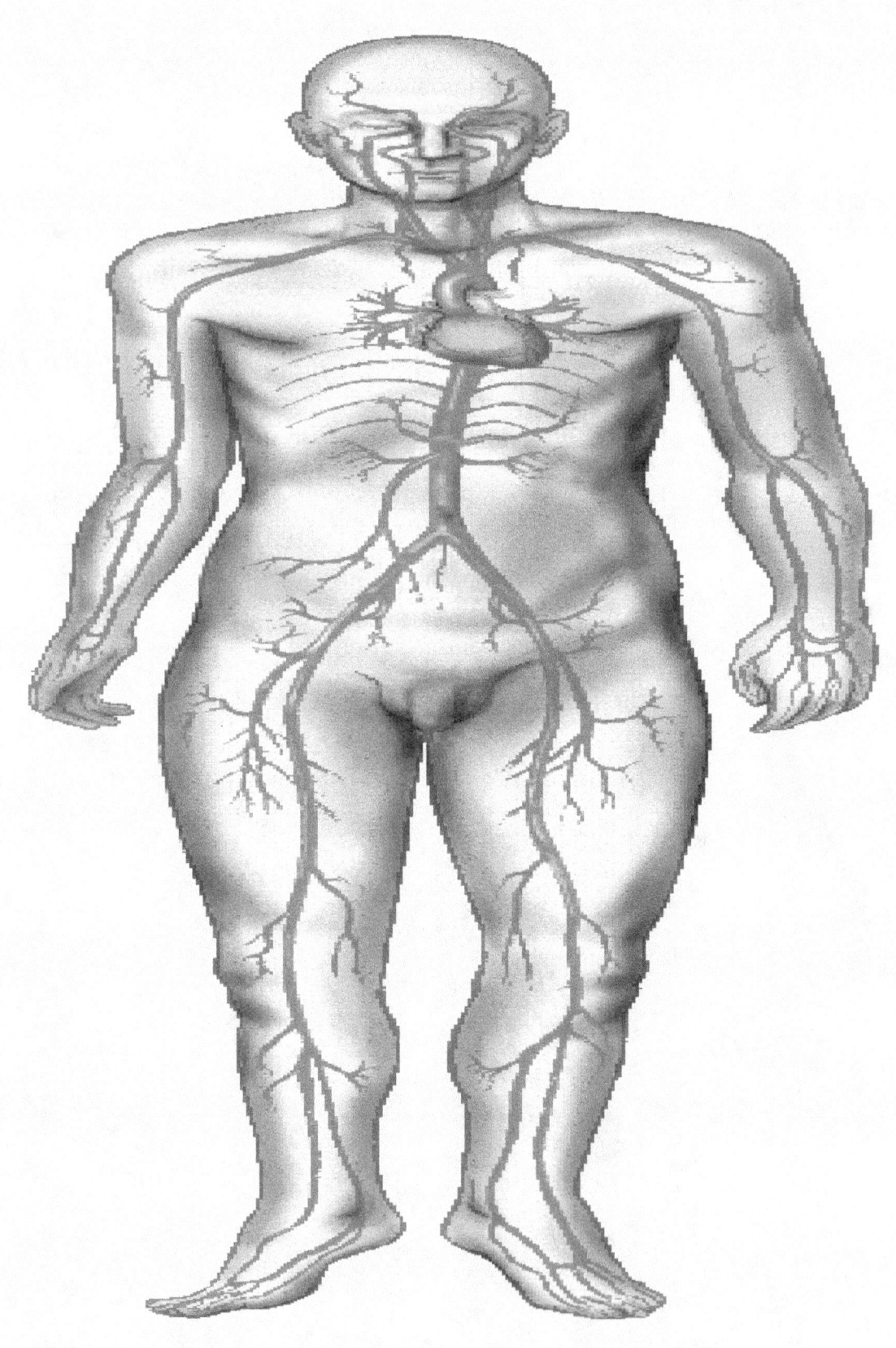

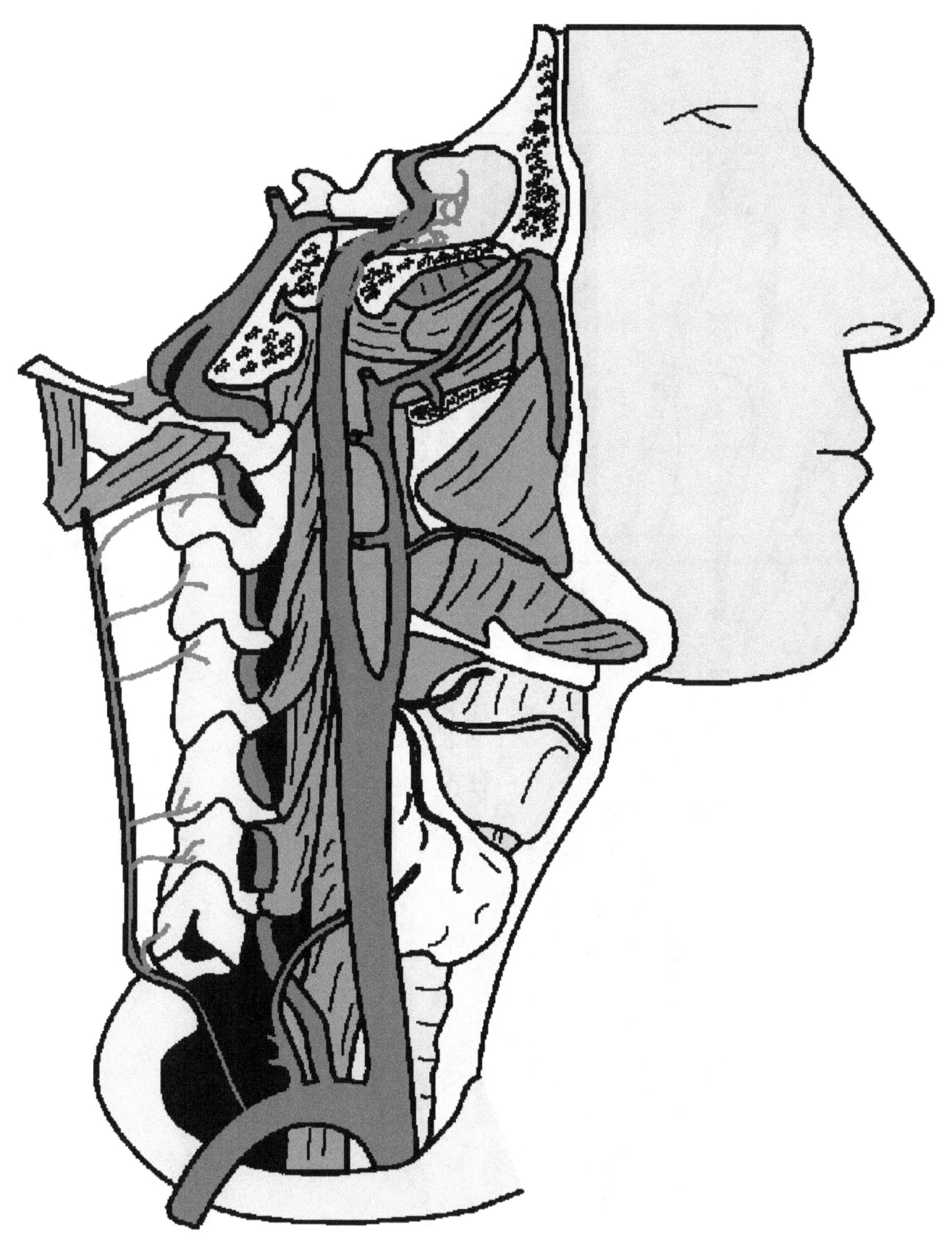

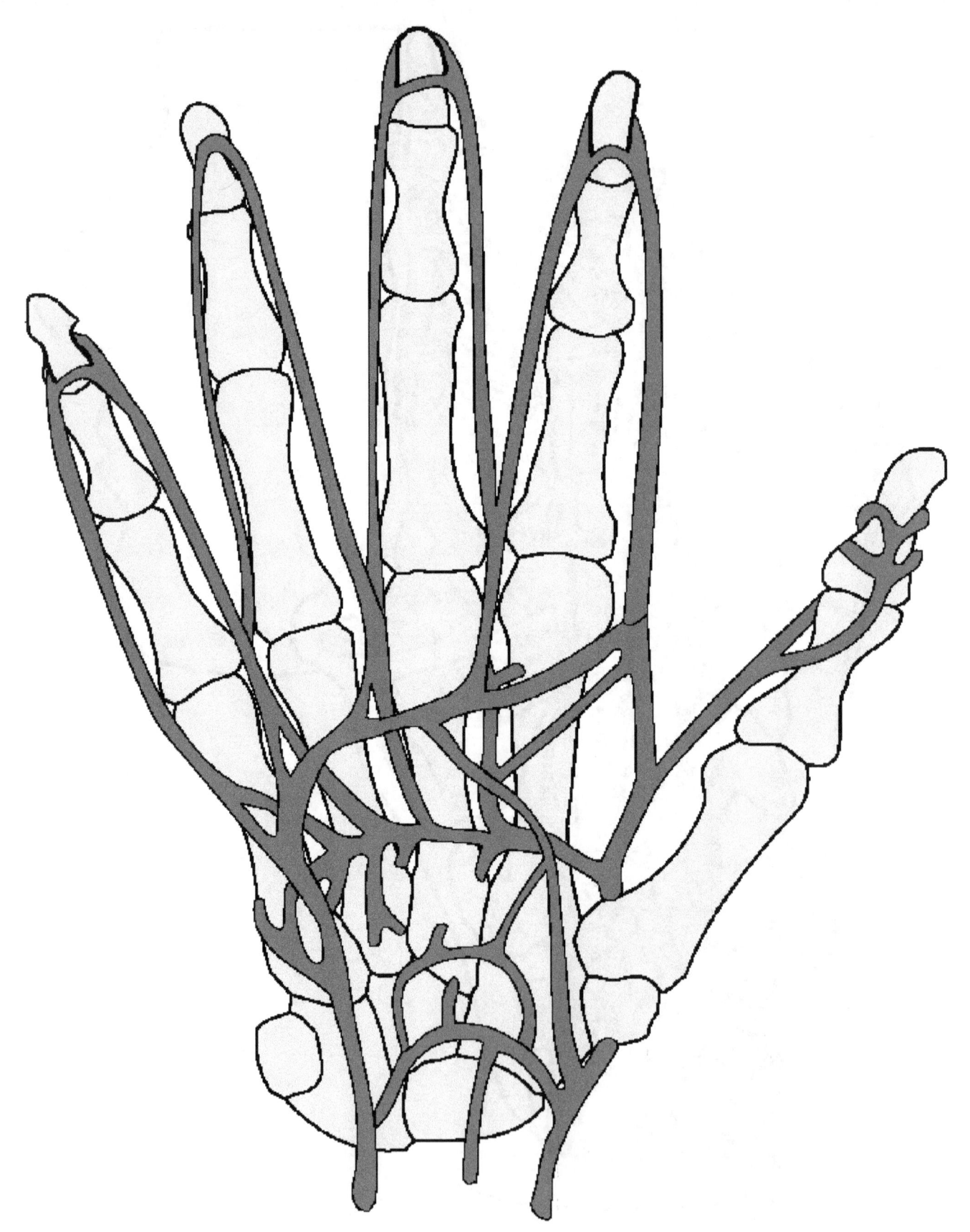

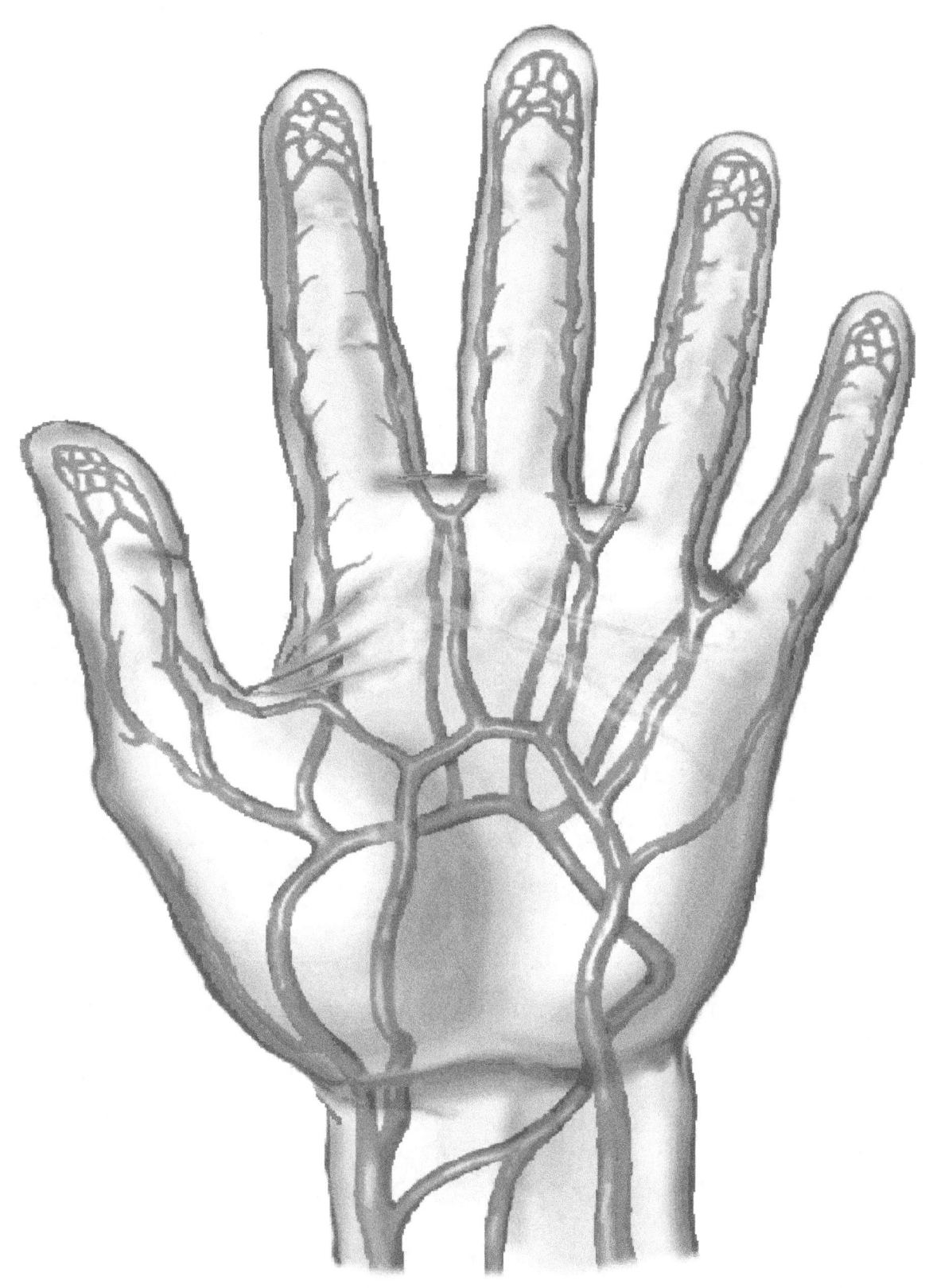

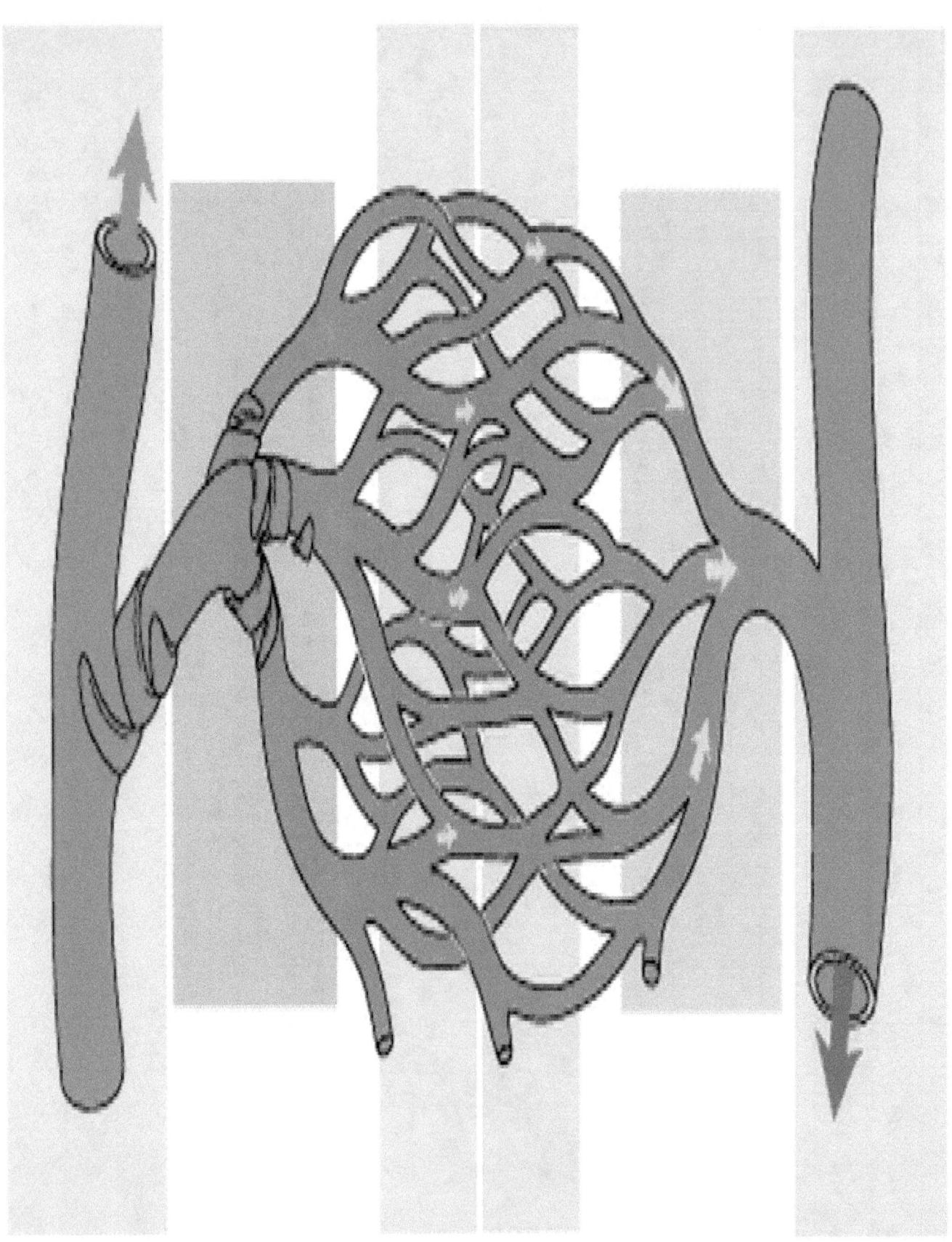

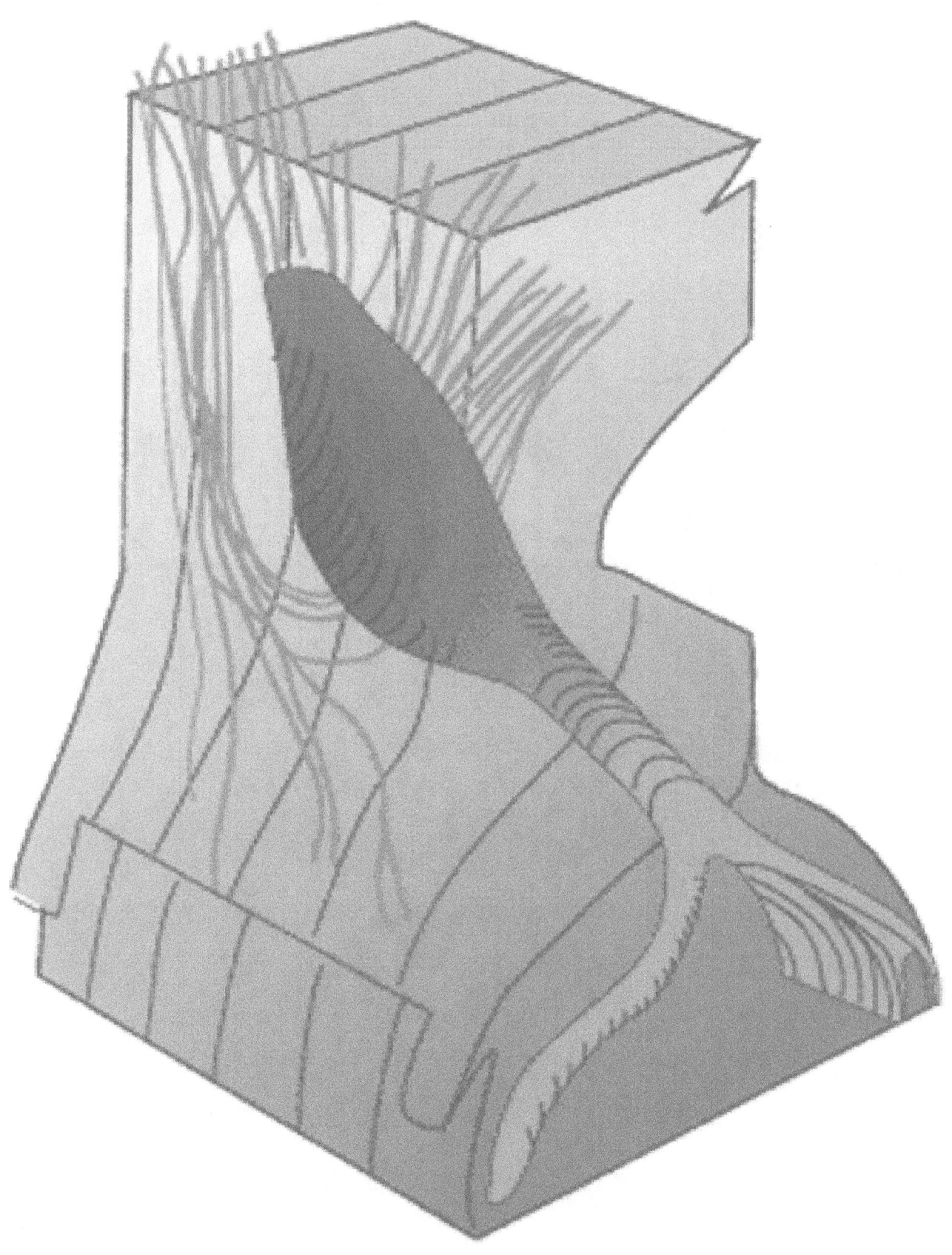

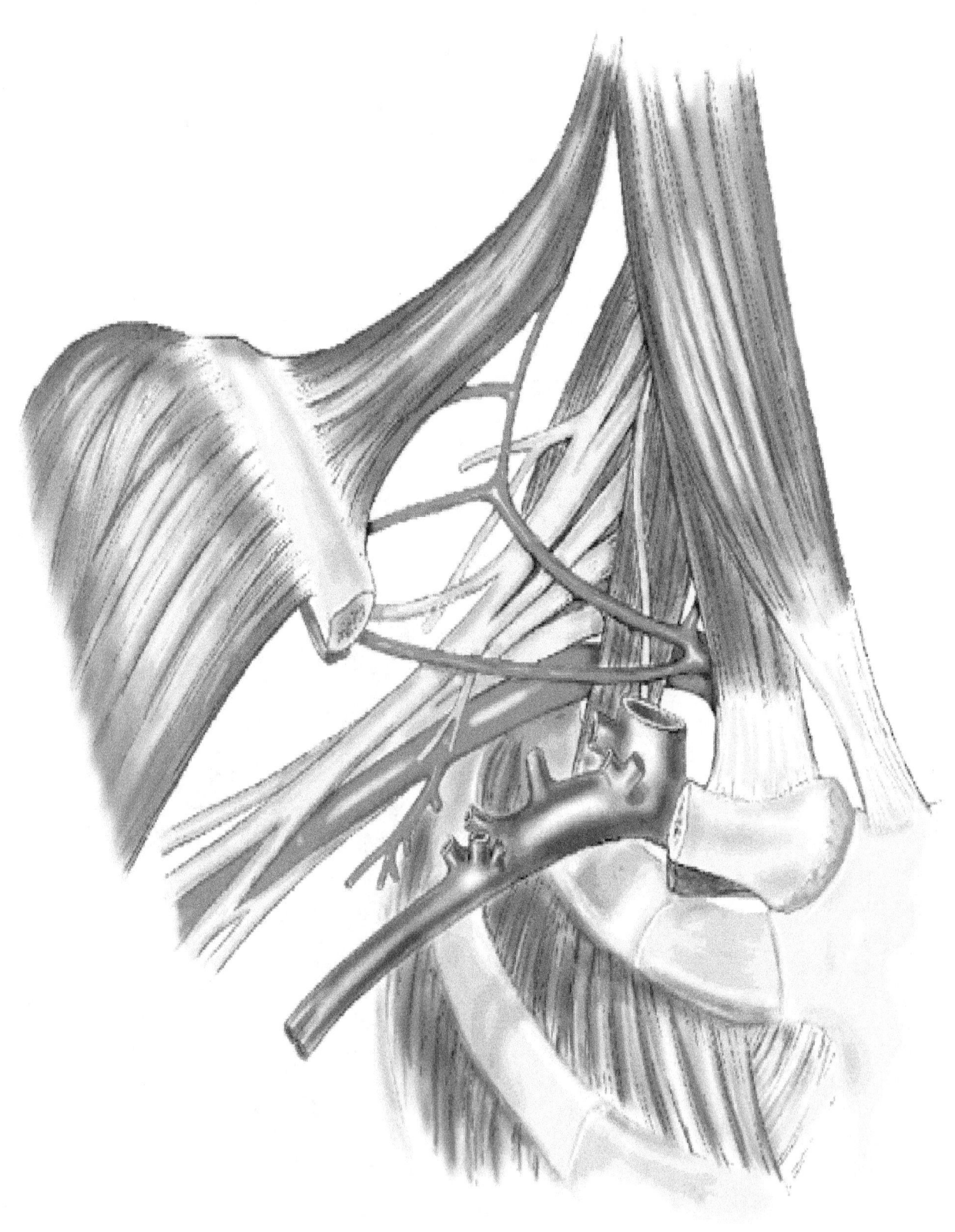

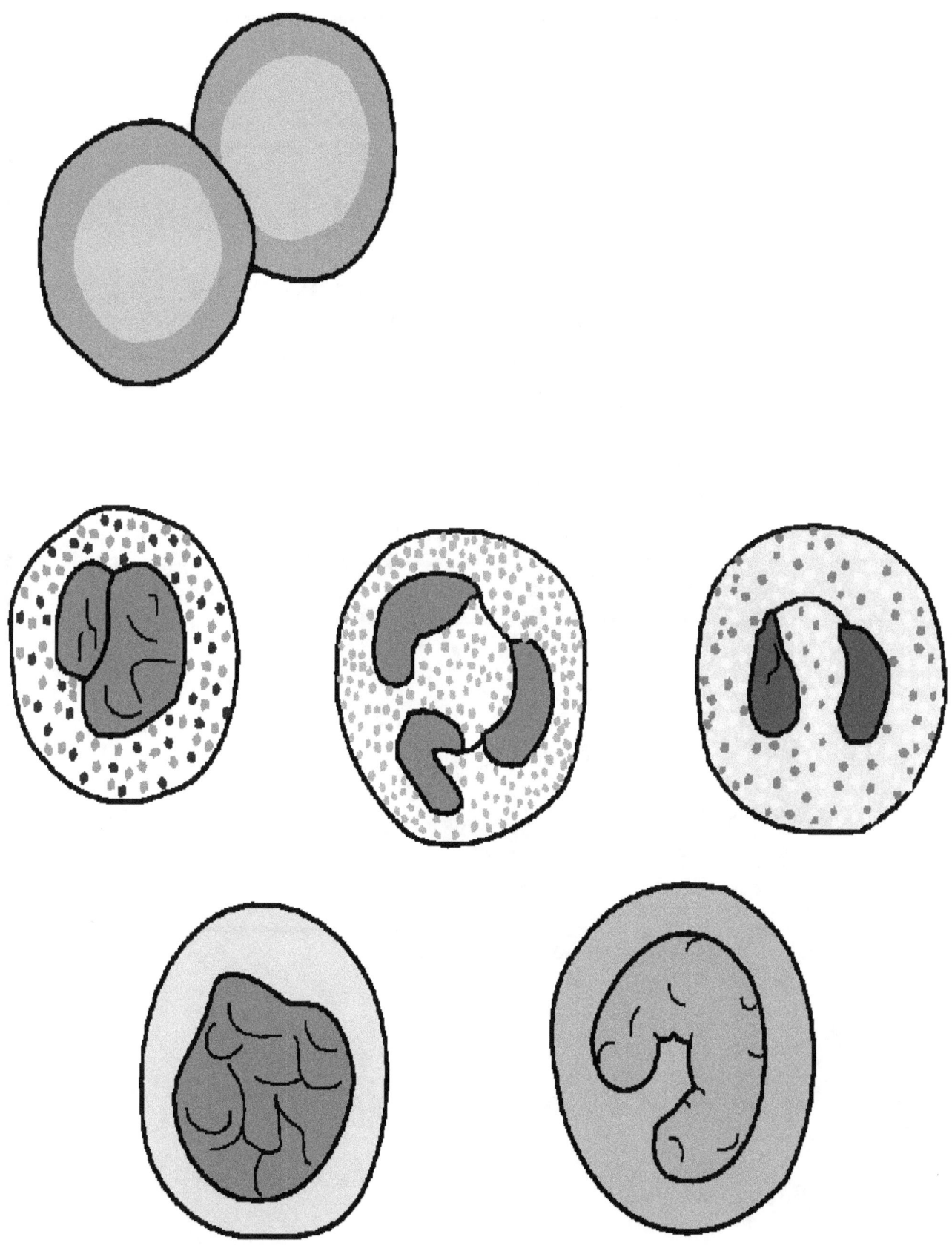

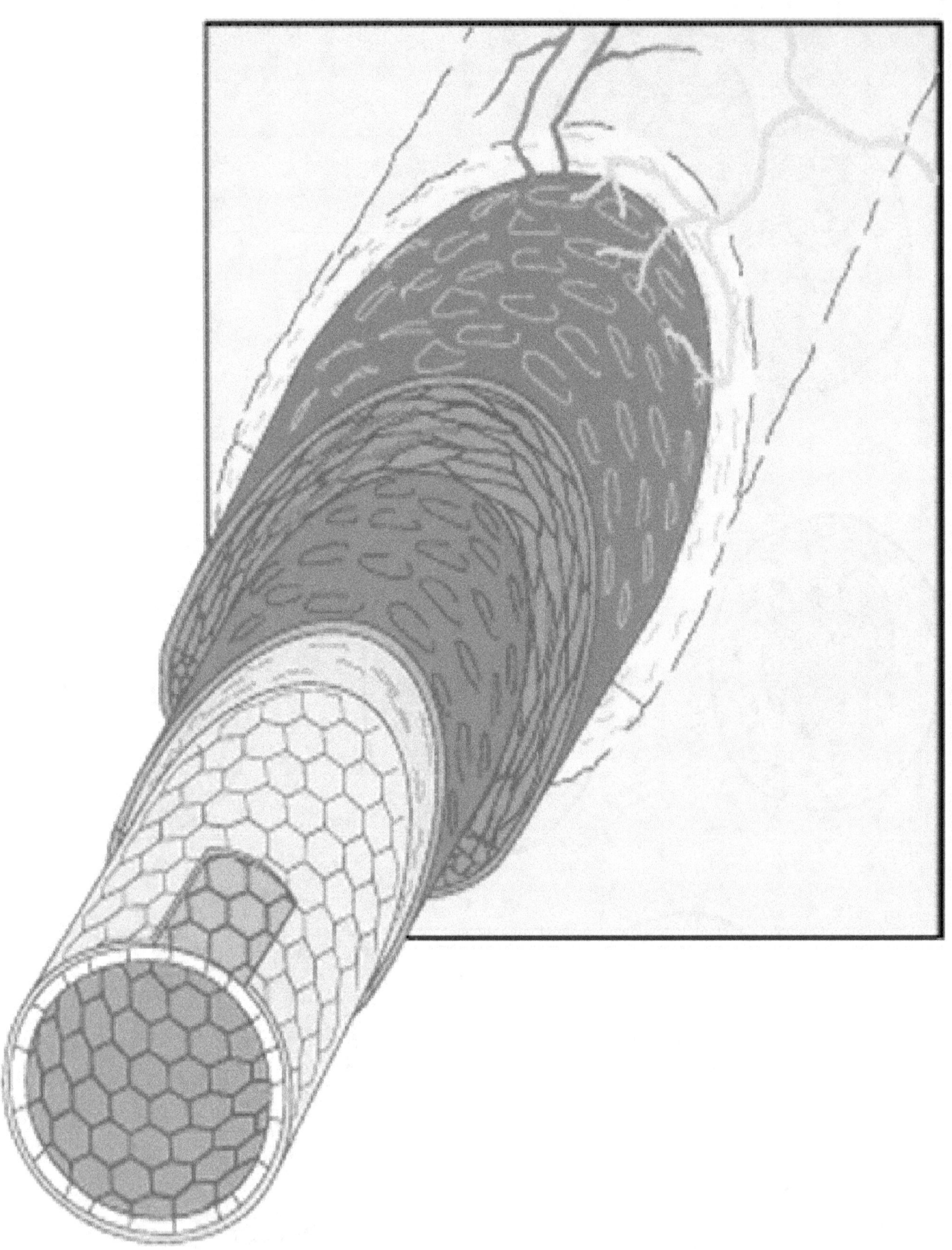

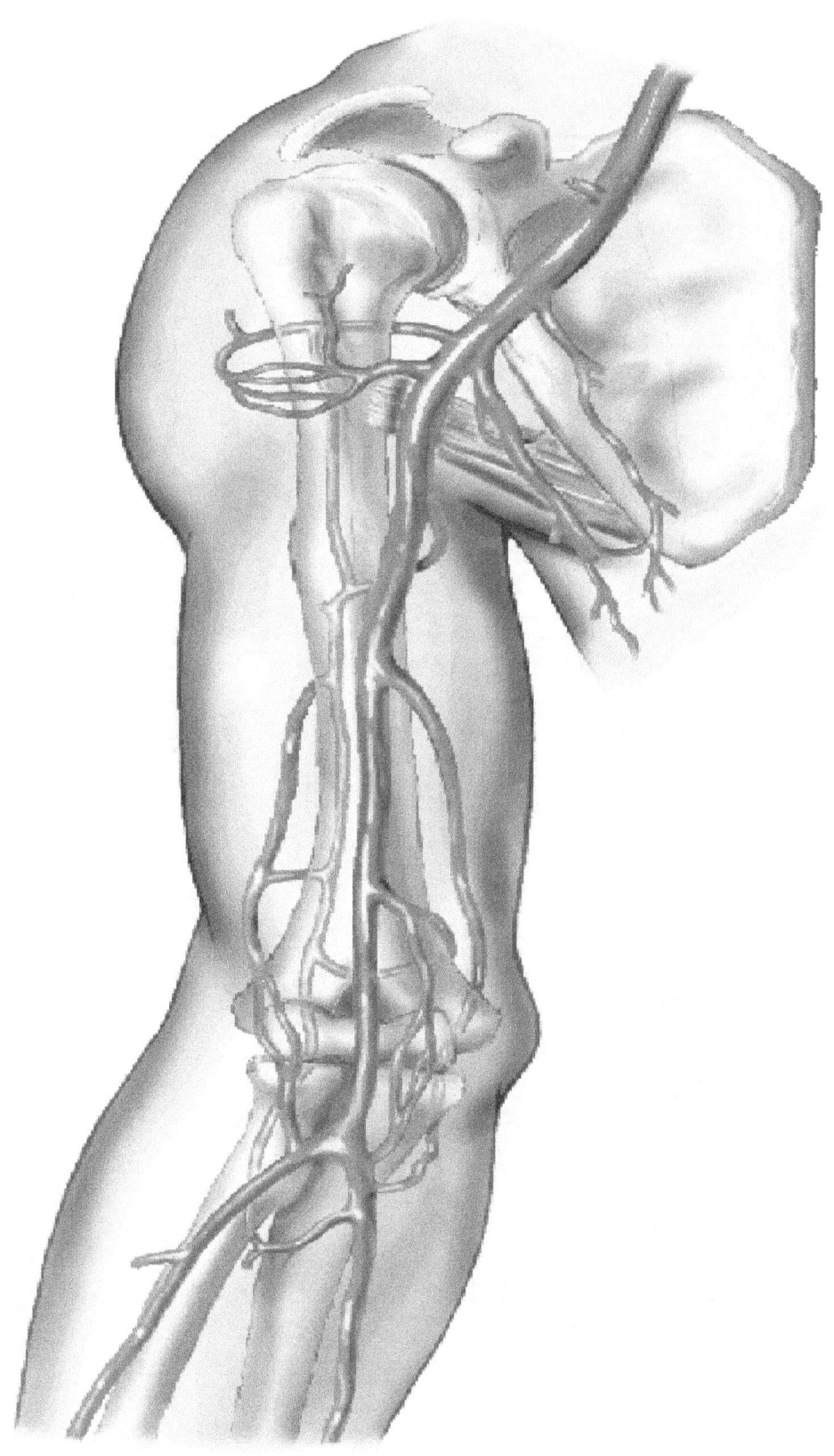

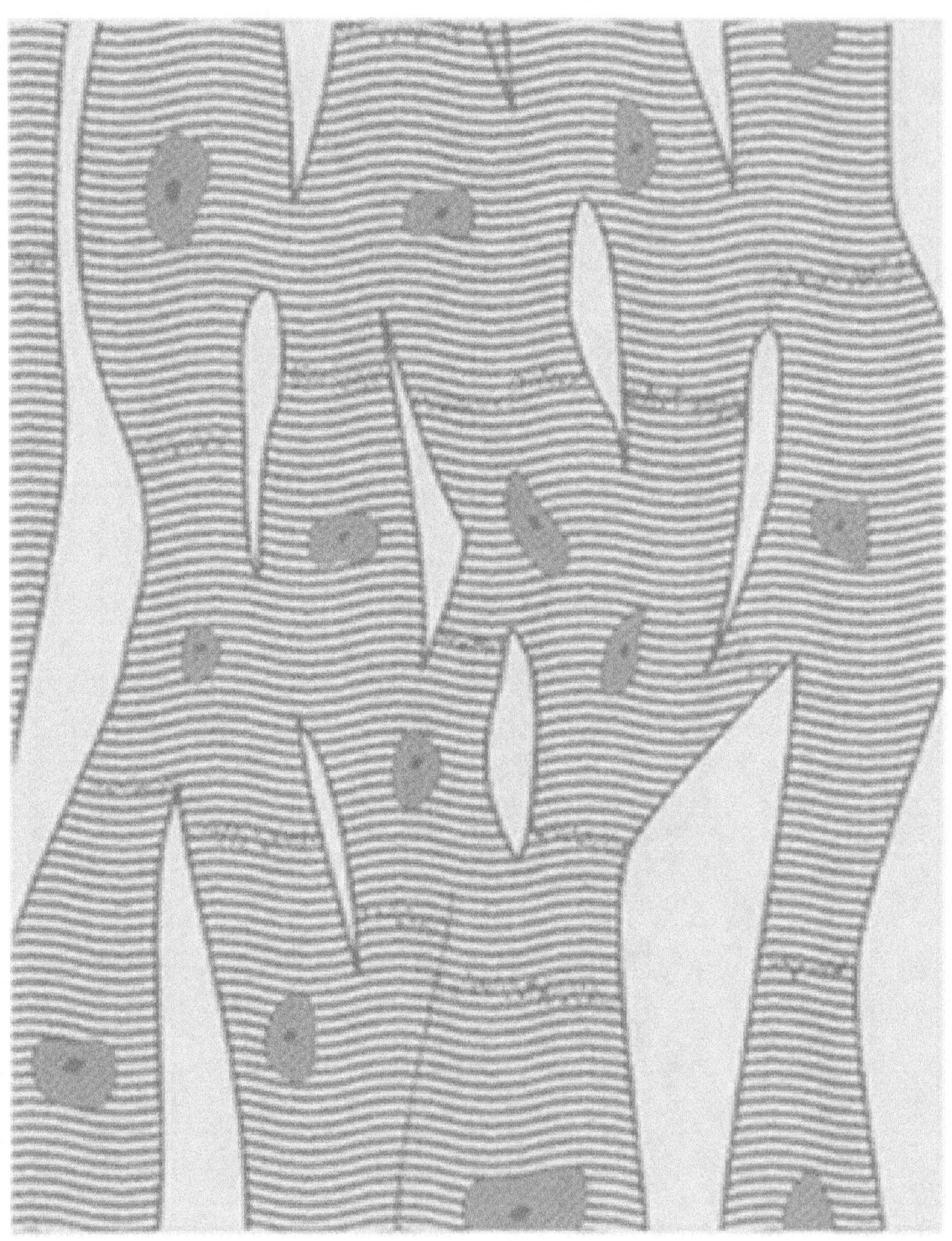

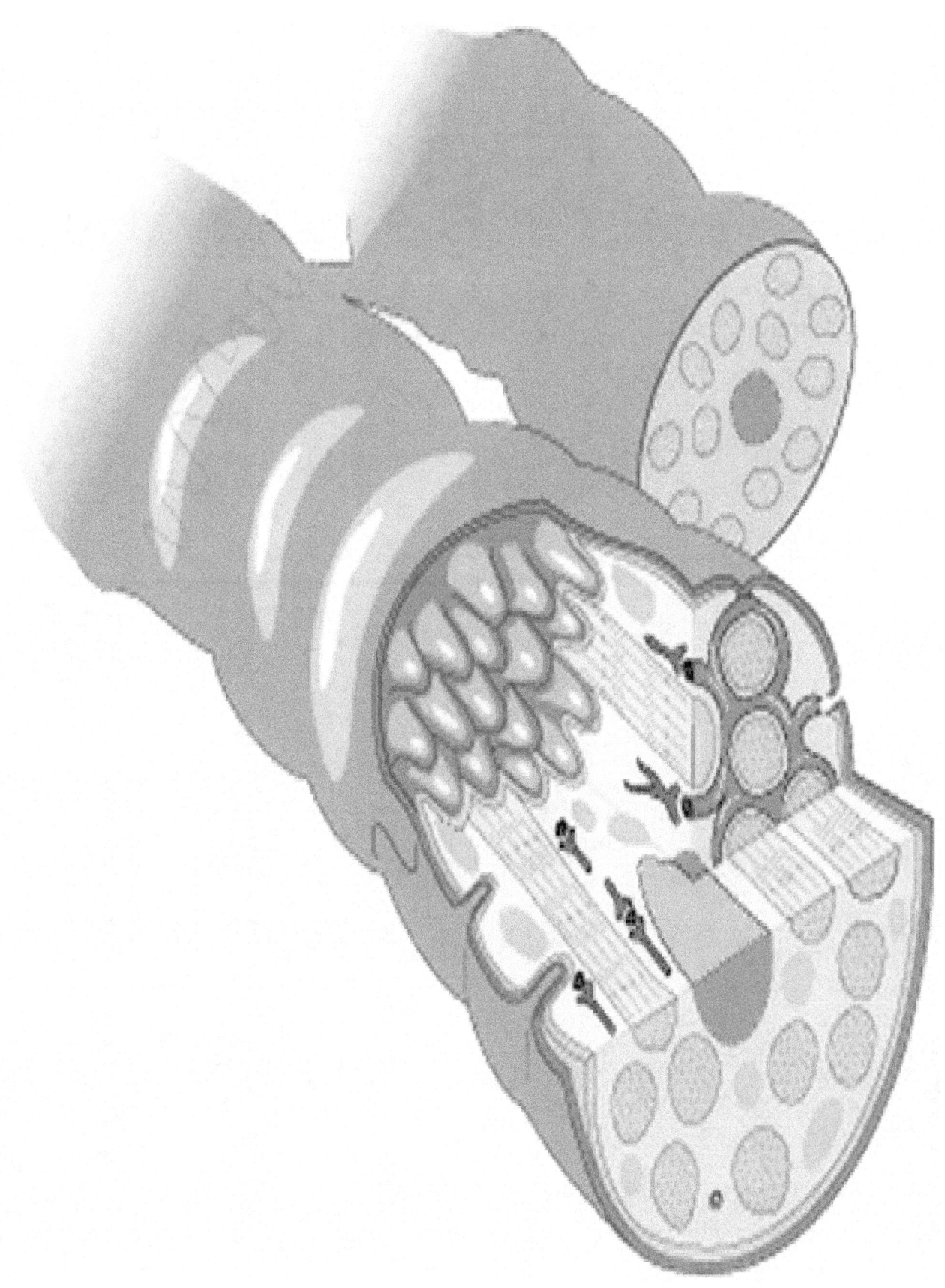

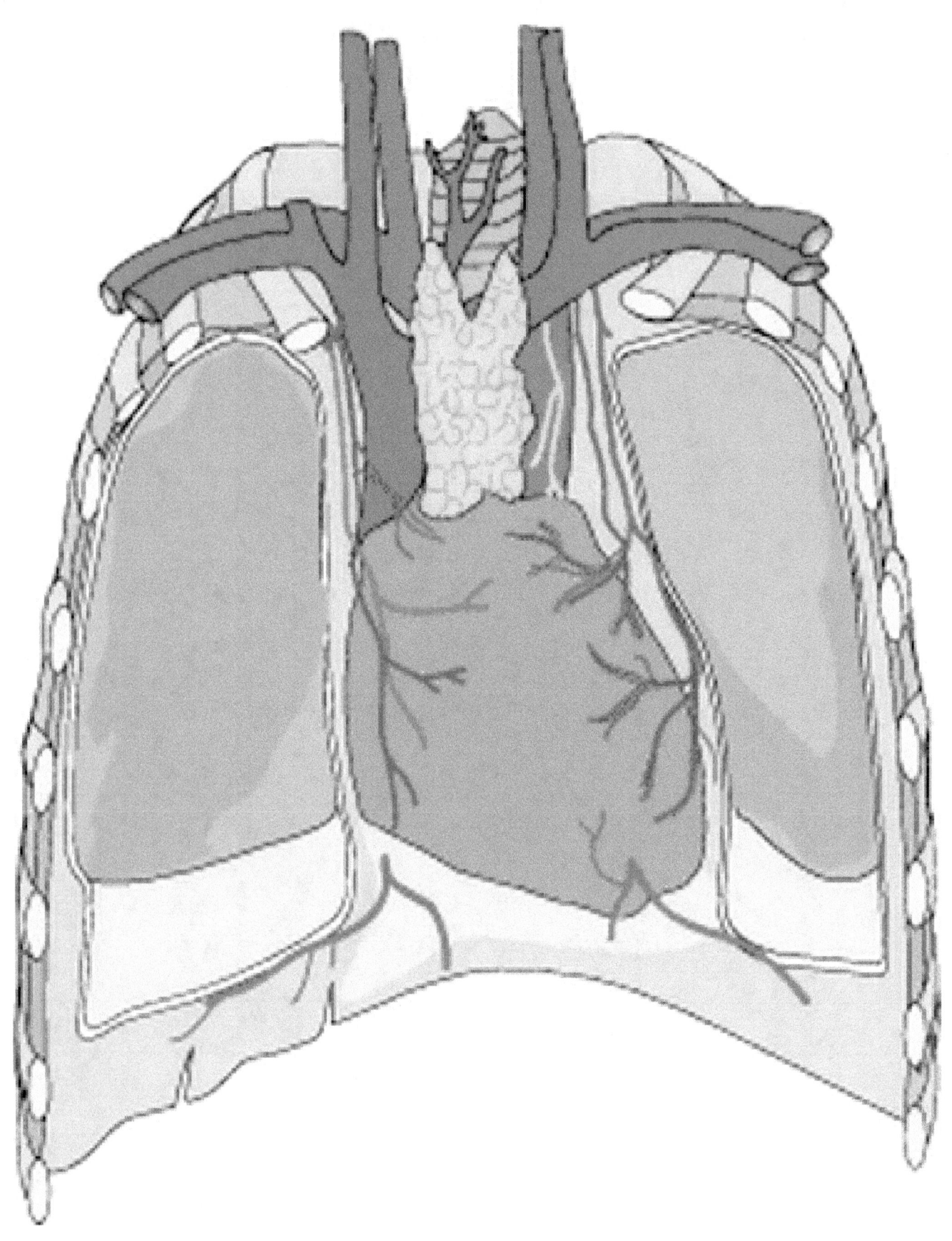

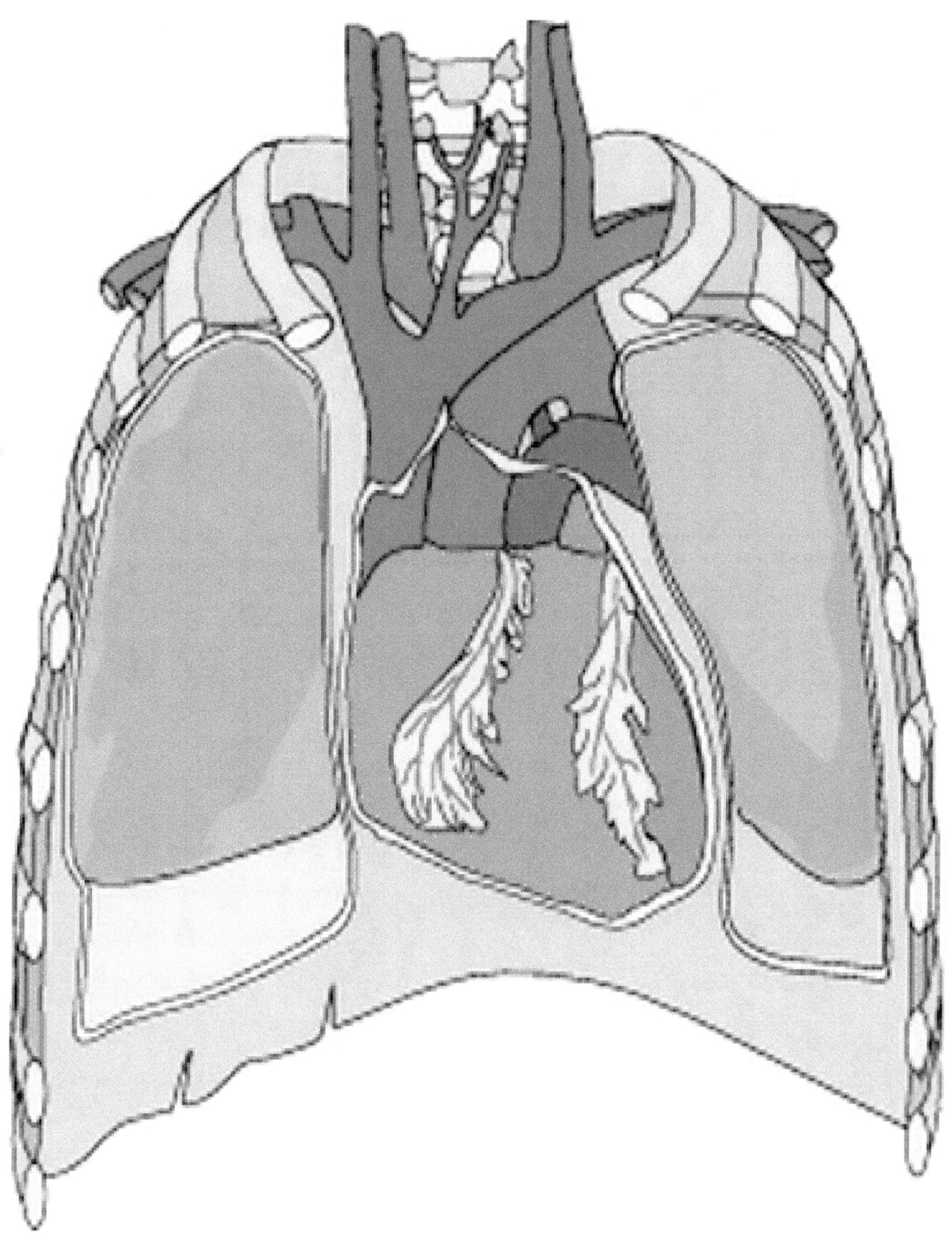

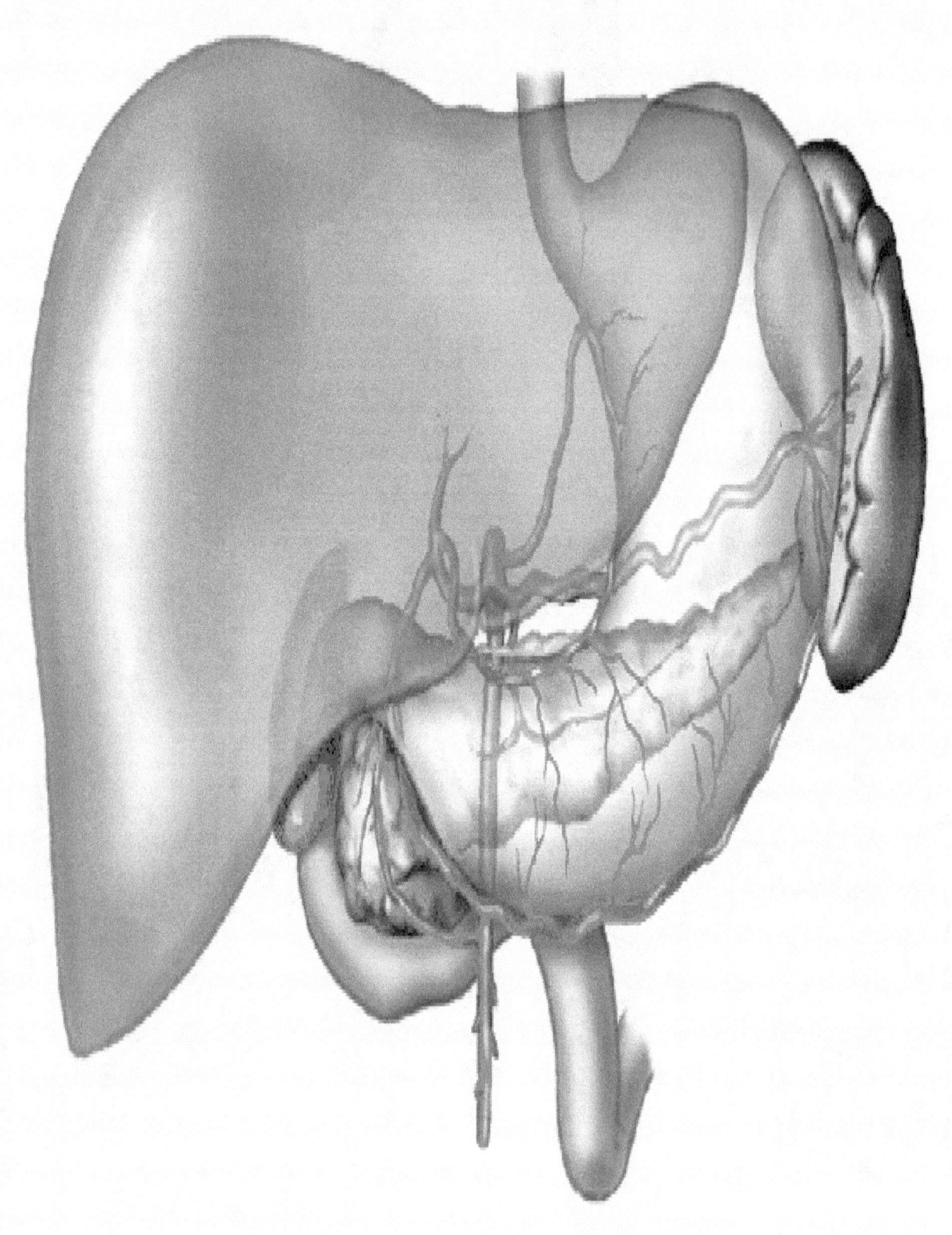

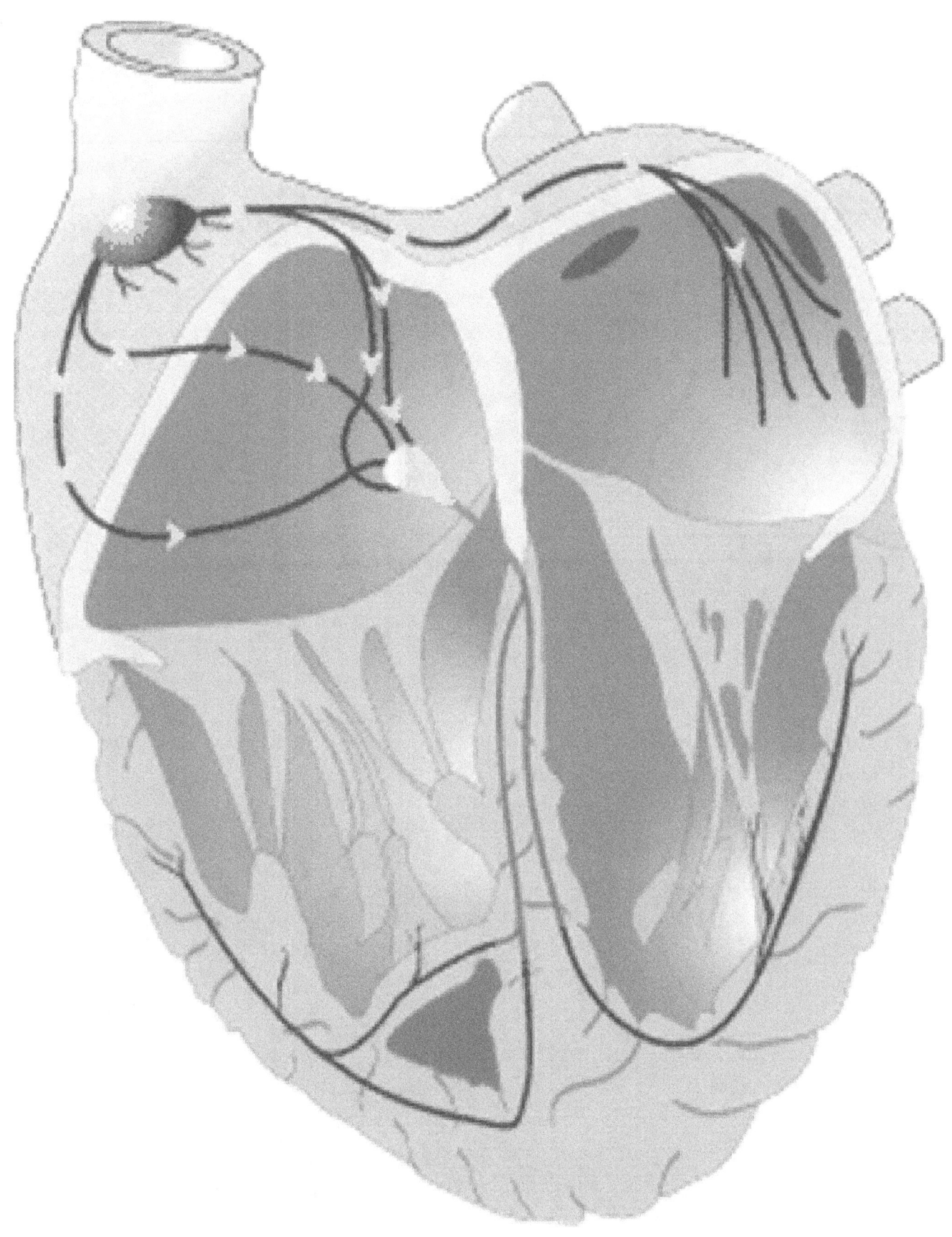

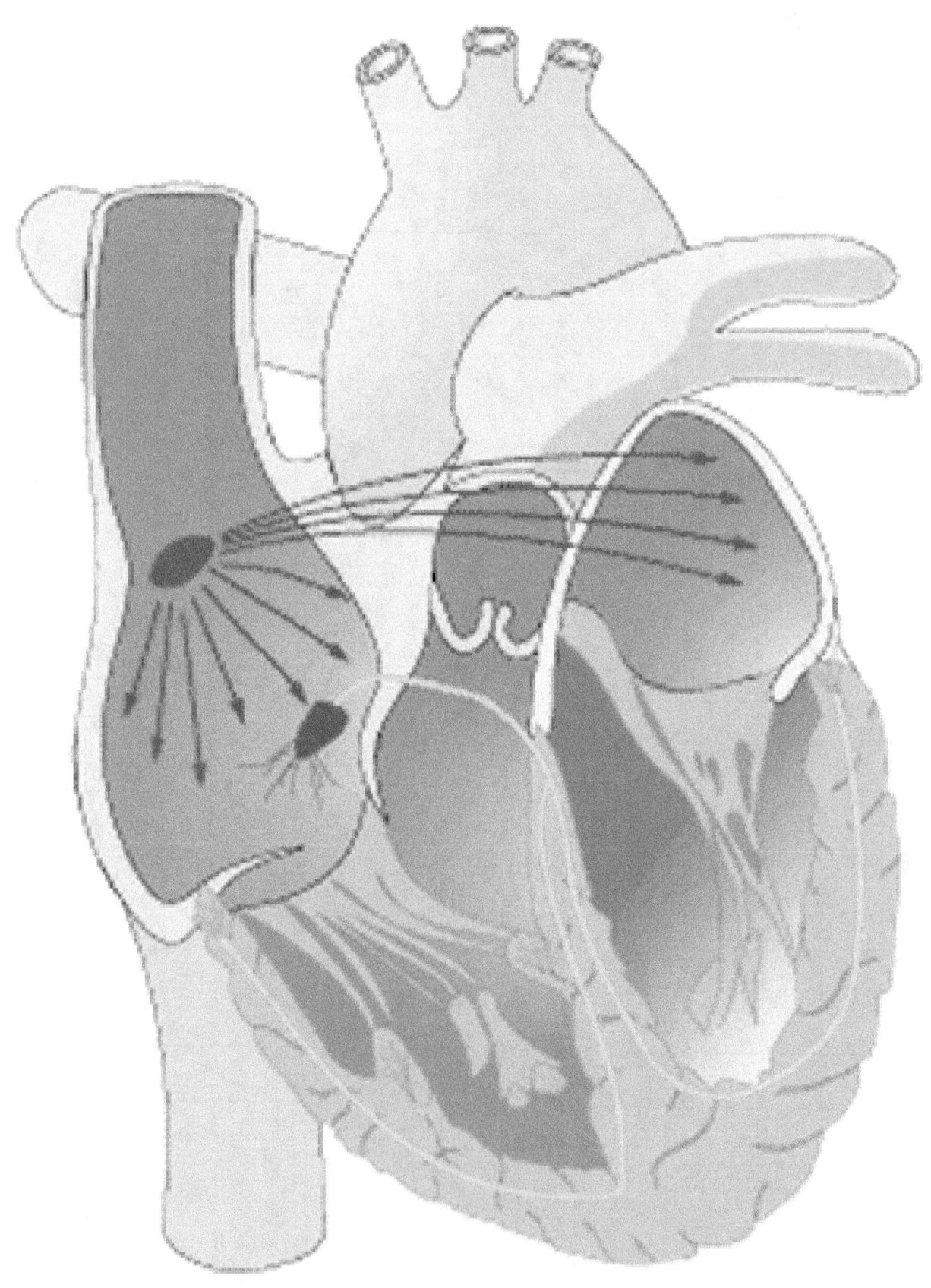

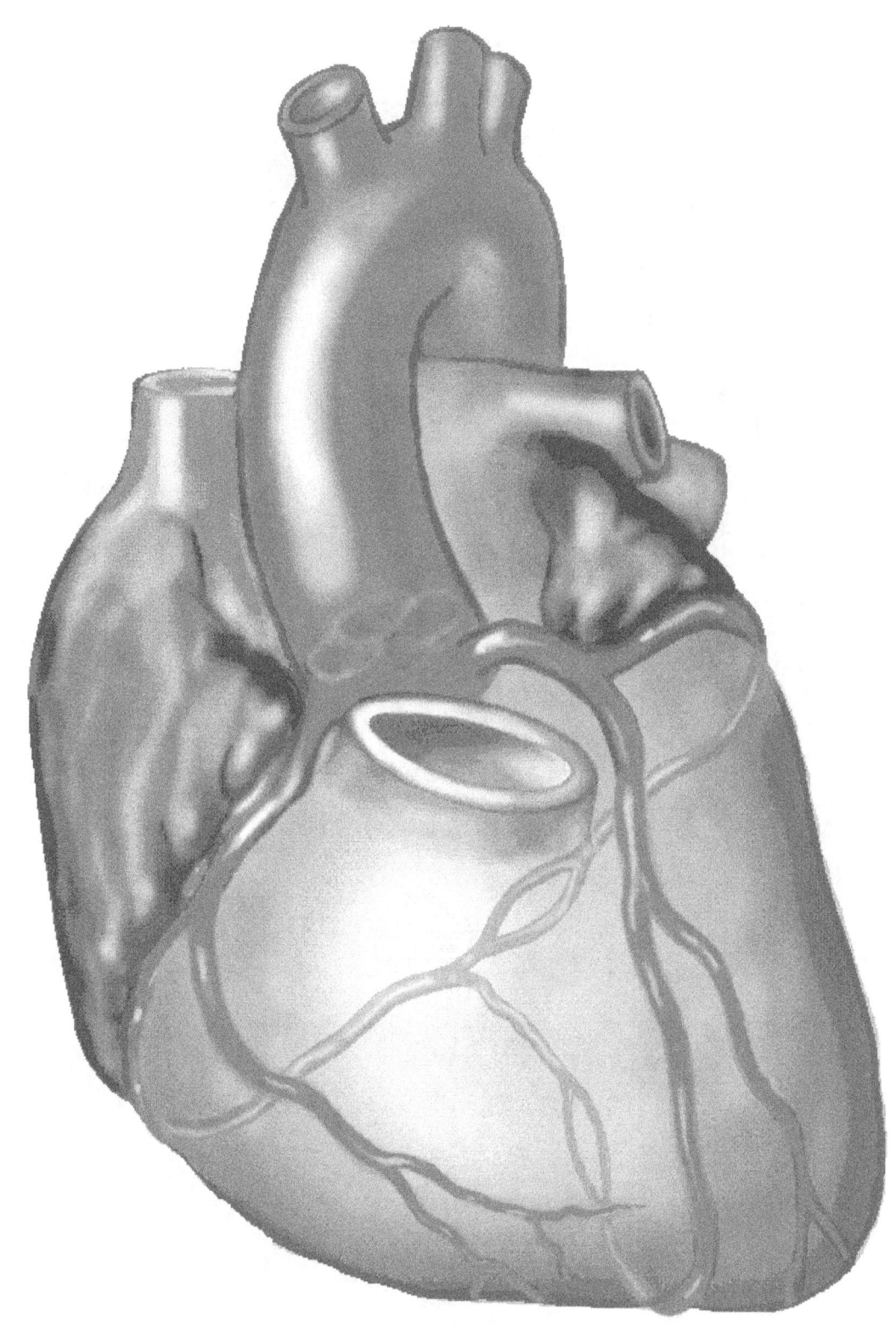

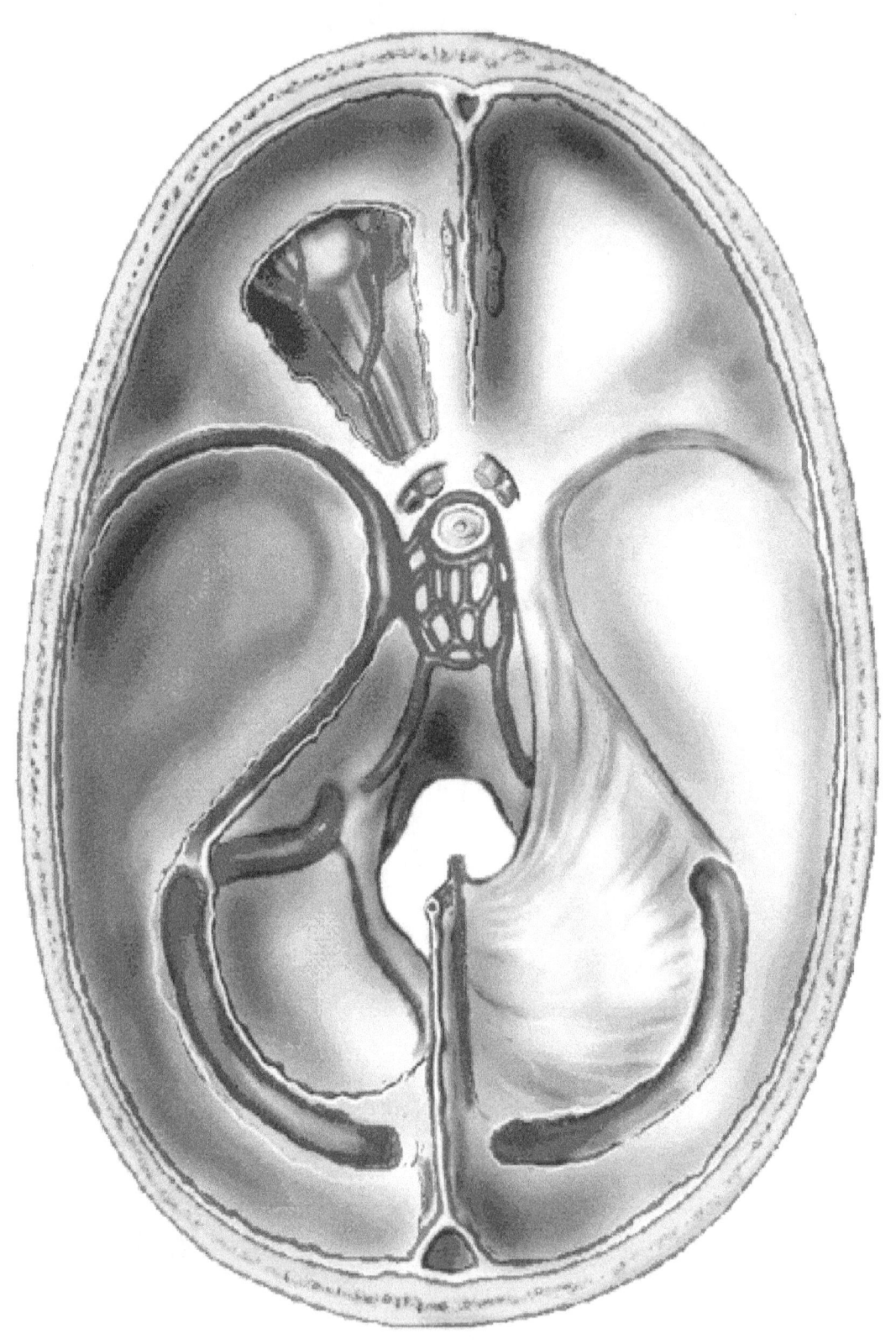

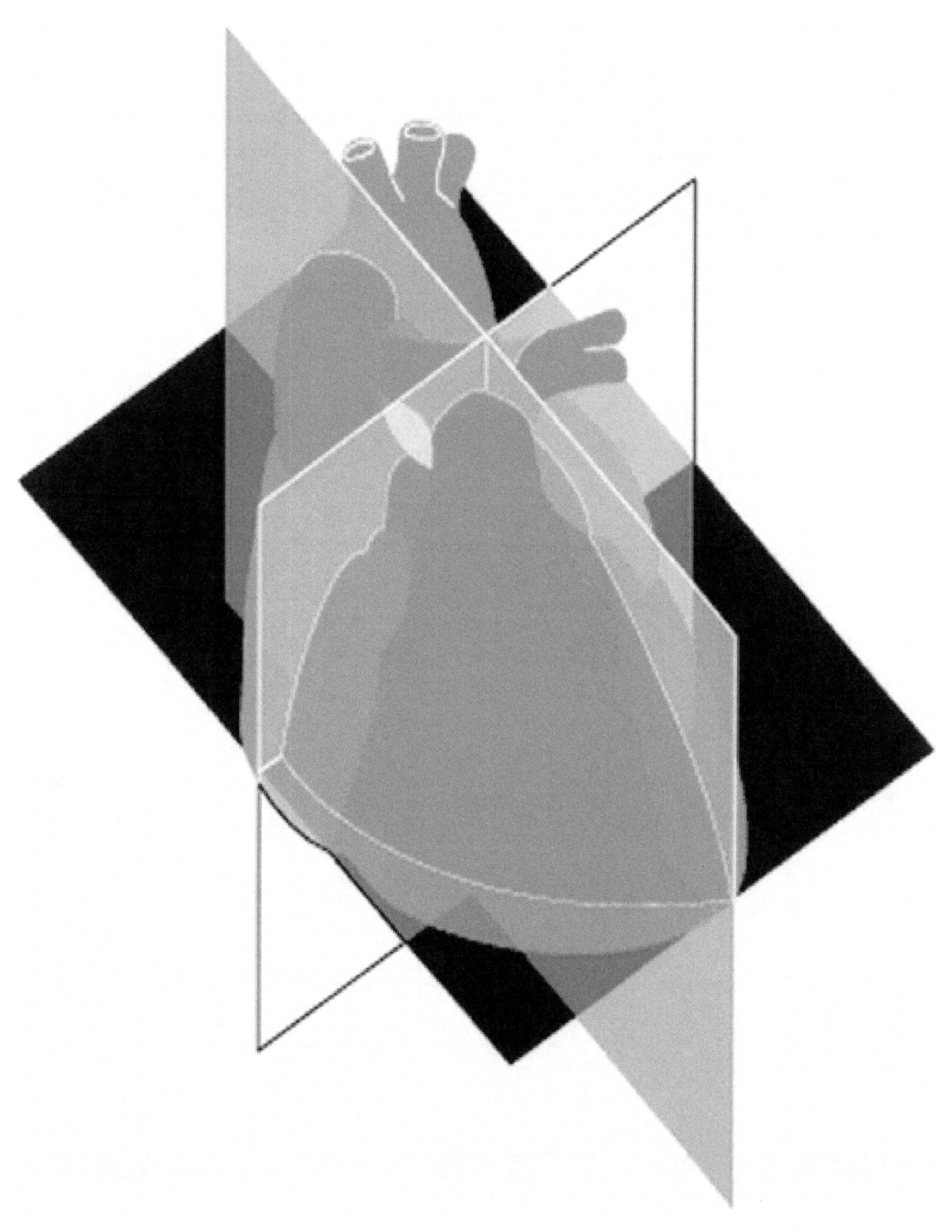

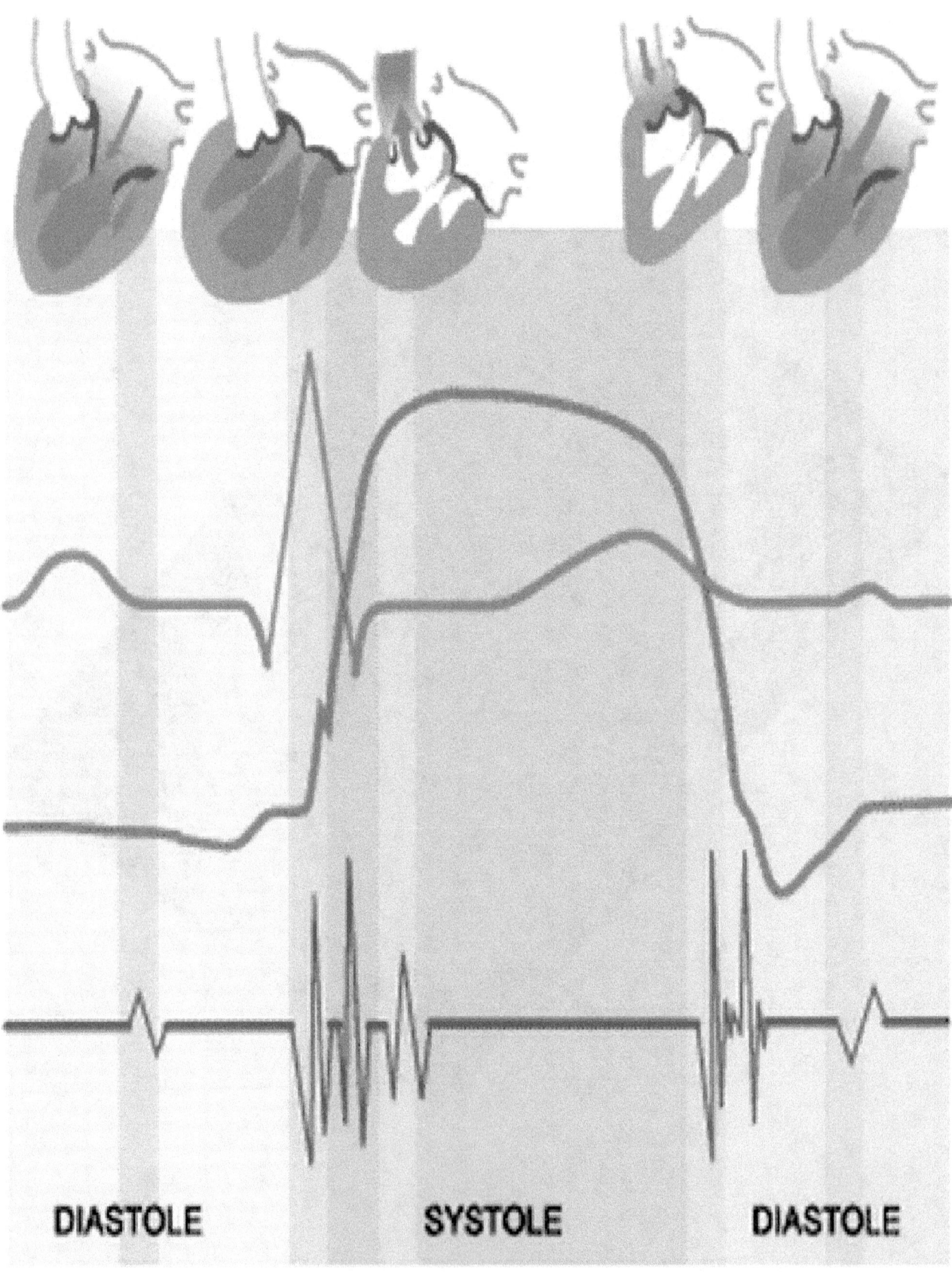

DIASTOLE   SYSTOLE   DIASTOLE

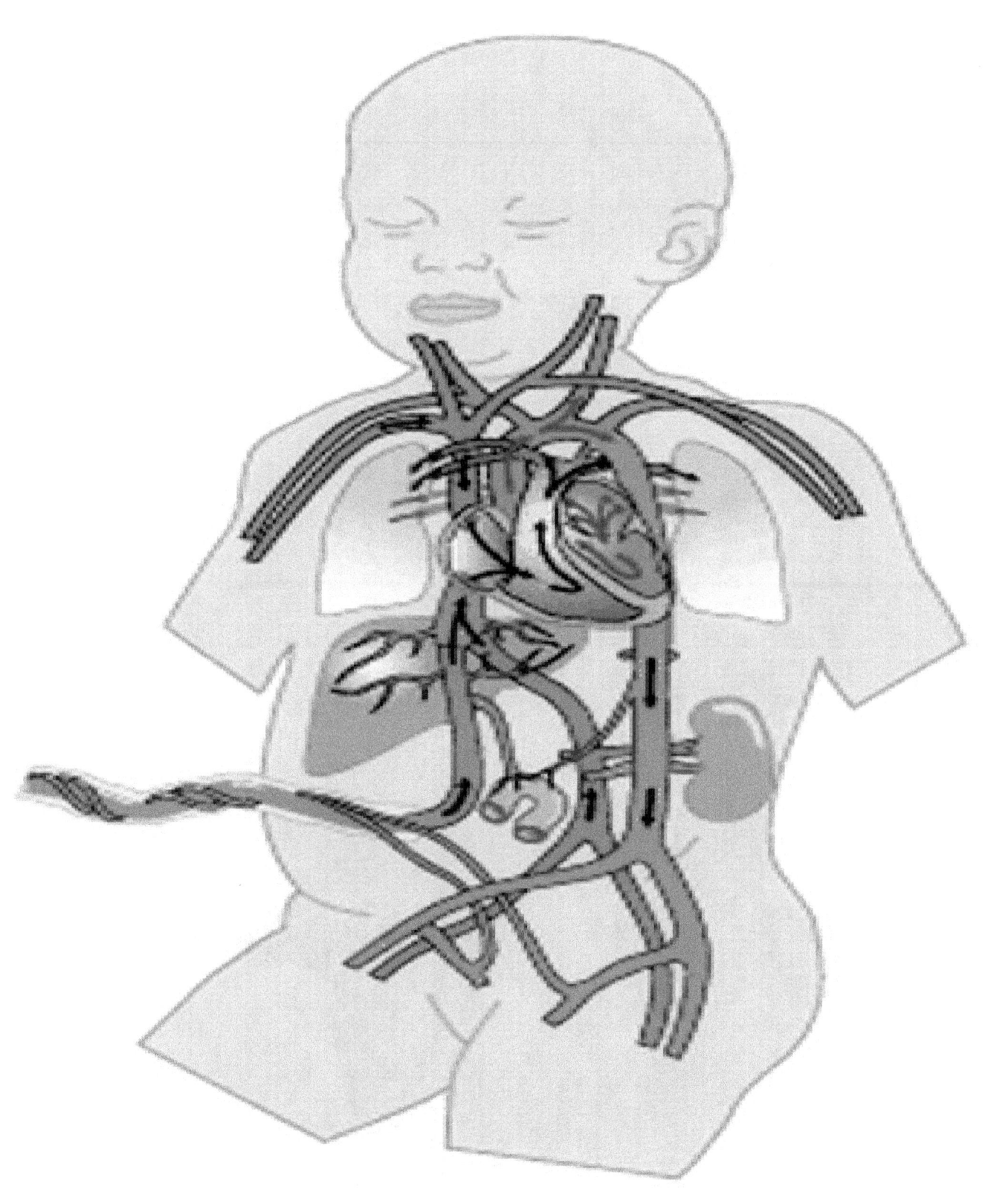

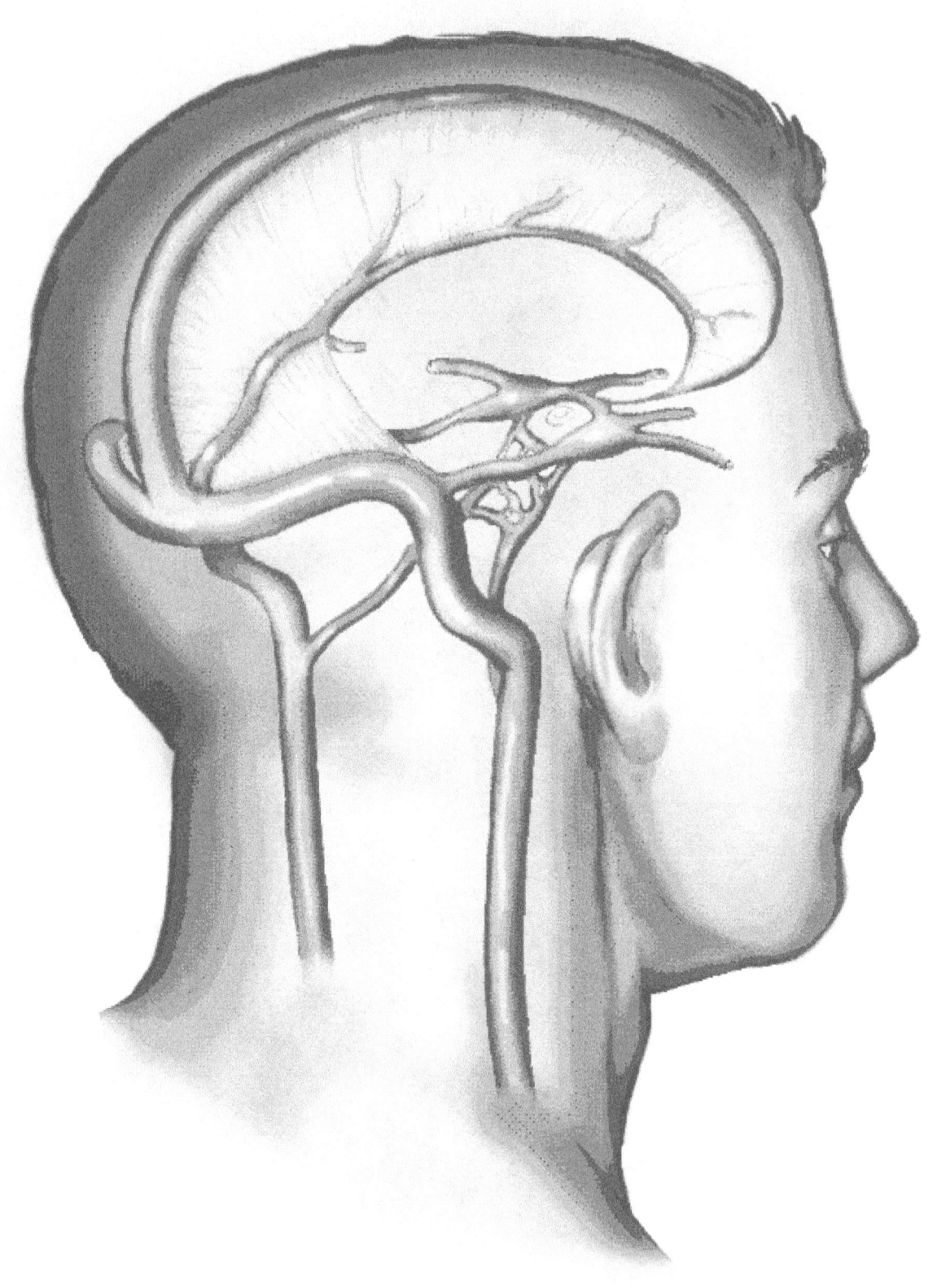

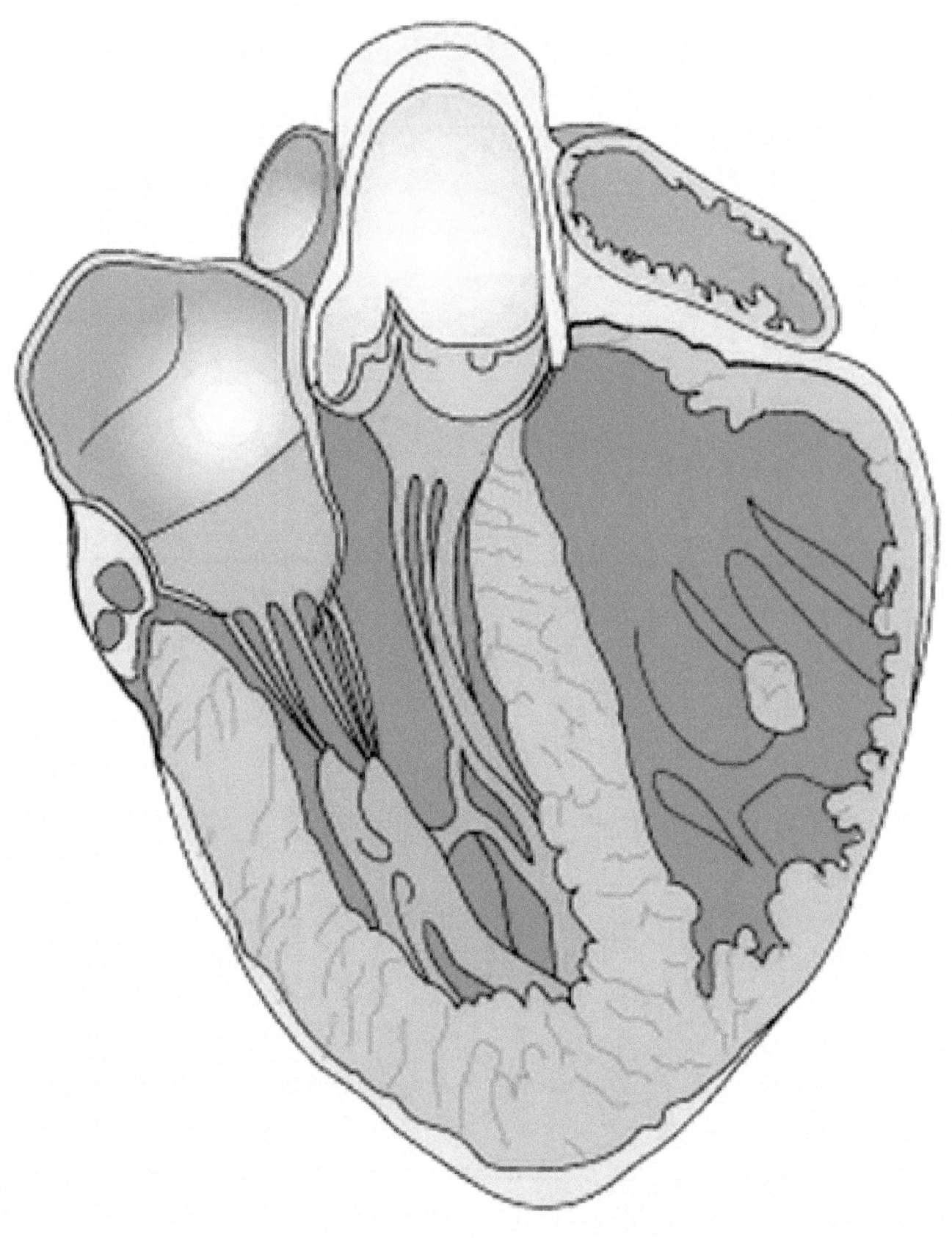

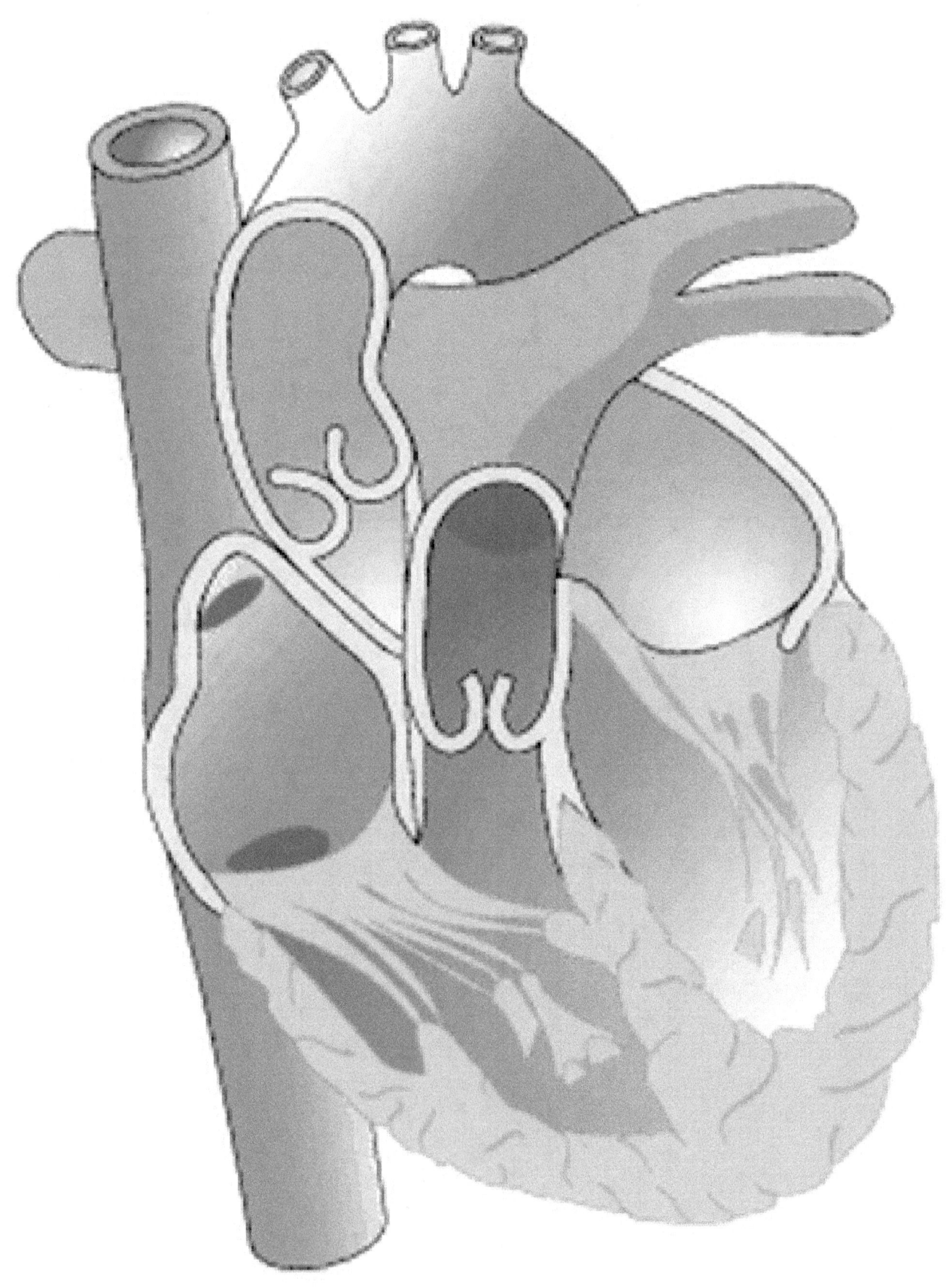

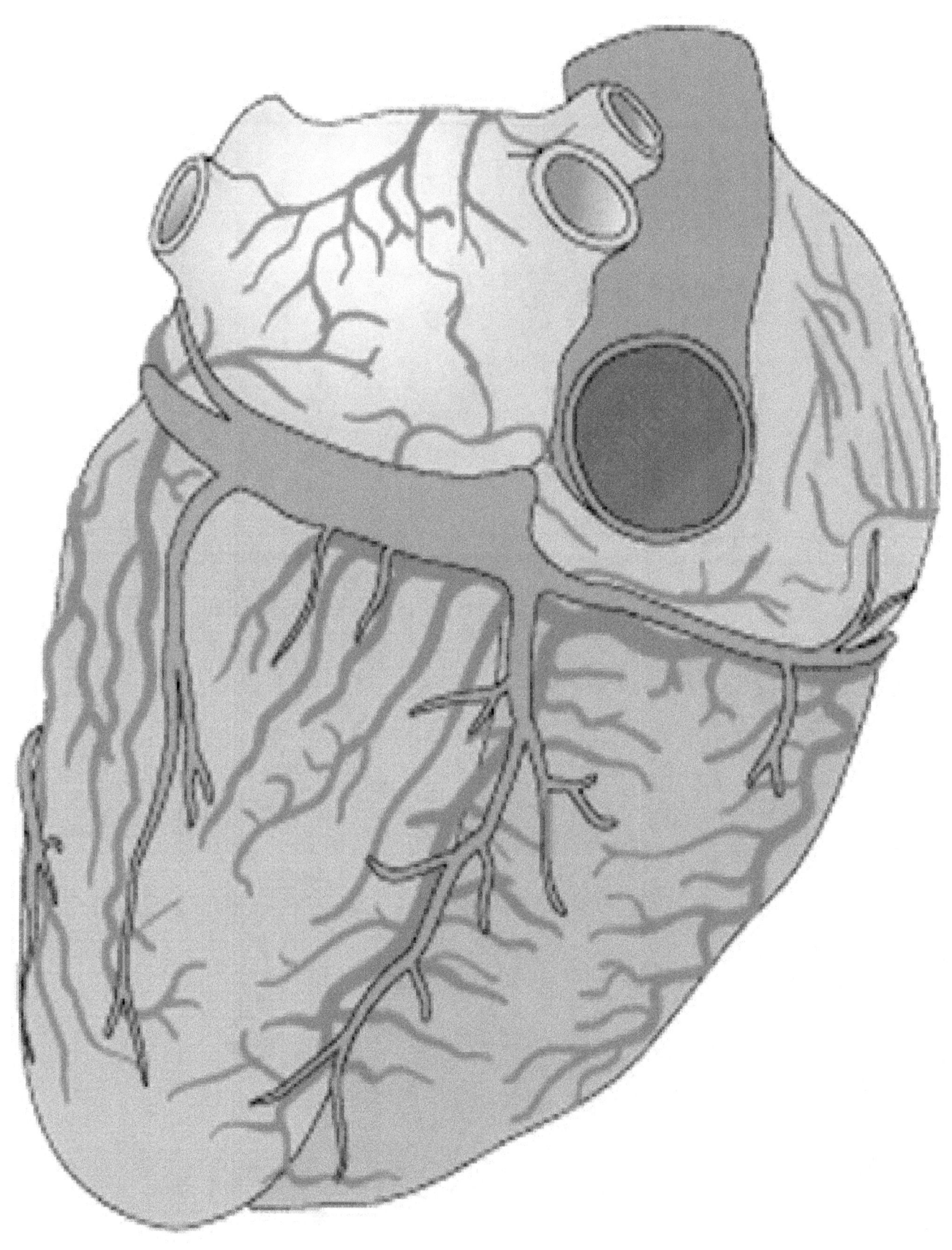

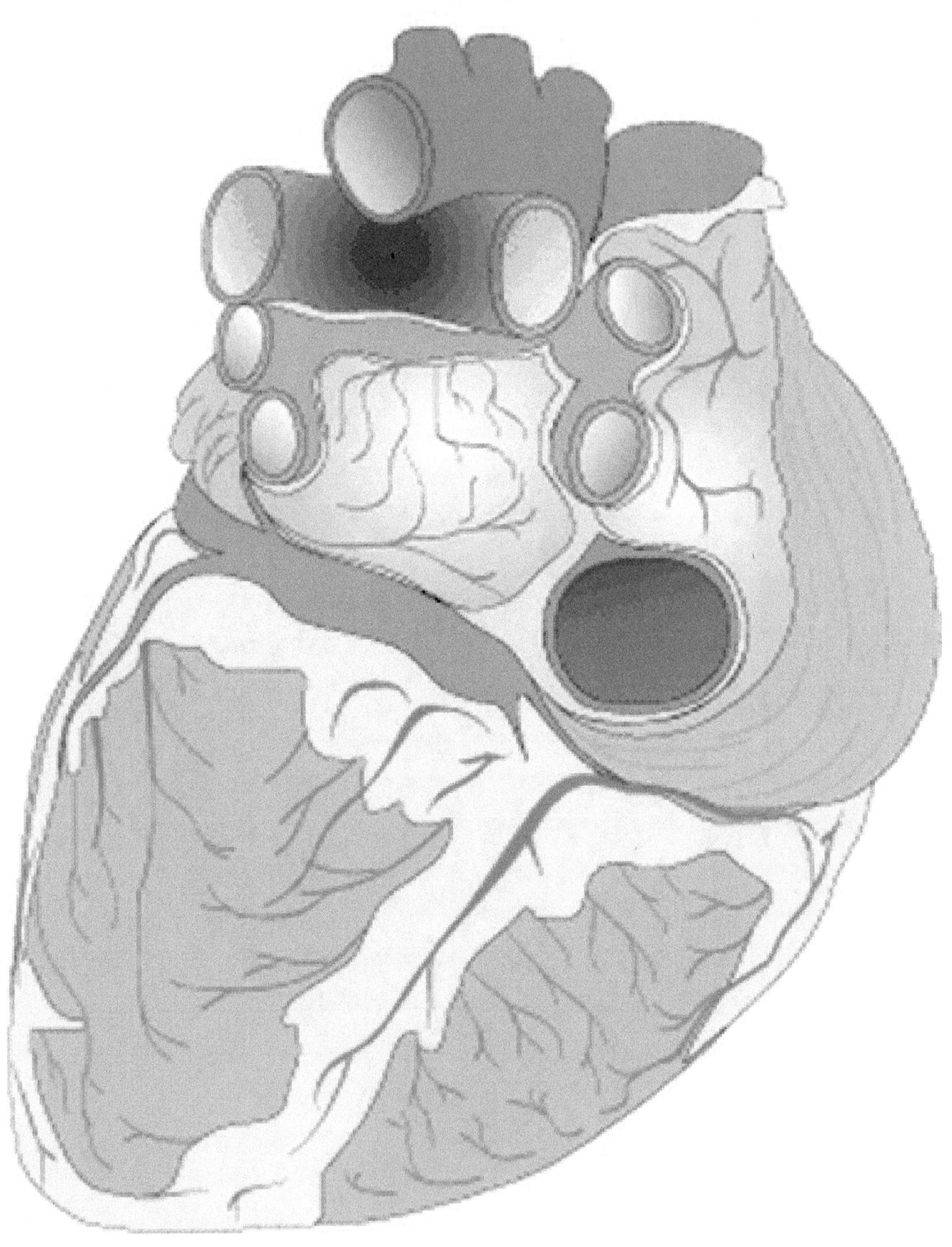

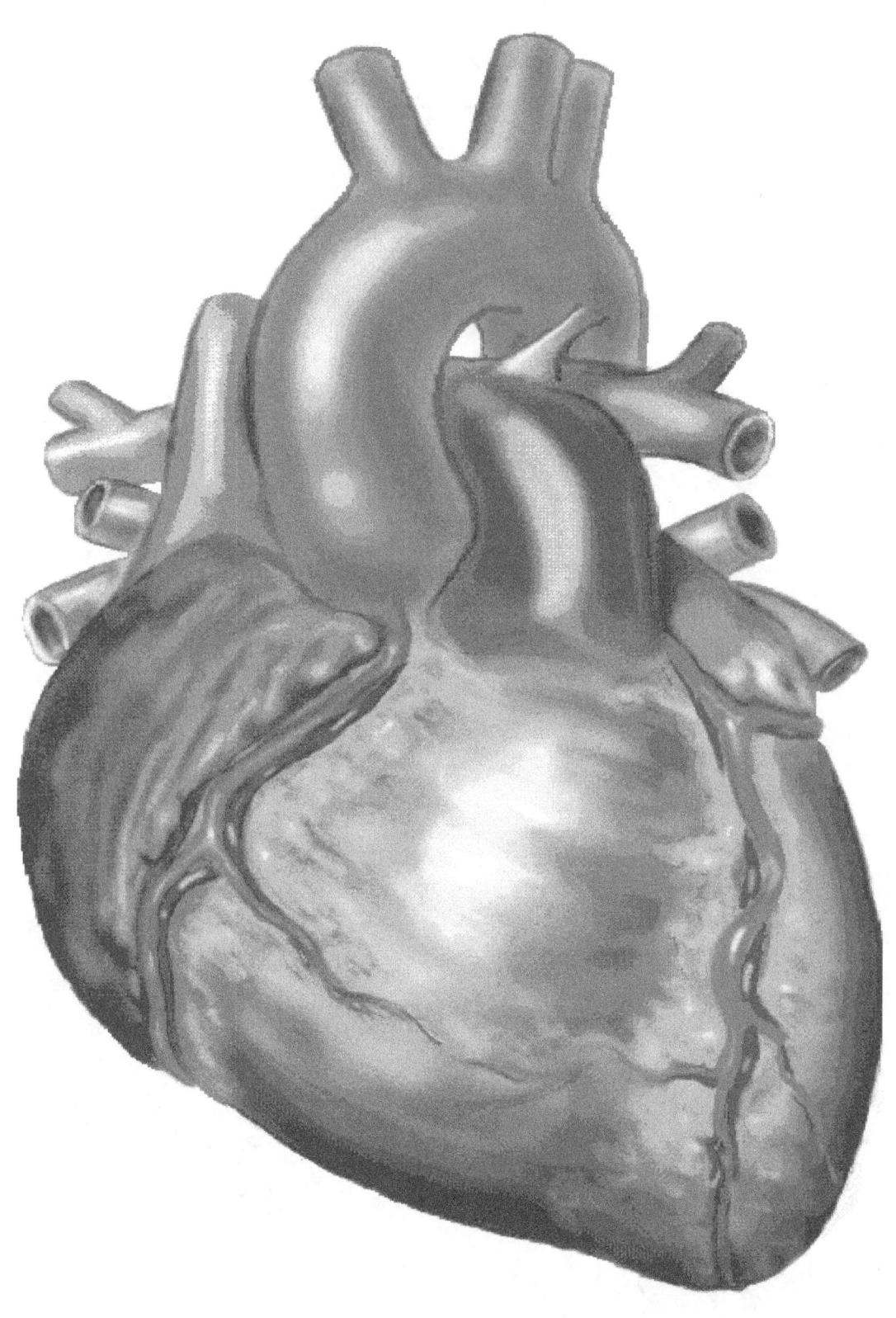

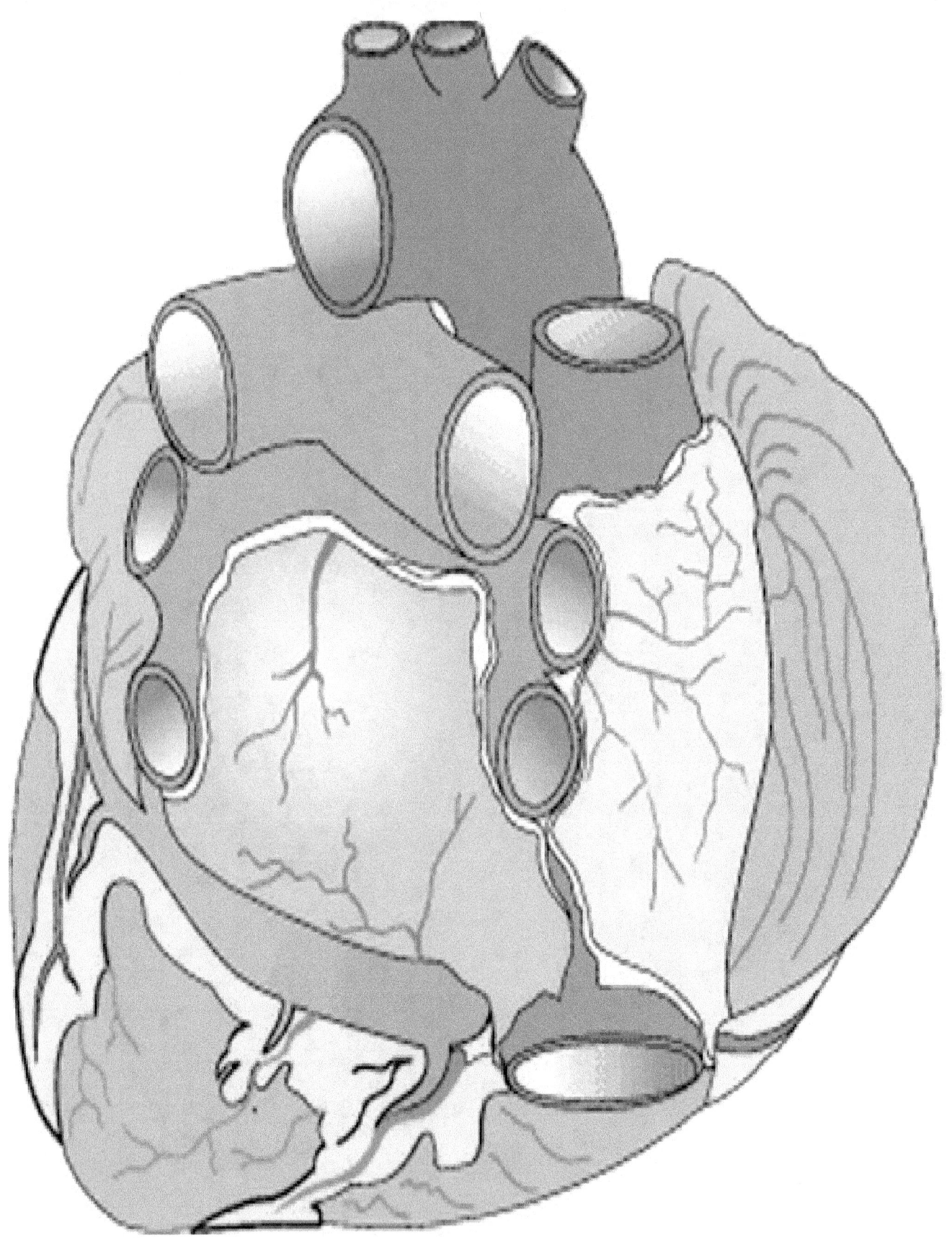

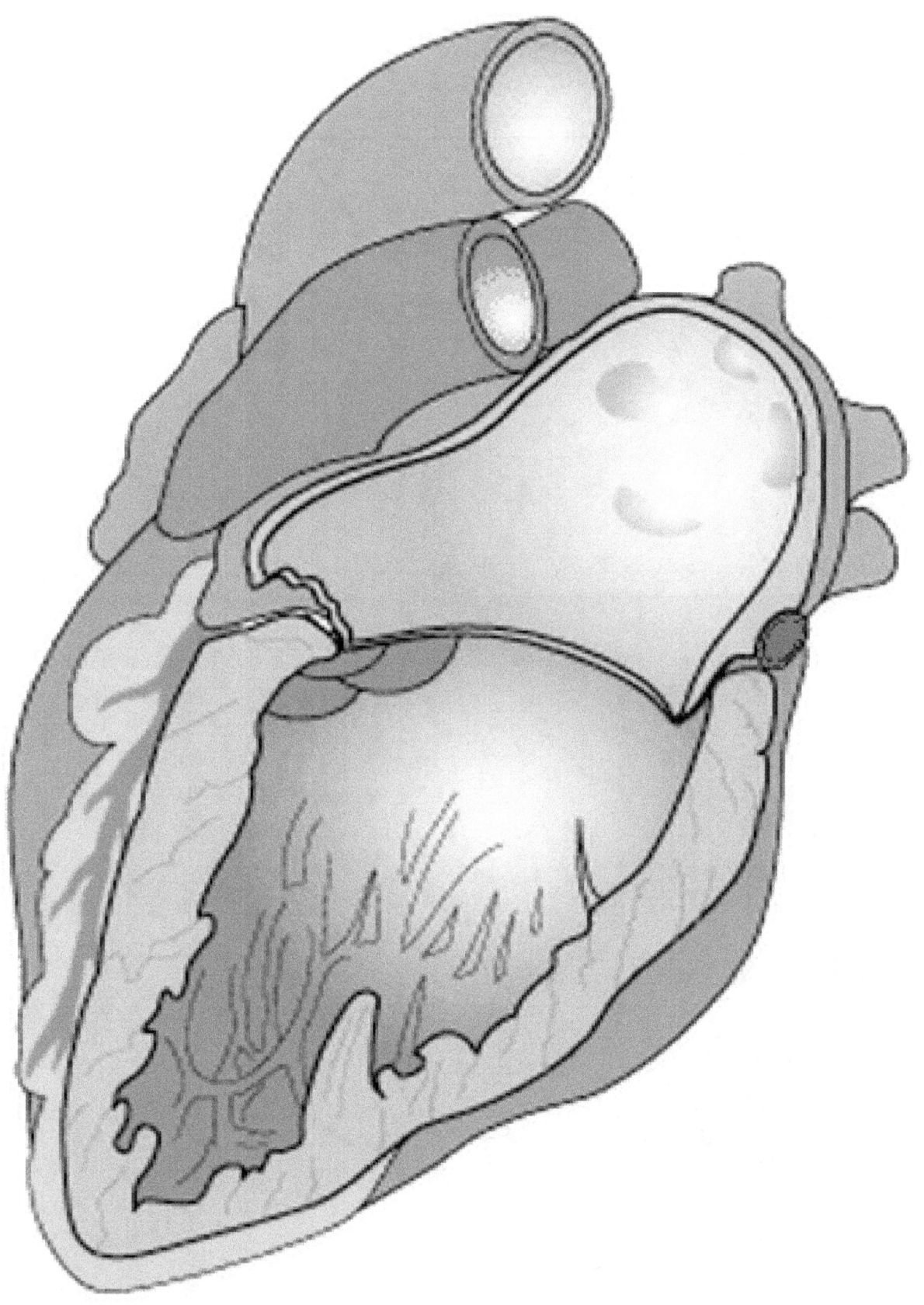

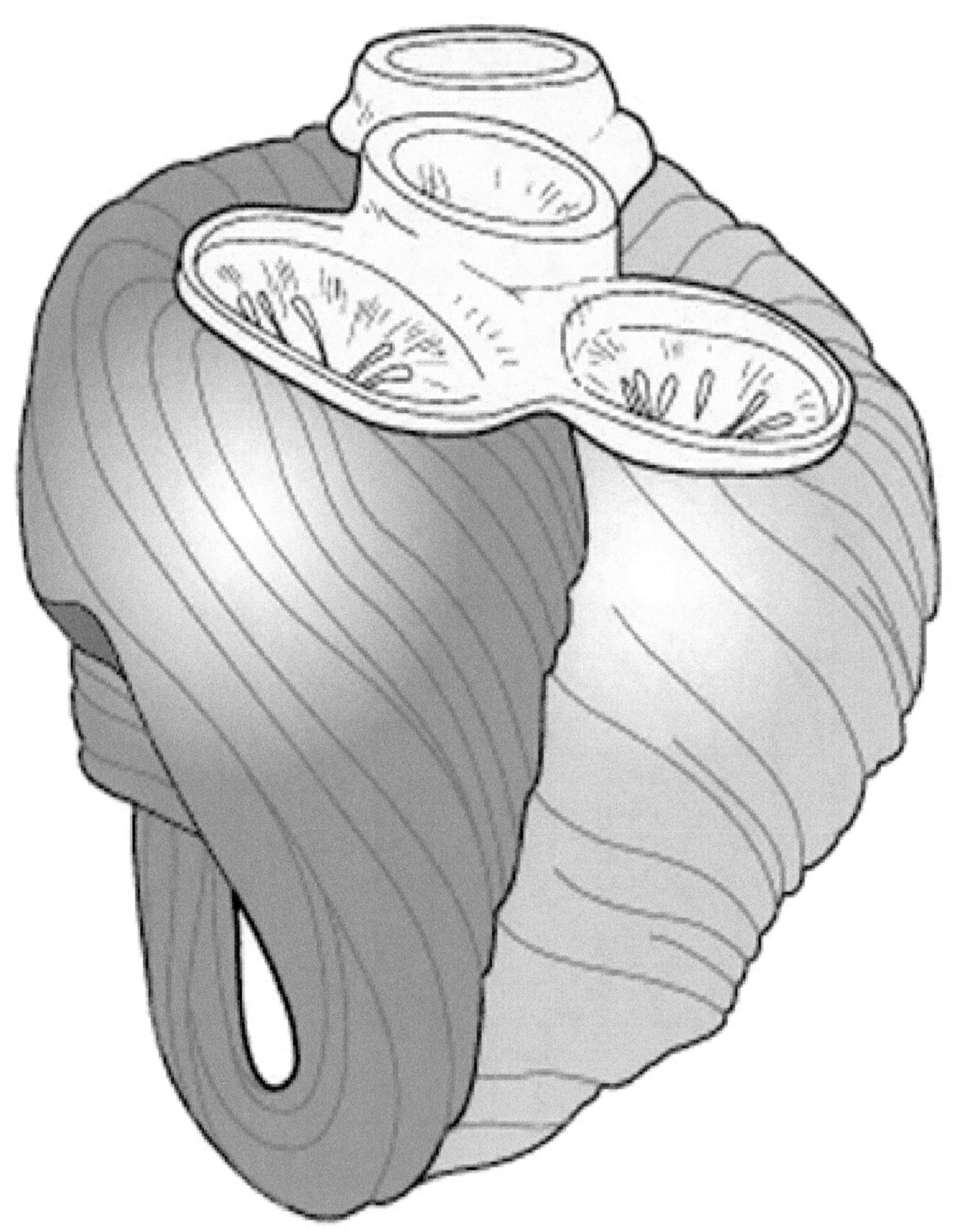

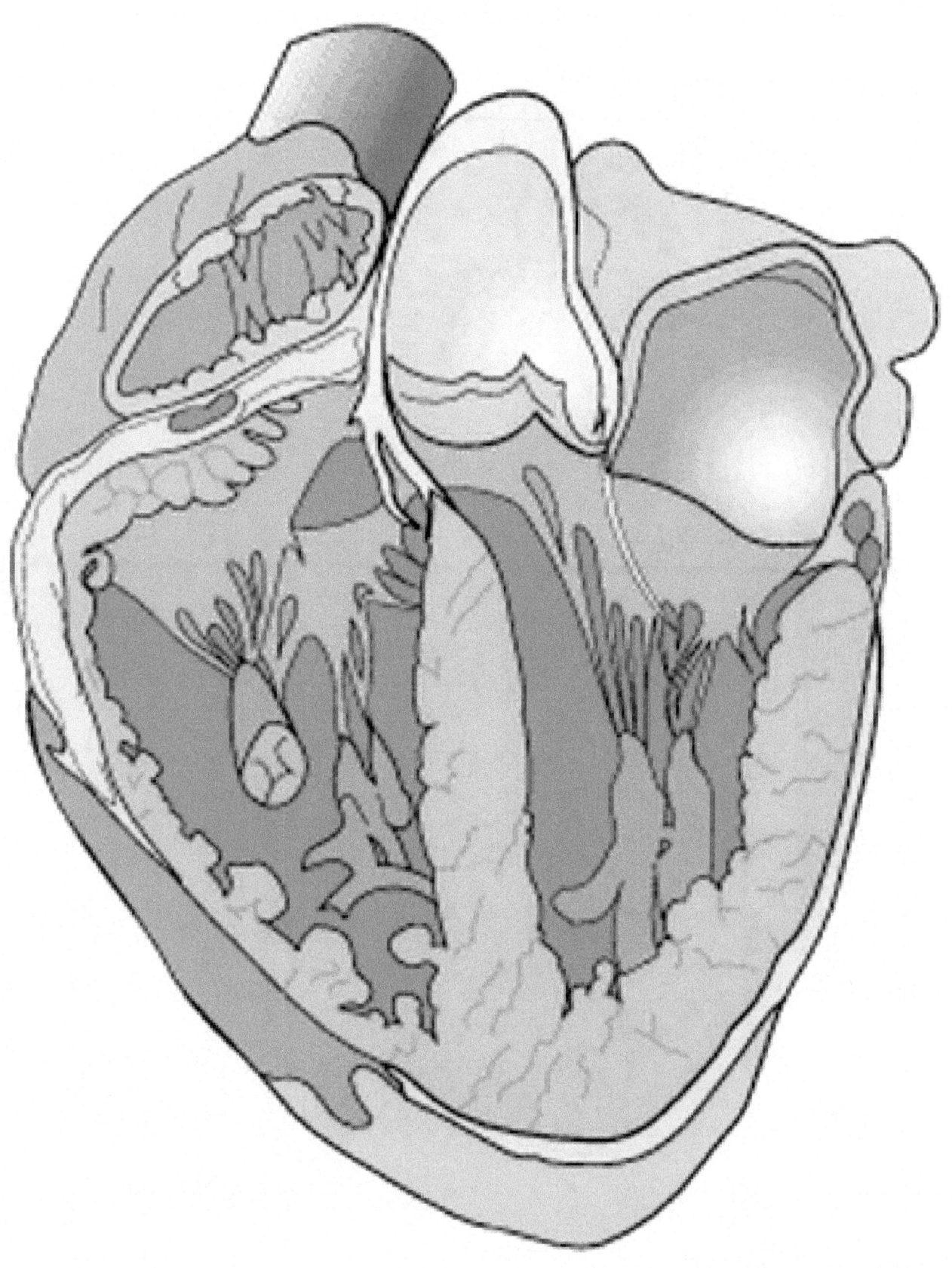

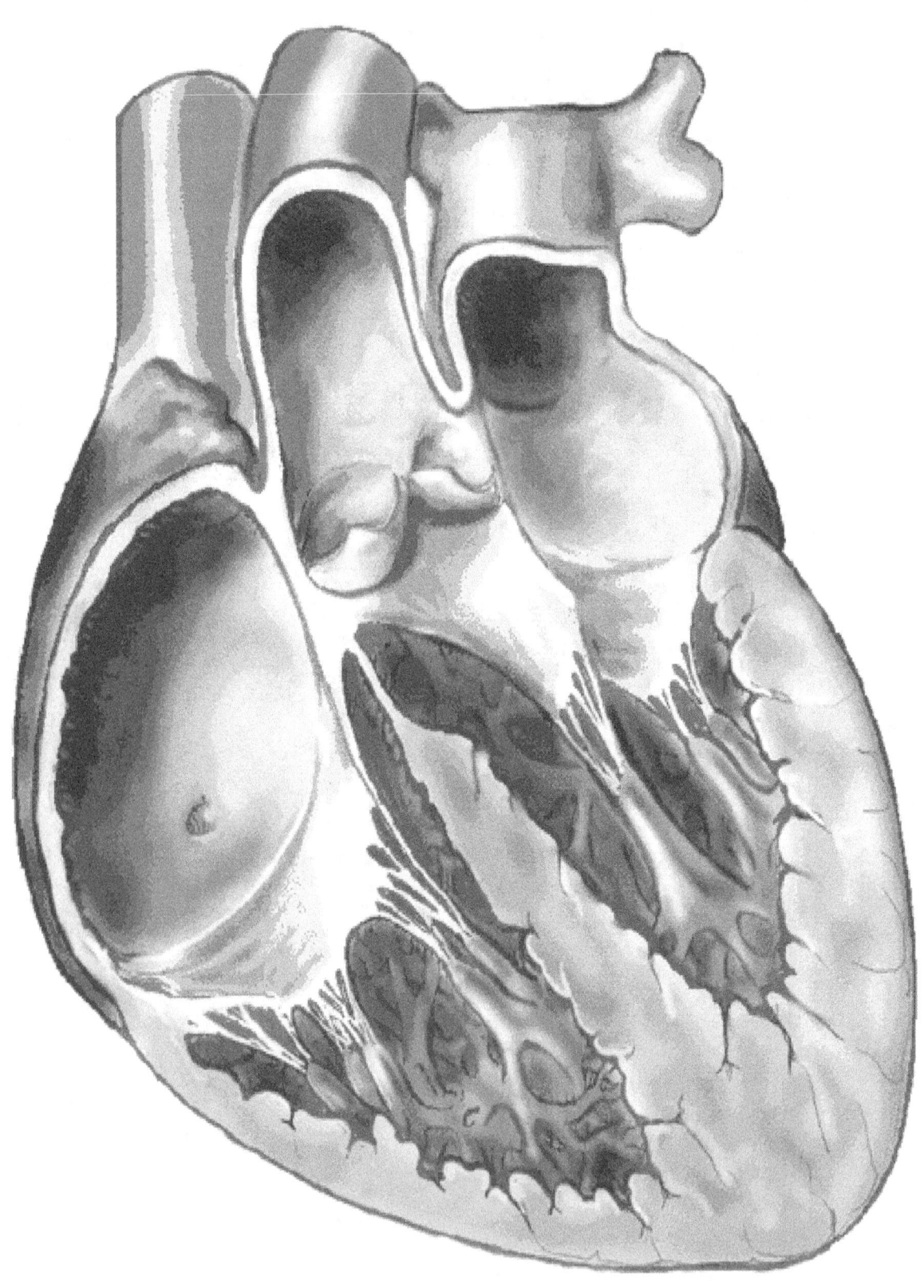

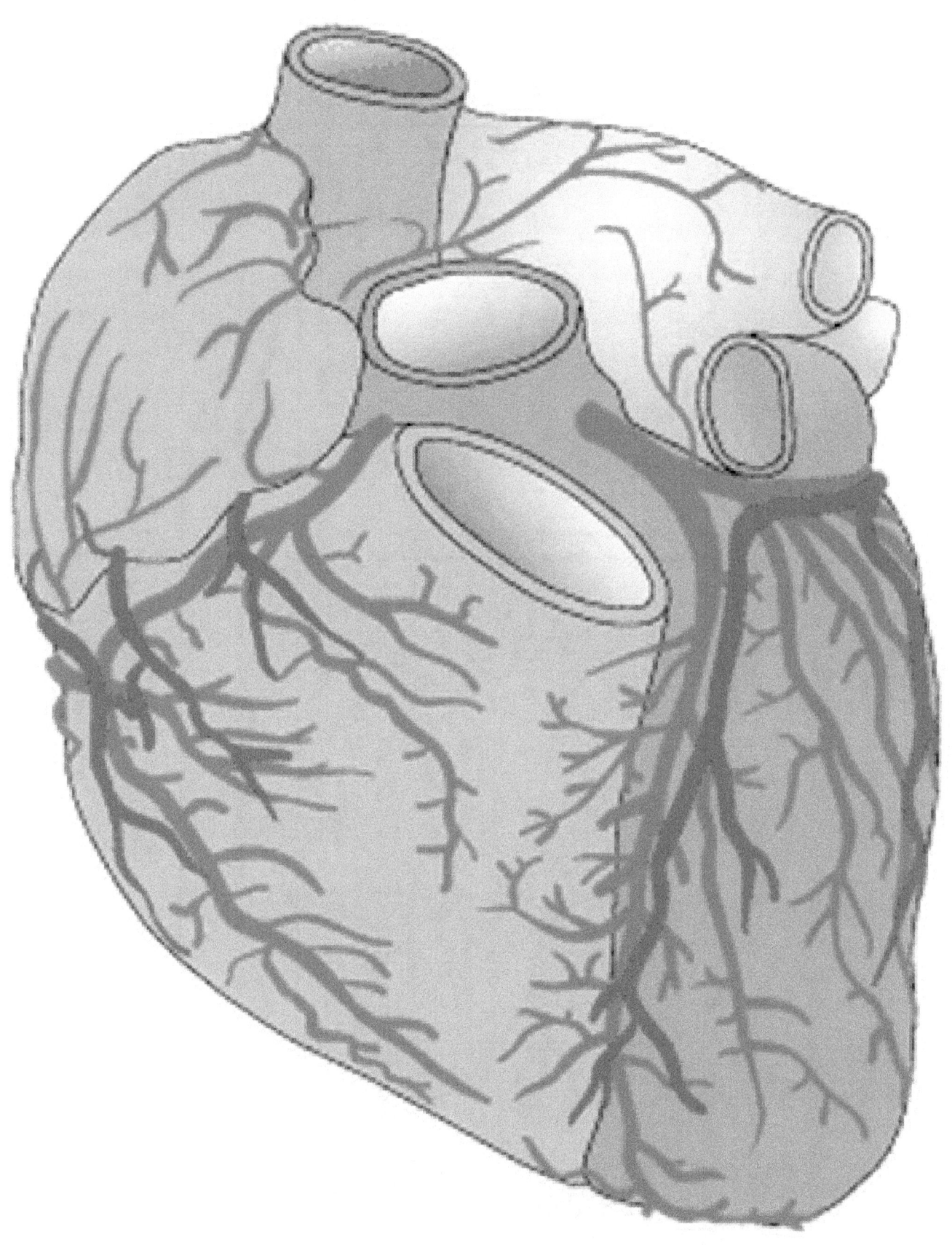

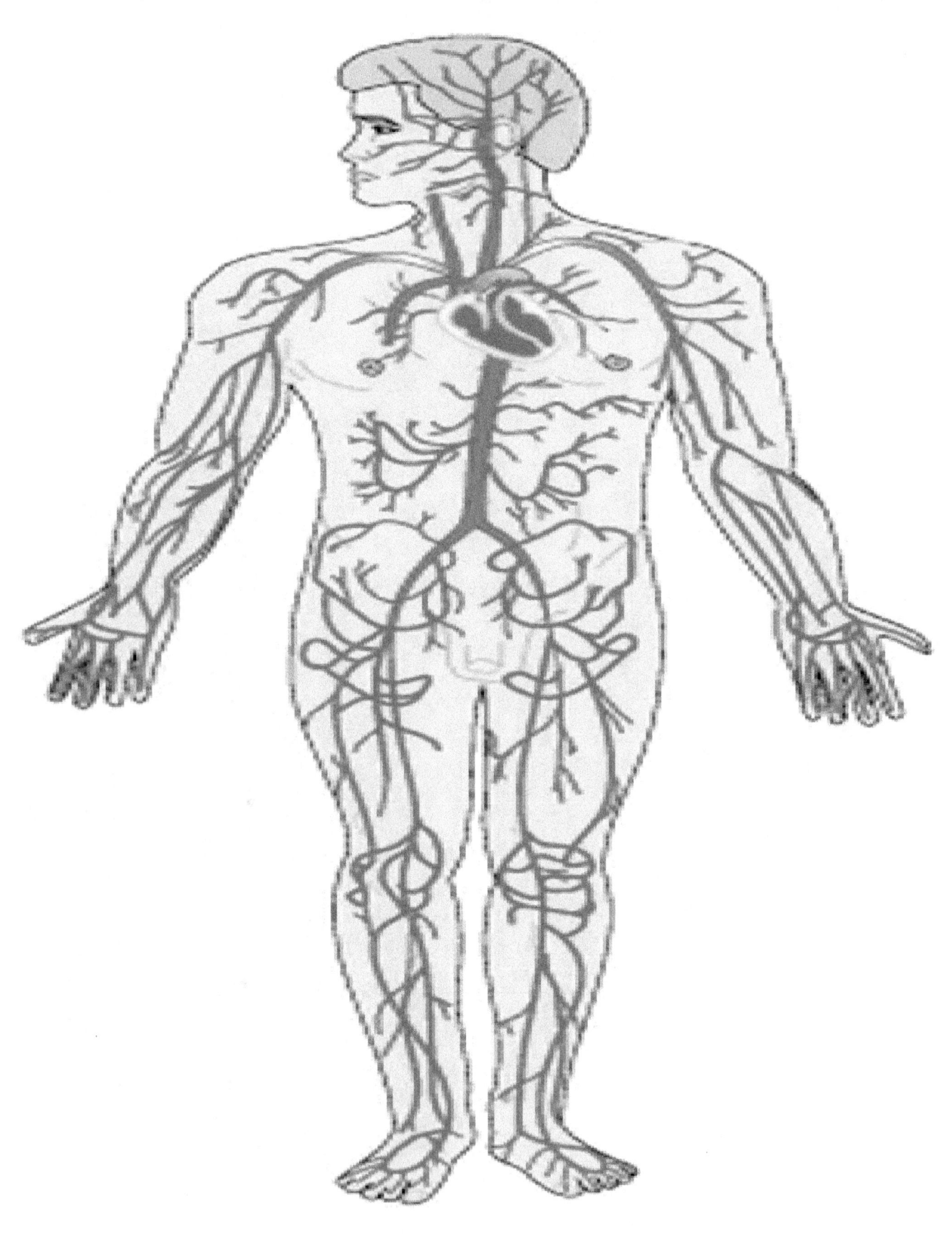

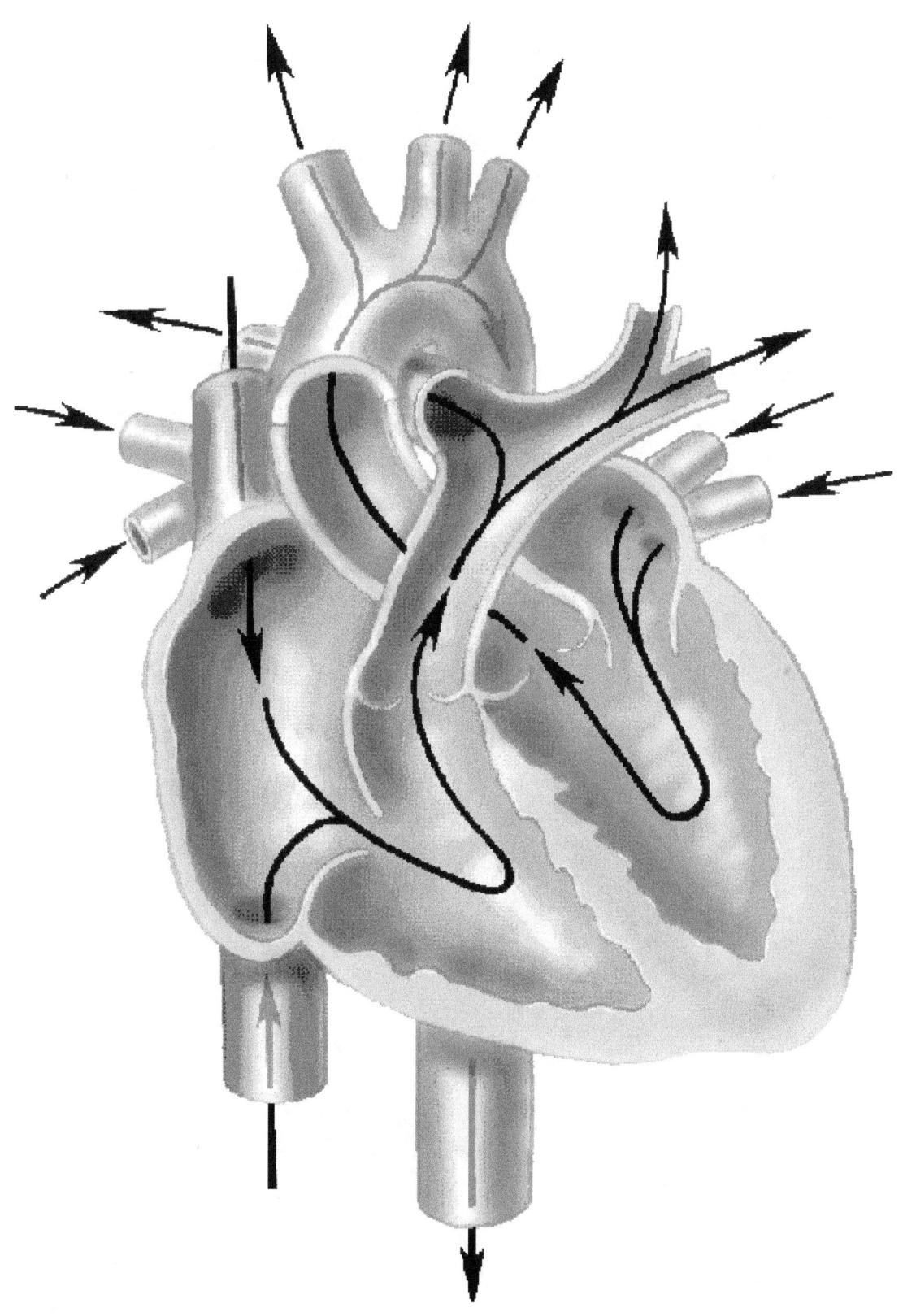

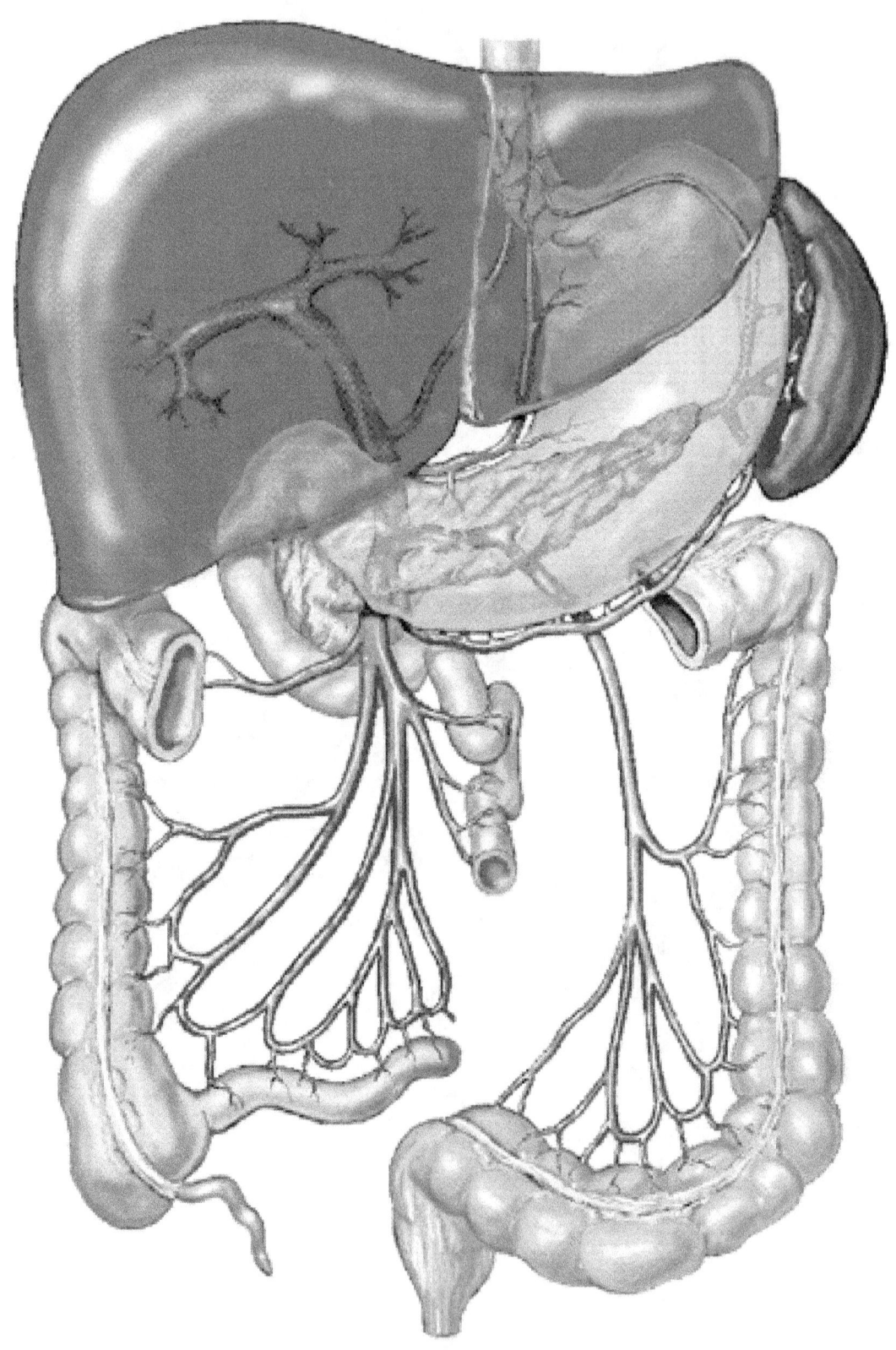

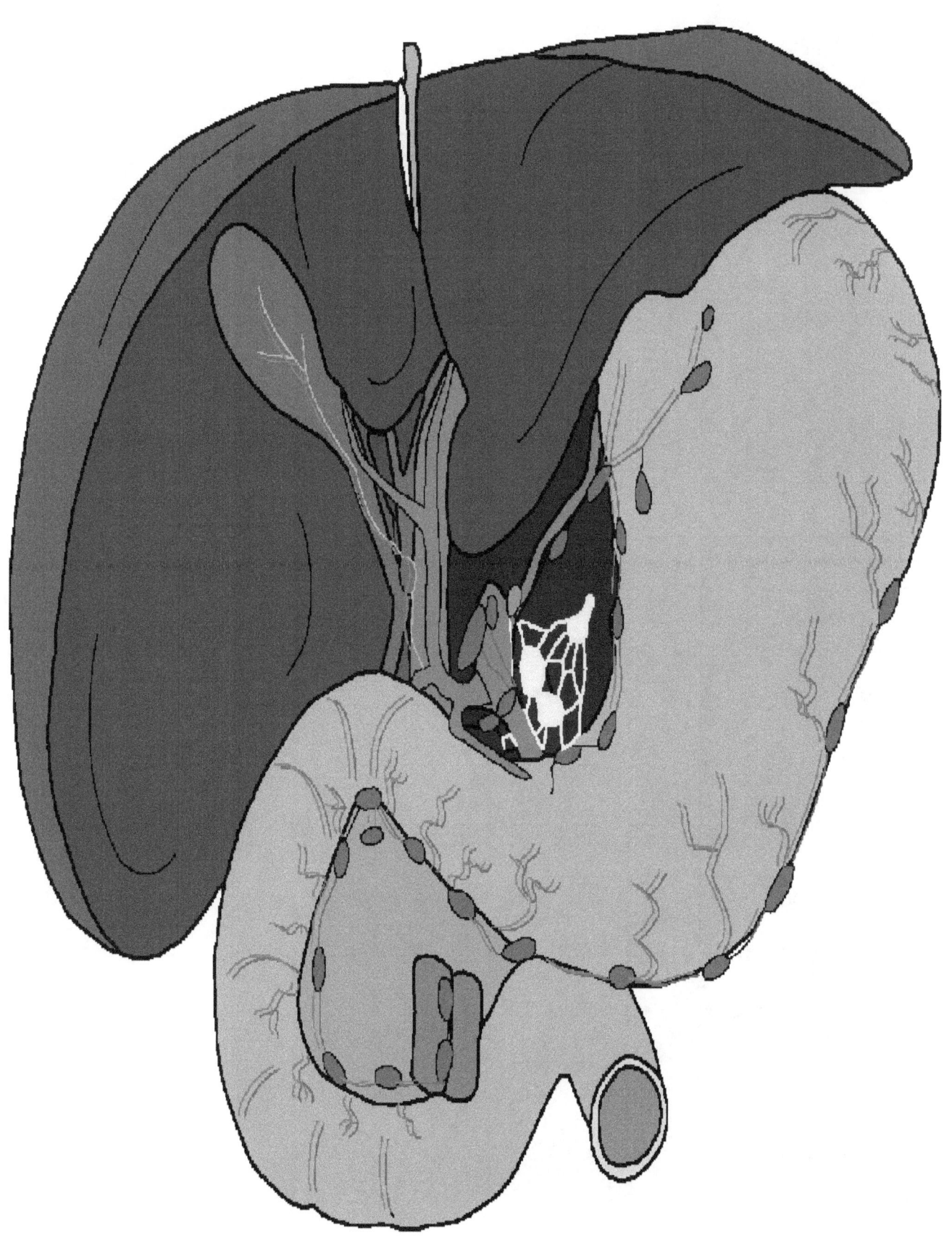

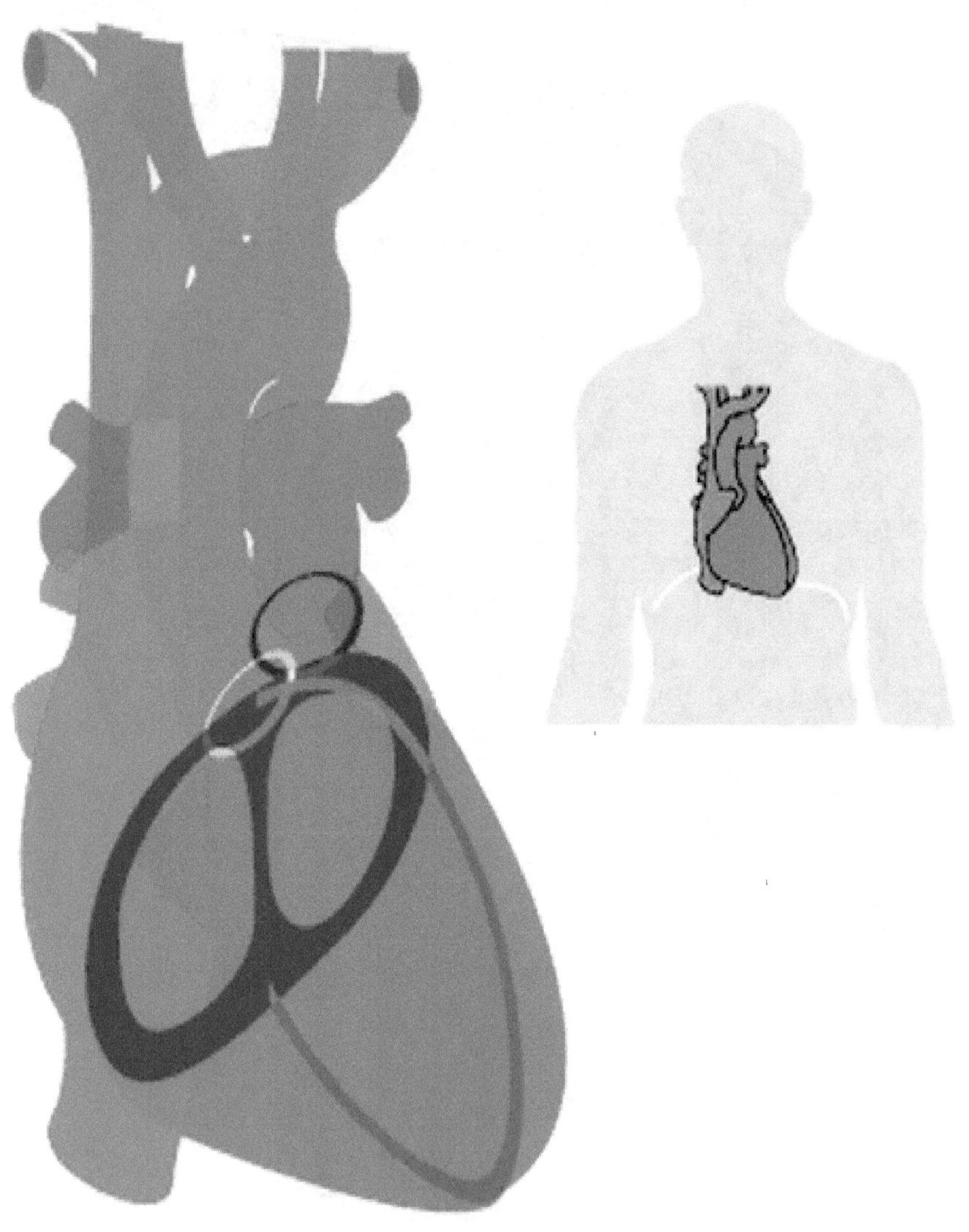

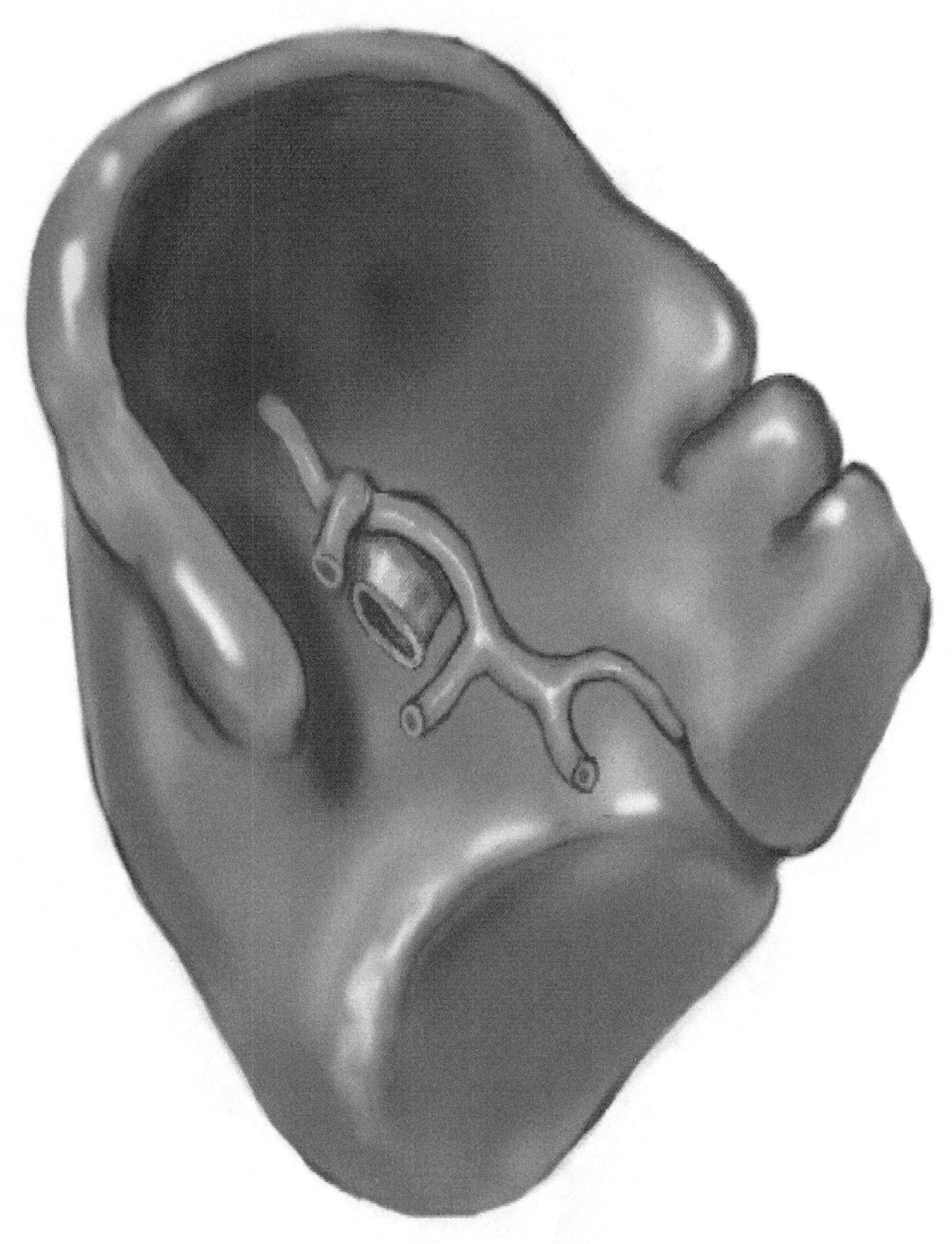

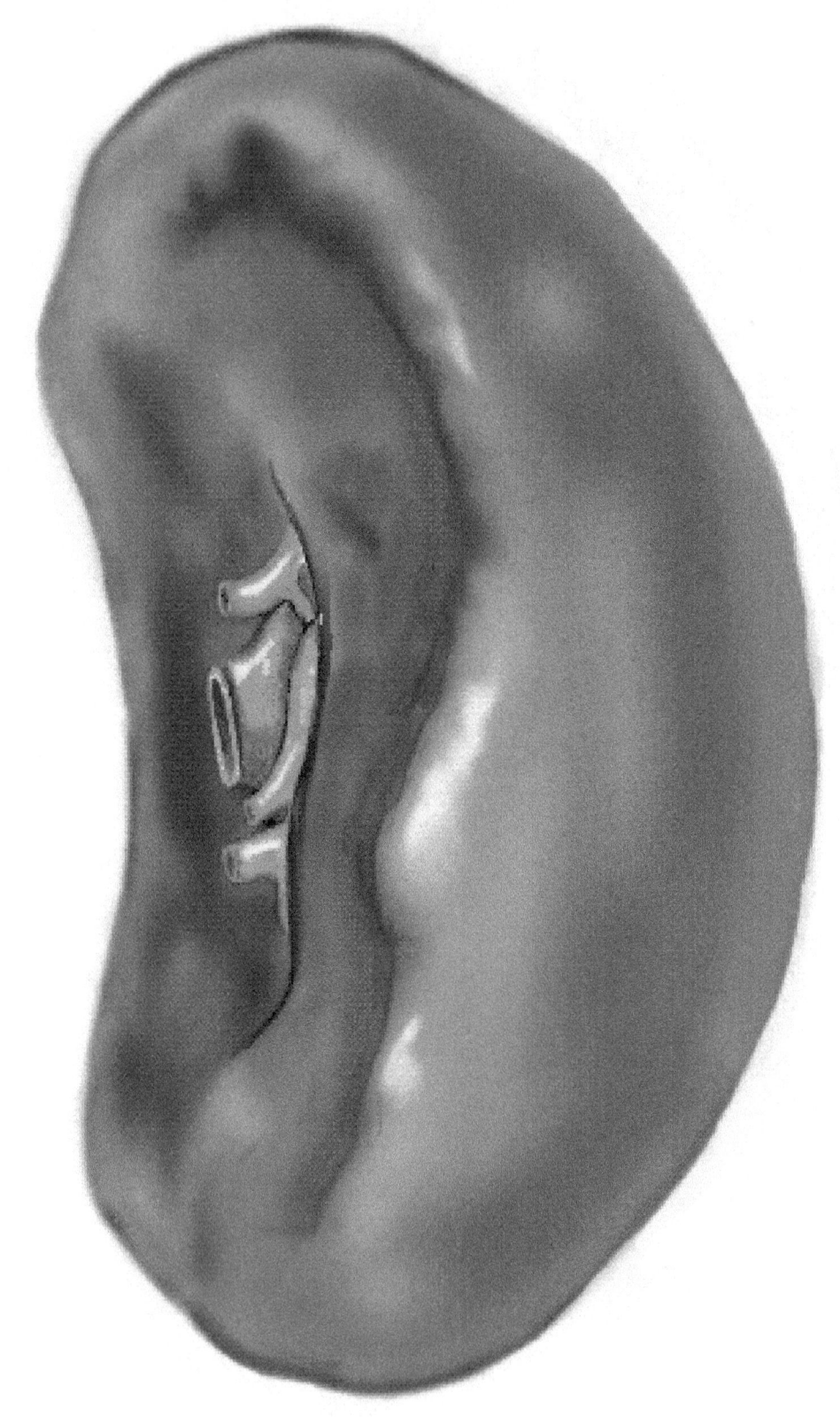

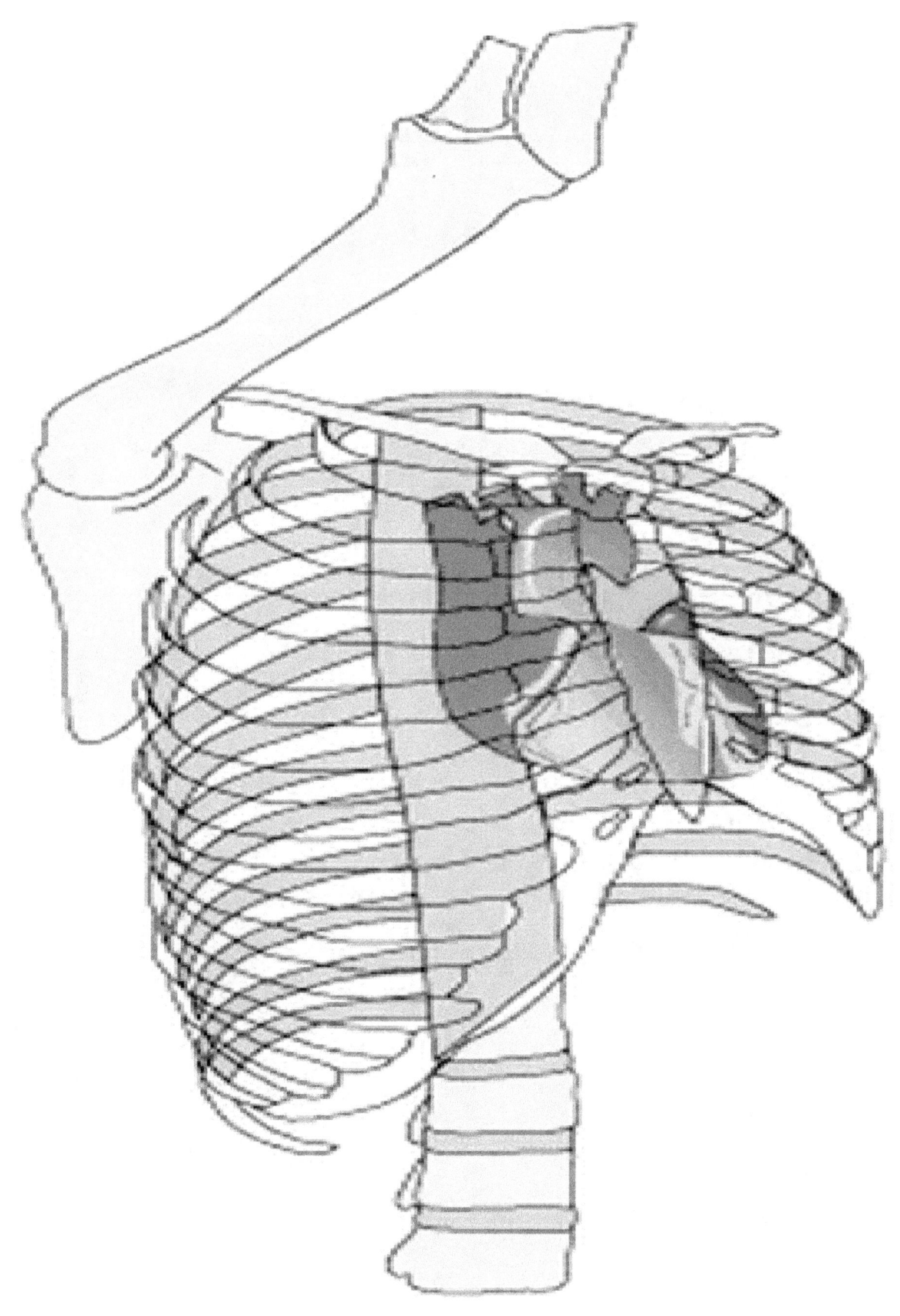

317

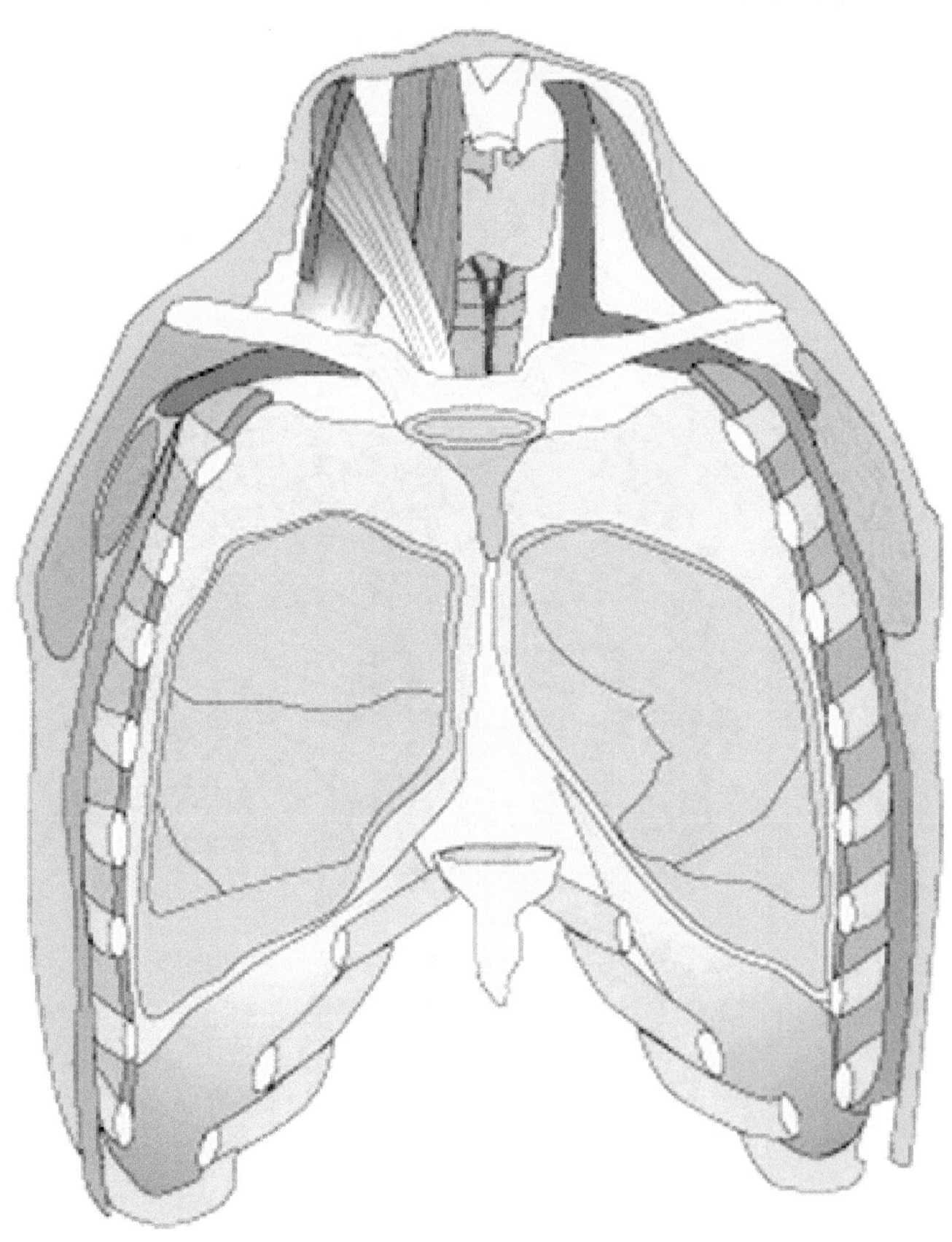

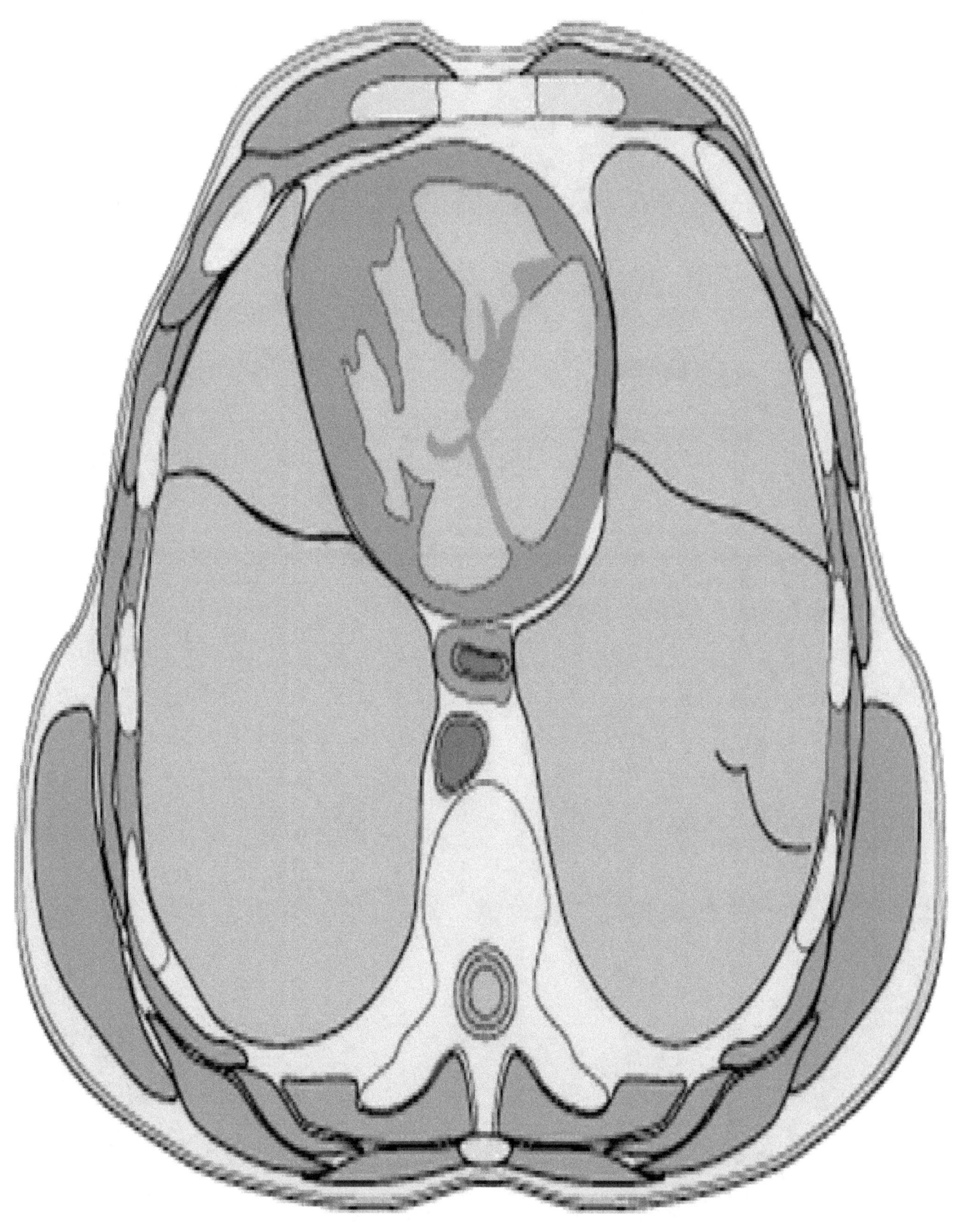

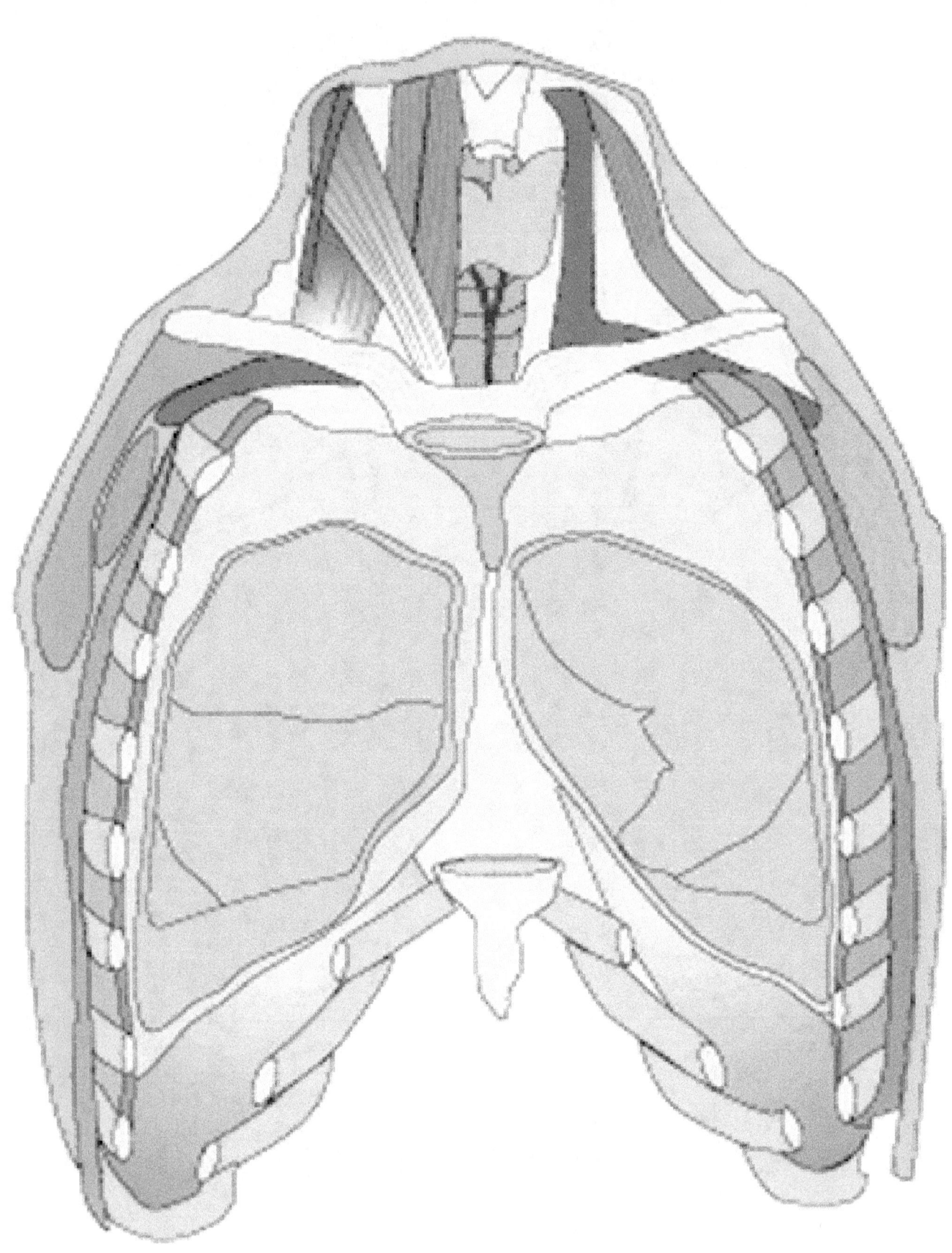

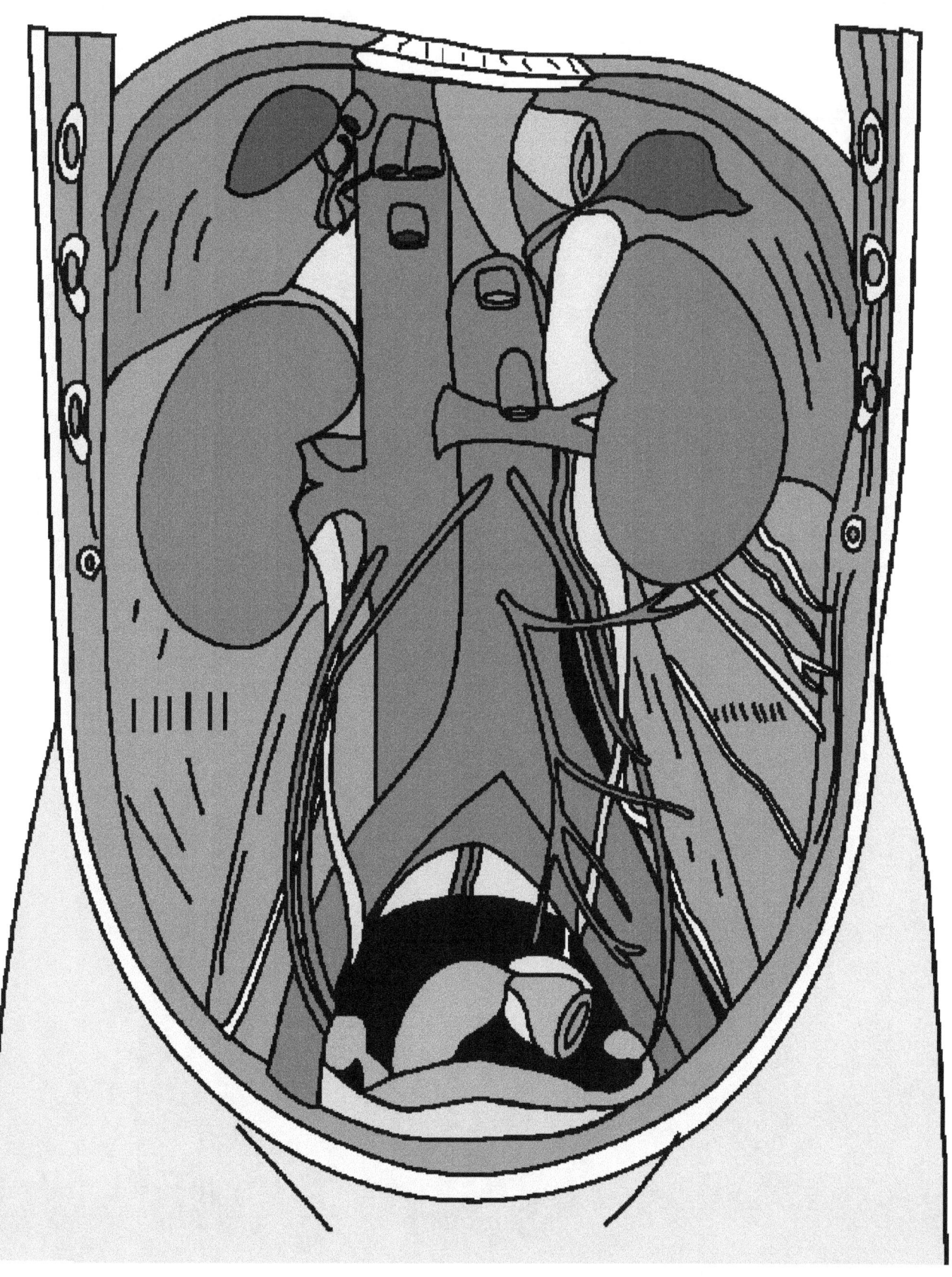

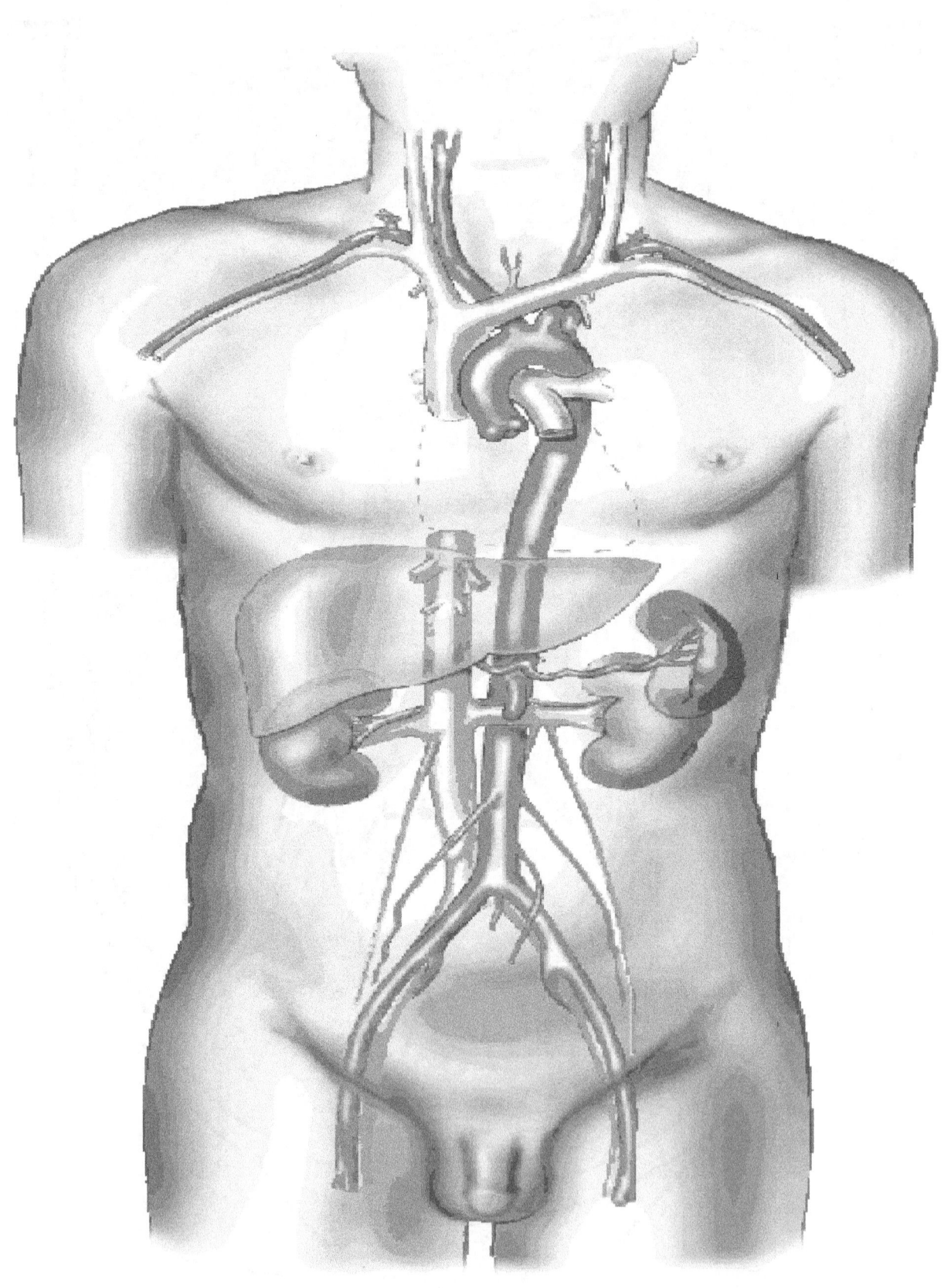

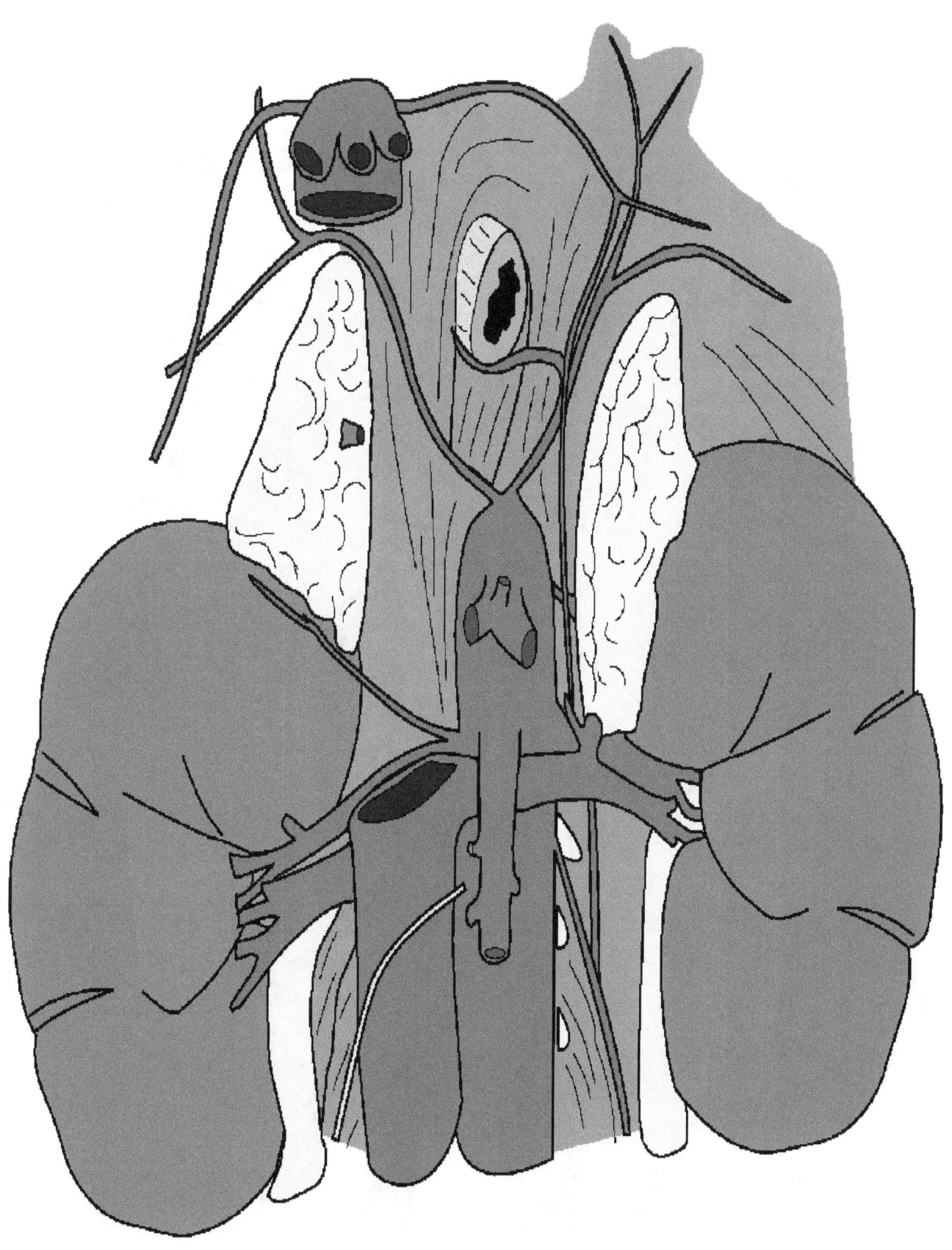

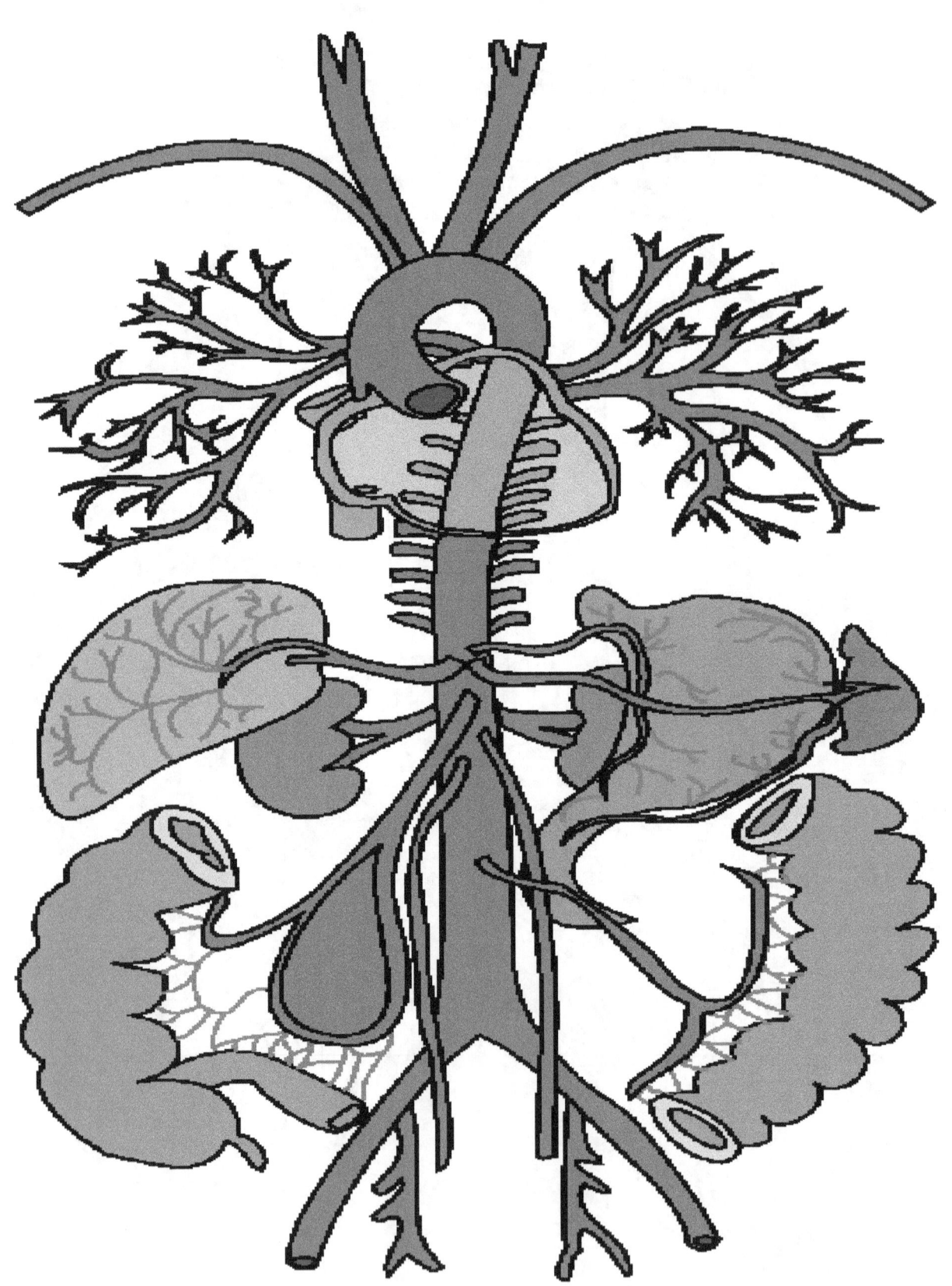

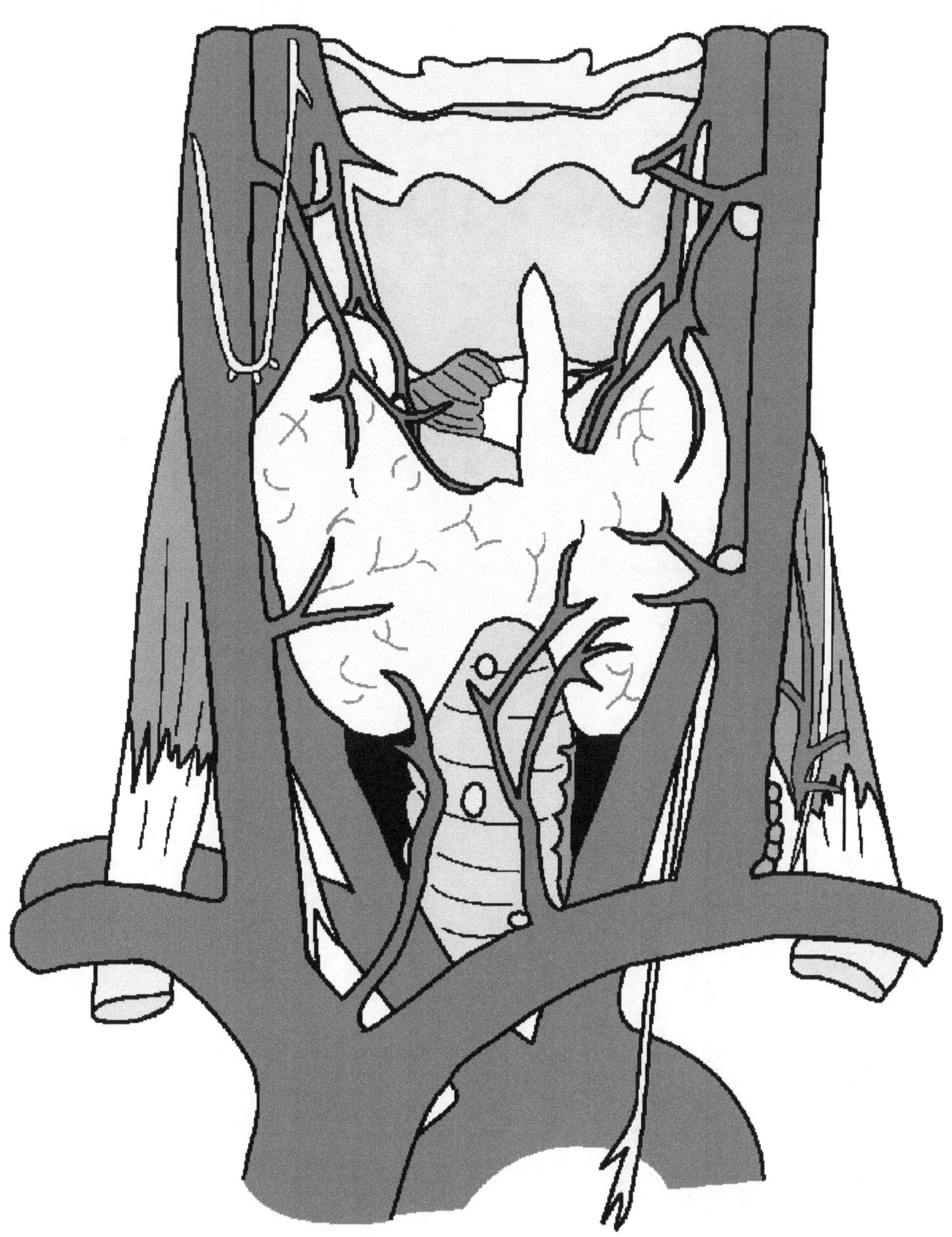

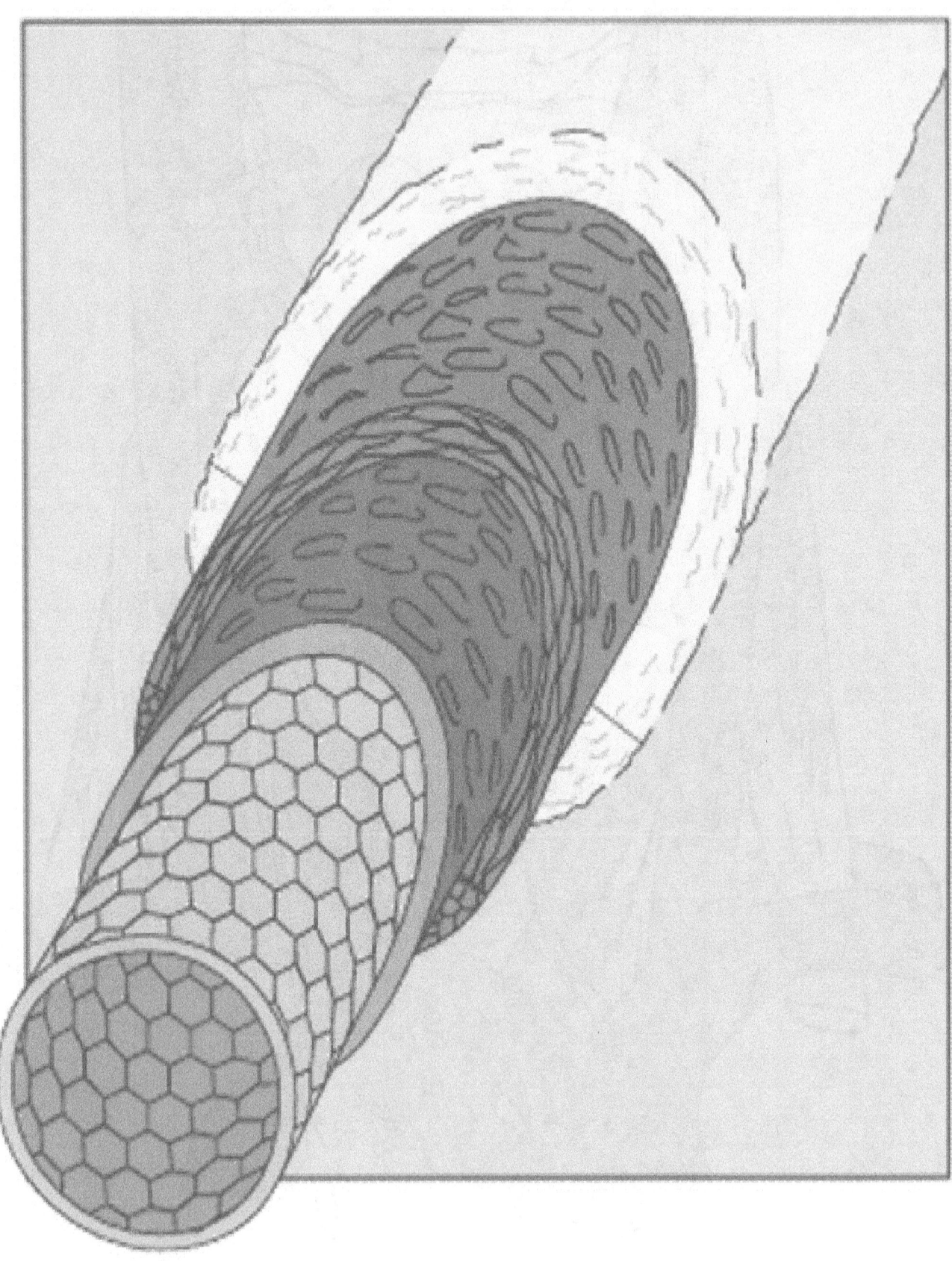

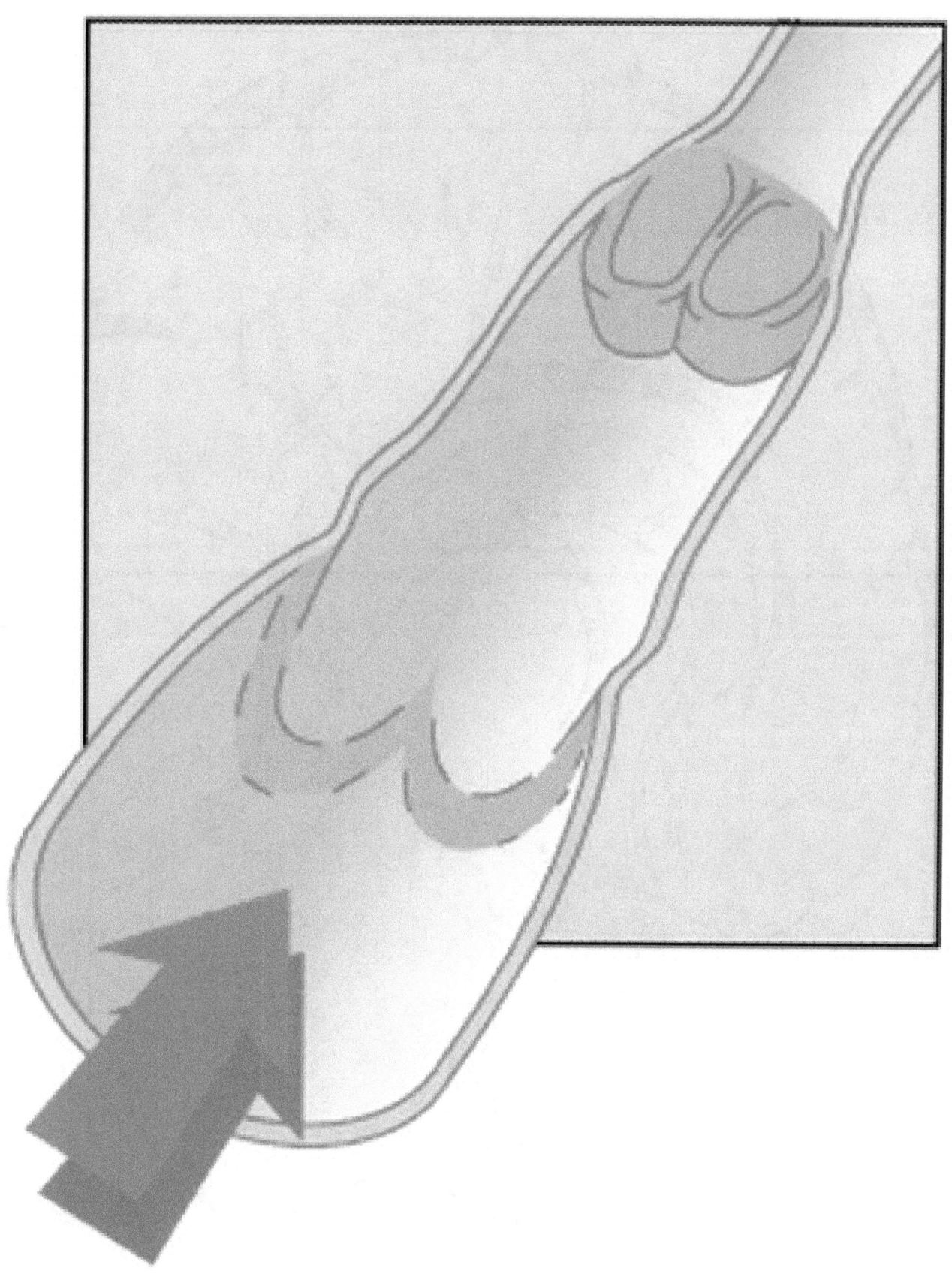

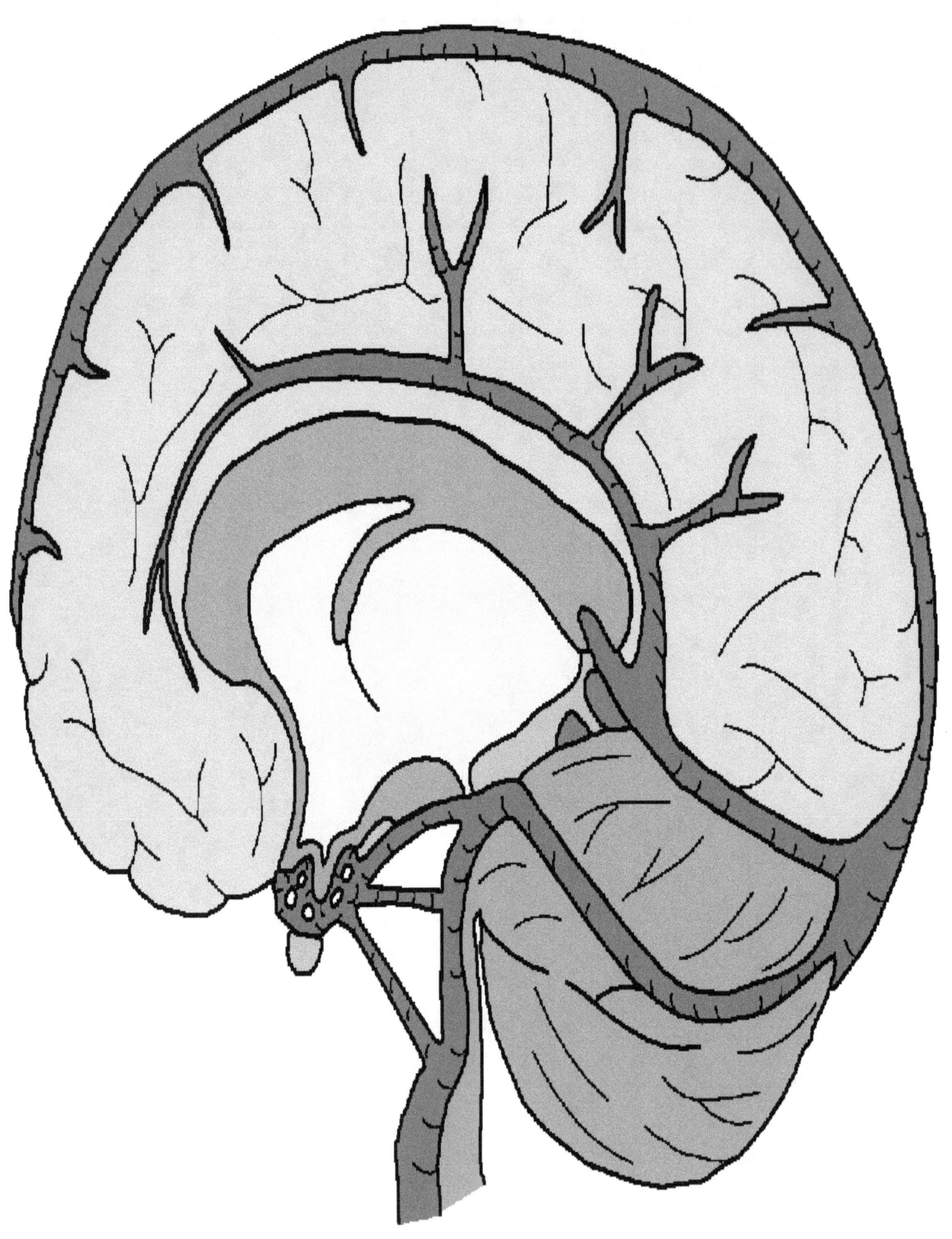

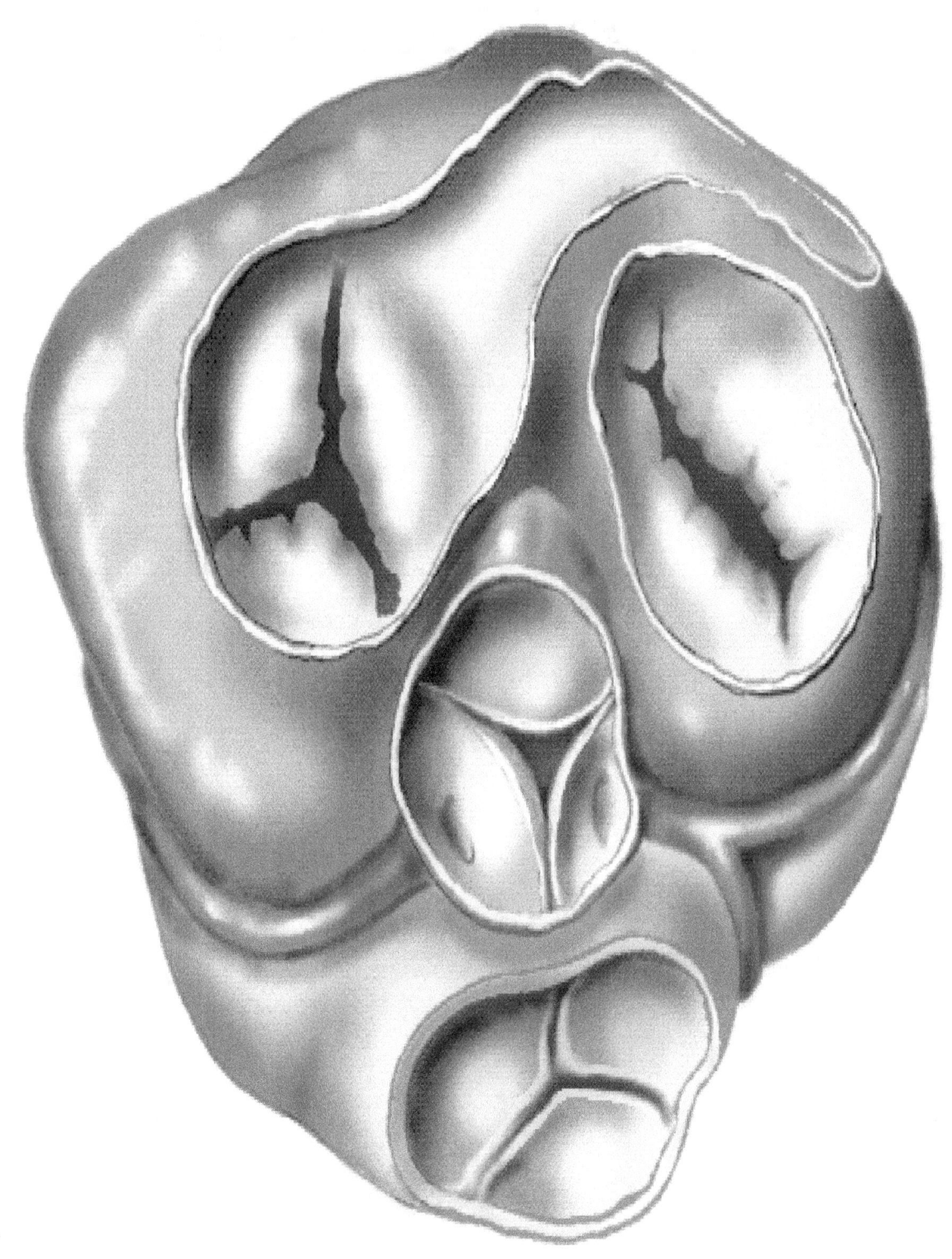

Eyes And Ears 334-344

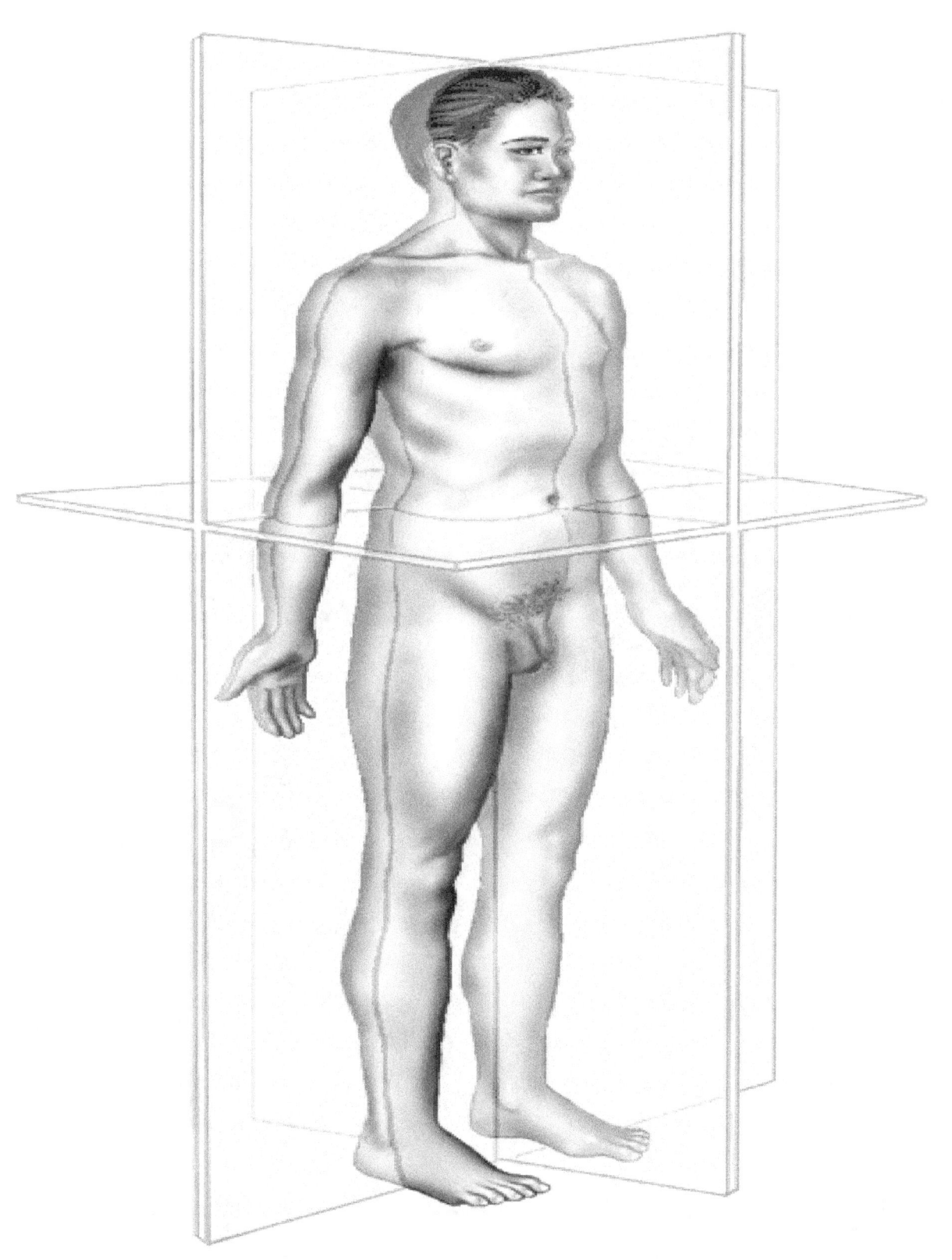

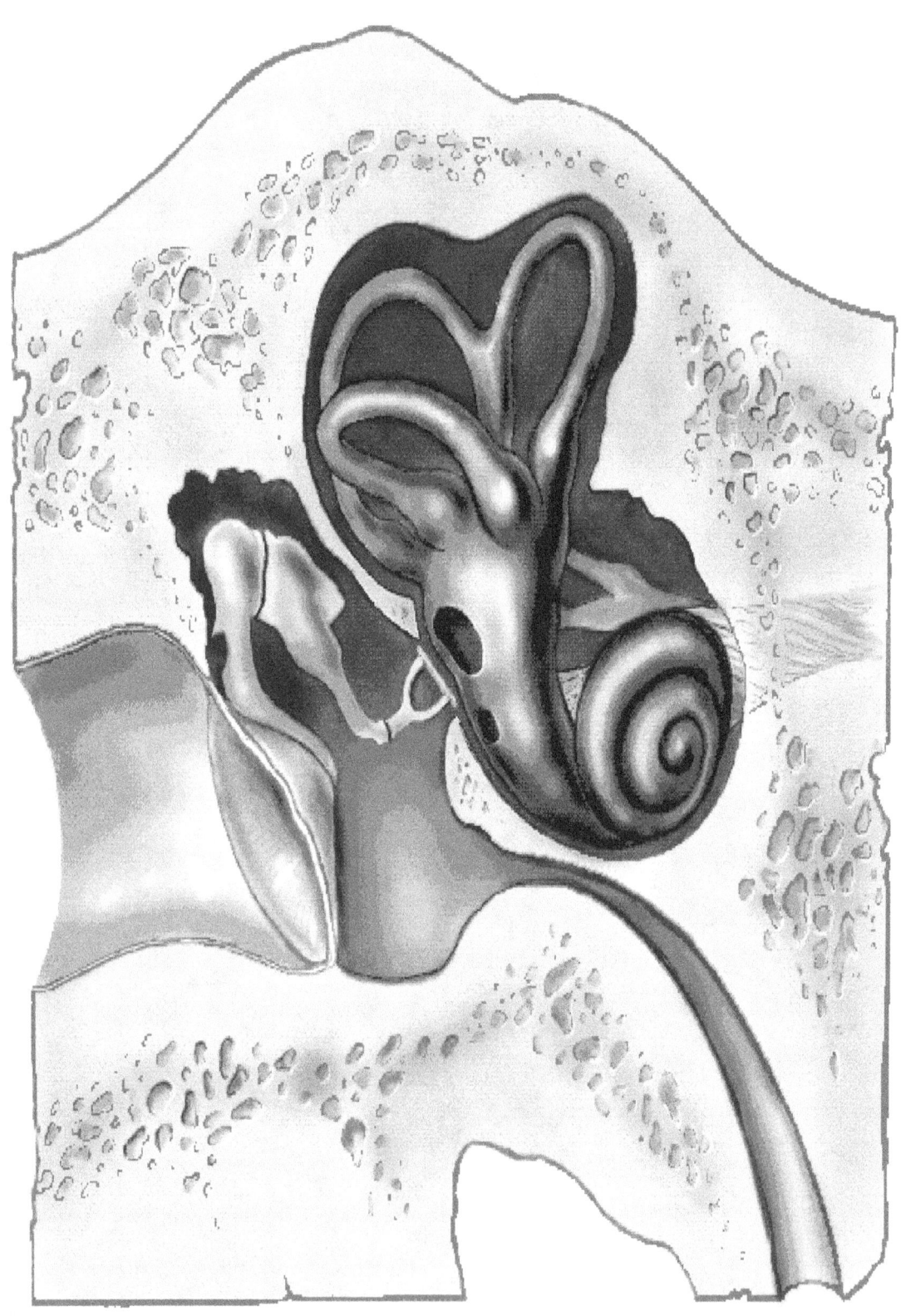

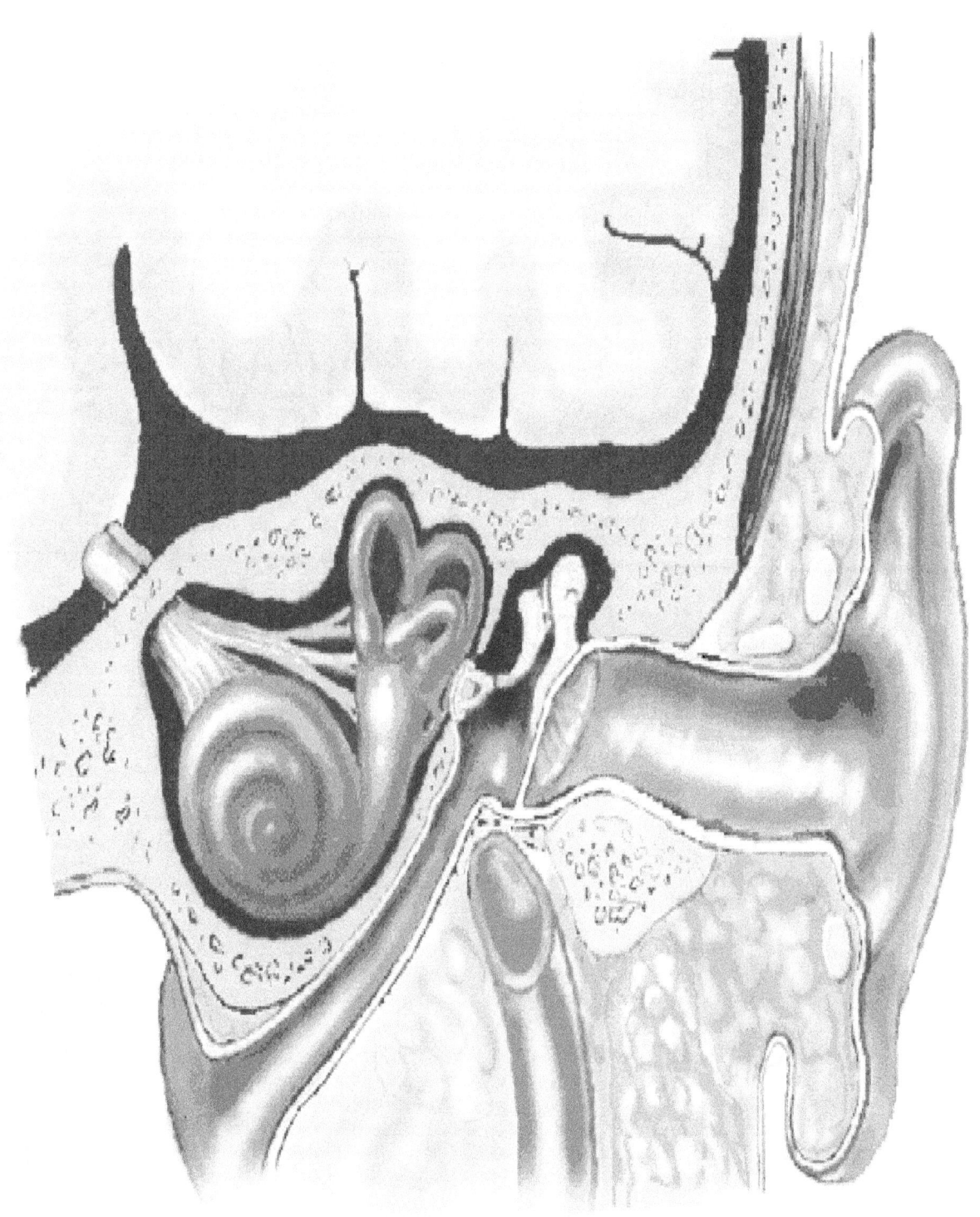

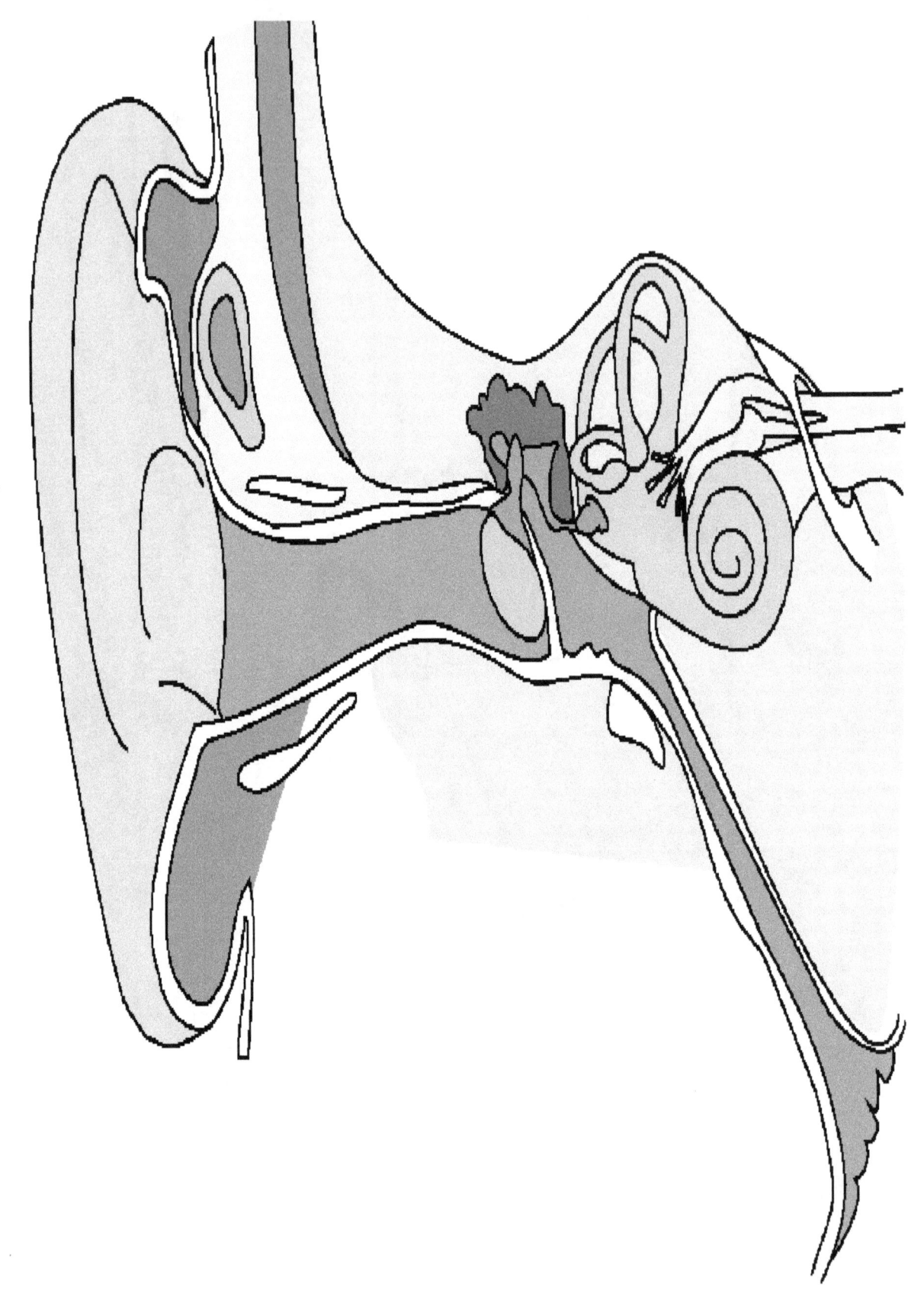

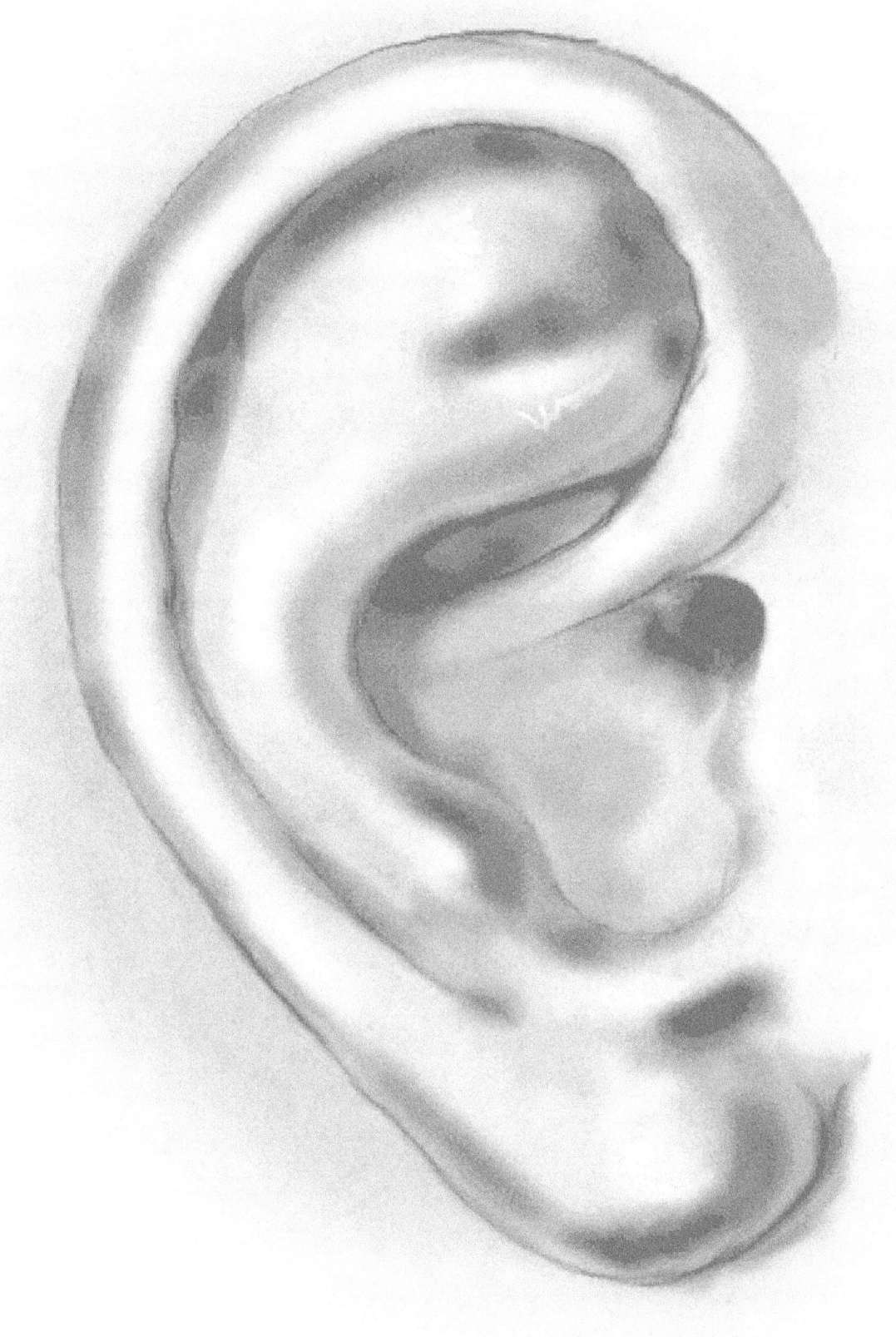

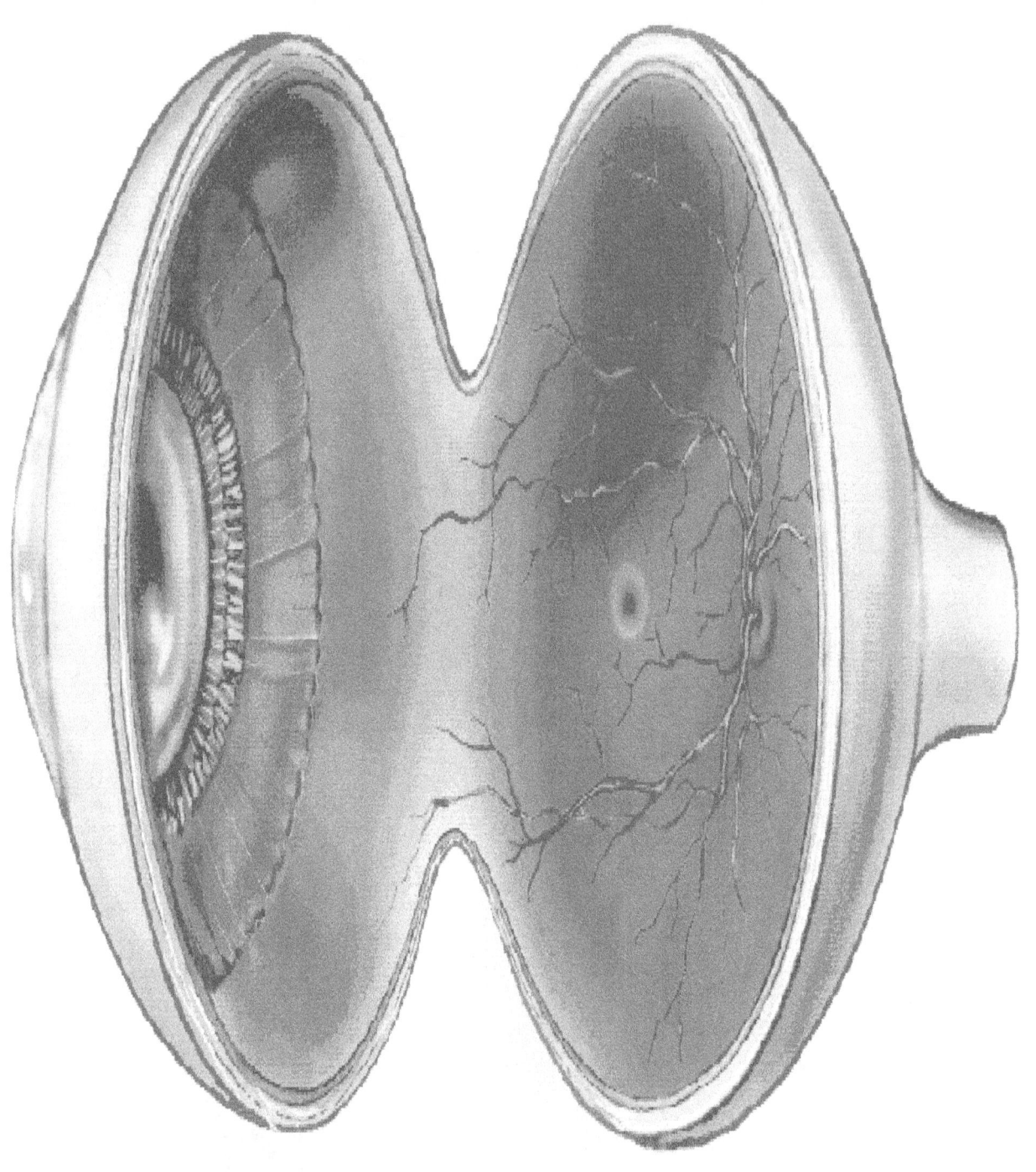

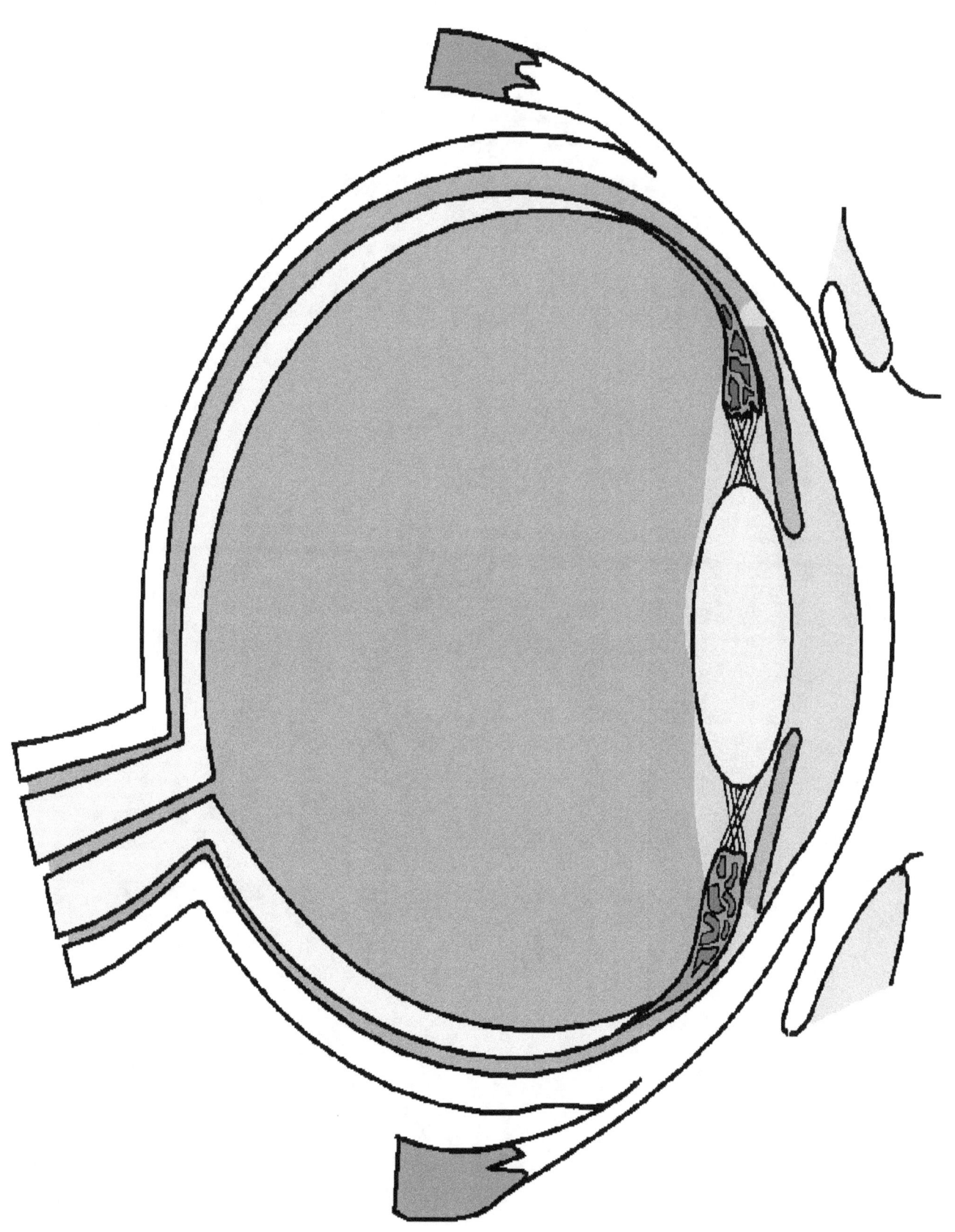

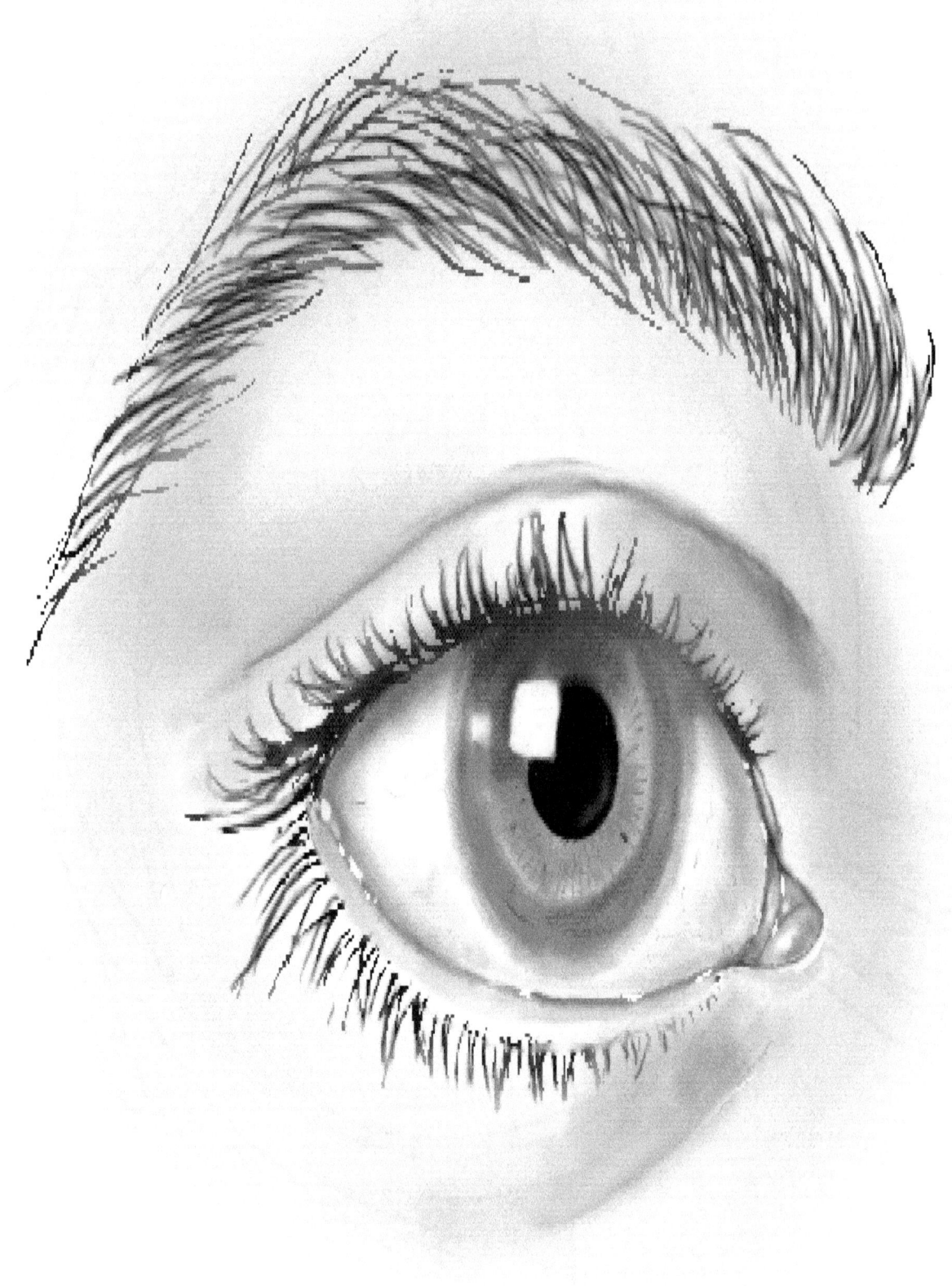

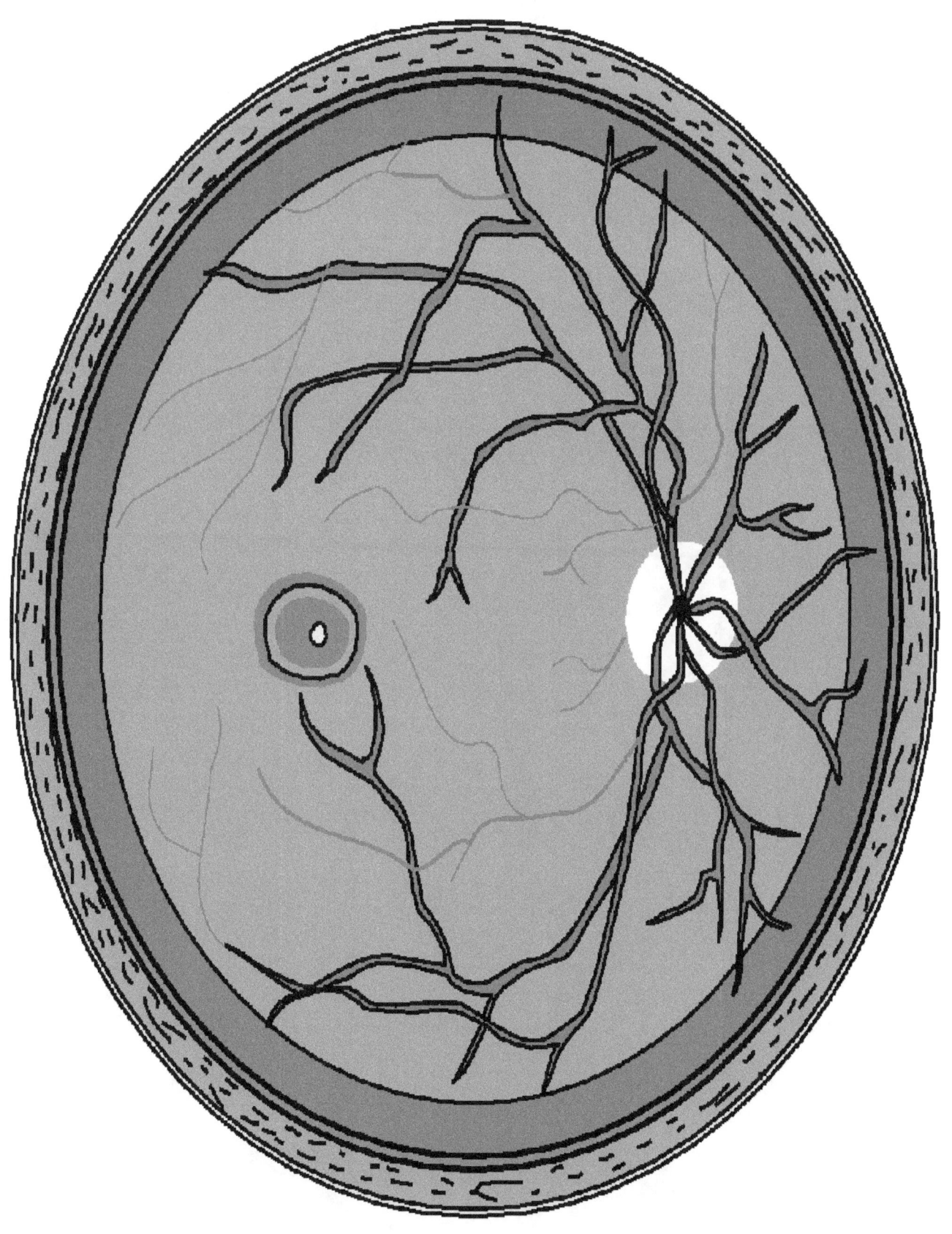

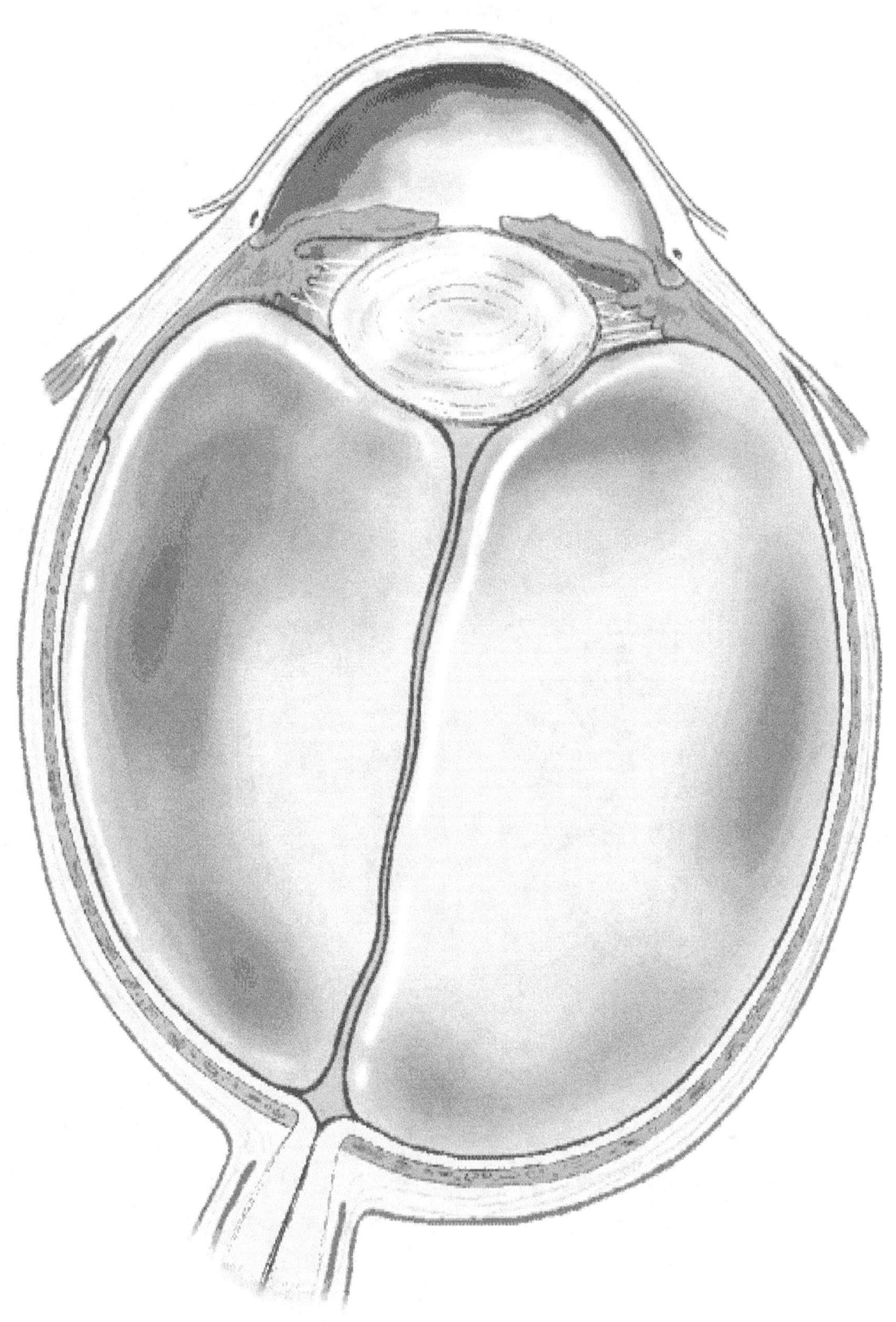

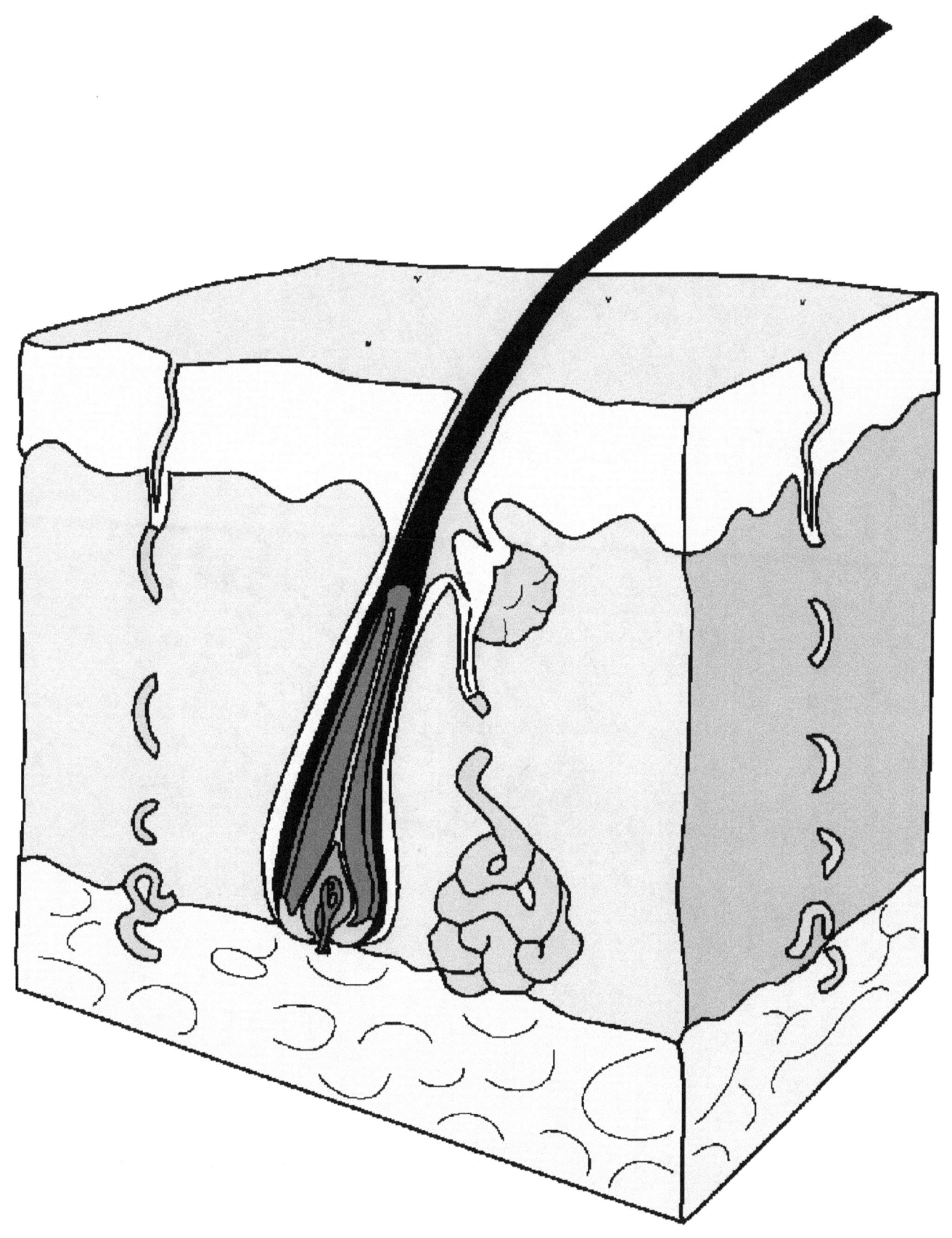

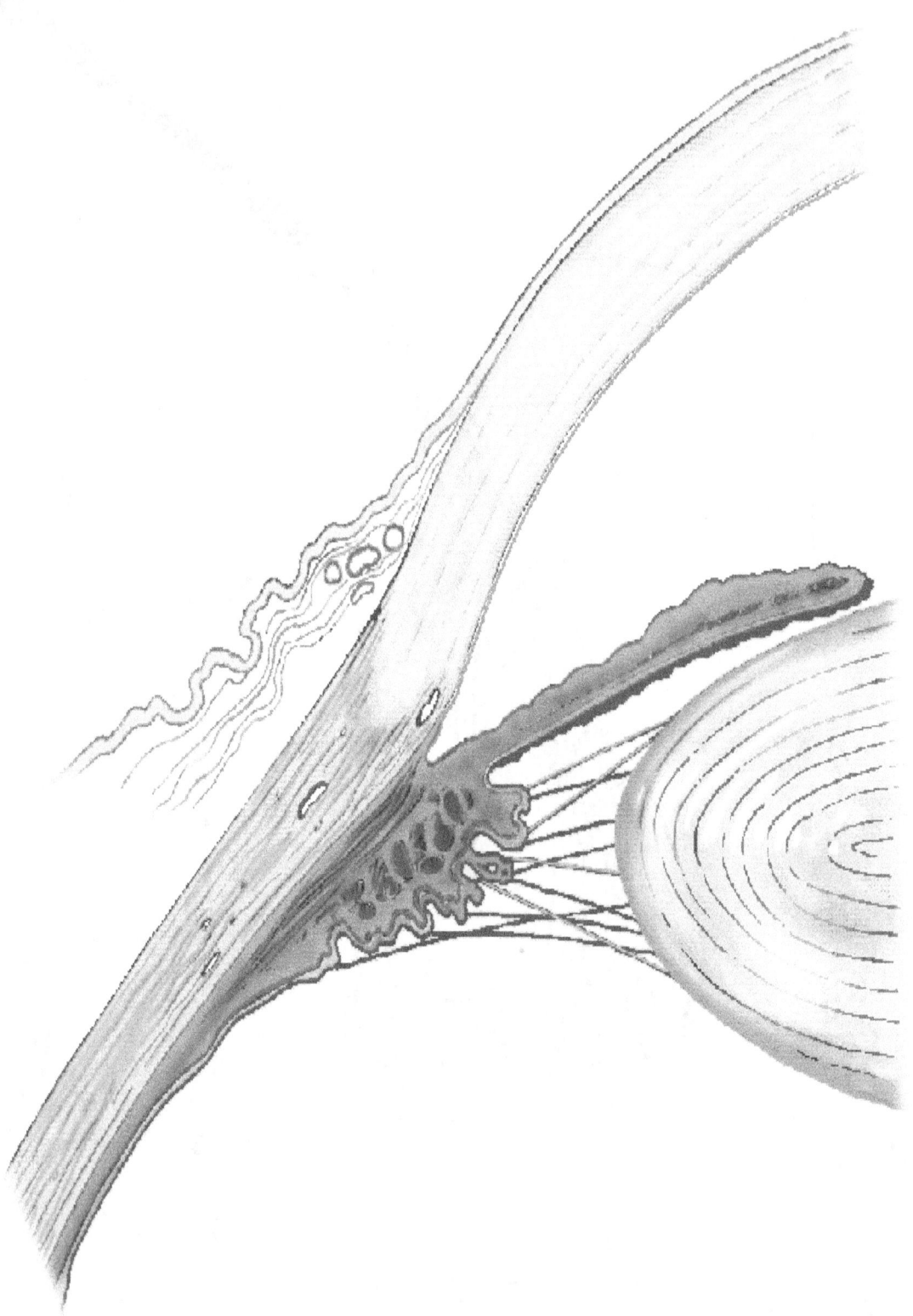

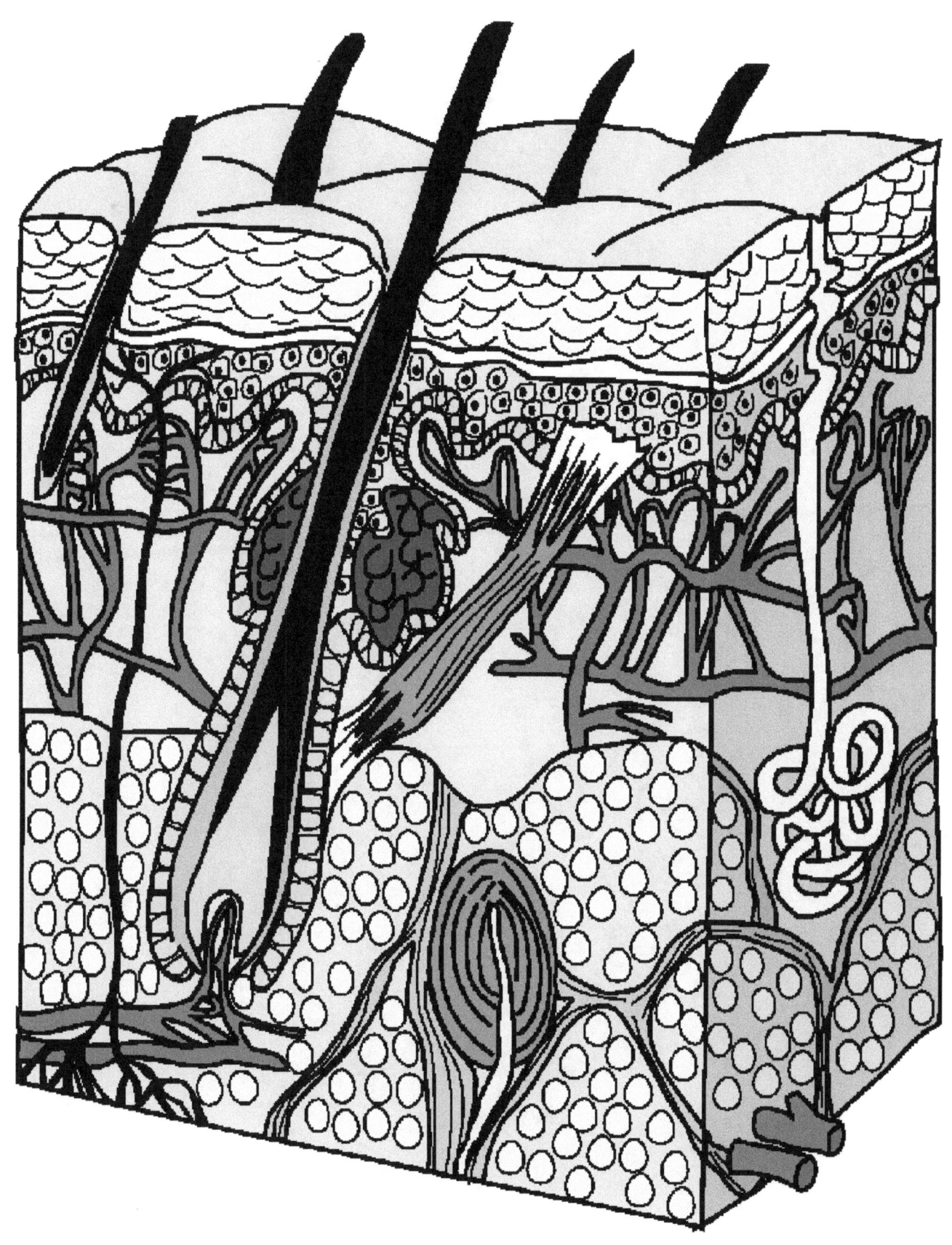

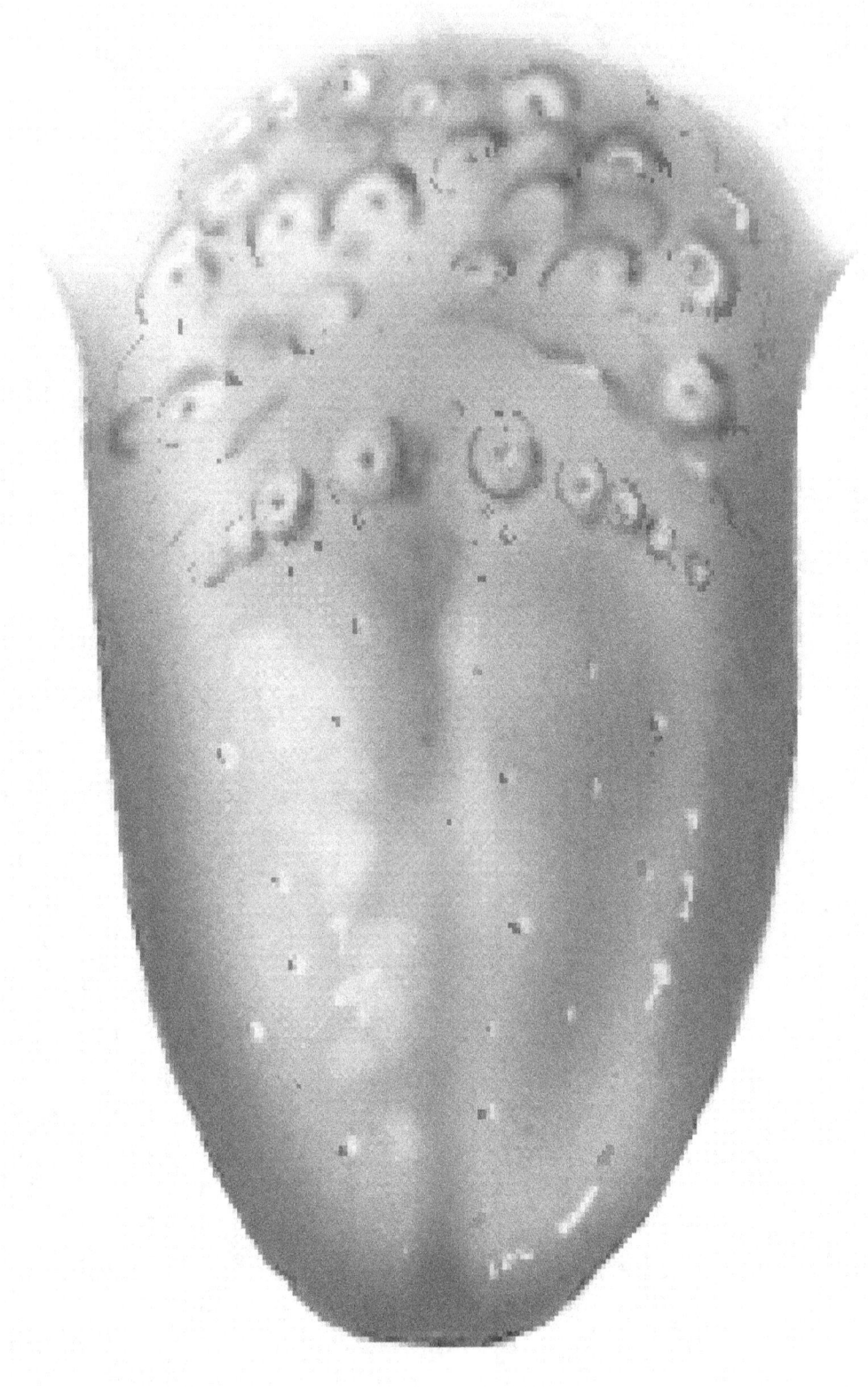

Other Anatomy System Label Practice <u>Books Available on Amazon</u>

1. Cardiovascular System
2. Digestive & Endocrine System
3. Muscular System
4. Nervous System
5. Respiratory System
6. Skeleteal System
7. Surface Anatomy & Senses
8. Urogenital System

www.ingramcontent.com/pod-product-compliance
Lightning Source LLC
Chambersburg PA
CBHW080650190526
45169CB00006B/2049